Intensive Care Nursing

Especially written for qualified nurses working in intensive care nursing units, this comprehensive text has been developed to be as accessible as possible. This fourth edition has been revised throughout to ensure the evidence base is completely up to date and the content reflects contemporary best practice.

Intensive Care Nursing is structured in user-friendly sections. The chapters contain sections outlining the "fundamental knowledge" needed to understand key chapters, "implications for practice" boxes, further reading and resources overviews, "time out" sections for revision and clinical scenarios with questions included. Reviewed throughout by experienced practitioners and teachers, it covers:

- patient-focused issues of bedside nursing;
- the technical knowledge necessary to care safely for ICU patients;
- the more common and specialised disease processes and treatments encountered;
- how nurses can use their knowledge and skills to develop their own and others' practice.

Written by a practice development nurse with a strong clinical background in intensive care nursing and experience of teaching nursing, *Intensive Care Nursing* is essential reading for nurses and health professionals working with seriously ill patients, particularly those undertaking post-registration training in the area.

Philip Woodrow is Practice Development Nurse in Critical Care at East Kent Hospitals University Foundation Trust, UK.

Intensive Care Nursing

A Framework for Practice

Fourth Edition

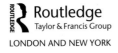 Philip Woodrow

Routledge
Taylor & Francis Group

LONDON AND NEW YORK

Fourth edition published 2019
by Routledge
2 Park Square, Milton Park, Abingdon, Oxon OX14 4RN

and by Routledge
711 Third Avenue, New York, NY 10017

Routledge is an imprint of the Taylor & Francis Group, an informa business

First edition published by Routledge 2000
Second edition published by Routledge 2006
Third Edition published by Routledge 2011

British Library Cataloguing-in-Publication Data
Names: Woodrow, Philip, 1957– author.
Title: Intensive care nursing : a framework for practice / Philip Woodrow.
Description: Fourth edition. | Abingdon, Oxon ; New York, NY : Routledge,
2018. | Includes bibliographical references and index.
Identifiers: LCCN 2018011153| ISBN 9780815385936 (hardback : alk.
paper) | ISBN 9781138713802 (pbk. : alk. paper) | ISBN 9781315231174
(ebook : alk. paper)
Subjects: | MESH: Critical Care Nursing--methods | Critical Illness—nursing
Classification: LCC RT120.15 | NLM WY 154 | DDC 610.73/6—dc23
LC record available at https://lccn.loc.gov/2018011153

Library of Congress Cataloging-in-Publication Data
Names: Woodrow, Philip, 1957– author.
Title: Intensive care nursing : a framework for practice / Philip Woodrow.
Description: Fourth edition. | Abingdon, Oxon ; New York, NY :
Routledge, 2018. | Includes bibliographical references and index.
Identifiers: LCCN 2018011153| ISBN 9780815385936 (hardback : alk. paper) |
ISBN 9781138713802 (pbk. : alk. paper) | ISBN 9781315231174
(ebook : alk. paper)
Subjects: | MESH: Critical Care Nursing—methods | Critical Illness—nursing
Classification: LCC RT120.15 | NLM WY 154 | DDC 610.73/6—dc23
LC record available at https://lccn.loc.gov/2018011153

ISBN: 978-0-8153-8593-6 (hbk)
ISBN: 978-1-138-71380-2 (pbk)
ISBN: 978-1-315-23117-4 (ebk)

Typeset in Sabon and Futura
by Florence Production Ltd, Stoodleigh, Devon, UK

To the States or any one of them, or any city of the States,
Resist much, obey little,
Once unquestioning obedience, once fully enslaved,
Once fully enslaved, no nation, state, city, of this earth,
ever afterwards resumes its liberty.

Walt Whitman

Fashion, even in medicine.

Voltaire

Contents

Part IX

■ **Metabolic** 435

Part X

■ **Professional** 459

x

Figures

Tables

Preface

This book is for ICU nurses. Intensive care is a diverse speciality, with many sub-specialities. Even within a single ICU, the range of pathologies and treatments seen may vary considerably. No text can hope to cover every possible condition readers may see, and general texts cannot cover topics comprehensively. My aim for this edition, as in the previous ones, is to offer nurses working in general ICUs an overview of the more commonly encountered pathologies and treatments. This text will probably be most useful about six to 12 months into ICU nursing careers, so assumes that readers are already qualified nurses, with experience of caring for ventilated patients, but wish to develop their knowledge and practice further. Because some knowledge is assumed, "fundamental knowledge" is listed at the start of many chapters for readers to pursue any assumed aspects of which they are unsure. "Further reading" at the end of each chapter identifies some useful, and usually relatively easily accessible, resources for readers to pursue. Definitions of some technical terms can be found in the glossary – where these terms appear in the text they are italicised, although italics are sometimes used for other reasons – for example, standard practices of italicising names of publications and micro-organisms is followed.

This book focuses on nursing care of Level 3 patients. Level 2 patients are the focus of a companion volume (Woodrow, 2016). Some overlap between the two is inevitable, but where reasonably possible I have attempted to make the books complementary. Some topics relevant to Level 3 patients are included in the other text – for example, intrapleural chest drains and non-invasive ventilation. The title and terminology, "intensive care unit (ICU)", has been retained, rather than replaced with the often used "critical care unit (CCU)", largely to avoid confusion with coronary care units (also CCUs).

This fourth edition has provided the opportunity to update and develop contents; the structure remains essentially unchanged from the third edition. Much more could be covered, but a larger book would be less affordable, more unwieldy and less used. My priority in revising this book has therefore been to identify core issues within a similar-length text. Some links made to incorporate topics into chapters are tenuous, but I hope that their presence justifies this approach.

Many aspects are inevitably relevant to various chapters; as most readers are likely to "dip in" to parts of this book, there is some repetition. I have also cross-referenced to chapters in both this book and Woodrow (2016). The index and glossary are also useful resources for expanding knowledge of many aspects.

The amount of evidence continues to increase, together with increased accessibility through the internet. Increased numbers of meta-analyses and systematic reviews means that some sources are more comprehensive than were generally available when developing the first edition of this book. Conversely, the quantity of dubious evidence has also proliferated. Searching literature is therefore necessarily selective, heavily reliant on guidelines, meta-analyses and publications from key organisations, as well as being influenced by serendipity. I have tended to follow UK standards and guidelines; for example, biochemistry references ranges follow the UK's Pathology Harmony. Readers outside the UK should check standards in their own country. References to statute and civil law are usually English and Welsh law, so readers in Scotland and Northern Ireland and those outside the United Kingdom should check applicability to local legal systems. Selection and interpretation from this wealth of resources is mine, and like any other selection and interpretation is inevitably subjective.

Many controversies are identified, but all aspects of knowledge and practice should be actively questioned and constantly reassessed. I have tried to minimise errors, but some are almost inevitable in a text this size; like any other source, this text should be read critically. If this book encourages further debate among practising nurses it will have achieved its main purpose. My hope remains that this book benefits readers, and so contributes to delivering quality patient care.

Philip Woodrow, 2018

Acknowledgements

Any book is inevitably a collaborative effort, and I am grateful to everyone who has contributed towards this text. Previous editions have benefitted in particular from advice of John Albarran and Jane Roe. Jane Roe also developed the scenarios used in the first edition, these have largely been retained in this edition. Reviewers and contributors towards text development include Grace McInnes (Commissioning Editor), Carolina Antunes (Editorial Assistant), Christina O'Brien (Production Editor), Josh Curtis and Richard Sanders (Project Management), Hugh Jackson (Copy-Editor), and Susan Leaper (Typesetting and Design Production).

The text has also been influenced by input from many other people, including reviewers, colleagues in the British Association of Critical Care Nurses, and East Kent Hospitals University NHS Foundation Trust – especially the staff of its three ICUs at Kent & Canterbury (Canterbury), Queen Elizabeth the Queen Mother (Margate) and William Harvey (Ashford) hospitals. I am especially grateful to the team at Routledge/Taylor & Francis for commissioning this fourth edition and supporting it throughout its development.

Abbreviations

<	less than
>	more than
2,3 DPG	2,3-diphosphoglycerate: a chemical in erythrocytes which aids oxygen dissociation from haemoglobin
ACS	acute coronary syndromes (see Chapter 29)
ACT	activated clotting times (normal 120–150 seconds)
AF	atrial fibrillation
AIDP	acute inflammatory demyelinating polyneuropathy
AIDS	acquired immunodeficiency syndrome
AMAN	acute motor axonal neuropathy
ANCA	antineutrophil cytoplasmic antibodies (test for renal vasculitis)
ANF	atrial natriuretic factor (also called atrial natriuretic peptide = ANP)
ANP	atrial natriuretic peptide (also called atrial natriuretic factor = ANF)
APACHE	acute physiology and chronic health evaluation
APRV	airway pressure release ventilation
ARC	AIDS-related complex
ARDS	acute respiratory distress syndrome (see Chapter 27)
ASV	adaptive support ventilation
ATP	adenosine triphosphate
AV	atrioventricular
BE	base excess
bpm	depending on context, "beats per minute" (heart rate) or "breaths per minute" (respiratory rate)
BSD	brainstem death
CCO	Critical Care Outreach
CABG	coronary artery bypass graft(s)
CCP	cerebral perfusion pressure
CD4, CD8	CD = cluster designation; type of surface antigen; numbers refer to different types
CIDP	chronic inflammatory demyelinating polyneuropathy
CK	creatine kinase
CMV	controlled mechanical ventilation *or* cytomegalovirus

COP	colloid osmotic pressure
COPD	chronic obstructive pulmonary disease
CPAP	continuous positive airway pressure
CPE	carbapenemase-producing *enterobacteriacae*
CPP	cerebral perfusion pressure
CRE	*Carbapenem-resistant enterobacteriaceae*
CRP	C-reactive protein (see Chapter 21)
CRRT	continuous renal replacement therapy, blanket term used to describe any mode
CSF	cerebrospinal fluid
CT	computerised tomography (scan)
cTnI	(cardiac) troponin I
cTnT	(cardiac) troponin T
CVVH	continuous veno-venous haemofiltration
CVVHDF	continuous veno-venous haemodiafiltration
Da	daltons: a unit of molecular weight
DCD	donation after circulatory death
DIC	disseminated intravascular coagulation
DKA	diabetic ketoacidosis
DSa	digital subtraction angiography
DVT	deep-vein thrombosis
E. coli	*Escherichia coli,* a species of gram-negative bacteria, one of the major gut commensals; presence of *E. coli* in the blood (or wounds) is an infection
$ECCO_2R$	extracorporeal carbon dioxide removal
ECLS	extracorporeal lung support
ECMO	extracorporeal membrane oxygenator
EfCCNa	European Federation of Critical Care Nursing Associations
eGFR	estimated glomerular filtration rate; normal > 90 ml/min/1.73m^2
ELSD	Extracorporeal liver support devices
ESBL	extended spectrum beta-lactamases: enzymes producing cross-resistance to many antibiotics
$etCO_2$	end-tidal carbon dioxide
ETT	endotracheal tube
EVAR	endovascular aneurysm repair
FDP	fibrin degradation product
FEV	forced expiratory volume (so FEV_1 = forced expiratory volume at one second)
FFP	fresh frozen plasma
FiO_2	fraction of inspired oxygen (expressed as a decimal fraction, so FiO_2 1.0 = 100% or pure oxygen)
FRIII	fixed-rate intravenous insulin infusion
FVC	functional ventilatory capacity
GBS	Guillain-Barré Syndrome
GCS	Glasgow Coma Scale
GFR	see eGFR

GRE	glycopeptide-resistant *Enterococci* (previously called *VRE*)
GTN	glyceryl trinitrate
HAI/HCAI	healthcare-associated infection
HAS	human albumin solution (i.e. albumin for infusion)
HbA	adult haemoglobin
HbF	foetal haemoglobin (abnormal after three months of age)
HBV	hepatitis B virus
Hct	haematocrit (also called "packed cell volume")
HCV	hepatitis C virus
HDL	high density lipoprotein
HELLP	Haemolysis elevated liver enzymes and low platelets
HHS	hyperosmolar hyperglycaemic state (= HONKS)
HITTS	heparin-induced thrombocytopenia and thrombosis syndrome
HIV	Human immunodeficiency virus (see Chapter 25)
HONKS	hyperosmolar non-ketotic state (= HHS)
HUS	haemolytic uraemic syndrome
Hz	hertz
I.C.N.	International Council of Nurses
I.C.S.	Intensive Care Society.
ICP	intracranial pressure
Ig	immunoglobulin (e.g. IgA = immunoglobulin A)
IL	interleukin
iLA	interventional lung assist
INR	international normalised ratio (measures clotting time – see Chapter 21)
iu	international units
IVI	intravenous infusion
IVIG	intravenous immunoglobulin
kDa	kiloDaltons (molecular weight), = 1000 daltons (Da)
kJ	kilojoule
LBBB	left bundle branch block
LDL	low density lipoprotein
LMW	low molecular weight (when prefixed to heparin)
MDMA	3–4 methylenedioxymethamphetamine (ecstasy)
MetHb	methaemoglobin
MIDCAB	minimally invasive direct coronary artery bypass grafting
mmol	millimole
MODS	multi-organ dysfunction syndrome
MRI	magnetic resonance imaging
MRSa	meticillin-resistant *Staphylococcus aureus*, also called *multi-resistant Staphylococcus aureus*; originally spelled "methicillin"
NAFLD	non-alcoholic fatty liver disease
NASH	non-alcoholic steatohepatitis
NIRS	near infrared spectroscopy
NIV	non-invasive ventilation
NPi	neurological pupil index

NSAID	non-steroidal anti-inflammatory drug
NSTEMI	non-ST elevation myocardial infarction
O_2Hb	fraction of total haemoglobin combined with oxygen
OPCAB	off-pump coronary artery bypass
$PaCO_2$	arterial carbon dioxide (from blood gas)
PaO_2	partial pressure of arterial oxygen
PAV	proportional assist ventilation
PCI	percutaneous coronary intervention
PCP	*Pneumocystis carinii* pneumonia (now retitled *Pneumocystis jirovici* pneumonia)
PCV	packed cell volume (also called "haematocrit")
PDIs	phosphodiesterase inhibitors
PE	pulmonary embolus
PEA	pulseless electrical activity
PEEP	positive end expiratory pressure
PERTL	pupils equal (and) react to light
PFC	perfluorocarbon
PGI_2	prostaglandin I_2 (also called "prostacyclin")
PJP	*Pneumocystis jirovici* pneumonia
pPCI	primary percutaneous coronary interventions
PPE	personal protective equipment
PPI	proton pump inhibitors
PS	pressure support
PSV	pressure support ventilation
PTT	prothrombin time
PUFAs	polyunsaturated fatty acids
QALYs	quality adjusted life years
QTc	QT interval corrected to what it would be if heart rate were 60 bpm
RBBB	right bundle branch block
RCT	randomised controlled trial
RNA	ribonucleic acid
ROS	reactive oxygen species (see oxygen radicals)
RR	respiratory rate
SA	sinoatrial (node)
SBE	standardised base excess
SD plasma	solvent detergent plasma
SDD	selective digestive decontamination
SIADH	syndrome of inappropriate antidiuretic hormone
SIMV	synchronised intermittent mandatory ventilation
SjO_2	jugular venous bulb saturation
SOD	selective oral decontamination
STEMI	ST elevation myocardial infarction
StO_2	saturation of tissues (venous blood) by oxygen
SV	stroke volume
SVT	supraventricular tachycardia

TBI	traumatic brain injury
TIA	transient ischaemic attack
Tn	troponin
TNF	tumour necrosis factor
TNFα	tumour necrosis factor alpha
t-PA	tissue plasminogen activator, also called recombinant tissue plasminogen activator (rt-PA)
TTP	thrombotic thrombocytopenia purpura
TV	tidal volume (also written at V_t)
UA	unstable angina
V/Q	(alveolar) ventilation to (pulmonary capillary) perfusion ratio; minute volume compared with cardiac output. Normal V/Q = 0.8
VALI	ventilator-associated lung injury (see VILI)
VAP	ventilator-associated pneumonia
VILI	ventilator-induced lung injury (see VALI)
VRE	vancomycin-resistant *Enterococci* (former name for *GRE*)
V_t	tidal volume (also written at TV)
VT	ventricular tachycardia
W/m^2	watts per square metre
WBC	white blood cells (in this text called "white cell count")
WCC	white cell count (see Chapter 21)

Part I

Contexts of care

Nursing perspectives

Contents

Introduction

This book is about nursing care of critically ill (Level 3 – see Table 1.1) patients; a companion book (Woodrow, 2016) focuses on Level 2 patients.

The 60 years of intensive care units (ICUs) have seen various technologies, drugs and protocols developed to treat problems of critical illness. While many have found a valid niche, initial hopes have often been largely disappointed. What has been constant is the contribution of nurses and nursing to outcomes for critically ill patients. So what is the purpose of nurses in ICU? What does critical illness, and admission to intensive care, cost patients and their families? In the busyness of everyday practice, these fundamental questions can be too easily forgotten. Nursing is expensive, costing more than one quarter of acute trust budgets, and although ICU staffing costs vary, high nurse:patient ratios necessitate the need for ICU nurses to clarify their value (Bray *et al.*, 2009). This book explores issues for ICU nursing practice; this section establishes core fundamental aspects of ICU nursing. To help readers articulate the importance of their role, this first chapter explores what nursing means in the context of intensive care, while Chapter 2 outlines two schools of psychology (Behaviourism and Humanism) that have influenced healthcare and society.

A recurring theme of pathologies described are two responses:

- inflammation
- stress

These are innate defensive/protective responses. Balanced responses (appropriate to the threat) often help resolve non-critical illness. Critical illness typically occurs with imbalanced responses – insufficient response means disease can cause death, while excessive responses themselves become pathological.

Table 1.1 Levels of care

Level 0	Patients whose needs can be met through normal ward care in an acute hospital.
Level 1	Patients at risk of their condition deteriorating, or those recently relocated from higher levels of care, whose needs can be met on an acute ward with additional advice and support from the critical care team.
Level 2	Patients requiring more detailed observation or intervention including support for a single failing organ system or post-operative care and those "stepping down" from higher levels of care.
Level 3	Patients requiring advanced respiratory support alone or basic respiratory support together with support of at least two organ systems. This level includes all complex patients requiring support for multi-organ failure.

Source: D.O.H., 2000a; I.C.S., 2015

Technology

Intensive care is a young speciality. Ibsen is widely credited with creating the first "modern" ICU in 1953 (Reisner-Senelar, 2011). The first purpose-built intensive care unit (ICU) in the UK opened in 1964 (Ashworth, personal communication). ICUs offer potentially life-saving intervention during acute physiological crises, with emphasis on medical need and availability of technology.

Technology facilitates monitoring and treatment but can also be dehumanising (Almerud *et al.*, 2007). Patients, not machines, should remain the focus of care (Bagherian *et al.*, 2017). Nurses should ensure that the use of technology is compatible with the safety, dignity and rights of people (I.C.N., 2012). ICU patients, often disempowered by their disease and drugs, are confronted with environments designed for medical and technical support which can create barriers for patients and their care (Eriksson *et al.*, 2010), so advocacy remains a fundamental nursing role (Williams *et al.*, 2016). Nurses should develop therapeutic and Humanistic environments which help the patient as a whole person towards their recovery (Almerud *et al.*, 2007). For patients, caring behaviour and relieving their fear and worries are the most valuable aspects of nursing (Hofhuis *et al.*, 2008a).

The patient . . .

Patients are admitted to intensive care because potentially reversible physiological crises threaten one or more body systems, and life (Crunden, 2010). Care therefore needs to focus primarily on supporting failed systems. This book discusses various aspects of technological and physiological care, many chapters focusing on specific systems and treatments. But these aspects should be placed in the context of the whole person. People are influenced by, and interact with, their environment. Extrinsic needs for:

- dignity
- privacy
- psychological support
- spiritual support

define each person as a unique individual, rather than just a biologically functioning organism.

Uniquely among healthcare workers, nurses are with the patient throughout their hospital stay. A fundamental role of nurses is to be with and be for the patient, as a whole person (McGrath, 2008). Person-centred care is widely cited in strategic documents, policy statements and organisational values, but its evaluation tends to be narrow and reductionist (Manley and McCormac, 2008).

. . . Their relatives . . .

Relatives are an important part of each person's life (Wong *et al.*, 2015), giving patients courage to struggle for survival (Bergbom and Askwall, 2000).

So, caring for relatives is an important part of patient care (Davidson *et al.*, 2017). Of all staff, nurses are best placed to meet relatives' needs, and are a valuable source for updating relatives about progress (Iverson *et al.*, 2014; Wong *et al.*, 2015).

In contrast to the often-high-tech focus of staff, families of intensive care patients often focus on fundamental aspects of physiological needs, such as pain relief and communication (Tingle, 2007). Rather than ruminate by bedsides, afraid to touch their loved ones in case they interfere with some machine, relatives should be offered opportunities to be actively involved in care (Davidson *et al.*, 2017).

Physiological crises for patients often create psychological crises for their relatives (Wong *et al.*, 2015). Holistic patient care should include caring for their families (Bagherian *et al.*, 2017).

Relatives experience a range of emotions, including anxiety, anger and frustration (Turner-Cobb *et al.*, 2016). They are usually angry at the disease, but it is difficult to take anger out on a disease. Instead, anger, complaints or passive withdrawal may be directed at those nearby, who are usually nurses (Maunder, 1997). Relatives may blame themselves, however illogically, for their loved one's illness. They place low priorities on their own physical and physiological needs, such as rest and food (Padilla, 2014). Facilities for relatives should include a waiting room near the unit, somewhere to stay overnight and facilities to make refreshments (NHS Estates, 2003; B.A.C.C.N., 2012).

Relatives need information, both to cope with their own psychological crisis and to make decisions (Padilla, 2014; Gaeeni *et al.*, 2015). Relatives, and patients, may seek information from the internet, often immediately available through mobile telephones and tablets. While many internet resources are reliable, some are not and can be a source for misinformation and confusion. Nurses should therefore clarify relatives' understanding of pathological conditions, treatments and other aspects.

Relatives often have a psychological need for hope (Bagherian *et al.*, 2017), but with nearly one fifth of patients dying on the unit (Vincent *et al.*, 2009), and additional post-discharge mortality and morbidity, there may be little hope to offer. If death seems likely, relatives need to know so they can start grieving (Wright, 2007). Relatives often anticipate more positive outcomes than physicians (Lee Char *et al.*, 2010), so may be unconvinced when bad news is broken. Changes in critical illness may be rapid and unpredictable. Where possible, both the nurse caring for the patient and a senior doctor should inform the family of anticipated outcomes, away from the patient's bedside, preferably in a room where discussion will not be interrupted by others. The door should be closed for privacy, but access to doors should not be obstructed in case distressed relatives need to escape. Everyone should sit down, as family members may faint, and staff should not stand above relatives. Posture, manner and voice should be as open as possible. Tissues should be available. Having witnesses is useful in case relatives later complain. Detailed records of discussions should be recorded.

Relatives should be given time to think about information, express their emotions and ask anything they wish, and be offered opportunities for further discussions if they wish. An information book, including details of who to contact and support groups (such as CRUSE), is useful. Further discussion about end-of-life care can be found in Woodrow (2016).

... And the nurse

Nurses monitor and assess patients. But nurses also provide care. Assessment is fundamental to providing care, but excessive paperwork can hinder care. Nursing assessments should therefore remain patient-focused, enabling nurses and others to deliver effective care. Proliferation of policies, protocols and competencies is often intended to ensure quality and parity of care wherever patients are admitted and whoever cares for them. But each patient is an individual and needs individualised nursing care. While guidance and safeguards can be useful, increasing protocols does not correlate with either compliance or reducing patient mortality (Sevransky *et al.*, 2015). Rather than introduce more proformas, nurses need to maintain and develop knowledge and skills to be able to adapt care to individualised patient needs.

Nurses should collaborate with other professions (N.M.C., 2015). Nurse-to-patient ratios for Level 3 patients should be 1:1 (I.C.S., 2015). The UK faces specific challenges: UK ICU patients are sicker than in most countries (Mandelstam, 2007), there are fewer ICU beds per 100,000 population (Adhikari *et al.*, 2010) than in other developed, and many Third World, countries. There is also disparity between the four UK countries: I.C.S. (2015) cite England as having seven beds per 100,000 population, compared with 3.2 in Wales and Scotland and 4.7 in Northern Ireland. For Level 2 patients, nurse:patient ratios should be 1:2 (I.C.S. 2015). These levels may reflect acuity of disease but often fail to reflect nursing workload: a conscious but delirious Level 2 patient often requires more nursing time than a fully sedated Level 3 patient. Decreasing staffing levels increase complication rates (EfCCNa, 2007) and mortality (Cho *et al.*, 2008; West *et al.*, 2009).

Nurses, and nursing, have valuable roles within intensive care. But staff are an expensive commodity. Even if economic pressures are ignored, the global shortage of nurses and ageing workforce (Crisp and Chen, 2014) limit supply. A pragmatic solution to both economic and recruitment limitations has been to develop support worker roles. Most units employing support workers have found they provide valuable contributions to teamwork. B.A.C.C.N. guidelines should protect patients, nurses and support workers from inappropriate delegation (Bray *et al.*, 2009).

Deterioration of acutely ill patients, and need for ICU admission, is often preventable (Hogan *et al.*, 2012; NHS Improvement, 2016). Comprehensive Critical Care (D.O.H. 2000a) recommended that acute hospitals should have a Critical Care Outreach service to prevent the avoidable deterioration of ward patients, and to facilitate their timely admission if ICU is needed. They also follow up on ICU patients after discharge back to wards, and sometimes post-hospital discharge through "ICU clinics". CCO forms an important part of the ICU team, and concerns during discharge to wards should be escalated to them.

Stress

Stress is frequently experienced by patients in ICU (Samuelson *et al.*, 2007), but it can also be a problem for relatives and staff. For staff, stress can lead to burnout, potentially causing staff to change careers and suffer mental ill health. Moss *et al.* (2016) suggest that burnout is especially common in staff caring for critically ill patients, although arguably stressors of nursing in other areas, while different, are potentially greater.

Stress is both a psychological and physiological phenomenon; psychology and physiology interact. Critically ill patients suffer physiological stress from their illness, and psychological stress from negative emotions, such as fear. Stress responses are defensive, activating the hypothalamic–pituitary–adrenal (HPA) axis (Chrousos, 2009; Steptoe and Kivimäki, 2012). The pituitary gland responds by releasing adrenocorticotrophic hormone (ACTH), which stimulates adrenal gland production of adrenaline (epinephrine) and noradrenaline (norepinephrine), with increased production of other hormones, including cortisol. This "fight or flight" response, discussed further in Chapter 31, increases:

■ heart rate
■ stroke volume
■ systemic vascular resistance
■ respiration rate
■ blood sugar
■ thrombolysis
■ fluid retention.

While protective for healthy people facing acutely life-threatening confrontation, all factors are frequently detrimental with critical illness. Caring for both physical and psychological needs, nurses can add a humane, holistic perspective into patient care, transcending an often-hostile environment (McGrath, 2008).

Duty of care

Nurses' primary duty of care should be to their patients. This includes a duty to maintain confidentiality (N.M.C., 2015). If patients are unable to express their wishes, and what information they wish shared with others, nurses should be cautious about sharing information even with close relatives and friends. Usually, if patients are unconscious, information will be given to the identified next of kin, who will usually be asked to liaise with other family and friends. Next of kin may identify a password to enable information to be shared with trusted people. Sensitive information should not be disclosed to anyone not directly involved in their patient's care, or if it is unnecessary to do so. Special care should be taken with telephone conversations, both because the other person may not be who they claim to be and because reactions are unpredictable. Requirements of the Mental Capacity Act (2005 – see Chapter 3) should be observed. If in doubt, advice should be sought, if necessary from the trust's legal department.

Implications for practice

■ nurses need technical knowledge and skills, but nursing is more than being a technician;
■ ICU nurses have a unique role in providing holistic, patient-centred care that can humanise a hostile environment for their patients;
■ nurses have a professional duty of confidentiality to their patients, which remains after patients die;
■ physiology and psychology interact, so although physiological crises necessitating ICU admission remain the focus of treatment, holistic care includes meeting physical and psychological needs. Reducing psychological distress reduces stress responses, so promoting physiological recovery;
■ relatives experience psychological distress. Holistic patient care should include care of relatives and significant others;
■ nursing values underpin each nurse's actions; clarifying values and beliefs helps each nurse and each team increase self-awareness;
■ patient experiences are central to ICU nursing, so consider what patients are experiencing.

Summary

Much of this book necessarily focuses on technological/pathological aspects of knowledge needed for ICU nursing, but the busyness of clinical practice brings dangers of paying lip service to psychological needs in care plans and course assignments, while not meeting them in practice. Psychological care is not an abstract nicety; it affects physiology and so remains fundamental to nursing care. This chapter is placed first to establish fundamental nursing values before considering individual pathologies and treatments; nursing values can (and should) then be applied to all aspects of holistic patient care.

Intensive care is labour-intensive; nursing costs consume considerable portions of budgets. ICU nursing needs to assert its value by:

■ recognising nursing knowledge
■ valuing nursing skills
■ offering holistic patient/person-centred care.

Person-centred care involves responding to patients' individual needs (Sharp *et al.*, 2015) – nurses being there for each patient, rather than the institution.

Having recognised the primacy of the patient, nurses can then develop their valuable technological skills, together with other resources, to fulfil their unique role in the multidisciplinary team for the benefit of patients. ICU nurses should value ICU nursing on its own terms: to humanise the environment for their patients. Relatives are an important part of the person's life and have valuable roles to play in holistic care. But relatives also have needs, which are often exacerbated by their loved one's critical illness and may remain unmet. The beliefs, attitudes and philosophical values of nurses will ultimately determine nursing's economic value.

Further reading

I.C.S. (2015) provide authoritative guidance for most aspects of critical care. Societies such as the Intensive Care Society and the British Association for Critical Care Nurses provide guidance on many aspects of critical care, including relatives (B.A.C.C.N., 2012). US guidelines for family-centred care (Davidson *et al.*, 2017) are also valuable. Similar societies exist in many countries and, although guidance from abroad needs to be interpreted in local contexts, much is often transferable. Relatives' needs have been studied over many years; Turner-Cobb *et al.*'s (2016) study identifies issues that persist, making much older literature still relevant.

Clinical questions

Q1. Identify environmental, cultural, behavioural and physiological factors from your own clinical area that may contribute to the suffering and dehumanisation of patients in the ICU.

Q2. Outline specific resources and nursing strategies, which can minimise suffering and dehumanisation of patients.

Q3. Reflect upon assessment of patient dependency in your own clinical area, and how far this considers:

- patients' need for nursing interventions;
- medical interventions;
- level of technology.

Humanism

Contents

Introduction

We are products of history. Nursing and healthcare have developed significantly in recent years, and the applicability of evidence from a decade or more ago is rightly questioned. But this does risk jettisoning awareness of philosophies that have influenced practice. Passive acceptance of philosophy can be dangerous, as philosophy affects our values – how we approach patients and patient care. Our values may be either explicit or implicit, and influence both individual attitudes and the culture we work in (Sarvimaki and Sanderlin Benko, 2001). Chapter 1 identified the need to explore values and beliefs about ICU nursing. Karlsson *et al.*'s (2011) suggestion that the ICU environment needs to be humanised for relatives can be extended to patients.

The label "Humanism" has been variously used through human history, probably because its connotations of human welfare and dignity sound attractive. The Renaissance "Humanistic" movement included such influential philosophers as Erasmus and More. This chapter describes and contrasts two influential twentieth-century philosophies, one of which called itself "Humanism", to supply a context for developing individual beliefs and values. This is not a book about philosophy, so descriptions of these movements are brief and simplified; readers are encouraged to pursue their ideas through further reading.

The Humanist movement, sometimes called the "third force" (the first being psychoanalysis, the second Behaviourism), was a reaction to Behaviourism. This chapter therefore begins by describing Behaviourism. Two World Wars, and other traumatic events of the twentieth century, have replaced some of Humanism's classical optimism with an emphasis on recovering humane values from the impersonality of bureaucratic and technological systems (Walter, 1997).

Behaviourism

Behaviourist theory was developed largely by Watson (1924/1998), drawing on Pavlov's famous animal experiments: if each stimulus eliciting a specific response could be replaced by another (associated) stimulus, the desired response (behaviour) could still be achieved ("conditioning"). Behaviourism therefore focuses on outward, observable behaviours. Behaviourist theory enabled social control, so became influential when society valued a single, socially desirable, behaviour. For Behaviourists, learning *is* a change in behaviour (Reilly, 1980).

Holloway and Penson (1987) suggested that nurse education contains a "hidden curriculum" controlling behaviour of students and their socialisation into nursing culture; nearly quarter of a century later Benner *et al.* (2008) called for nurse education to move from focusing on socialisation and role-taking to formation. Through Gagné's (1975, 1985) influence, a Behaviouristic competency culture pervades nursing, without nurses necessarily being aware of its philosophical framework. Hendricks-Thomas and Patterson (1995) suggest that Behaviouristic philosophy is often covert, masked under the guise of

Humanism. Increasingly, learner-centred teaching (Carter, 2009) and reflection (Edwards, 2017) have replaced didactic education, enabling nurses to respond to individual patients and situations.

Protocols and policies are arguably a means to extend control when their originators are not present, with implicit commands and requirements. While prevalent in ICU practice, protocol compliance is often poor, and their existence does not reduce length of stay or mortality (Sevransky *et al.*, 2015). Their benefits, as well as their motives, are therefore questionable.

Behaviourist theory derives largely from animal experiments, but humans do not always function like animals, especially where cognitive skills are concerned. Focus on outward behaviour does not necessarily change inner values. People can adopt various behaviours in response to external motivators (e.g. senior nursing/medical staff) but, once stimuli are removed, behaviour may revert; when no external motivator exists, people are usually guided by internal motivators, such as their own values. So, if internal values remain unaltered, desired behaviour exists only as long as external motivators remain.

Behaviourism relies on rewards and punishments to motivate individuals to conform to desired behaviour. Rewards and punishments used by Behaviourism are public, external to the individual, such as essay grades, job promotion, salary or loss of privileges. Humanism also uses rewards and punishments but relies on internal ends, such as self-actualisation and individual conscience. Humanism is therefore dependant on the individual valuing a moral code.

Behaviourism in practice

Delirium (discussed further in Chapter 3) poses a major challenge for managing care in ICU. In the first decade of this century it was believed that haloperidol could help "cure" the acute delirium often experienced by ICU patients (e.g. Devlin *et al.*, 2008). More recent evidence demonstrates that haloperidol only controls problem behaviour; it does not resolve underlying causes (Page *et al.*, 2013). Controlling "problem" behaviours is compatible with Behaviourism, while attempting to understand patient-centred causes and enabling the patient to make informed choices would be a Humanistic approach. Where the patient behaviour poses a threat to themselves or others, safety may necessitate a Behaviouristic approach (haloperidol), but if underlying causes are not resolved then problem behaviours may recur.

No philosophy is ideal for all circumstances, and few are without some merit. In situations such as the above, Behaviourism may "buy time" until underlying pathophysiology is resolved or reduced. Behavioural approaches can be useful, but they can also be harmful, dehumanising others to lists of task-orientated responses. Pre-registration courses emphasise learning outcomes, creating passive learners (Romyn, 2001), while healthcare structures sometimes emphasise targets and a "tick-box" mentality at the cost of patient-centredness and caring. Protocols and care/treatment algorithms are widely used, and can help guide practice, especially among less experienced staff, but they can also become restrictive, favouring a Behaviouristic approach to care. Analysing values and beliefs, understanding the implications they have for practice, and selecting appropriate approaches to each context enable nurses to give Humanistic, individualised care.

Humanism

In this text, "Humanism" is a specifically twentieth-century movement in philosophy, led primarily by Abraham Maslow (1908–1970) and Carl Rogers (1902–1987). The Humanist movement was concerned that Behaviourism overemphasised animal instincts and attempted to control outward behaviour. People who are controlled too often learn to become helpless (Seligman, 1975). Humanism emphasises inner values that distinguish people from animals, a "person-centred" philosophy. Rather than emphasising society's needs, Humanism emphasised the needs of the individual self. Simplistically, Behaviourism can be viewed as attempting to control, whereas Humanism attempts to empower. Seeing patients as human beings, and placing them at the centre of care, is therefore fundamental to nursing (Hofhuis *et al.*, 2008a). Maslow's *Motivation and Personality* (1954/1987) popularised the concept of "holism" (the whole person). Humanists believe people have a psychological need to attempt to achieve and realise their maximum potential. Maslow (1954/1987) described a hierarchy of needs, self-actualisation being the highest. Roper *et al.* (1996) adopted Maslow's hierarchy into their nursing model, although arguably to Behaviouristic ends.

Humanist educators concentrate on developing and/or attempting to change inner values. Values that are internalised will continue to influence actions after external motivators are removed. Arguably, the Humanist alternative to Behaviouristic policies would be guidelines (i.e. advice rather than commands).

Concern for inner values and holistic approaches to care makes Humanism compatible with many aspects of healthcare and nursing, although familiarity with terms can reduce them to levels of cliché. Patients believe empowerment helps their recovery (Williams and Irurita, 2004). Facioli *et al.* (2012) describe how "narrative medicine", communicating on a human level, benefitted a mechanically ventilated patient. Humanism has much to offer nurses analysing their philosophies of care and practice, but no ideas should be accepted uncritically.

Lifelong learning

Where Behaviourist education aims to achieve conformity, Humanist education seeks to promote individuality; this reflects the training versus education debate. Training seeks to equip learners with a repertoire of behaviour responses to specific stimuli, usually with a "hidden curriculum" of indoctrinating conformity. Such training is often time-limited. In animals, stimulus–response reactions are often simple (as with Pavlov's dogs). Training equips learners to react to problems (stimuli) rather than proactively anticipate and prevent problems occurring. Conditioned responses can be life-saving during a cardiac arrest, but "training" fails to develop higher skills to work constructively through actual and potential human problems.

Facts and ideas are quickly outdated (Rogers, 1983), so are less valued by Humanists than the development of skills to enable personal growth (Maslow, 1971) and learning (Rogers, 1983). Humanism seeks to develop higher cognitive and affective skills to analyse issues according to individual needs, most valuable human interactions occurring above stimulus–response levels. For healthcare, Humanism promotes a person-centred philosophy that enables learning to continue beyond designated courses; each clinical area becomes a place for learning, and nurses should be extending and developing their skills through practice.

Many nursing actions have (literally) vital effects. Professional safety is necessary (Rogers, 1951), and most countries have professional regulatory bodies (e.g. N.M.C.), but emphasis on individualised learning (e.g. learning contracts), reflection and regular learning (N.M.C., 2015) recognises that learning processes must be meaningful for each individual rather than determined by Behaviourist objectives and outcomes. Attendance at study days does not ensure learning has occurred.

Evidence

Humanism and person-centred care have a weak research base (Traynor, 2009), so acceptance or rejection of its philosophy remains largely subjective. Arguably, research-based approaches conflict with Humanism's fundamental beliefs in individualism; Rogers's early work did attempt to adapt traditional scientific research processes to Humanism, but his later work adopts more discursive, subjective, approaches. Much has been written about "values", but values largely resist quantification and analysis. Promotion of patients' views and experiences into policies, planning and education attempt to promote empathy.

Much learning occurs through making mistakes; individualistic learning necessarily means making mistakes. Accepting the possibility of mistakes involves taking risks. Human fallibility should be recognised – expecting that mistakes will not occur, and so treating them as unacceptable, is unrealistic (D.O.H., 2000a). Errors with critically ill patients can cause significant, potentially fatal, harm. ICU staff, especially managers, need to achieve the difficult balance between facilitating positive learning environments and maintaining safety for patients and others.

Implications for practice

- philosophy (beliefs and values) influences practice, so to understand our practice, we need to understand our underlying beliefs and values;
- changing inner values, rather than just outward behaviour, ensures continuity when external stimuli are removed;
- healthcare, nursing and ICU retain Behaviouristic legacies that can undermine individualistic, patient-centred care;

- Humanism emphasises inner values and individualism, so Humanistic nursing helps humanise ICU for patients by placing them at the centre of care;
- nurses should seek to humanise the potentially alien environments and practices of ICU for their patients;
- humans are fallible, so mistakes will occur. Accepting this fallibility encourages errors to be acknowledged and learned from, and so limit future risks.

Summary

Philosophy is not an abstract theoretical discipline but something underlying and influencing all aspects of practice, so is relevant to each chapter in this book. Our beliefs, even if we are unaware of their source, influence our practice. Nurses can humanise care by:

- being there
- sharing
- supporting
- involving
- interpreting
- advocating.

(Andrew, 1998)

This chapter has outlined two influential and opposing philosophies; applying these beliefs to nursing values (see Chapter 1) helps clarify our own and others' motivation.

Further reading

Many texts identified in Chapter 1 reflect (often unacknowledged) Humanistic philosophy, but the best resources remain the classic texts that developed Behaviourism and Humanism. Skinner (1971) gives interesting late perspectives on Behaviourism, while Gagné's (1975, 1985) influence entrenched Behaviourism in a generation of nurse education. Maslow (1954/1987) is a classic text of Humanistic philosophy. Rogers is equally valuable, and more approachable; his 1967 text synthesises his ideas, while his 1983 book valuably discusses educational theory. Benner *et al.* (2008) outlines US proposals for changes to nurse education that largely reject Behaviourism in favour of Humanistic values.

Patient experiences of critical care provide useful perspectives on staff values. A recent example is Awdish (2017).

Clinical scenarios

Mr Oliver is a 35-year-old who was admitted to ICU with a GCS of 6 (E = 1 V = 2 M = 3) following an unsuccessful attempt at suicide. He is invasively ventilated but without sedation in order to facilitate the weaning process. He continually reaches towards his oral endotracheal tube (ETT). This behaviour causes the nurse to respond.

Q1. Describe a "Behaviourist" response by the nurse to Mr Oliver reaching for his ETT.

Q2. Explain how a "Humanistic" response would differ from a "Behaviourist" response in this situation. Consider the values that underpin each response, for example safety, duty of care, autonomy, motivation of Mr Oliver and needs of Mr Oliver.

Q3. Review your own practice and evaluate typical responses to this patient's gesture. What are your own and others' motivating values? How might the presence of a nurse with Mr Oliver influence his and the nurse's responses? Reflect on how the presence of relatives frequently modifies patients' behaviour, and what factors you think may cause such changes.

Chapter 3

Psychological care

Contents

Fundamental knowledge

Sensory receptors and nervous system;
Motor nervous system;
Autonomic nervous system;
Stress response (see Chapter 1);
Psychological coping mechanisms – e.g. denial.

Introduction

In the busyness of attempting to resolve acute physiological crises, psychological care can be consigned to afterthoughts. But physiology and psychology interact; psychological stressors cause physiological stress responses (see Chapters 1 and 31):

■ tachypnoea
■ tachycardia
■ hypertension
■ hyperglycaemia
■ thrombolysis
■ immunocompromise
■ oedema formation

– all usually complicating critical illness.

Anxiety, delirium and post-traumatic stress disorder (PTSD) are common, and often related, problems for ICU patients, and adversely affect morbidity and mortality (Jackson *et al.*, 2012; Wolters *et al.*, 2013). Since Ashworth's classic 1980 study, ICU nurses have been aware of problems from psychoses, and it has been given many names, but, while progress has been made, many challenges remain.

Delirium

One third of critically ill patients, and the majority of mechanically ventilated patients, suffer delirium (acute confusion) (N.I.C.E., 2010a; Pandharipande *et al.*, 2013; Page *et al.*, 2013; Builic *et al.*, 2014; Klouwenberg *et al.*, 2014). Delirium increases morbidity and mortality, causing psychological stress to patients and families, reducing motivation and prolonging recovery (N.I.C.E., 2010a; McCusker *et al.*, 2011; Pandharipande *et al.*, 2013; Builic *et al.*, 2014; Klouwenberg *et al.*, 2014; Salluh *et al.*, 2015).

Delirium may be:

■ hyperactive
■ hypoactive
■ mixed.

Hyperactive delirium is usually fairly easy to identify – the person behaves out of character in extrovert and bizarre ways, or says bizarre things. Unfortunately, most episodes of delirium are hypoactive (Lloyd *et al.*, 2012), where the person withdraws into themselves, becoming quiet and passive. Hypoactive delirium is often unrecognised (Eeles *et al.*, 2010). Hyperactive and mixed delirium often causes bizarre actions, but hypoactive delirium more often causes withdrawal, remaining quiet, passive and unnoticed.

All ICU patients should be assessed for delirium (Builic *et al.*, 2014). CAM-ICU is the most reliable screening tool (Luetz *et al.*, 2010), but quantifying delirium does not in itself treat problems; assessment tools are only useful if findings influence action.

Delirium is difficult to manage but can be reduced by:

- patient orientation
- communication
- mobilisation
- analgesia
- rationalising drugs.

(Page, 2010)

Alcohol withdrawal can be treated with chlordiazepoxide or benzodiazepines. Sedation may provide anxiolysis (see Chapter 6) but it is also (chemical) restraint, so is not a substitute for nursing care. While drugs may change behavioural responses (delirium), they do not change underlying causes. Active observation and proactive nursing can do much to humanise care and environments, removing many factors which contribute to delirium. The previous belief that haloperidol modifies the course of delirium is no longer supported (Page *et al.*, 2013). Compared with other sedatives used in ICU, dexmedetomidine may reduce risk of delirium (Ahmed and Murugan, 2013; Barr *et al.*, 2013; Su *et al.*, 2016), although non-pharmacological interventions remain preferable.

Time Out 1

ICU environments are abnormal. Using your senses – sight, hearing, touch, taste, smell. – take two to three minutes to list your own impressions of your current environment; complete this before reading any further. Repeat this exercise on your ICU.

Review your lists, noting down beside each item whether impressions were perceived through sight, hearing, touch, taste or smell. Some items may be perceived by more than one sense. How often was each sense used?

Most items are probably listed under sight, followed by a significant number under hearing. Touch is probably a poor third, with few (if any) under taste or smell. This reflects usual human use of senses: most input is usually through sight and hearing, with very limited inputs perceived from other senses.

Time Out 2

Imagine yourself as a patient in your own ICU. Jot down under each of the five senses any inputs you are likely to receive.

When finished, review your lists, analysing how many of these inputs are "normal" for you. Remember most people usually rely on visual and auditory inputs.

Sensory input

Even if eyes are open, ICU patients often have distorted *vision* from:

■ drugs, e.g. opioids may cause blurred vision
■ absence of glasses (if normally worn)
■ restricted visual field from positioning of head or equipment such as ventilator circuits.

Absence of vision may be caused by:

■ periorbital oedema (preventing eye opening)
■ exposure keratopathy (see Chapter 11).

Walls and ceilings are usually visually unstimulating; overhead equipment may be frightening. Waking to this alien environment, and trying to rationalise it, is likely to cause bizarre interpretation. Staff watching overhead monitors detracts from eye contact (non-verbal communication) and becomes dehumanising. Nurses should actively develop non-verbal skills (e.g. open body language, quality touch). Windows with views help maintain orientation to normality, so views should not be obscured by blinds, or beds placed so that patients are unable to see out of windows.

Hearing is often unaltered by critical illness; over half of ICU patients remember nurses speaking to them (Margarey and McCutcheon, 2005), so staff and visitors should assume patients can hear normally. It is important to communicate verbally with unconscious patients (Alasad and Ahmad, 2005). Communication is fundamental to nursing care, yet aural communication may be impaired because:

■ patients are unable to respond to cues;
■ hearing aids are missing, faulty or not switched on;
■ the cochleal nerve is damaged by ototoxic drugs (e.g. gentamicin, furosemide);
■ English is not understood, or is not the person's first language.

Conversation is too often confined to either instructions or others' conversation (e.g. medical/nursing/team discussions, sometimes spoken across patients, often in jargon). Instructions, although valid in themselves, should be supplemented by quality conversation. Family are a valuable source for "normal" conversation, and should be encouraged to talk to their loved one.

Touch is a major means of non-verbal communication, especially for those with impaired vision. Most touch in ICU remains task-orientated. Task-orientated touch is necessary but reduces individuals to commodities, reinforcing their dehumanisation. Caring touch reduces stress responses (Henricson *et al.*, 2008), and is valued by patients (Henricson *et al.*, 2009), yet is frequently underused in ICU. Overload of abnormal tactile sensations may be caused by:

- unfamiliar bedding (e.g. people used to duvets)
- pulling from tubes/drains/leads
- oral endotracheal tubes
- endotracheal suction
- pressure area care, passive movements and body positioning.

Patients may appreciate their pillow being turned or their hand being held. Human touch is valuable, especially if provided by loved ones.

Various receptors sense information about the body's internal and external environment. Proprioceptors in the musculoskeletal system provide information about body movement. Prolonged intervals between movement, common in most unconscious patients, results in lack of signals. Any movement sensed, such as movement in hoists or for procedures, may cause abnormal proprioceptive stimulation.

Barrier nursing, and reverse barrier nursing, can reduce infection but has negative psychological effects (Antonio and Jensen, 2014) and can reduce staff input and actions, such as delaying weaning (Wenham and Pittard, 2009). Isolation also reduces surveillance by staff and can result in higher rates of falls (Maben, 2009). Social isolation may be overt (e.g. gowns and masks, emphasising subhuman "untouchable" status, restricting visiting) or covert (e.g. avoidance of patients who have nit infestation, or depriving patients of quality touch and meaningful conversation).

Warm environments (above 24°C) contribute to poor sleep, as probably experienced by readers during warm summer nights. Ambient temperature in most ICUs usually exceeds 24°C.

Few ICU patients receive oral diets, so *taste* is limited to thirst and drugs (e.g. metronidazole causes a metallic taste) and anything remaining in the mouth:

- blood
- vomit
- mucus
- mouthwash/oral drugs
- toothpaste
- fungal infections (*Candida albicans* – "thrush"), stomatitis.

Being thirsty is one of the commonest memories of ICU patients (Margarey and McCutcheon, 2005). Taste relies largely on smell, so reduced olfactory input (from intubation) reduces perception of taste.

Air turbulence over the four nasal conchae (or tubinates) exposes *smells* to olfactory chemoreceptors. Intubation bypasses this mechanism, so sense of smell is usually reduced, although not absent. ICU smells are often abnormal:

- "hospital" smells (disinfectant, diarrhoea, body fluids)
- human smells (perfume, body odours)
- putrefying wounds
- nasogastric feeds.

Making sense of environments

The reticular activating system, near the medulla, filters information from the senses. Normally nearly all information is blocked, with only the few meaningful (for the individual) stimuli reaching the cerebral cortex, where we make sense of our environment. Removing irrelevant stimuli prevents sensory overload, keeping us sane. Reticular activating system dysfunction may be caused by "psychedelic" drugs (e.g. ketamine, lysergic acid – LSD, ecstasy – see Chapter 46) or:

- reduced sensory input
- relevance deprivation
- repetitive stimulation
- unconsciousness.

(O'Shea, 1997)

Responses depend on both *reception* (sensory stimuli) and *perception* (sensory transmission to, and interpretation by, higher centres). Hallucinations vary, often being vivid, and usually terrifying. Sensory deprivation can cause acute psychoses, delusions, severe depression and post-traumatic stress disorder (Åkerman *et al.*, 2010; Pandharipande *et al.*, 2013; Wade *et al.*, 2013), which may persist for many days, months and possibly years.

Intubation prevents ICU patients from speaking, and conscious ICU patients often have psychomotor weakness, which makes writing difficult. Patients find not being able to communicate extremely stressful (Wenham and Pittard, 2009; Khalaila *et al.*, 2011). Gestures, facial expression and physiological signs (e.g. tachycardia) may be attempts to communicate, or indicate comfort, pain or anxiety. Conscious intubated patients often mouth words, but the effectiveness of this varies with their mouthing and others' ability to lipread. Speaking valves and devices exist for patients with tracheostomies.

Understanding patients' perceptions and interpretations is not always possible but can make sense of hallucinations and bizarre actions. Reported experiences often suggest profound fear; nurses (and other healthcare professionals) may become devils/tormentors, so nurses attempting to explore fears or reassure patients may meet resistance.

Explanations may reduce anxiety and psychological (and so physical) pain (Hayward, 1975). But, like any physiological intervention, reality orientation is not beneficial for all situations, while quality and quantity affect its effectiveness. Inappropriate reality orientation can provoke aggression.

Noise

ICUs are noisy (Stafford *et al.*, 2014). Much noise is unavoidable, inevitably continuing overnight, but this can disturb sleep (Lawson *et al.*, 2010; Basner *et al.*, 2014) and contribute to cardiovascular disease (Basner *et al.*, 2014). Nurses should actively reduce unnecessary noise, especially overnight (Alway *et al.*, 2013).

Circadian rhythm

Circadian rhythm, the body's daily rhythm (*circa dias* = Latin for "around the day"), is a "clock" regulated by the suprachiasmatic nuclei, in the hypothalamus. Inevitably it is individual to each person, with normal slight variations between each day, but is strongly linked to light (Craig and Mathieu, 2017), and in ICUs is too often disrupted by excessive light at night (Durrington, 2017). Circadian rhythm regulates release of many hormones; for example, endogenous nor-adrenaline release is reduced overnight, contributing to reduction in blood pressure. Critical illness and abnormal environments (ICU) can severely disrupt circadian rhythm (Gazendam *et al.*, 2013). Bjovatn *et al.* (2012) found shift work increased psychological ill health in ICU nurses working shifts, while Vyas *et al.* (2012) linked circadian rhythm to increased risk of myocardial infarction and stroke. Historically, most major disasters involving human error have occurred at night (Rajaratnam and Arendt, 2001), so unnecessary high-risk actions (e.g. extubation) should be avoided overnight when they and other staff are likely to be less alert. During this ebb, reduced peripheral circulation may cause ischaemia (e.g. "night cramps"). Sedation, unlike normal sleep, is not circadian (Grounds *et al.*, 2014), and so sedation lacks many restorative functions of normal sleep.

Circulating catecholamine and cortisol levels peak around 6 am (Chassard and Bruguerolle, 2004). Sympathetic stimulation makes the cardiovascular system hyperdynamic – tachycardia, vasoconstriction. Peak time for myocardial infarctions and strokes is 6 am to 10 am (Scheer and Shea, 2014), so early-morning stimulation (e.g. washes) is best avoided with vulnerable patients.

Sleep

Sleep is essential to physical and psychological health; sleep deprivation increases mortality (Pulak and Jensen, 2016) and delirium (Petrovsky *et al.*, 2014), yet many ICU patients sleep poorly (Elliott *et al.*, 2013; Pulak and Jensen, 2016). Sleep cycles are usually about 90 minutes, with the final stages (especially *rapid eye movement – REM*) being the most restorative (Wenham and Pittard, 2009;

Kamdar *et al.*, 2012; Pulak and Jensen, 2016). Mechanically ventilated patients often suffer reduction of REM sleep (Grounds *et al.*, 2014), but for many patients sleep in ICU is often suboptimal; some inhibitory factors have been mentioned above, but sleep is most commonly disturbed by pain, anxiety and fear (Krotsetis *et al.*, 2017).

ICU nurses should facilitate sleep by:

■ ensuring night-time environments are as quiet and dark as reasonably and safely possible;
■ minimising interruptions, and allowing 90–120 minutes between interventions likely to disturb sleep;
■ providing earplugs/eyeshades if desired (Daneshmandi *et al.*, 2012; Alway *et al.*, 2013; Stafford *et al.*, 2014);
■ assessing effects of any night sedation used;
■ individual assessment of sleeping pattern/needs.

While earplugs and eye masks improve quality of sleep in disruptive environments, they reduce symptoms rather than resolve underlying problems. Nurses should therefore also attempt to facilitate environments conducive to sleep. Dimming lights mimics day/night cycles, but "dimmed" lighting often exceeds levels most nurses would choose for their own bedrooms at night, although some patients may find some light comforting.

The pineal hormone melatonin facilitates sleep (Ganz, 2012). Released during hours of darkness, ICU patients typically have low levels (Kamdar *et al.*, 2012). Lack of melatonin during daylight hours results in short sleep episodes and more wakefulness (Luckhaupt, 2012). Commercially available melatonin has been used in various contexts (Auld *et al.*, 2017) but at present there is no clear evidence of benefit for ICU patients (Bellapart and Boots, 2012). Afternoon rest periods of 90–120 minutes provide the opportunity for patients to recuperate from often physically tiring morning activities.

Patient diaries

Memories of ICU are often incomplete and compressed. "Missing time" can be psychologically traumatic. "Patient diaries", recording significant events during their illness which patients may want to find out about, have been promoted as a means of coming to terms with "missing time" (Åkerman *et al.*, 2010; Garrouste-Orgeas *et al.*, 2012; I.C.S., 2015), reducing post-traumatic stress disorder (Jones *et al.*, 2010) and helping relatives cope (Nielsen and Angel, 2016; Davidson *et al.*, 2017), but evidence for their benefits or potential harm remains weak, and there is insufficient evidence to support their use (Ullman *et al.*, 2014).

Nursing staff are the primary authors of patient diaries (Ullman *et al.*, 2014). Professional duties of confidentiality, other ethical issues, and workload (Åkerman *et al.*, 2010) may limit staff keeping patient diaries, and this may not be the best use of limited nursing time, but entries can be made by families, who are more likely to record what would interest patients. Where diaries are used, opportunities for follow-up discussion and explanations should be available. Follow-up can be provided through:

- Critical Care Outreach
- return visits to the unit
- ICU follow-up clinics.

Much initial literature about ICUs' follow-up clinics was enthusiastic, although Cuthbertson *et al.* (2009) suggest that nurse-led follow-up clinics are neither effective psychologically nor cost-effective. Ramsay *et al.* (2014) identify that following discharge patients have psychiatric and psychological needs, while Herridge *et al.* (2016) suggest that families suffer similar PTSD, so should be included in follow-up programmes. Whether through follow-up visits on wards or through clinics, Critical Care Outreach and other support services help reduce relocation stress for patients, as well as providing "safety nets" in case of physiological deterioration.

Safety

Patient safety is central to healthcare, being enshrined in all professional codes, national bodies such as the Care Quality Commission, and such classic resources as Nightingale (1859/1980) and Roper *et al.* (1996). Confused patients may cause harm to themselves. While the law expects that healthcare professionals will act in patients' best interests (Dimond, 2015), how far "best interests" includes restraining confused patients from harming themselves is ethically and legally debatable. The five key principles of the Mental Capacity Act (2005) identify that:

- staff must presume capacity to make decisions until proved otherwise;
- staff must support people to make their own decisions using "all practical means";
- staff must not treat people as lacking capacity to make decisions because their decision is unwise;
- patients' best interests are paramount;
- decisions by others must interfere least with rights and freedom of action of those lacking capacity.

Rights of the incapacitated are enforceable through the Court of Protection, but when confused patients attempt to self-extubate there is not time to seek guidance from courts or lawyers. The Mental Capacity Act is law in England and Wales; for Scotland, the Adults with Incapacity (Scotland) Act 2000 makes similar provisions.

Restraint is sometimes necessary to prevent patients harming themselves (e.g. self-extubation), but means used must be proportional to the harm (Musters,

2010), and restraint may actually increase problem behaviours (Hulatt, 2014) such as self-extubation rates (Chang *et al.*, 2008) and falls (Tzeng and Yin, 2012). Physical restraints are marketed, but ICUs should be cautious about introducing them as they may cause more harm than good (Hine, 2007). Where physical restraints are used, local protocols should be developed (Bray *et al.*, 2004) to protect both staff and patients. Physical restraint should be a last resort (R.C.N., 2016). Traditionally, the UK has preferred chemical to physical restraint, although ethical and legal differences between the two are also debatable (Bray *et al.*, 2004). Sedatives are discussed further in Chapter 6.

Recovery

Despite complications, most ICU patients survive critical illness. Having become used to 1:1 and 1:2 nursing, transfer to reduced staffing ratios and reduced monitoring of wards can be stressful for both patients and family (Guest, 2017), at a time when they are coping with "Postintensive Care Syndrome" (Harvey and Davidson, 2016). Weaning care by reducing:

- time spent with patients, and
- monitoring (equipment, frequency)

helps adjustment to non-intensive care environments ("de-ICU-ing"). Ongoing physical and psychological deficits are common; over half of ICU survivors suffer long-term cognitive impairment (Wolters *et al.*, 2013).

Implications for practice

- many ICU patients suffer delirium, post-traumatic stress disorder, and other psychological problems;
- psychology affects health; psychological ill health increases mortality and morbidity;
- psychological problems are not always obvious and may remain undetected;
- good psychological care can prevent problems;
- sensory imbalance is a symptom of psychological pain, provoking a stress response; alleviating pain provides both humanitarian and physiological benefits, so should be fundamental to nursing assessment and care.
- Sensory imbalance can be reduced by

  - creating environments that minimise sensory monotony or overload;
  - providing patients with explanations, and helping them to understand what they are experiencing;
  - where patients are able to participate in care, encouraging them to take active roles.

- monitors should be sited unobtrusively;
- facilitating sleep is usually the nurse's most important role overnight;

- patient diaries can be a useful means for patients to come to terms with "missing time" and post-traumatic stress disorder, but there should be opportunities for patients to discuss these after ICU discharge;
- with recovery, care should be weaned to prepare patients for ward environments ("de-ICU-ing").

Summary

The significance of psychology is often acknowledged in academic assignments, but not so often translated into practice. Critical care nurses necessarily prioritise resolving physiological crises. But psychological problems are common and complicate recovery. Nurses can valuably humanise environments for patients and help promote psychological well-being.

Further reading

N.I.C.E. provides guidance for post-ICU rehabilitation (2009) and delirium (2010a). At the time of writing, Intensive Care Society guidelines for delirium are scheduled for review; their guidelines on sedation (Grounds *et al.*, 2014) are recent. The R.C.N. (2016) discusses physical, but not chemical, restraint.

Clinical scenarios

Mr Robert Duke is 67 years old and was admitted to the ICU 26 days ago following emergency abdominal surgery. His past medical history includes COPD, smoking and heavy alcohol use. Mr Duke has a tracheostomy and his respiratory support has been weaned to high-flow nasal oxygen. He continues to have copious secretions requiring clearance, and twice-daily 5 mg nicotine patch applications. Mr Duke refuses to cooperate with nursing care and avoids eye contact with everyone except his wife. He appears sleep-deprived, often napping, but totalling three hours sleep recorded in 24 hours.

Q1. In what ways can Mr Duke's psychological state be monitored? Consider effects of mood, anxiety, understanding, consent to treatments, pain and discomfort. How can Mr Duke's communication abilities and understanding be assessed?

Q2. Identify risk factors associated with development of sensory imbalance and delirium in the ICU for Mr Duke. How can these risks be minimised?

Q3. How might his experience of ICU be improved? Include specific interventions for psychological and physical comfort.

Part II

Fundamental

Chapter 4

Artificial ventilation

Contents

Fundamental knowledge

Respiratory anatomy and physiology
Normal (negative pressure) breathing and mechanics
    of normal breathing
Dead space and normal lung volumes
Experience of nursing ventilated patients
Local weaning protocols/guidelines

Introduction

Ventilation is the process by which gases move in and out of the lungs. When self-ventilation is, or is likely to be, inadequate owing to disease or drugs, artificial ventilation may be required. Artificial ventilation may fully replace patients' own ventilation, or support self-ventilation.

Intensive care units developed from respiratory units. Providing mechanical ventilation, and so caring for artificially ventilated patients, is fundamental to intensive care nursing. Nurses should have a safe working knowledge of machines and modes they use – manufacturers' literature, websites and company representatives are usually good sources for information. This chapter discusses

Table 4.1 Commonly used abbreviations and terms

AMV	assisted mandatory ventilation
APRV	airway pressure release ventilation
APV	adaptive pressure ventilation
ASV	assisted support ventilation
barotrauma	damage to alveoli from excessively high (peak) airway pressure
CMV	controlled mechanical ventilation
FiO_2	fraction of inspired oxygen (expressed as a decimal fraction, so FiO_2 1.0 = 100% or pure oxygen)
I:E	inspiratory to expiratory ratio (on ventilator)
MMV	mandatory minute ventilation
open lung strategies	strategies to keep alveoli constantly open, and so prevent atelectasis
PAV	proportional assist ventilation
permissive hypercapnia	tolerating abnormally high arterial carbon dioxide tensions ($PaCO_2$) to enable smaller tidal volumes
pressure support	self-ventilating (triggered) breaths have volume augmented by the ventilator until preset airway pressure is reached
PRVC	pressure regulated volume control
PS	pressure support
Respiratory failure	Type 1: oxygenation failure – hypoxia ($PaO_2 < 8$ kPa) with normocapnia ($PaCO_2 < 6$ kPa); Type 2: ventilatory failure – hypoxia ($PaO_2 < 8$ kPa) with hypercapnia ($PaCO_2 > 6$ kPa)
SIMV	synchronised intermittent mandatory ventilation
trigger	when patient-initiated breaths generate sufficient negative pressure, trigger initiates inspiratory phases through ventilators
V/Q	(alveolar) ventilation to (pulmonary capillary) perfusion ratio; normal V/Q = 0.8
VALI	ventilator-associated lung injury (see VILI)
VILI	ventilator-induced lung injury (see VALI)
volutrauma	damage from alveolar distension (excessive volume); also called "volotrauma"

the main components of ventilation, more commonly used modes, and identifies complications of positive pressure ventilation on other body systems. Table 4.1 lists commonly used abbreviations and terms, but terminology of modes varies between manufacturers and authors. Prone positioning is discussed in Chapter 27, and further ventilatory options, including ECMO, are discussed in Chapter 28. Negative pressure ventilation is rarely used in ICUs, so is not discussed in this book.

Frequently used ventilator settings are discussed, but different diseases need different supports, and the variety of adjustments that can be offered means that different practitioners will often prefer different options. Anaesthetists normally decide ventilator settings, although experienced nurses may make adjustments. If in doubt about any settings, nurses should always seek further advice.

Invasive ventilation can be life-saving, but dying sedated and intubated on a busy ICU is not dignified. Invasive ventilation should therefore only be used for potentially recoverable conditions. When patients cannot make competent decisions for themselves, nurses (as patients' advocates) should contribute actively to multidisciplinary decisions. A useful ethical maxim is whether proposed interventions are likely to prolong life or prolong death.

Ventilator-associated pneumonia (VAP) is discussed in Chapter 15.

Respiratory failure

There are two types of respiratory failure:

■ Type 1: oxygenation failure – hypoxia (PaO_2 < 8 kPa) with normocapnia ($PaCO_2$ < 6 kPa);
■ Type 2: ventilatory failure – hypoxia (PaO_2 < 8 kPa) with hypercapnia ($PaCO_2$ > 6 kPa).

(British Thoracic Society – B.T.S., 2002)

Gas exchange in lungs is determined by three factors:

■ ventilation (V) – breath size;
■ perfusion (Q) – pulmonary blood flow;
■ diffusion – movement of gases across tissue between pulmonary blood and alveolar air.

Healthy, resting, average-sized adults breathe about four litres each minute, and have cardiac outputs of about five litres. This creates ventilation:perfusion (V/Q) ratios of 4:5, or 0.8. Perfusion without ventilation is called a *shunt*. Shunting can also occur at tissue level (reduced oxygen extraction).

Carbon dioxide is much more soluble than oxygen. In health, the distance between alveolar air and pulmonary blood is minuscule – 0.2–0.4 micrometres (erythrocyte diameter is about 7 micrometres). So, in health, poorer solubility of oxygen is insignificant. Diseases increasing distance between alveolar air and pulmonary blood (such as pulmonary oedema) inhibit oxygen transfer, causing type 1 respiratory failure.

Air contains virtually no carbon dioxide (0.04%). Carbon dioxide is a waste product of cell metabolism. Provided metabolism and carbon dioxide production remain constant, blood levels depend on removal, which is mainly affected by breath size, flow and frequency (rate). Type 2 respiratory failure may be caused by any disease which limits breath size, such as neuromuscular weakness (e.g. Guillain-Barré Syndrome), bronchoconstriction (chronic obstructive pulmonary disease) or extensive alveolar damage (emphysema, ARDS). Carbon dioxide production can be affected by nutrition – feeds such as Pulmocare produce less carbon dioxide than standard feeds.

Artificial ventilation

Artificial ventilation attempts to temporarily replace or support patients' own ventilation. This may be planned as part of post-operative care or necessitated by existing or potentially imminent severe respiratory failure.

Ventilators have various safety features, including apnoea backup, which changes self-ventilating modes to mandatory ones if apnoea persists beyond preset limits, often 20 seconds.

Oxygenation relies on functional alveolar surface area, so is determined by:

- mean airway pressure
- inspiration time
- PEEP
- FiO_2
- pulmonary blood flow.

Carbon dioxide removal requires active tidal ventilation, so is affected by:

- tidal volumes
- expiratory time
- frequency and flow of breath
- resistance to expiration ("gas trapping").

Manipulating these factors can optimise ventilation while minimising complications.

Positive pressure ventilation is often life-saving but it can also cause lung damage from excessive airway pressure (barotrauma) and volume (volutrauma) – in diseased lungs often, but not always, essentially the same problem, causing biotrauma – the release of toxic mediators (Slutsky, 2015). As awareness of ventilator-induced lung injury (VILI) developed, so "lung-protective" strategies evolved (see below). Many other developments in ventilation have been to reduce other problems, making ventilators more "patient-friendly", so allowing lighter sedation and earlier extubation.

Modes of ventilation

Historically, positive pressure ventilators were classified by their cycles:

■ time (controlled by rate or I:E ratio);
■ volume (delivers gas until preset tidal volume is reached);
■ pressure (delivers gas until preset airway pressure is reached);
■ flow (rarely used).

Such classifications are now over-simplistic; most modern ventilators use elements in these cycles in an often-bewildering variety of modes. Choice of modes depends partly on options available, partly on preference and partly on need. For example, effects of ventilation on sleep were discussed in Chapter 3.

Originally, positive pressure ventilation was usually *controlled mandatory ventilation (CMV)* – the minute or tidal volume together with a respiratory rate was set by the operator, then fully controlled by the machine. This would be distressing for conscious patients, necessitating deep sedation. CMV is usually still available on ventilators but is rarely used in ICUs. With self-ventilating modes, almost all ventilators will have a default mode, so that if patients become apnoeic they continue to be ventilated. CMV is often the default mode of modern ventilators. On modern ventilators, CMV will almost invariably be tempered by pressure limits, to prevent barotrauma. This therefore mixes time, volume and pressure cycles.

Pressure control (PC) developed from paediatric use, where cuffed endo-tracheal tubes used not to be used until about eight to 12 years of age (see Chapter 13). With adult ventilation, pressure control is usually an adjunct to prevent excessive pressure (and so barotrauma) in other modes.

Some of the more commonly available modes on ventilators include:

■ *pressure regulated volume control (PRVC)*, also called *adaptive pressure ventilation (APV)*
■ *synchronised intermittent mandatory ventilation (SIMV)*
■ *adaptive support ventilation (ASV)*
■ *neuronally asssisted ventilation (NAVA)*
■ and various "self-ventilating" modes such as
  ● *airway release pressure ventilation (ARPV)*
  ● *pressure support ventilation (PSV)*
  ● *continuous positive airway pressure (CPAP)*
  ● *bilevel positive airway pressure (BiPAP, bilevel)*
  ● *proportional assist ventilation (PAV)*

PRVC controls volume, so is essentially CMV, but ceases if maximum preset pressure is reached (to prevent barotrauma – see below). Self-ventilating breaths are often difficult (but vary between manufacturers), so this mode is not suitable for weaning.

SIMV was an early weaning mode, reducing the frequency of ventilator breaths while synchronising with patient-initiated breaths to prevent hyper-inflation and barotrauma.

Relatively rarely used now, it is usually combined with pressure regulation (to limit barotrauma) and pressure support (see below) – PSIMV. It should not now be used for weaning (Brignall and Davidson, 2009).

ASV adjusts various aspects (mandatory rate, tidal volume, inspiratory pressure, inspiratory time, I:E ratio) to maintain preset minute volume. ASV may be useful for weaning (Petter *et al.*, 2003) or to replace conventional ventilation (Iotti *et al.*, 2010).

NAVA uses the patient's own electrical activity of the diaphragm (Edi), detected through a modified nasogastric tube (Tane *et al.*, 2015), to trigger ventilation. Advocates claim this improves ventilator synchrony (Di Mussi *et al.*, 2016; Navalesia and Longhini, 2015), but most studies found it less effective than other patient-led options (Moerer *et al.*, 2008; Delisle *et al.*, 2011). Patient intolerance to feeding tubes presumably invalidates this mode.

Airway Pressure Release Ventilation (APRV) sets target minute volumes as a percentage in relation to ideal body weight, usually derived from height (O'Brien *et al.*, 2009c). Pressures are set as high pressure (P High) for much of the cycle, with periodic release to a lower pressure (P Low). P High achieves an "open lung" approach, recruiting alveoli and maintaining patency in open alveoli, while periodic P Low facilitates carbon dioxide clearance. APRV facilitates weaning, as reducing percentage of minute volume, or pressure difference, encourages spontaneous ventilation.

Facchin and Fan (2015) suggest that APRV creates inverse ratio ventilation, so should be avoided with ARDS. Studies comparing outcome against ARDSNet protocols show mixed results, Kollisch-Singule *et al.* (2015) finding that APRV caused less lung damage, while Zhou *et al.* (2017) found APRV improved outcomes. Davies *et al.* (2015) reported worse neurological outcomes with APRV, but Marik *et al.*'s (2012) case report suggested that APRV was safe with neurological pathologies.

PSV is a self-ventilating, flow-cycled, mode. Once a breath is triggered, pressure support delivers gas until preset pressure is reached, adding volume to weak breaths, so compensating for respiratory muscle weakness. Although often available as a mode in its own right, it is also often used as an adjunct with other modes (pressure support – PS). Pressure support is often commenced at 20 cmH$_2$O, then weaned usually by increments of 2; once pressure support is 8–10 cmH$_2$O extubation is often possible. Pressure support ventilation is the most widely used weaning mode (Brignall and Davidson, 2009), but it is less conducive to sleep than assist–control ventilation (Figuerosa-Ramos *et al.*, 2009), so may not be an ideal choice for night-time. Pressure support is often available in other modes to increase size of patient-initiated breaths.

CPAP is a self-ventilating form of PEEP (see below), and is available on many ventilators, although more often bilevel modes (see below) are used. CPAP stabilises and recruits alveoli, enables gas exchange to continue between breaths, and can resolve pulmonary oedema. Expired positive airway pressure (EPAP) of bilevel modes has similar benefits to CPAP.

Bilevel positive airway pressure is like two alternating levels of CPAP: higher pressure on inspiration (inspired positive airway pressure – IPAP) and lower during expiration (expired positive airway pressure – EPAP). EPAP provides all the benefits of PEEP/CPAP, while higher inspiratory pressures increase tidal volume. Though often colloquially called BiPAP, this is a brand name, so ventilators may use various terms for this option, usually including the letters "PAP" (positive airway pressure). Although technically not NIV, high-flow humidified nasal oxygen generates 2–8 cmH$_2$O pressure in the oropharynx (Corley *et al.*, 2011), is better-tolerated than CPAP or BiPAP (Price *et al.*, 2008; Turnbull, 2008), and may prevent need for NIV (Maggiore *et al.*, 2014). NIV is often useful for:

- attempts to avoid intubation (e.g. Guillain-Barré Syndrome);
- patients who have been deemed not suitable for invasive ventilation ("ceiling treatment");
- weaning, especially for patients with COPD (Burns *et al.*, 2009; Ferrer *et al.*, 2009).

NIV is discussed further in Woodrow (2016).

PAV allows ventilators to adjust (proportion) airway pressure according to patients' effort (Hess, 2002), thus compensating for changes in lung compliance and resistance. It is currently not available on many ventilators.

Settings

Within each mode, various settings can "fine-tune" ventilation, although not all options are available in all modes. Different modes and ventilators offer different options, but core options are:

- tidal volume
- minute volume
- respiratory rate
- oxygen.

Increasing one or more of the first three usually clears more carbon dioxide. Additional options usually include:

- PEEP
- I:E ratio
- trigger.

Tidal volume (Vt) affects gas exchange but can also cause shearing damage to lungs; settings therefore balance gas exchange against limiting lung injury.

Patients at greatest risk from alveolar trauma usually have poor compliance, low functional lung volumes, and hypoxia. The Acute Respiratory Distress Syndrome Network (ARDSNet, 2008) recommends initial tidal volumes of 8 ml/kg predicted body weight, reducing quickly to 6 ml/kg (420 ml for 70kg patients), which may necessitate accepting permissive hypercapnia. Larger tidal volumes risk ventilator-induced lung injury (see below); even slight increases escalate mortality with ARDS (Needham *et al.*, 2015). Gas exchange may be improved through adjusting other aspects (e.g. inspiratory flow, mean airway pressure, PEEP).

Minute Volume is the sum of tidal volume multiplied by respiratory rate (if both are constant):

$$\text{minute volume} = \text{tidal volume} \times \text{respiratory rate}$$

Setting two of these components on any ventilator necessarily sets the third. All three are usually monitored.

Respiratory rate is usually set between eight and 16 breaths per minute if ventilation is fully controlled, but reducing respiratory rate is a useful means of weaning. If treatment is withdrawn, rate will usually be set at eight.

Oxygen is usually adjusted according to PaO_2 and saturation targets, although other aspects (e.g. PEEP) also affect oxygenation. In ICUs, oxygen is usually recorded as FiO_2; this means "fraction of inspired oxygen", so pure (100%) oxygen is an FiO_2 of 1.0, while 50% oxygen is an FiO_2 of 0.5.

Like any drug, oxygen can be toxic. Prolonged use of high-concentration oxygen (probably > 50% for > 24 hours, although precise figures remain unknown) can cause excessive release of oxygen radicals (also called reactive oxygen species – ROS), which cause lung and other tissue damage (Gomes *et al.*, 2012). Maintaining normal oxygen levels, rather than hyperoxic, levels, hastens recovery from critical illness and improves survival (Eastwood *et al.*, 2016).

Positive end expiratory pressure (PEEP):

- prevents atelectasis;
- recruits collapsed alveoli; and
- facilitates oxygen exchange during expiratory pause, so improving oxygenation.

Increasing PEEP can therefore be an alternative or supplement to increasing inspired oxygen. High PEEP is sometimes used for "open lung strategies" to prevent ventilator-associated lung injury (VALI).

Respiratory muscles normally relax passively with expiration, leaving residual gas within airways, usually exerting 2–2.5 cmH_2O pressure and so maintaining alveolar patency. This is variously called "auto-PEEP", "intrinsic PEEP", "natural PEEP", "air trapping" and "breath stacking". Intubation prevents upper (but not lower) airway closure, so measured airway pressure returns to *zero-PEEP* at the end of expiration.

Increased intrathoracic pressure can:

- cause barotrauma;
- cause gas trapping and hypercapnia;
- reduce venous return (increasing cardiac workload);
- increase work of breathing on self-ventilating modes, by increasing resistance to expiration.

High PEEP (e.g. 10 cmH$_2$O) may increase extravascular lung water (Maybauer *et al.*, 2006), so with ARDS, and many other conditions, optimal PEEP is generally 5 cmH$_2$O (Caironi *et al.*, 2015). The Acute Respiratory Distress Syndrome Network (2008) recommends increasing PEEP according to FiO$_2$. With conditions such as asthma, where gas trapping from bronchospasm is a major problem, minimal or zero-PEEP is used (Brenner *et al.*, 2009).

Inspiratory:expiratory (I:E) ratio. Breaths have three active phases:

- inspiration
- pause/plateau/inspiratory pause
- expiration

and a fourth passive phase:

- expiratory pause.

Normal I:E ratios are about 1:2, with plateau usually being adjusted separately. I:E ratio cannot be regulated in self-ventilating modes.

Awake patients are unlikely to tolerate significantly different ratios. Reduced airflow (poor lung compliance, e.g. ARDS), necessitates relatively longer inspiratory time. Oxygen transfer occurs primarily during inspiration and plateau; incomplete expiration (e.g. short expiratory phase; gas trapping) increases alveolar carbon dioxide concentrations, reducing diffusion from blood. Changing the inspiration to expiration (*I:E*) ratio therefore manipulates alveolar gas exchange. Prolonging pause/plateau time has similar effects to PEEP – increasing gas exchange, but also increasing intrathoracic pressure. Bronchospasm (e.g. asthma) reduces expiratory flow, needing longer expiratory time.

Trigger senses patient-initiated breaths. Making trigger levels less negative makes it easier to initiate breaths through the ventilator, so can be useful for weaning. With many modes, triggered breaths are additional to preset volumes.

At rest, self-ventilation negative pressure is approximately –3 mmHg; trigger levels below this can cause discomfort (fighting). Settings close to zero are usually used (e.g. 0.5–2). Settings of zero can cause autocycling, the ventilator triggering itself at the end of each expiratory phase. Trigger/sensitivity settings normally allow for PEEP (but check manufacturers' information), so trigger of –0.5 cmH$_2$O with PEEP of 5 allows triggering at +4.5 cmH$_2$O.

Self-ventilating modes rely on patient-initiated breaths. If patients are gas trapping (e.g. asthma), they may generate insufficient negative pressure to trigger ventilators.

Airway pressure is created by flow through the airways. High pressure can cause lung tissue damage (barotrauma), so peak pressure limits should ideally be below 30 cmH$_2$O (ARDSNet, 2008; Petrucci and De Feo, 2013). Maximising mean arterial pressure while limiting peak pressure optimises volume, and so oxygenation. Adjusting modes and aspects of modes can affect both peak and mean pressures, which is why it is useful to record both on observation charts. Generally, *peak pressure limits* alarms should be set at 30 cmH$_2$O, although sometimes compromises between ventilation needs and barotrauma risks necessitate other limits. Ventilators halt flow once peak pressure limit is reached, so preset tidal volumes may not be achieved if airway pressures are high.

Inverse ratio ventilation (IRV) uses ratios of 1:1 or below, making expiratory time abnormally short. Potential advantages of IRV are:

- alveolar recruitment from prolonged inspiration time;
- alveolar stabilisation from shorter expiratory time (like PEEP);
- increased mean airway pressure (increased ventilation) without raising peak pressure (barotrauma).

IRV is physiologically abnormal, so it can only be used with mandatory ventilation and usually necessitates additional sedation and often paralysis. IRV further increases intrathoracic pressure, compromising cardiac output. Enthusiasm for IRV has waned, possibly due to increasing concerns that ventilatory dyssynchrony may increase mortality and morbidity (Blanch *et al.*, 2015).

Independent lung ventilation

With single-lung pathology, patients may benefit from different modes of ventilation being used to each lung. Independent lung ventilation requires double-lumen endotracheal tubes, one lumen entering each bronchus. Independent ventilators, each using any available mode, may then be used for each lung.

Independent lung ventilation may be impractical owing to:

- insufficient available ventilators;
- increased costs and workload (e.g. ventilator observations are doubled);
- danger to safety (access to patient, consuming more nursing time).

Care of ventilated patient

Ventilators are usually complex machines and can be a source of fear for many nurses new to ICU, but, while technical skills are essential, the focus of care should remain the individual patient as a person. Care should be patient-centred, holistic, respectful and dignified – themes underlying many chapters in this book. Artificial ventilation causes potential problems with:

- safety
- replacing normal functions (see Chapter 5)
- system complications.

Safety

Individual patient handover is usually at the bedside. During handover, and frequently during their shift, nurses should observe their patients'

- general appearance (e.g. colour, position, facial expression);
- level of sedation;
- comfort (signs of pain, body position/alignment, coughing/gagging from tube).

Following handover, respiratory observations include:

- chest wall movement (bilateral);
- lung auscultation to identify air entry (see Chapter 17) and lung sounds. If secretions (rattles) are heard, suction is usually needed;
- ETT size and position;
- cuff pressure (see Chapter 5);
- effectiveness of sedation and analgesia (usually through scoring systems).

Additional observations should be individualised to the patient, but may include:

- Glasgow Coma Scale;
- arterial blood gases;
- ventilator and capnography waveforms.

Following handover, the ventilator should be checked for:

- all settings, and whether they are appropriate for the patient;
- alarm limits;
- what effort/breaths (if any) the patient is making, and size of self-ventilating tidal volumes;
- ventilator waveforms (see Chapter 17).

Layout of bed areas should minimise nurses having to turn their backs on their patients. Alarms do not replace the need for nursing observation but are useful adjuncts, so should be narrow enough to provide early warning of significant changes, but with sufficient leeway to avoid causing patients or family unnecessary distress.

Safety equipment and backup facilities in case of ventilator, power or gas failure should include:

- manual rebreathing bag, with suitable connections;
- full oxygen cylinders;
- reintubation and suction equipment (check suction equipment works).

Additional safety equipment may also be needed (e.g. tracheal dilators). Nurses should check all safety equipment at the start of each shift.

System complications

All body systems are affected by artificial ventilation. Managing artificial ventilation focuses on avoiding or limiting ventilator-induced damage rather than achieving "normal" gases. Generally higher pressures create more complications, so the ideal pressure is the lowest one that achieves the aims – generally it is best to start low and increase pressures according to needs (R.C.P., 2008).

Respiratory. The main complication, ventilatory-associated lung injury (VALI), is discussed below. Other respiratory complications include:

- increased work of breathing (in self-ventilating modes/breaths) from narrow, rigid tubes;
- induced diaphragmatic weakness, from potentially as little as 18 hours diaphragmatic rest (Tobin *et al.*, 2010).

Artificial support should therefore be increased if patients show signs of exhaustion or become tachypnoeic with low tidal volumes. Ventilatory support may be increased overnight to facilitate sleep. Optimal ventilation will be individual to each patient, with modes and settings varying between clinicians. If severe respiratory muscle causes prolonged weaning, patients may benefit by "resting" overnight on ventilator-initiated modes, to resume weaning the following day.

Cardiovascular. Normal respiration aids cardiac return through negative intrathoracic pressure. Conversely, positive pressure ventilation:

- impedes venous return
- increases right ventricular workload
- reduces stroke volume.

So, positive pressure ventilation increases venous while reducing arterial pressures, potentially causing:

- oedema (including pulmonary)
- hypoperfusion/failure of all organs.

Oedema may be caused by:

■ venous congestion
■ renin–angiotensin–aldosterone response
■ antidiuretic hormone secretion
■ atrial natriuretic peptide.

Liver dysfunction from:

■ diaphragmatic compression (raised intrathoracic pressure)
■ portal congestion and hypertension (impaired venous return)
■ ischaemia (arterial hypotension)

reduces:

■ albumin production
■ drug, hormone and toxin metabolism
■ clotting factor production
■ complement production (infection control),

so contributing to:

■ reduced colloid osmotic pressure (hypovolaemia, hypotension, oedema)
■ toxicity (e.g. ammonia can cause coma)
■ coagulopathy
■ opportunistic infection.

Neurological. Reduced cerebral blood flow predisposes to confusion/delirium.

Ventilator-associated lung injury (VALI)

Identification of VALI has led to various strategies including:

■ open lung strategies: PEEP + prone position (Slutsky and Ranieri, 2013)
■ semi-recumbent position (Drakulovic *et al.*, 1999; Rose *et al.*, 2010)
■ low tidal volumes (ARDSNet, 2008)
■ pressure-limited ventilation (Amato *et al.*, 2015)
■ extracorporeal membrane oxygenation (see Chapter 28).

Lung volume and pressure are indirectly linked; artificial ventilation can be optimised by maximising mean airway pressure while limiting peak pressure, achievable through monitoring on ventilators, including pressure:volume waveforms (see Chapter 17).

The I.C.S. (2015) endorses lung-protective strategies of:

■ tidal volumes of 6 ml/kg (ideal body weight)
■ plateau pressure limited to 30 cm/H_2O.

Lung protection may necessitate accepting parameters outside normal physiological ranges:

■ tachypnoea
■ acidosis
■ lower oxygenation.

Lung protection reduces duration of mechanical ventilation (Imanaka *et al.*, 2010) and increases survival (Needham *et al.*, 2012; Serpa Neto *et al.*, 2012).

Weaning

With severe respiratory failure, artificial ventilation may be life-saving. But prolonging ventilation unnecessarily is costly, both to patients (morbidity, risks – especially ventilator-associated pneumonia – see Chapter 15) and to ICUs (workload, financial). Judging the optimal time for weaning is therefore challenging. If weaning is likely to be slow, tracheostomy increases success and survival (Wu *et al.*, 2010; Jubran *et al.*, 2013). Prolonged (18–69 hours) of complete diaphragmatic inactivity damages muscle fibres, so should be avoided if possible (Tobin *et al.*, 2010).

Daily "sedation holds" (see Chapter 6) help assess likely success of weaning/extubation.

Debate persists over optimal weaning criteria, but EfCCNa (2012) suggest:

■ improvement in the patient's underlying problem;
■ adequate respiratory rate and gas exchange;
■ stable cardiovascular function;
■ an acceptable state of consciousness.

Specific respiratory parameters may include:

■ PEEP 5, FiO_2 < 0.5; pressure support 8–10;
■ arterial blood gases pH 7.3–7.45, PaO_2:FiO_2 ratio > 26.

Modes used for weaning are less important that the multidisciplinary team process (Rose *et al.*, 2011; EfCCNa, 2012). Boles *et al.* (2007) recommend a spontaneous breathing trial of initially 30 minutes, using either a T-piece or low-level pressure support; if the trial fails, pressure support or assist–control ventilation are recommended modes, with NIV being considered to reduce intubation time. Brignall and Davidson (2009) favour pressure support ventilation for weaning. Various weaning protocols have been developed and recommended, claiming to reduce both number of ventilator-dependent days and length of ICU stay. Girard *et al.* (2017) favour weaning protocols, but these were written in the context of US healthcare. Weaning requires great skill (Crocker, 2009), and over-rigid use of protocols may delay more proactive, and equally (or more) successful, weaning using skilled clinical judgement

(Blackwood *et al.*, 2004; Krishnan *et al.*, 2004). Care given is more important than weaning mode used (Wu *et al.*, 2010). Psychological factors, such as communication and sleep, significantly influence success (Brignall and Davidson, 2009). Weaning should therefore be individualised to each patient and is best managed by experienced nurses (Crocker, 2009). With the array of weaning options available on most ventilators, locally preferred weaning methods are more likely to succeed (Blackwood *et al.*, 2004), and modes that are effective for one patient are not always effective for another. Some ventilators include automatic weaning loops, but Rose *et al.*'s (2013) Cochrane review found mixed results about whether they reduced weaning time. If initial short-term weaning plans fail, slower weaning plans should be instigated. Occasionally patients may need referral to centres specialising in long-term ventilation.

One-year survival for patients needing artificial ventilation for more than 14 days is poor (Damuth *et al.*, 2015), so, where further aggressive intervention would be inappropriate, teams may plan a "one-way wean". This may be part of terminal care or with hope of survival but recognising futility of reintubation, raising ethical issues about certainty of prognosis and value of life. Ideally, patients would participate in decision making, but this is not always possible. Where expected outcome of a one-way wean is rapid death, withdrawal of life-prolonging treatment should not mean withdrawal of all treatment. Terminal care, however brief, should aim to provide patients with the best possible death that can reasonably, and legally, be offered. What makes a "good death" is value-laden, so may vary greatly between patients – some patients might choose to die fully sedated and analgesed, while others might choose consciousness even at the cost of possible pain.

Implications for practice

- critically ill (Level 3) patients usually need mechanical ventilation;
- nurses have a central role in managing ventilation, so need technical knowledge of equipment to care safely and effectively for their patients;
- any machine can be inaccurate or fail; nurses should check all alarms and safety equipment at the start of each shift; ventilator function should be checked through recorded observations and continuously by visual observation and setting appropriate alarm parameters (often within 10%); remember that alarms may also fail;
- check the patient – air entry, appearance, and effectiveness of ventilation (SpO_2, tidal volume, ABGs). ABCDE is a useful structure for assessment;
- ventilators include default settings – know your machine and check that settings are appropriate for your patient;
- positive pressure ventilation affects all body systems; function of other systems should be continuously and holistically assessed;
- unless other positions are specifically indicated, patients should be nursed semi-recumbent;
- ventilated patients depend on nurses to provide fundamental aspects of care (e.g. hygiene, mouthcare);

- all intubation/mask equipment can cause damage – ties/tapes can occlude venous flow or cause direct trauma (e.g. tapes can damage lips and eyes); NIV masks and endotracheal cuffs can cause pressure sores;
- in addition to maintaining safe technological environments, nurses should provide psychological care through explanations and reassurance;
- Weaning necessitates close monitoring and observation, revising plans if patients appear to tire.

Summary

Breathing is vital to life. Patients rely on nurses and others to maintain safety. When breathing is wholly or partly replaced by mechanical ventilation, maintaining safety includes ensuring adequate ventilation.

Most ICU patients need ventilatory support. Many modes and options are available, although not all modes discussed are available on all machines. Choice should be adapted to individualised patient needs, which relies on nurses to continually monitor and assess their patients. Nurses therefore need a working knowledge of equipment on their unit and should be familiar with local protocols.

Positive pressure ventilation compromises function of other body systems. Nurses should assess complications from artificial ventilation, preventing risks where possible, minimising risks that cannot be avoided and replacing lost functions through fundamental care.

Further reading

Readers should familiarise themselves with manuals for ventilators used on their units. Slutsky (2015) provides an interesting and useful history of mechanical ventilation. Intensive Care Society guidelines for weaning are scheduled for review. Vincent *et al.* (2017) summarise oxygen toxicity.

Clinical scenarios

Mr Robert Hook is 32 years old with acute pancreatitis, bilateral pleural effusions, hypoxia, metabolic acidosis, tachypnoea and renal impairment. He was admitted to ICU for mechanical ventilation following four days of non-invasive ventilation and worsening respiratory function. He is orally intubated, weighs 106 kg, has copious white secretions via ETT and is draining thick sinus fluid into his oropharynx.

Ventilator settings

Mode APRV	Respiratory rate 26 breaths per minute
IBW 65 kg	TV 710–750 ml
130% minute volume	MV 18 to 19.5 litres/minute
FiO$_2$ 0.6	Peak/Mean Airway pressures 28/16 cmH$_2$O
PEEP 10 cmH$_2$O	

Arterial blood gas result	*Other blood results*	*Vital signs*
pH 7.41	Hb 98 grams/litre	Heart Rate 118 bpm
PaO$_2$ 14.5 kPa	WCC 15.5 × 10^9/litre	BP 140/55 mmHg
PaCO$_2$ 6.69 kPa	Platelets 32 × 10^9/litre	SpO$_2$ 100%
HCO$_3^-$ 27.6 mmol/litre	Albumin 13 grams/litre	Temperature 39.6°C
BE 4.5 mmol/litre	CRP 83 mg/litre	
SaO$_2$ 97%	Phosphate 1.23 mmol/litre	
	Magnesium 0.6 mmol/litre	

Q1. With this mode of ventilation, list other parameters which may be set, and specify what alarm limits you would set. What other observations should be documented?

Q2. Interpret Robert's results and suggest changes to the ventilator settings. Using ARDSNet (or your local) criteria, what should his tidal volumes ideally be? Identify potential complications of mechanical ventilation and strategies to minimise these for Robert.

Q3. Assess Robert's readiness to wean and identify your rationales. Devise a weaning plan for Robert including modes, parameters and indicators of success.

Chapter 5

Airway management

Contents

Fundamental knowledge

Glossopharyngeal nerves
Oropharynx, and proximity of oesophagus to trachea
Tracheal anatomy, mucociliary mechanism ('ladder')
Cricoid anatomy
Carina + positions of right and left main bronchi
Differences between paediatric and adult trachea
Alveolar physiology
Dead space

Introduction

Ventilatory support usually necessitates insertion of endotracheal tubes (*ETTs*) or formation of a tracheostomy. ICU nurses caring for intubated patients are responsible for ensuring patency of, and minimising complications from, artificial airways. This chapter describes types of tubes usually used in ICU, main complications of intubation and controversies surrounding endotracheal suction.

Intubation

Traditionally intubation could be:

- oral
- nasal
- tracheostomy.

Oral tubes cause gagging but are relatively easy to insert, so are usually used initially. Nasal tubes are narrow, increasing airway resistance, and cause sinusitis, so are rarely used unless oral intubation is contraindicated (e.g. dental or head/neck surgery). Tracheostomies are more comfortable for patients, and useful for weaning, but are not usually used initially.

To ventilate both lungs, ETTs should end above the carina (see Figure 5.1); this should be checked by:

- auscultating for bilateral air entry;
- ensuring chest movement is bilateral.

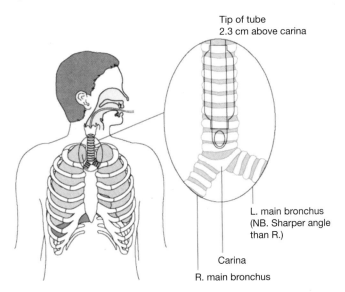

Tip of tube
2.3 cm above carina

L. main bronchus
(NB. Sharper angle
than R.)

Carina

R. main bronchus

Figure 5.1 ETT just above carina

Accidental single bronchus intubation is more likely to occur in the right main bronchus, as it is more vertical to the trachea than the left main bronchus. Misplaced tubes should be repositioned by anaesthetists and reassessed.

Endotracheal tubes are manufactured in a single (long) length, so almost invariably require cutting to minimise ventilatory dead space, usually to 21 cm (female) and 23 cm (male). Children's airways differ from adults and are discussed in Chapter 13.

Most ETTs used in ICU are bacteriostatic (Gupta, 2015; Naidu et al., 2015). Many tubes have subglottic drainage ports; subglottic drainage reduces colonisation and ventilator-associated pneumonia (Muscedere et al., 2011; Wang et al., 2012; Damas et al., 2015) and is recommended by the Intensive Care Society (Hellyer et al., 2016), although it neither reduces length of ICU or hospital stay nor mortality (Wang et al., 2012; Caroff et al., 2016).

Nurses may be required to assist with intubation. Intubations in ICU are often emergency procedures, due to desaturation, leaving little time for pre-planning. The person intubating should follow a safety checklist (Cook et al., 2011); failure to do so increases risks of something being forgotten, exposing patients to risk at vulnerable stages of hypoxia. Equipment should be prepared and checked, including:

- tubes
- laryngoscopes with blades and working lights
- gel
- syringe
- tube ties
- ambubag with oxygen working
- yankauer suction catheter with working suction.

Various drugs will also be required, typically including:

- sedation
- paralysing agent
- analgesia
- emergency drugs, e.g. metraminol.

Saturation should be monitored during the procedure, and end-tidal carbon dioxide monitoring be ready (I.C.S., 2011a). The ventilator should be prepared and checked before the procedure is commenced. If the bedside nurse is the anaesthetist's assistant, they should place themselves on the anaesthetist's dominant side (i.e. right side if the anaesthetist is right-handed). As the bedside nurse will probably be assisting the doctor near the patient's head, at least one other member of nursing staff should be available to fetch any requested equipment. As medical staff will probably be focused on the procedure, either the bedside nurse or assistant should be observing respiratory function.

Nurses assisting with intubation may be asked to apply cricoid pressure. Cricoid cartilage (C5–C6 – just below the "Adam's apple") is the only complete ring of cartilage around the trachea, so cricoid pressure (pressing cricoid cartilage down with three fingers towards the patient's head) compresses the pharynx against cervical vertebra, preventing gastric reflux and aspiration. Although not always effective, this should compress the oesophagus, preventing aspiration (McNarry and Patel, 2017). Pressure is maintained until the endotracheal tube cuff is inflated.

Whereas intubations are usually unplanned, tracheostomy insertion is usually a planned procedure. The same principles apply to both, but planned procedures allow more time to ensure safety.

During insertion of either endotracheal tubes or tracheostomies, doctors' priorities are rightly establishing an airway, which frequently results in overinflation of cuffs. An early nursing priority after the procedure should be to check cuff pressure. Respiratory function should be continuously monitored, and a blood gas will usually be checked 20 minutes after insertion.

Extubation

Planned extubation should occur once:

- patients can adequately self-ventilate;
- cough reflex is sufficient to maintain a clear airway,

although extubation is generally best avoided at evening/night. If not already identified by medical plans, nurses should check that medical staff are satisfied for patients to be extubated.

The usual procedure in extubation is:

- inform patient; assemble equipment; hand hygiene;
- endotracheal suction, to remove any significant airway secretions;
- subglottic aspiration if available;
- orotracheal suction, to remove secretions on top of cuff;
- deflate ETT cuff, cut tube holder/tapes;
- endotracheal suction; remove ETT with suction catheter;
- offer patient mouthwash;
- commence oxygen via facemask, usually with slightly more oxygen than used with ventilation;
- continuous pulse oximetry, with ABG 20–30 minutes after extubation.

During extubation subglottic secretions may be aspirated, causing pneumonitis, pneumonia, and possibly extubation failure (Hodd *et al.*, 2010). Hodd *et al.* (2010) identify alternative methods to clear secretions:

- adjusting PEEP on ventilators;
- extubate with cuff inflated;
- asking patients to cough;
- but acknowledge that effectiveness remains unproven.

Extubation stridor

If bronchospasm is anticipated, cuffs should be deflated before extubation. Normally this would create an air leak, usually audible, and causing loss of tidal volume; if bronchospasm is present, no air leak will be heard/measured, so extubation should not proceed, and an anaesthetist should review the patient. Laryngeal oedema often causes hoarseness following extubation, making voice often temporarily weak or absent. Children, having smaller airways, are especially liable to oedematous obstruction. Post-extubation oedema is less common in ICU than theatre but can still occur (Shaikh *et al.*, 2016; Yıldırım, *et al.*, 2016). Stridor may be treated with:

- nebulised adrenaline (1 mg in 5 ml saline)
- steroids
- Heliox (see Chapter 28).

If stridor cannot be rapidly reversed, reintubation is usually necessary.

Tracheostomy

Tracheostomy avoids many complications of oral and nasal intubation. They halve dead space, so should make the work of breathing, and so weaning, easier. Many intensivists perform early tracheostomy; Andriolo *et al.* (2015) suggest that early tracheostomy probably reduces mortality but caution against the poor quality of evidence. Young *et al.* (2013) argue early tracheostomy is not beneficial.

Tracheostomies are usually formed percutaneously rather than surgically (Nolan and Kelley, 2011), as percutaneous insertion is quicker and has fewer complications. The Intensive Care Society (I.C.S., 2014) recommends surgical tracheostomy with:

- difficult anatomy;
- proximity to site of recent surgery or trauma;
- potential instability;
- severe gas exchange problems;
- children under 12 years of age.

Percutaneous stomas take seven to 10 days to become established, so tubes should not routinely be replaced before then (I.C.S., 2014).

Emergency bedside equipment should include:

- tracheal dilators;
- spare tubes: one the same size and one a half-size smaller;
- suction;
- syringe.

Tracheostomies are seldom stitched into skin, but if they are a stitch cutter is also needed. Nurses caring for patients with a tracheostomy should check this emergency equipment is easily accessible at the start of their shift.

Frequency of tracheostomy dressing depends on both the wound and the type of dressing used. If the stoma looks infected, it should be redressed. Otherwise, most tracheostomy dressings should be replaced daily or according to local protocols.

Because tracheostomies reduce dead space, decannulation significantly increases the work of breathing (Dumas and Martin, 2016). Weaning from a tracheostomy should be carefully planned and staged to minimise need for recannulation:

■ remove or minimise PEEP and pressure support (typically, PEEP 5 cmH$_2$O, PS 8 cmH$_2$O);
■ initially use a T-piece ("Swedish Nose") rather than tracheal mask; T-pieces provides some PEEP and a reservoir of oxygen-rich gas.

Minitracheostomies (crichothyroidotomy) are occasionally used to facilitate removal of secretions.

Problems from intubation

Intubation is often a necessary medical solution that creates various nursing problems.

Coughing is a protective mechanism, removing foreign bodies, including respiratory pathogens, from the airway. This reflex can also be triggered by oral endotracheal tubes and suction catheters, causing distress, possibly necessitating sedation.

Artificial airways can *damage tissue*, especially lips and gums. Condition of lips and gums should be assessed, and tissues protected as necessary – various commercial products can cushion pressure from tapes on lips. Tube position on the lips/gums should be changed at least daily.

Cuff pressures of about 20 cmH$_2$O reduce aspiration, and so ventilator-associated pneumonia (Pneumatikos *et al.*, 2009; Torres *et al.*, 2009); cuff pressure exceeding capillary occlusion pressure can cause *tracheal ulcers*. "High-volume low-pressure" "profile" cuffs (see Figure 5.2) reduce cuff pressure by exerting lower pressure over an extended area. Unlike pressure sores on skin, tracheal epithelium is not directly visible. Average capillary occlusion pressure is about 30 cmH$_2$O but can be lower (see Chapter 12), especially in hypotensive ICU patients. For tracheostomies, the Intensive Care Society (I.C.S., 2014) recommends a maximum pressure of 25 cmH$_2$O, which logically should also apply to endotracheal tube cuff pressures. Most cuff pressure manometers display a "safe" range of 25–30 cmH$_2$O, derived from Landis (1930), which does not comply with current evidence. Cuff pressures should be checked and recorded at least once each shift, and whenever cuff volume is changed.

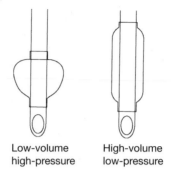

Low-volume   High-volume
high-pressure   low-pressure

■ *Figure 5.2* **High- and low-pressure ETT cuffs**

Impaired cough and swallowing reflexes may cause *aspiration* of saliva and gastric secretions. Profile cuffs rarely completely seal lower airways, making some aspiration almost inevitable, hence the promotion of subglottic drainage.

Although secured, ETTs can become displaced, rising up the airway. Each shift the length of the ETT at the lips should be recorded, and if tube movement is suspected, an anaesthetist informed.

Oral ETTs cause *hypersalivation* and all tubes impair swallowing reflexes, with drying of mucosa near the lips and saliva accumulation (and potential aspiration) in the throat. Audible "bubbling" indicates need to remove secretions and check cuff pressure.

Sympathetic nervous stimulation from intubation and suction initiates *stress responses* (see Chapter 1). Direct *vagal* nerve stimulation (anatomically close to the trachea) occasionally causes bradycardic dysrhythmias and heart-blocks, especially during intubation and suction.

Oral ETTs cause discomfort and *anxiety*; nasal tubes and tracheostomies are usually tolerated better. Patients' inability to speak due to intubation through their vocal cords should be explained.

Humidification

The upper airway:

- warms
- moistens
- filters

inhaled air (see Figure 5.3). Endotracheal intubation bypasses these normal physiological mechanisms, necessitating artificial replacement. Oxygen is a dry gas, so inadequate humidification dries exposed membranes (below the endotracheal tube), damaging cilia and drying mucus. Stickier, thicker mucus, and impaired cilial clearance reduces airflow and increases infection risks.

During inspiration, airways warm air to body temperature. By the time air reaches the oropharynx it has normally been warmed to 32–34°C, with relative

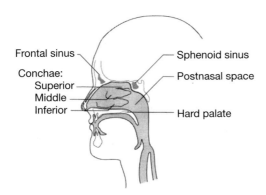

Frontal sinus

Conchae:
Superior
Middle
Inferior

Sphenoid sinus

Postnasal space

Hard palate

Figure 5.3 Nasal cavity

humidity close to 100% (Wilkes, 2011). Much warming and moistening of air occurs in the nasal cavity.

Humidification may be achieved by:

- heat moisture exchange (HME) filters;
- large-volume nebulisers ("cold water humidifiers");
- hot water humidifiers;
- nebulisers (e.g. saline).

Instilling bolus saline is not recommended (Ayhan *et al.*, 2015; Leddy and Wilkinson, 2015).

Heat moisture exchangers (HMEs) use hydrophobic membranes to repel airway moisture, are very efficient bacterial filters (95–100% efficacy (Lawes, 2003)), and reflect heat. They cause less infection risk than heated humidifiers (Torres *et al.*, 2009) but should be changed daily, or more frequently if soiled.

Heat moisture exchangers increase dead space (Wilkes, 2011), but Gillies *et al.*'s (2017) Cochrane review was unable to conclude whether or not they should be avoided with children.

Hot water humidifiers warm inspired air to preset temperatures, usually 37°C. Most systems are self-filling, avoiding need to break circuits. Like HMEs, significant technological improvements invalidate many early studies. Nurses should monitor and record humidifier temperature and keep fluid bags easily visible and replaced when empty. Circuits should be changed according to manufacturers' instructions. Historical concerns of increased infection risk from warm water pre-date the current generation of hot water humidifiers, and recent meta-analyses (Gillies *et al.*, 2017; Vargas *et al.*, 2017) comparing them with HMEs found no significant difference in infection rates, or tube occlusion.

Large-volume nebulisers (usually called "cold water humidifiers") provide less efficient humidification (B.T.S., 2017), but fewer risks from infection and tracheal burns. Water bottles should be replaced when empty and circuits changed according to manufacturers' instructions.

Nebulisation delivers particles initially into airways, so where drugs effects are desired primarily within airways, such as bronchodilation (e.g. salbutamol) or pulmonary vasodilators (prostacyclin), nebulisation is often the best route, although may create the paradox that drugs mainly reach open parts of lungs, whereas effect may be needed most in collapsed airways. This makes nebulisation a poor choice for antibiotics. Nebulising saline (2–5 ml) delivers droplets directly to airway epithelium, and is an efficient means of humidification (B.T.S., 2017), and may help mobilise secretions.

Different types of nebulisers create different sized droplets. To reach alveoli and smaller airways, droplets need to be 1–5 micrometres (Rello *et al.*, 2017), necessitating a gas glow rate of 6–8 litres per minute if flow meters are used. Ultrasonic nebulisers deliver smaller droplets (below one micron).

Nebulisers should ideally be placed near the patient, just before the Y connection, with no HME between the nebuliser and the ETT. Most ventilators include nebuliser circuits. If not used for humidification, HMEs should be placed on return circuits to protect ventilators. Nebulisers should be replaced or cleaned and dried after each use (check manufacturers' instructions), as fluid is a medium for bacterial growth.

Suction

Endotracheal suction is usually necessary to remove accumulated secretions, but can cause:

- distress
- infection
- trauma
- hypoxia
- atelectasis,

so should be performed when needed, not routinely. Indications include:

- rattling/bubbling on auscultation
- sudden increases in airway pressure
- audible "bubbling"
- sudden hypoxia (e.g. in SpO_2).

Suction is painful (Arroyo-Novoa *et al.*, 2008), so warn patients before suctioning, and pass tubes steadily but not aggressively.

Negative pressure should be sufficient to clear secretions but low enough to minimise trauma. In the UK, suction pressure is usually measured in kilopascals (kPa) but sometimes in millimetres of mercury (mmHg). Most ICU staff limit negative pressure to 20 kPA, although, if a lower pressure is effective, that should be used.

Suction removes oxygen from airways and can cause atelectasis, so the procedure should be as brief as possible – maximum 10 seconds. Nurses are recommended to hold their own breath during each pass: when they need oxygen, so will their patient. Endotracheal suction can cause bronchoconstriction (sympathetic stress response) and possible hypoxia. If there is time, pre-oxygenate prior to suction; most ventilators have a time-limited facility for giving pure oxygen. Results of suction, together with any problems encountered, should be fully recorded, to help later staff decide how and when to suction.

Catheters

Oral secretions are often best removed with Yankauer catheters. Closed-circuit suction is almost always used with intubated ICU patients, "open" suction largely being limited to self-ventilating patients who have a tracheostomy but whose cough reflex is too weak to effectively clear secretions. Open suction is discussed further in Woodrow (2016). Closed-circuit systems maintain ventilation and PEEP when passing catheters, enabling slower (less traumatic) catheter introduction. In-line circuits should be changed according to manufacturers' instructions.

Many texts (usually anecdotally) recommend that catheters should not exceed half to two thirds ETT diameter, although it is probably better to individualise selection to patient need – using the smallest size that will remove secretions. Smaller catheters cause less trauma but remove fewer secretions. For adults, standard catheter sizes are French Gauge (FG) 10 (black), 12 (white) and sometimes FG 14 (green). Watery secretions can usually be easily removed with FG 10, but thicker secretions usually need larger sizes; it is usually best to commence with FG 12, and change size as necessary. Smaller sizes will be needed for children (NB some colours are similar to adult sizes).

Implications for practice

- nurses assisting with intubation may have to perform cricoid pressure, so should be familiar with how to perform it;
- ETT cuff pressures should be checked each shift, and whenever any change in pressure is suspected. Pressures should not exceed 25 cmH$_2$O (3.3 kPa);
- airway humidification is essential to maintain effective mucociliary clearance;
- suction should never be "routine" but performed when indicated;
- negative pressure during suction should not exceed 20 kPa.

Summary

Intubation remains a medical intervention, but nurses monitor and manage artificial airways, so should:

- maintain safe environments, including ensuring safety equipment;
- replace lost/impaired physiological functions, including humidification and clearing secretions;

    ▪ individually assess each patient for risk factors caused by intubation; and

    ▪ plan individualised care accordingly. No aspect of airway management is routine. Respiratory assessment, including breath sounds, is discussed in Chapter 17.

Further reading

Tracheostomy care is discussed in greater detail in Woodrow (2016); I.C.S. (2014) and N.C.E.P.O.D. (2014) provide guidelines for tracheostomy care. Although not developed for ICU, B.T.S. (2017) guidelines for oxygen therapy provide valuable evidence. Gillies *et al.* (2017) provide a Cochrane review of HMEs. Other topics discussed in this chapter lack current national guidelines for ICU practice, but resources cited provide potentially useful material.

Clinical scenarios

Tony Richards is 45 years old, very hirsute with a thick, bushy beard and weighing 160 kg. He was admitted to ICU following elective surgery for closer airway management. He was a difficult intubation (Grade 3) and mechanically ventilated via a size 9.0 ETT, with length 21 cm marking at his lips and cuff pressures of 28 cmH₂O. Tony is ready for extubation and biting on his ETT.

Q1. List the equipment and process used to prepare Tony for extubation. Identify the most suitable type of respiratory support for Tony. Provide a rationale for your suggestion.

Fifteen minutes after extubation Tony develops an audible stridor with intermittent gurgling noises from his throat. His respiratory rate changes from 18 bpm to 28 bpm.

Q2. What may cause Tony's added airway sounds and changed respiratory rate? Interpret the significance of these results and implications for his airway management.

On expectoration, Tony's sputum is thick, with brown discolouration. He has a weak cough with high risk of sputum retention.

Q3. How can sputum be mobilised and cleared from both lower and upper airways? What methods would you choose, and why?

Chapter 6

Sedation

Contents

Fundamental knowledge

Psychological distress in ICU (see Chapter 3)

Introduction

Critical illness, many interventions used in intensive care, and the intensive care environment itself can all cause distress and psychoses (see Chapter 3). Traditionally, sedation was usually used to facilitate invasive ventilation. But sedation also deprives individuals of their autonomy, and to some extent their current awareness of being alive. In the Intensive Care Society guidelines, Grounds *et al.* (2014) argue that amnesia increases risks of delusional memories, anxiety and post-traumatic stress disorder. Improved ventilator technology makes invasive ventilation more tolerable for conscious patients. Sedative drugs are "chemical restraint" (Whitehouse *et al.*, 2014), an intervention only justified when there is a specific indication, and within the limits of that indication.

Adverse effects vary between sedatives, but problems include (Barr *et al.*, 2013; Grounds *et al.*, 2014):

- hypotension;
- reduced gut motility (malabsorption, constipation), especially opioids;
- preventing REM sleep;
- amnesia;
- delirium and post-traumatic stress disorder.

Although drugs are mentioned, this chapter focuses on nursing assessment and care, including for neuromuscular blockade (paralysing agents). As with any other drug, use outside of manufacturers' licences makes individual users potentially legally liable for any harm caused (I.C.S., 2009a).

Drugs

Opioids (e.g. morphine, fentanyl, alfentanil, remifentanil)

Used primarily for analgesia, opioids also have sedative effects. Although they should not normally be used primarily for sedation, this "side effect" is often useful for ICU management. Preferred opioids vary between units; morphine remains widely used, but the more expensive fentanils cause less accumulation and fewer detrimental side effects. Opioids are discussed in Chapter 7.

Benzodiazepines (diazepam, lorazepam, midazolam)

Once the mainstay of ICU sedation, benzodiazepines stimulate GABA receptors. Gamma-aminobutyric acid (GABA) is the main cerebral cortex inhibitory neurotransmitter, so GABA stimulation induces sedation, *anxiolysis* and hypnosis (Grounds *et al.*, 2014). Anxiolysis may be desirable, but Weich *et al.*'s (2014) community study suggests increased seven-year mortality from anxiolytic and hynoptic psychotropic drugs, a finding which may, or may not, be transferable to short-term use in ICU.

Midazolam has largely superseded other benzodiazepines in ICU because it acts relatively rapidly and has the shortest half-life. Midazolam is largely hepatically metabolised and renally excreted, metabolism produces an active metabolite (α1-hydroxymidazolas), making half-life variable, especially with poor renal/hepatic function (Grounds *et al.*, 2014). After some days, midazolam appears to accumulate in tissues, resulting in prolonged clearance time.

The antagonist for benzodiazepines is flumazenil. Flumazenil's effect is far shorter than benzodiazepines (half-life under one hour) so, although useful to assess underlying consciousness, sedation is likely to return rapidly.

Anaesthetic agents (e.g. propofol, ketamine)

Propofol and midazolam are the most widely used ICU sedatives (Shehabi *et al.*, 2012). Propofol's lipid emulsion easily crosses the blood–brain barrier, giving rapid sedation. This, together with its metabolites being inactive, makes its half-life short – Grounds *et al.* (2014) suggest a start of activity half-life of two to three minutes, with an elimination half-life of 30–60 minutes. Propofol (like benzodiazepines and barbiturates) reduces cerebral metabolism, so is useful for treating status epilepticus (Grounds *et al.*, 2014). Propofol is available in both 1% and 2% concentrations, so staff should check what strength is being used; although most units standardly use just one strength, both may be available.

The most significant side effect of propofol is usually hypotension from peripheral vasodilatation, and negative inotropic and chronotropic effects (Grounds *et al.*, 2014), often necessitating noradrenaline. Krajcova *et al.* (2015) and Mirrakhimov *et al.* (2015) raise concerns about "propofol syndrome": myopathy, rhabdomyolysis, hyperkalaemia and acute kidney injury. Alternative sedatives often entail greater risks. Propofol can also cause greenish urine, which, although probably clinically insignificant, may make relatives anxious.

It contains no preservative but its lipid base may facilitate bacterial growth; Loveday *et al.* (2014) recommend dedicated lumens and daily changing of lines for lipid-based infusions. Propofol has no analgesic effect (Barr *et al.*, 2013), so concurrent analgesia should be given.

Ketamine can cause nightmare-like hallucination, so should not be used as the only opioid for an ICU patient (Grounds *et al.*, 2014), but it can be a useful adjunct.

Most anaesthetic agents, including propofol and midazolam, impair inflammation, so predisposing to infection (Cruz *et al.*, 2017).

Alpha 2 Agonists (e.g. clonidine, dexmedetomidine)

Alpha 2 antagonists can be useful for controlling both hypertension and agitation (Ahmed and Murugan, 2013; Barr *et al.*, 2013; Grounds *et al.*, 2014; Whitehouse *et al.*, 2014; Constantin *et al.*, 2016). Antihypertensive effects should be remembered if used for sedation in hypotensive patients.

Whitehouse *et al.* (2014) suggest the half-life of clonidine is six to 24 hours, although the summary of product characteristics data sheet (Boehringer Ingelheim, 2015) cites 10–20 (mean 13) hours, so if used for agitation it should usually be weaned cautiously.

Dexmedetomidine is eight times more powerful than clonidine (Ahmed and Murugan, 2013), often enabling ICU patients to be comfortable and awake (Grounds *et al.*, 2014). Metabolised by the liver, with normal liver function it has a half-life of three hours (Barr *et al.*, 2013). Compared with many other sedatives, dexmedetomidine facilitates earlier extubation and discharge, induces anxiolysis (Mo and Zimmermann, 2013), while causing less delirium (Constantin *et al.*, 2016). Like clonidine, it can cause bradycardia and hypotension, potentially limiting its usefulness for many ICU patients. Dexmedetomidine should be administered via infusion, not as a bolus (Grounds *et al.*, 2014).

Some ICUs have increasingly adopted no-sedation regimes (Strøm *et al.*, 2010). Avoiding sedation avoids side effects, such as induced hypotension, which so often necessitates noradrenaline infusions. Many ICUs using no-sedation also use physical restraints to prevent removal of devices such as endotracheal tubes (Hevener *et al.*, 2016). Few UK ICUs have adopted this strategy, and Grounds *et al.* (2014) suggest that some of the patients in Strøm's "no-sedation" group did receive sedation, making Strøm's findings questionable. Samuelson *et al.* (2007) suggest that use of physical restraints without sedation increases incidence of post-traumatic stress disorder. Whether chemical restraint is ethically different from physical restraint is debatable. There may also be ethical differences between levels of physical restraint – for example, mittens verses immobilisation of arms.

Assessing sedation

Over- and undersedation are relative concepts, open to subjective interpretation. Oversedation delays weaning and recovery, compromises perfusion to, and so function of, all organs, and increases financial costs. Undersedation arguably exposes patients to pain and stress. Achieving optimum sedation is a humanitarian necessity; professional autonomy and accountability make each nurse responsible for ensuring their patients are appropriately (i.e. not over- or under-) sedated. All ICU patients should be assessed for sedation level (Barr *et al.*, 2013) to facilitate titration of drugs to achieve optimal sedation.

How assessment is undertaken is much debated. Subjective assessments, such as gently brushing tips of eyelashes, can usefully identify if someone is sedated deeply enough to tolerate traumatic interventions (e.g. intubation), remain useful. Many scoring systems and methods have been developed to try to achieve objective assessment. Some technologies, such as BIS, are also available, but if used these should be adjuncts to, not replacement for, clinical scoring (Whitehouse *et al.*, 2014). Many scales are used in practice, most being relatively simple lists, usually variants of the Ramsay scale. Some units use sedation protocols, although protocols alone do not guarantee improved patient outcomes (O'Connor *et al.*, 2010; Curley *et al.*, 2012).

Paralysis, whether from paralysing agents or pathology, prevents patients expressing awareness, invalidating almost all means of assessing sedation.

So, infusions of any paralysing agents should be stopped long enough before sedation assessment to ensure they will not influence results.

Sedation scoring

The Ramsay scale (Ramsay *et al.*, 1974), originally designed for drug research, was one of the earliest sedation scoring systems. Although now rarely used, its simple numeric scoring formed the basis for most subsequent scoring systems, including the Sedation–Agitation Scale (Riker *et al.*, 2001) and the Richmond Agitation–Sedation Scale (Ely *et al.*, 2003). Many other sedation scales have been developed, but Barr *et al.* (2013) recommend using either:

- the Sedation–Agitation Scale (SAS) or
- the Richmond Agitation–Sedation Scale (RASS).

Quantifying sedation is only useful if it results in improved care.

Sedation holds

Stopping sedation daily enables thorough assessment of:
- neurological state;
- effectiveness of and need for sedation and analgesia;
- readiness to wean.

Benefits claimed for sedation holds include reduced delirium and earlier discharge (Barr *et al.*, 2013). Burry *et al.*'s (2014) Cochrane review found no evidence of significant benefits from sedation holds. Improved (patient-friendly) ventilator technology reduces need for any sedation, so minimal or no sedation is increasingly becoming the norm (Strøm *et al.*, 2010). Sedation holds should be carefully planned to ensure adequate comfort for procedures such as physio-therapy and insertion of any invasive devices, and be long enough for effects of sedatives previously given to fade. Time of sedation holds and observed effects should be recorded.

Sedation holds are usually excluded with:

- head injury, to avoid increases in intracranial pressure (Grounds *et al.*, 2014);
- paralysis (from drugs or disease);
- patients in prone positions or on kinetic beds;
- patients awaiting procedures, such as CT scans or tracheostomy insertion;
- problematic ventilation (Grounds *et al.*, 2014).

Neuromuscular blockade

Improved ventilator technology has largely removed the need to prevent patients making respiratory effort. Neuromuscular blockade (chemical paralysis) is usually only used if there is a specific indication to prevent muscle work, such as raised intracranial pressure (see Chapter 36).

Paralysing agents ("muscle relaxants") cannot cross the blood–brain barrier, so have no sedative or analgesic effects. Paralysed patients cannot alert staff if they are awake, distressed or in pain; any memories are usually distressing (Whitehouse *et al.*, 2014). Tasaka *et al.* (2016) suggest that up to one in 10 patients paralysed in ICU are inadequately sedated; deep sedation should be achieved before using paralysing agents (Annane, 2016).

Blocking release of acetylcholine (a neurotransmitter) at the neuromuscular junction causes skeletal (but not smooth) muscle relaxation. Paralysing agents may be classified as:

- depolarising or
- non-depolarising.

Depolarising drugs act on motor end plates, whereas non-depolarising drugs act on the post-synaptic end plate. Whichever site is affected, acetylcholine transmission is blocked, causing muscle paralysis. Suxemethonium is a depolarising muscle relaxant; most other paralysing agents used in ICU are non-depolarising.

Most paralysing agents are metabolised hepatically or excreted unchanged in urine, giving them a relatively long duration of effect. Atracurium and suxamethonium hydrolyse spontaneously in plasma, so are relatively short-acting. Atracurium is the most widely used paralysing agent in ICU and is relatively short-acting – often about half an hour following bolus intravenous injection. Rocuronium paralysis can, but not always will, be limited to relatively few minutes. Duration of action of all muscle-paralysing agents is therefore unpredictable, varying between drug, dosage and individual characteristics (Soares and Esteves, 2016).

Paralysing agents should be stopped to assess sedation but stopped before sedatives. Once muscle movement is identified, sedatives can then be safely stopped.

Assesssing neuromuscular blockade

With paralysis, effectiveness of neuromuscular blockade should be assessed, but debate persists about the best way to achieve this. Paralysis is typically tested by absence of reflexes. The extrinsic eye muscle is the first muscle affected by paralysing agents, and the first to recover (Rang *et al.*, 2007), so brushing eyelids may indicate effectiveness.

Peripheral electrical nerve stimulation uses relatively low (non-painful) voltage to stimulate nerve reflexes. Before using this, nurses should be shown how to use the stimulator and are recommended to try testing themselves first so they know what they are inflicting on their patients. Shocks are usually applied on either the ulnar nerve or the temporal artery on the face (Bouju *et al.*, 2017), and assessed by the "train of four":

- four or three twitches = under-paralysed
- two or one twitch = well-paralysed
- 0 twitches = over-paralysed

(Bouju *et al.*, 2017)

Barr *et al.* (2013) recommend the Bispectral Index (BIS), which uses a forehead sensor for adapted EEG monitoring, deriving a numerical level of sedation between 1 and 100:

Awake patients	90–100
Conscious sedation (responds to noxious stimuli)	60–80
General anaesthesia	50–60
Deep hypnotic state	< 40
Very deep sedation	< 20
Absence of any brain activity	0

Although many ICU patients will be managed in the 60–80 range, < 60 is usually desirable if patients are paralysed. Similar EEG adaptations include evoked potentials, cerebral function monitors (CFMs) and cerebral function analysing monitors (CFAMs). Tasaka *et al.* (2016) recommend BIS for assessing neuromuscular blockade, although Avidan *et al.*'s (2008) large-scale study found that patients remained aware during anaesthesia despite target-range BIS.

Implications for practice

- undersedation and oversedation cause complications, so sufficient sedation should be provided to achieve comfort;
- nurses should assess efficacy of sedative and paralysing agents for their patients at least once every shift;
- there is no ideal sedation score; all staff should be familiar with whichever score is used on their unit;
- daily sedation holds enable thorough reassessment, so should only be omitted by team decision;
- the sedation needs of each patient should be individually reviewed daily by the multidisciplinary team to meet each patient's need, evaluating:

  - humanitarian needs, to ensure patient comfort;
  - therapeutic benefits, to facilitate interventions;
  - that side effects (e.g. hypotension) are minimised;

- for brief procedures (e.g. intubation), absence of blink reflexes confirms patients are adequately sedated;
- paralysing agents should be stopped for sufficient time prior to assess sedation;

■ nerve stimulators are potentially painful/uncomfortable, so if used nurses should try tests on themselves (where safe to do so) so they are aware what they are subjecting their patients to;

■ BIS is the recommended means of assessing sedation with paralysis.

Summary

Sedation can relieve much psychological trauma caused by ICU admission, potentially providing physiological as well as humanitarian benefits. Conversely, hypotension and other side effects can cause problems, while deep coma inhibits orientation and compliance with requests, removes patient autonomy and may contribute to post-traumatic stress disorder.

Although chemical sedatives are prescribed by doctors, they are (normally) given by nurses, so the professional accountability of each nurse ensures that patients receive adequate (but not excessive) sedation.

Use of paralysing agents has declined; where used, there are usually specific therapeutic indications. If used, nurses should monitor and assess their effects.

Further reading

UK (Grounds *et al.*, 2014; Whitehouse *et al.*, 2014) and US (Barr *et al.*, 2013) guidelines provide comprehensive reviews of sedation (including dosing) and related topics. They are discussed in other chapters of this book (psychology, analgesia). As with most drugs, the B.N.F. and pharmacology texts provide useful information. Murray *et al.*'s (2016) US guidelines for neuromuscular blockade provide some useful cautions together with information about some paralysing agents.

Clinical scenarios

Peter Renton is a 30-year-old builder who was admitted to ICU 10 days ago with crush injuries from an industrial accident. He has multiple lung contusions, causing problems with ventilation. During his time on ICU he develops acute respiratory distress syndrome, acute kidney injury and sepsis. In order to facilitate ventilation and other interventions, Peter has been sedated with intravenous infusions of:

Morphine	5 mg/hour;
Propofol	250 mg/hour for three days.

After three days the propofol is changed to:

Midazolam	10 mg/hour.

Peter also received intravenous atracurium, initially as boluses, and from day four as an infusion.

Q1. List the significant side effects (short and longer-term) that these drugs can have, and identify nursing actions to identify and reduce detrimental effects.

Q2. Evaluate appropriateness of sedation holds for Peter. Plan how these are best managed, for example time of day, reduction in infusion rates, order in which to stop infusions, which infusions should continue, assessment of sedation level, and goals of sedation.

Q3. Review the actions (pharmacodynamics) of these drugs against those available on your ICU. What changes would you recommend to managing Peter's sedation? Provide rationales for your suggestions. From reading this chapter, are there any other drugs or strategies you might suggest, including those which may not be available on your unit?

Chapter 7

Acute pain management

Contents

Fundamental knowledge

Anatomy and physiology of the nervous system, including
   sympathetic and parasympathetic, central and peripheral,
   motor, sensory
Spinal nerves – position of thoracic and lumbar nerves
Stress response (see Chapter 1)
Pain as a physical and psychological phenomenon
Local protocols/policies for epidural and PCA management

Introduction

Pain is undesirable, a physical and psychological phenomenon that can cause physiological as well as psychological complications. Physiological problems caused by pain include:

- stress responses (see Chapter 1);
- reluctance to breathe deeply (if self-ventilating), contributing to atelectasis and respiratory failure;
- immunosuppression (Barr *et al.*, 2013).

Most ICU patients experience pain (Puntillo *et al.*, 2010; Barr *et al.*, 2013; Gélinas *et al.*, 2014; Grounds *et al.*, 2014). Alleviating and relieving pain is fundamental to nursing care, yet pain is often underestimated and undertreated (Hartog *et al.*, 2010; Wu and Raja, 2011; Joffe *et al.*, 2013), especially in older people (Ahlers *et al.*, 2010; Abdulla *et al.*, 2013) and people with COPD (Christensen *et al.*, 2016). Nurses therefore should understand:

- physiological and psychological processes of pain;
- how to assess pain;
- how to control pain.

Nurses should be familiar with indications, contraindications, usual doses, preparation, benefits and adverse effects of drugs they use. Much literature on pain management focuses on pharmacology, and specific information can be found in manufacturers' summaries of product characteristics (SPC) and pharmacopoeias (e.g. British National Formulary), both of which should be available in all clinical areas. This chapter discusses some drugs but focuses mainly on mechanisms and assessment of pain.

Causes of acute pain may be obvious (e.g. surgery) but patients may also suffer pre-existing chronic pain (e.g. arthritis). Chronic pain is usually less amenable to analgesia, and drugs that do work often create complications, such as immunosupression. Many interventions can cause pain (Grounds *et al.*, 2014), including:

- suctioning (the most commonly reported cause of pain in intubated patients);
- line insertion;
- drain removal;
- repositioning;
- physiotherapy.

Individual nursing assessment may identify ways to minimise discomfort, information which should be shared with colleagues (verbally, nursing records).

Many ICU patients are unable to perform even fundamental activities of living, so managing pain should include comfort measures, such as:

- smoothing creases in sheets;
- relieving prolonged pressure;
- turning pillows over;
- limb placement (e.g. with arthritis);
- reducing noise and light;
- touch, explanations, reassurance, empowerment.

Physiology

Pain signals, which may originate from physical or psychogenic stimuli, are transmitted to and received by the cerebral cortex, where they are perceived (interpreted) by higher centres in the brain. Pain is therefore necessarily individual to each sufferer, a complex interaction between physiology and psychology. Pain relief can therefore block either reception or perception of pain signals.

Pain from physiological causes is sensed by nociceptors, specialised nerve endings found throughout the body, especially skin and superficial tissues. Two main types of nerves (A and C fibres) transmit pain signals. A fibres have myelin sheaths that conduct signals rapidly, whereas C fibres are unmyelinated and so conduct impulses slowly (Macintyre *et al.*, 2010). C fibres transmit dull, poorly localised, deep and prolonged pain signals, causing guarding movements and immobility. Sharp impulses from the fast A delta fibres are superseded by slower, dull and prolonged impulses from C fibres.

Melzack and Wall (1988) describe a "gate" (in the substantia gelatinosa capping grey matter of the spinal cord dorsal horn), which may be:

- open
- closed
- blocked.

When open, impulses pass to higher centres (where they are perceived). A closed gate prevents impulses passing, leaving nothing to perceive. Endogenous chemicals control this gate (e.g. serotonin increases pain tolerance), so manipulating, supplementing or replacing these chemicals can control pain. The gate can also be blocked by other signals. A delta and C fibres share pathways, so A delta stimulation (e.g. skin pressure) can block the slower, dull, prolonged C fibre pain. Hence, scratching itches, pressure bracelets and transcutaneous electrical nerve stimulations can relieve pain.

Pain may be referred (e.g. phantom limb pain, cardiac pain in left arm, appendix pain in loin – see Figure 7.1) where embryonic nerve pathways were shared or where residual nerve pathways remain intact.

Psychology

Perception of signals received is influenced by various psychological factors, including:

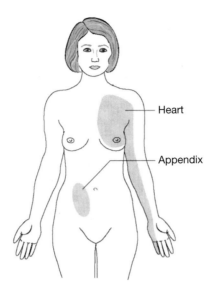

Heart

Appendix

■ *Figure 7.1* **Referred pain**

■ culture;
■ anticipation – e.g. past experience, misinterpretation;
■ emotional vulnerability – e.g. fear;
■ distraction.

The word "pain" derives from the Latin "poena" (= punishment); perceiving pain as retribution may be partly a psychological coping mechanism but also encourages physiologically harmful stoic attitudes of endurance. Culture also influences whether, when and how it is acceptable to admit to pain.

While recognising cultural influences, especially when pain is denied, stereotyping people is unhelpful and dehumanising. For example, older people may require less analgesia owing to slower metabolism of analgesics and reduced pain sensation, but also grew up when stoicism was more widely expected, and often report less pain than younger people (Jabusch *et al.*, 2015). They are also more likely to suffer chronic conditions, such as arthritis. Arthritis may be visually apparent but individual assessment may identify other needs, enabling nurses to avoid inflicting accidental pain. Even if pain impulses were comparable, pain experiences are unique to each individual, necessitating individual assessment.

Anticipation is influenced by previous exposure to similar stimuli (e.g. endotracheal suction) and expectations. Readers may experience anticipation for themselves when visiting dentists, or with patients who are needle-phobic.

Critically ill patients are vulnerable. They feel, and are, disempowered. Fear can create self-fulfilling prophecies (something hurts because we expect it to hurt), but uncertainty increases fear, so clear, honest explanations before actions, warning them how long they will have to endure it, help patients prepare for pain. Hayward's (1975) classic study found information reduced pain, analgesia needs and recovery time.

Distraction may help people cope with pain by blocking the gate. Distraction and guided imagery can be useful nursing strategies, although impaired consciousness and verbal responses can limit their value in ICU.

Assessing pain

Pain relief and providing comfort are fundamental to nursing. Many pain assessment tools have been developed. Ideally, assessment of pain and effectiveness of pain management begins by asking patients, but communication may be limited by intubation, sedation, impaired psychomotor skills and sometimes denial. The Critical-Care Pain Observation Tool (CPOT; Gélinas et al., 2006) and the Behavioral Pain Scale (BPS; Payen et al., 2001) were designed for assessing patients when verbal communication is problematic. Rijkenberg et al. (2015) favours CPOT over BPS, but assessments are only useful if they result in improved care.

Where patients are conscious, discussing individual needs and preferences can provide nurses with valuable information and empower patients and reassure them. Where possible, open rather than closed questions should be used. Family/friends and nursing/medical notes may provide useful information, especially about chronic pain and individual coping mechanisms.

Pain experiences and analgesia needs frequently change significantly, necessitating frequent reassessment. If patients are able to respond, they should be asked about their pain:

■ site (including any radiation);
■ type (intensity, frequency, duration, radiation);
■ whether anything triggers it;
■ whether anything relieves it.

Nurses should observe whether pain is related to any activity, such as breathing (including artificial ventilation) or movement.

Ideally, pain assessment would rely primarily on patients own verbal reports, but this is not always practical or possible in ICU. Changes in vital signs, such as:

■ tachycardia
■ hypertension
■ tachypnoea
■ vasoconstriction (clammy, pale peripheries)
■ sweating

may indicate acute pain, but can also have other causes, so should not form the only means of assessing pain (Barr et al., 2013). Assessment tools include:

- numerical scales (e.g. 0–3, 0–10, with higher numbers indicating worse pain);
- "faces" (originally paediatric tools, but adapted for ICU by McKinley *et al.* (2003));
- behavioural scales.

For patients who are unable to self-report, Gélinas *et al.* (2014) recommend numeric scales but impaired vision can make visual tools, whether numbers or faces, difficult to use (Bird, 2003).

Non-verbal cues such as:

- facial grimacing – clenched teeth, wrinkled forehead, biting lower lip, wide open or tightly shut eyes;
- position – doubled up, "frozen", writhing;
- facial grimacing;
- pupil dilatation (Blenkharn *et al.*, 2002; Murdoch and Larsen, 2004).

can suggest pain, and have been adapted into various assessment tools, such as the Behavioral Pain Scale (Payen *et al.*, 2001) and the Critical-Care Pain Observation Tool (Arbour *et al.*, 2011).

The Behavioral Pain Scale Tool assesses facial expression, upper limb movements and compliance with ventilation, so is useful for assessing pain in ventilated patients (Aïssaoui *et al.*, 2005; Young *et al.*, 2006; Ahlers *et al.*, 2010), although weakness/immobility and pathology may mask any or all of these signs, some of the criteria for assessing tolerance of ventilation are questionable, and it necessarily assumes that patients are conscious enough to move limbs. The variant Behavioral Pain Scale – Non-Intubated (BPS-NI) is effective (Chanques *et al.*, 2009).

Managing pain

Opioids rightly remain the mainstay of acute pain management, but pain may be relieved through alternative or supplementary means. Pain is individual to each patient, so pain management should be individualised. Some generalisations can be made, provided practitioners remember to adapt generalisations to meet individual needs. Options will also be limited by what is available.

Opioids

Morphine remains the "gold standard" opioid against which others are judged. It suppresses impulse from C fibres, but not A delta, so relieves dull, prolonged pain. Its relatively long effect makes bolus administration feasible, which also reduces problems from accumulation. Morphine, and most opioids, can be reversed with naloxone (Narcan); with a half-life of 30–90 minutes (Calás *et al.*, 2016), effects of morphine will outlast reversal. It should also be remembered that reversing respiratory depression from morphine also reverses analgesia.

Diamorphine (heroin) is metabolised to morphine. Its use in the UK is largely confined to palliative care.

Fentanyl acts rapidly – within five to seven minutes (Lovich-Sapola *et al.*, 2015). Although more potent than morphine, it does not cause histamine release, so causes less hypotension. Fentanyl derivatives include alfentanil and remifentanil. Although available as transdermal patches, these are seldom used in ICU, as they will not have significant effect for 24 hours, and prevent short-term titration.

Alfentanil's shorter duration (one to two hours) makes continuous infusion safer. It is mainly metabolised in the liver (Grounds *et al.*, 2014), making it useful for patients with kidney injury, although liver failure prolongs its half-life.

Remifentanyl is rapidly metabolised (by plasma), so has few, if any, complications from accumulation. It is relatively expensive.

Ketamine can be useful for uncontrolled pain and, unlike most opioids, increases blood pressure (Chumbley, 2011; Hopper *et al.*, 2015), which can be useful with cardiovascular instability. Ketamine can cause nightmare-like hallucinations (Avidan *et al.*, 2017), although this is often not problematic with low doses (Lovich-Sapola *et al.*, 2015).

Pethidine is rarely used because it is very short-acting, produces the neurotoxic metabolite norpethidine, is highly addictive and provides no greater pain relief than morphine (Macintyre *et al.*, 2010).

Epidurals

Epidural opioids are usually more effective than intravenous (Marret *et al.*, 2007). Infusions usually combine opioids (fentanyl) with local anaesthetic (bupivacaine). Local anaesthetics prevent nerve conduction of pain signals, so produce an opioid-sparing effect.

The most common side effect of epidural analgesia is probably hypotension (Weetman and Allison, 2006), so when first mobilising patients it is usually advisable to use a hoist. Other common opioid-related side effects include pururitis (itching) from histamine release (Weetman and Allison, 2006). Nearly half of epidurals fail, including a significant minority from misplacement or becoming dislodged (Hermanides *et al.*, 2012). Effectiveness and level of block should therefore be tested regularly. Level of block is often tested with cold spray or ice, although cotton wool has also been used. Block should be sufficiently high to analgese, but not unnecessarily high or uneven. Blocks reaching T4 (nipple area) may paralyse respiratory muscles, so should be stopped immediately. Hypotension should *not* be managed by tilting head-down, as this allows drugs to travel up the spine.

Each shift, nurses should check the epidural site – any infection is likely to be from skin-surface organisms, such as *Staphlococcus aureus* (Darouiche, 2006). In addition to vital signs,

- pain
- nausea

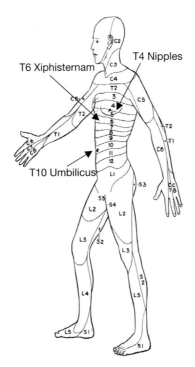

T4 Nipples

T6 Xiphisternam

T10 Umbilicus

Figure 7.2 Dermatomes

- sedation level
- level of sensory block (see below)

should be assessed hourly. Dermatomes (see Figure 7.2) show levels affected by each spinal nerve. The epidural site should be checked at least once each shift.

For safety, epidural lines and equipment are colour-coded yellow (N.P.S.A., 2010). No other infusions should be attached to epidural lines. Drugs manufactured, and labelled, for epidural use should not be given through any other route.

Removing epidural lines can cause infection and haematoma, so removal should be aseptic and only when clotting time is normal. The tip should be inspected to check it is intact; it is coloured (often blue) to make it distinctive. Heparin should usually be avoided before and after removal – times should be identified in local trust policies.

Patient-controlled analgesia (PCA)

Giving patients control over their own opioid administration, within maximum preset lock-out limits (typically, five minutes), usually achieves effective analgesia (Lovich-Sapola *et al.*, 2015; McNicol *et al.*, 2015). PCAs usually contain morphine, although other opioids can be used. PCA is usually unsuitable if patients have:

- impaired psychomotor function
- muscle weakness
- visual deficits
- confusion or if they forget how to control the machine.

Unsuccessful attempts (demand within lock-out time, displayed on pump screens) indicate that analgesic needs are not being fully met, and so regimes should be reviewed.

PCAs should normally be attached to a dedicated lumen, to avoid flushing opioid when other drugs are given.

Non-opioids

Non-opioids, such as paracetamol, inhibit the neurotransmitter prostaglandin E_2 (PGE_2). Some non-opioids (but not paracetamol) are anti-inflammatory, making them effective against musculoskeletal pain. Synergistic effects enable lower doses of opioids (Maund *et al.*, 2011; Barr *et al.*, 2013), and so reducing side effects, such as constipation and itching. NSAIDs (e.g. ibuprofen) are mainly used for chronic musculoskeletal pain but are sometimes used for post-operative pain. They can cause kidney injury.

Neuropathic pain

Up to 7–8% of people suffer neuropathic pain. (Deng *et al.*, 2016), so pain resistant to other analgesics may be neuropathic. Caused by damage to central or peripheral nerves, neuropathic pain is often difficult to control, but N.I.C.E. (2010b) recommends amitriptyline and gabapentin, while Barr *et al.*, (2013) recommend gabapentin and carbamazepine. Pregabalin reduces opioid need and thus side effects (e.g. vomiting) but increases risk of visual disturbances (Zhang *et al.*, 2011; Baiyda *et al.*, 2011). Other drugs worth trying include tramadol (N.I.C.E., 2010b). Most neuropathic pain analgesics take days to become effective.

Anti-emetics

Opioids, given by any route, may induce nausea, both through delayed gastric emptying and by directly stimulating the vomiting centre in the brain. Nurses should observe for signs of nausea, assess likely causes and give appropriate prescribed anti-emetics. Most commonly used anti-emetics, such as ondansetron, cyclizine and prochlorperazine, primarily affect the vomiting centre. Meto-clopramide primarily increases gastric motility, so is useful where nausea is caused by gastric contents but less useful when nausea is caused by vomiting centre stimulation (e.g. post-operative nausea and vomiting).

Implications for practice

- promoting comfort and removing/minimising pain are fundamental to nursing;
- pain is a complex phenomenon involving both physiological transmission of pain signals and cognitive interpretation;
- nociceptor signals (reception) are interpreted as pain in the cerebral cortex (perception); pain can be managed by removing either component;
- pain is individual to each person, so requires individual nursing assessment;
- currently there is no ideal pain assessment tool for ICU, but verbal questions and visual observations can indicate comfort;
- good pain management involves teamwork, so means of assessing and managing pain should be shared by the team. Where possible, this team should include the patient – discussing options and effectiveness, and offering PCA;
- opioids remain the mainstay of ICU analgesia, but supplementary ways to relieve pain and provide comfort should also be used;
- simple analgesics, such as paracetamol, have opioid-sparing effects, reducing opioid need and so opioid-related side effects;
- analgesia should be given before tasks which are likely to cause pain;
- nurses should evaluate the effectiveness of pain relief to optimise its effect and minimise its complications;
- nurses should observe for signs of nausea, assess likely causes, and give appropriate prescribed anti-emetics.

Summary

Suffering is an almost inevitable part of critical illness, but this should not make pain acceptable. Pain is a complex phenomenon, involving both physiological transmission of pain signals and cognitive interpretation. It is culturally influenced and individual to each person, so should be assessed and managed individually. Promoting comfort and achieving effective pain management is fundamental to nursing, yet many patients continue to suffer unnecessary pain. Understanding physiological and psychosocial effects, together with pharmacology of drugs used, enables nurses to plan effective pain relief. Acute pain often needs opioids, although non-opioid drugs can provide useful synergy with opioids, and non-pharmacological approaches should be considered. Evaluating and documenting effectiveness of pain relief helps optimise its effect and minimise its complications.

Further reading

Classic books on pain management include Melzack and Wall (1988), McCaffery and Pasero (1999) and Hayward's (1975) study on post-operative pain. McMahon *et al.* (2013) have updated Wall and Melzack's classic comprehensive reference text. Macintyre and Schug (2014) provide a useful handbook, while the Australian guidelines (Macintyre *et al.*, 2010) provide a comprehensive review. ICU-specific guidelines are available from the USA (Barr *et al.*, 2013). Gélinas *et al.* (2014) review assessment tools. A Cochrane review (McNicol *et al.*, 2015) favours PCA analgesia, while acknowledging that evidence is weak. As with all drugs, the B.N.F. provides useful summaries.

Clinical scenarios

Ms Persad is a 38-year-old legal secretary who was admitted to ICU for respiratory management following her second bariatric weight loss surgical procedure. She has no immediate family in the area and has given her employer as next of kin. Ms Persad has a PCA of morphine sulphate 1 mg/ml; her pain is poorly controlled. Ms Persad had previously had her pain controlled with pethidine and developed an urticaric rash. She dislikes the PCA and is requesting additional pethidine and medication to relieve itchiness.

Q1. Identify the type, location and source of pain Ms Persad has been experiencing, along with other influencing factors. Select the most appropriate pain assessment tools to use.

Q2. Review the range of approaches used to administer analgesia in the ICU. Analyse the use of pethidine versus morphine in managing Ms Persad's acute pain and discuss alternative approaches and drugs which could be effective in managing her pain.

Q3. Consider other non-pharmacological interventions that can be implemented to effectively manage Ms Persad's pain.

Chapter 8

Thermoregulation

Contents

Fundamental knowledge

Thermoregulation – hypothalamic control, shivering, sweating and heat loss through vasodilatation

Introduction

Human bodies can only function healthily within narrow temperature ranges. Body temperature, normally 36–37.5°C (Augustine and Augustine, 2017), is controlled by the thermoregulatory centre in the hypothalamus, responding to central and peripheral thermoreceptors. If cold, vasoconstriction and shivering responses conserve and produce heat; if hot, sweating and vasodilatation responses increase heat loss. Core body temperature normally varies up to 0.5°C during each day (Faulds and Meekings, 2013).

Body heat is produced:

■ by metabolism
■ in response to pyrogens.

Metabolism (chemical reactions) produces heat, so temperature and metabolism both peak about 4 pm, with circadian rhythm (Blume *et al.*, 2017). Most post-operative pyrexia are caused by hypermetabolic tissue repair, not infection (Barone, 2009). Blood transfusion similarly usually causes low-grade pyrexia. With metabolic pyrexia people usually feel hot, as experienced during heavy exercise.

Infection causes pyrogens to be released; pyrogens (e.g. TNFα, interleukin-1) increase prostaglandins production, and prostaglandins increase the hypothalamus set point (Walter *et al.*, 2016), typically to higher temperatures than metabolism produces. As the hypothalamus attempts to increase heat production to match the higher set point, people usually feel cold/shivery, so attempt to conserve warmth (e.g. extra bedding/clothing).

Infants are especially prone to rapid pyrexial fluctuations, due to hypothalamic immaturity, higher metabolic rates, and having more brown fat (which generates heat). Thermoregulatory impairment may cause febrile convulsions, so pyrexial children should be monitored frequently. The body surface area of children is proportionately larger than adults, making them also prone to more rapid heat loss.

Older people (most ICU patients) have lower body temperatures (Güneş and Zaybak, 2008), making 20–30% afebrile despite having serious infections (Woodford, 2015). Similarly, immunocompromise or immunosuppressive drugs may prevent pyrexia occurring with infection. So, pyrexia may occur without infection, while infection may occur without pyrexia.

Pyrexia

The American Society of Critical Care Physicians (ACCP) defines clinically significant (i.e. probably from infection) temperatures as > 38.3°C (O'Grady *et al.*, 2008), although hypermetabolism can cause severe hyperpyrexia.

Pyrexia can be protective,

■ inhibiting bacterial and viral growth (Golding *et al.*, 2016) ("nature's antibiotic");

- inhibiting pro-inflammatory cytokines (Young and Saxena, 2014);
- promoting tissue repair through hypermetabolism,

but every degree centigrade also increases:

- oxygen consumption;
- metabolic waste – carbon dioxide, acids, water

by about 10% (Young and Saxena, 2014). With infection, pyrexia within 24 hours of admission to ICU is associated with reduced mortality (Young et al., 2012). Nurses should therefore assess likely cause of pyrexia and its cost to the patient, as well as benefits and burdens to "treating" pyrexia.

Hyperpyrexia (also called "heatstroke" and "severe hyperthermia") is a temperature above 40°C, high enough to cause cell death (Walter and Carraretto, 2016). At 41°C, convulsions occur and autoregulation fails, death usually following at about 44°C, necessitating urgent ("first aid") neuroprotective cooling.

Malignant hyperpyrexia

Malignant hyperpyrexia, a genetic disorder of calcium channels in skeletal muscle (Litman et al., 2018), may be triggered by drugs (e.g. suxamethonium, amphetamines) and stress (e.g. massive skeletal injury, strenuous exercise). Untreated malignant hyperpyrexia is fatal.

Precipitating causes should be removed. The only available drug to treat malignant hyperpyrexia is dantrolene sodium (1 mg/kg) (Hopkins, 2008), which blocks calcium channels, relaxing skeletal muscle. Dantrolene infusions require a filter, as crystals may not all dissolve (M.H.R.A. 2014). Neuromuscular blockade (paralysis) may be used to prevent shivering (heat production).

Measurement

"Core temperature", the temperature at the core of the body, is the ideal temperature to measure (Asadian et al., 2016). Core temperature normally remains stable throughout the day varying within ±0.6°C (Washington and Matney, 2008). The problem is how to measure it. Ideally, temperature would be measured at the hypothalamus, which contains the thermoregulatory centre, but as this is impractical any site chosen is necessarily a compromise between proximity to core and risks/benefits of invasiveness. Many sites, often called "core", are merely approximations. Crawford et al. (2005) suggest normal ranges for sites are:

- core: 36.8–7.9°C;
- tympanic: 35.6–37.4°C;
- forehead: 36.1–37.3°C;
- axilla: 35.5–37.0°C;

- rectal: 34.4–37.8°C;
- oral: 36.0–37.6°C,

although individual factors, critical illness and specific system function should also be considered.

Many thermometers and measurement sites are available, often provoking passionate and contradictory views. Evidence can be found to both favour and disparage each type of thermometer and each measurement site. Historically, temperature measurement was usually oral, rectal or axillary, often with mercury-in-glass thermometers. Mercury-in-glass thermometers are now clinically almost obsolete, as glass is hazardous and mercury neurotoxic, but many older studies compared other thermometers and sites with these, often unfavourably. Historically, rectal was considered a core site, although given impaired bowel perfusion and function of many critically ill patients this view is questionable. Rectal measurement is undignified and probably unreliable, so difficult to justify in ICU, yet Niven *et al.*'s (2015) meta-analysis recommends rectal over peripheral measurement. Thermometer technology has advanced, undermining findings of some older studies, but Black's (2016) doctoral thesis on thermometers concluded there is no ideal thermometer, and how staff use them is a significant source of error.

Axilla measurement is unreliable for ICU (Asadian *et al.*, 2016), but often used for disposable *chemical thermometers*. Chemical thermometers rely on visual interpretation, so can be subjective – Creagh-Brown *et al.* (2005) found that over three quarters of qualified nurses read them inaccurately. Black's (2016) review found significant discrepancies between chemical thermometers and other types.

Pulmonary artery temperature, measured through a pulmonary artery floatation catheter, is the standard control used in many late twentieth-century thermometers studies. Catheters being highly invasive, temperature measurement alone does not justify their use.

Forehead (temporal artery) may use direct touch ("deep forehead") or, more commonly, non-touch infrared beams. Harioka *et al.* (2000) suggested deep forehead thermometers were the best non-invasive device available, but Asadian *et al.* (2016) found forehead thermometry the least reliable of four methods they studied, although they failed to clarify whether they used deep forehead (tactile) or non-touch thermometers. Black (2016) found little evidence about non-touch devices but this was the one type of thermometer which she concluded were clinically unacceptable.

Tympanic measurement is widely used. The carotid artery supplies both the tympanic membrane and the nearby hypothalamus, so tympanic measurement is closer to core temperature than any other non-invasive device or site (Jefferies *et al.*, 2011; Asadian *et al.*, 2016; Bijur *et al.*, 2016). A common cause of under-readings is incomplete insertion. Dirty or damaged lenses also cause under-reading. Many tympanic thermometers offer optional adjustments of temperature to equivalents at other sites. Provided a tympanic (sometimes called "ear") option is available, it is logical to set this and ensure all thermometers are adjusted to the same setting, especially as "offsets" for adjustment to other sites vary significantly between firms and models.

Probes on urinary catheters can measure *bladder* temperature. One quarter of cardiac output flows through renal arteries, so if urine flow is good (60 ml/hour), bladder temperature indicates core temperature (Jung *et al.*, 2008). Accuracy is affected by urine flow (Sessler, 2008) so oliguria probably makes bladder thermometry unsuitable. Fallis (2005) found that urine flow did not significantly affect bladder thermometry but she was measuring effects of furosemide.

Nasopharyngeal and *oesophageal* probes provide relatively non-invasive measurement but cannot be recommended unless patients are deeply sedated. They are useful with hypothermia, which makes any near-surface site inaccurate.

Non-invasive skin probes, usually on patients' feet, measures *peripheral* temperature. Comparing differences between peripheral and central temperature indicates perfusion/warming – differences should be below 2°C if well perfused. Limb reperfusion should be monitored following vascular surgery to the leg.

While ICUs may have additional options for specific patient groups, the main thermometers used are often decided centrally by the hospital, not locally by the unit, and there are benefits from consistent practice within each hospital. Thermometer choice may be dictated by quality, but more often by cost. How significant differences are between different types of thermometers is questionable, especially as the significance of pyrexia in sepsis receives less emphasis in more recent guidelines, such as N.I.C.E. (2016a) and Rhodes *et al.* (2017). There are inevitably rogue machines in each type, but most should indicate trends.

Treatment

Too often, nursing interventions for pyrexia are based on institutional habit or ritualistic practices (Scrase and Tranter, 2011). Appropriateness of treating pyrexia necessitates individual assessment and evidence-based practice. With pyrexia of infective origin, micro-organisms can often be destroyed more safely by antibiotics than by endogenous pyrexia.

Cooling may be:

- central (altering hypothalamic set point);
- peripheral (increasing heat loss).

Peripheral cooling (reducing bedding, tepid sponging, fans) stimulate further hypothalamus-mediated heat production (shivering) and conservation (vasoconstriction). Shivering increases metabolism, increasing oxygen and energy consumption, while vasoconstriction traps heat produced in central vessels, creating hostile environments for major organs. Cooling also shifts the oxygen dissociation curve to the left, reducing oxygen delivery. Peripheral cooling is therefore fundamentally illogical. Paralysing and sedative drugs can reduce metabolism.

Antipyretic drugs (e.g. aspirin, paracetamol, non-steroidal anti-inflammatory drugs – NSAIDs) seem to inhibit prostaglandin synthesis (Niven and Laupland, 2013), so should restore normal hypothalamic regulation. Infective pyrexia should respond to antipyretic drugs, while pyrexia from hypermetabolism or hypothalamic damage do not. Whether antipyretic treatment benefits, does not benefit, or harms ICU patients is unclear (Lee et al., 2012; Niven et al., 2013; Young and Saxena, 2014).

Sweat evaporation, vasodilatation and increased capillary permeability cause hypovolaemia and hypotension, necessitating additional fluid replacement. Electrolyte and acid–base imbalances should be monitored and treated.

If infection is suspected, appropriate (e.g. blood) cultures should be taken and empirical antibiotics prescribed. Suspected sources of infection (e.g. cannulae) should be removed if possible. Samples usually take days to culture, so recording samples sent on microbiology flow sheets helps ensure results are promptly acted upon.

Hypothermia

Traditionally, mild hypothermia was defined as 32–35°C, but temperatures below < 36°C are now widely regarded as being hypothermic; for example, this is the trigger used by the National Early Warning Score (NEWS), a logical change within the context of approximations to core rather than oral measurement. Unless induced, significant hypothermia in ICU is very rare.

Problems from hypothermia (including therapeutically induced) include:

- reduced dissociation of oxygen from haemoglobin;
- peripheral shutdown, causing anaerobic metabolism;
- cardiac dysrhythmias (Bourdages et al., 2010);
- impaired liver detoxification (Lam and Strickland, 2014 p838);
- hyperglycaemia (Bernard and Buist, 2003).

Moderate to severe hypothermia (< 32°C) has high mortality. Patients should be rewarmed at 0.5–1°C/hour, or 1–2°C/day if intracranial hypertension exists (Varon and Acosta, 2008), although severe hypothermia may necessitate rewarming by 3° per hour (Farley and McLafferty, 2008). The main side effect of rewarming is shivering, which can be controlled with neuromuscular blockade (Varon and Acosta, 2008).

Targeted temperature management

Hypothermia reduces metabolism, so reducing cerebral oxygen demand and reperfusion injury (Nichani et al., 2012). Hypothermia may also inhibit inflammatory cytokines (Peake et al., 2008) and reduce release of the radical chemical hydrogen peroxide (Kuffler, 2012). Previously used for cardiac surgery, therapeutic hypothermia has been advocated for out-of-hospital cardiac arrests

(N.I.C.E., 2011), post VF arrest (Nichani *et al.*, 2012) and cerebral protection during neurological injury/surgery (Kuffler, 2012). Detrimental effects increasingly led to recommendations of only moderate temperatures (32–34°C) for therapeutic hypothermia for limited time (12–24 hours) (Varon and Acosta, 2008), while more recent major studies showed no reduction in mortality from therapeutic hypothermia with cardiac arrest (Nielsen *et al.*, 2013; Moler *et al.*, 2015), and even increased mortality if used for in-hospital arrests (Chan *et al.*, 2016). Current US traumatic brain injury guidelines (Carney *et al.*, 2016) are ambivalent, recognising potential to reduce injury but also problems from coagulopathy and immunosuppression.

Pyrexia does have metabolic costs, including increased oxygen demand; whether or not therapeutic hypothermia is beneficial remains debated, but avoidance of pyrexia is usually desirable. The term "targeted temperature management" has therefore been coined to include therapeutic hypothermia, and maintenance of normothermia. Doyle and Schortgen (2016) found conflicting evidence for efficacy of cooling methods, although suggest that surface cooling is more effective than paracetamol.

Implications for practice

- pyrexia is a symptom, not a disease. Pyrexia should be managed in the context of individual patients (cost/benefit analysis);
- current evidence for thermometers is limited and inconsistent;
- pyrexia may be metabolic or infective in origin;
- clinically significant pyrexia (infection) is usually > 38.3°C;
- pyrexia inhibits micro-organisms but increases oxygen and energy consumption, while increasing metabolic waste;
- infection should be treated with appropriate antibiotics;
- peripheral cooling of infective pyrexia is usually illogical and counter-productive;
- central cooling (antipyretic drugs) can restore normal hypothalamic thermoregulation;
- evidence for therapeutic hypothermia is controversial and conflicting.

Summary

Pyrexia is a symptom, not a disease. Patients, not observation charts, should be treated. Low-grade pyrexia may be beneficial, so managing pyrexia should be individually assessed for each patient – cause, cost, benefit. Clinically significant pyrexia (> 38.3°C) usually indicates infection, and excessive cost, so should usually be reversed with paracetamol, while infection is treated with antibiotics. Unidentified infections should be traced through culture.

Further reading

The evidence base for thermometry is often thin and dated. There are a number of comparative studies, such as Asadian *et al.* (2016), which provide useful information. Therapeutic hypothermia has generated much literature; with the weight of evidence mounting against its use, N.I.C.E. guidance (2011) will hopefully be updated. In 2016 *Critical Care* published a series of articles about pyrexia, including Doyle and Shortgen, Walter and Carraretto and Walter *et al.* Readers should be familiar with manufacturers' advice for thermometers on their units – information may be immediately available on units or held centrally by the hospital; manufacturers' websites usually contain useful information.

Clinical scenarios

Fiona Clarke, a 35-year-old known asthmatic was admitted to ICU with severe dyspnoea and rash on upper body and arms. Fiona's core (central) body temperature is 38.2°C, with shell (skin) temperature of 33°C. She has started to shiver.

Q1. a) List potential causes of her increased core temperature.
    b) Identify the blood cells and mediators responsible.
    c) Explain the shivering response and its effects on metabolism.
Q2. Compare various approaches to temperature assessment in your own clinical area; include common sites used in temperature assessment as well as the equipment available. Which would be the most appropriate method to monitor Fiona's core temperature (consider accuracy, time resources, safety, comfort, minimal adverse effects)?
Q3. Review effective nursing strategies for managing Fiona's temperature; select most suitable pharmacological interventions, laboratory investigations, physical cooling methods (their value, limitations, necessity) and comfort therapies.

Chapter 9

Nutrition and bowel care

Contents

Fundamental knowledge

Gut anatomy and physiology

Introduction

Nutrition is fundamental to health, yet Nightingale's (1859/1980) claim that thousands starve in hospitals continues to be relevant: Cahill *et al.* (2010) found that nutrition in intensive care is suboptimal. Starvation causes the body to use alternative energy sources – usually body protein (muscle), causing significant muscle wasting (Preiser *et al.*, 2015), which delays weaning and recovery and increases risks of sepsis (Ros *et al.*, 2009). Early nutrition improves survival from critical illness (McClave *et al.*, 2016).

Nitrogen (protein)

Metabolising (oxidising) protein produces nitrogen. Serum nitrogen is transported mainly as ammonia (NH_3), which the liver converts to urea. Measuring urinary nitrogen indicates protein metabolism. Unless diet is especially protein-rich, excessive protein metabolism indicates malnourishment-induced muscle atrophy. So:

■ neutral nitrogen balance = dietary nitrogen matches urinary loss;
■ negative nitrogen balance = excess urinary nitrogen catabolised for energy;
■ positive nitrogen balance = protein building (anabolism).

Protein is the most important macronutrient in critical illness, as it promotes wound healing, immunity and muscle-building (McClave *et al.*, 2016).

Energy

Cells need energy to function. The energy used is adenosine triphosphate (ATP), produced by cell mitochondria. In health, glucose metabolism is the main source of ATP:

$$C_6H_{12}O_6 + 6O_2 \rightarrow 36 \text{ ATP} + \text{waste } (6\ CO_2 + 6\ H_2O)$$

Some energy is also derived from fats. Fat metabolism is more complex – Krebs' or the "citric acid" cycle (Figure 9.1). Each stage of Krebs' cycle releases ATP and two carbon atoms. Carbon combines with coenzyme A, forming acetyl-CoA, which enables further reactions. Fat metabolism produces much energy but also much waste, each stage releasing acids (ketones, lactate), carbon dioxide and water. Carbon dioxide and water combine to form carbonic acid (H_2CO_3).

Hypoperfusion (shock) deprives cells of normal energy sources (oxygen and glucose) and waste removal. Anaerobic metabolism of alternative energy sources (such as fat) increases waste, causing hypercapnia and metabolic acidosis and creating increasingly hostile, acidic environments for cells.

Critical illness increases energy expenditure, a cost often not matched by the body's ability to use energy sources from food. Assessing nutritional needs is a complex task, usually undertaken by dieticians.

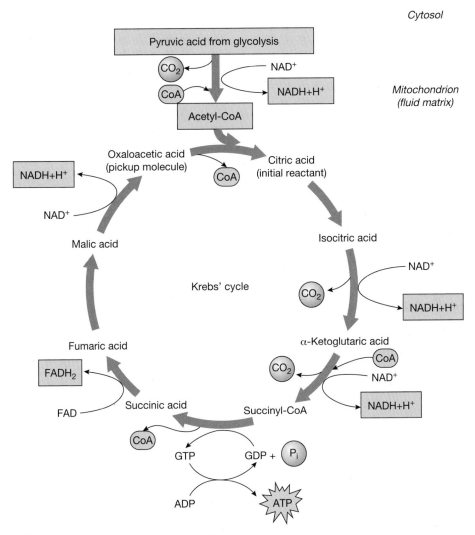

Figure 9.1 Krebs' (citric acid) cycle

Enteral nutrition

The gut contains many bacteria. Immunonutrition, addition of nutrients to improve the immune response, has been widely used, but to date there is insufficient evidence to show benefit (Preiser *et al.*, 2015). Translocation of gut bacteria into blood remains a major concern in critically ill patients, and, although the precise mechanism for this remains unclear, poor perfusion is a likely factor (Sertaridou *et al.*, 2015); enteral nutrition increases blood flow to the gut, preserving normal function and reducing infections such as pneumonia (McClave *et al.*, 2016).

Wide-bore gastric tubes (e.g. Ryles) are easier to insert than fine-bore tubes but cause more oesophagitis. Placement can be confirmed by:

- testing aspirate pH < 6.0 (N.I.C.E., 2006);
- radiography;
- ultrasound (e.g. Coretrak) (Gok *et al.*, 2015), although NHS England (2013) states that this is not an acceptable method for confirming position.

Gastric ulcer prophylaxis generally causes pH above the required 5.5, necessitating exposure to radiation (CXR). Nasal bridles reduce accidental tube removal (Gunn *et al.*, 2009).

Paralytic ileus typically affects the stomach first and small bowel last, so nasojejunal tube feeding should be considered if there is no little or no gastric motility (Compton *et al.*, 2014). Jejunal aspirate should be alkaline, making pH testing for placement invalid. Unless inserted with ultrasound, position should therefore always be checked by radiography, before removing guidewires. Jejunal tubes are frequently displaced (Berkelmans *et al.*, 2017), for example with coughing.

Gut surgery does not contraindicate enteral feeding (Hans-Geurts *et al.*, 2007). Bowel sounds only indicate contractility, not mucosal integrity, so absorption often occurs even if bowel sounds are absent (McClave *et al.*, 2016).

McClave *et al.* (2016) suggest that gastric residual volume (GRV), also called aspirate, should not be used to evaluate feed tolerance. European practice continues to favour GRV-guided feeding. The upper limit of aspirate which should be tolerated is often considered 200 ml, although European guidelines (Blaser *et al.*, 2017) recommend 500 ml over six hours. Fine-bore tubes can usually be aspirated, sometimes by injecting air to dislodge the tube from stomach folds. Gastric aspirate contains nutrients, digestive juices and electrolytes but is also needed to stimulate peristalsis and ileal secretions, so volumes of up to 200 ml are usually returned.

For patients in ICU, N.I.C.E. (2006) recommends continuous feeding over 16–24 hours, with 24 hours recommended if insulin is infused. Most UK ICUs feed continuously. These recommendations are ICU-specific and do not necessarily apply to patients in other areas. They also date from the era of tight glycaemic control; now this has been relaxed, it may be time to revisit this issue.

If nutrition cannot be achieved enterally, McClave *et al.* (2016) recommend "trophic" feeding, such as 10–20 ml/hour, to maintain gut integrity.

Type and rate of feeds should be prescribed by dieticians, although most ICUs have protocols for commencing standard feeds at incremental rates. Feeds available include:

- standard – carbohydrate-rich;
- fibre – may reduce diarrhoea;
- "respiratory" feeds – produce less carbon dioxide;
- "renal" feeds – produce less (nitrogen) waste;

■ pre-digested feeds – for malabsorption;
■ immune-modulating/enhancing feeds – contain substrates which alter immune/inflammatory responses – e.g. glutamine.

Risk of aspiration can be reduced by prokinetics (e.g. metoclopramide, low-dose erythromycin) (N.I.C.E., 2006; McClave *et al.*, 2016) and nursing patients at 30–45° (McClave *et al.*, 2016).

To reduce risks of confusion infusions, all enteral feeding equipment and lines should be purple (N.P.S.A., 2010).

Parenteral nutrition

While enteral nutrition is preferable (Blaser *et al.*, 2017), supplementary or (total) parenteral nutrition (PN) may be necessary to prevent muscle atrophy. If normal nutrition is unlikely to be achieved within three days, parenteral nutrition should be commenced within 24–48 hours of admission (Singer *et al.*, 2009), and if target enteral nutrition is not achieved within two days, it should be supplemented with parenteral (Singer *et al.*, 2009).

PN can cause:

■ gut atrophy, enabling translocation of gut bacteria;
■ infection;
■ hyperglycaemia;
■ hypertriglycidaemia;
■ impaired neutrophil function;
■ lipid agglutination in capillaries (increased afterload);
■ refeeding syndrome,

and is costly. Ideally, a dedicated lumen should be used for PN (Baker and Harbottle, 2014; Loveday *et al.*, 2014), so if possible a lumen should be reserved unused if need for parenteral nutrition is anticipated.

Refeeding syndrome

During starvation, the body uses alternative energy sources ("auto-cannibalism"). Refeeding provides glucose, the normal energy source. This stimulates insulin production, which causes loss of important electrolytes and micro-nutrients into cells – especially potassium, phosphate, magnesium and calcium (Sabol and York, 2018a). Complications can be reduced by introducing feeds slowly after prolonged starvation – half estimated requirement for 24–48 hours (N.I.C.E., 2006), with electrolyte and micronutrient supplements given where necessary. Prophylactic vitamin and phosphate supplements should be given (N.C.E.P.O.D., 2010a). While refeeding syndrome can occur with enteral feeds, it is more likely to occur with parenteral nutrition (McClave *et al.*, 2016).

Bowel care

In contrast to eating and oral care, bowel function is often a social taboo. Despite its importance for nursing care, it can often be given relatively low priority. ICU patients are prone to bowel dysfunction from:

■ immobility;
■ reduced peristalsis;
■ fluid imbalances;
■ effects of many drugs on the bowels (e.g. antibiotics, opioids, diuretics).

Commensal bacteria and yeasts in the colon assist digestion. Critical illness may facilitate their translocation across gut mucosa, causing endogenous infection. Translocation, and the controversial management of selective digestive decontamination, are discussed in Chapter 15.

Bowel care should include recording frequency, type and amount of faeces (Lewis and Heaton, 1997). The Bristol Stool Form chart provides objective descriptions and is widely used.

Diarrhoea

Many ICU patients develop diarrhoea (Tirlapur *et al.*, 2016). Diarrhoea is simply more fluid entering the colon than can be reabsorbed, and may be caused by:

■ antibiotics (destroy gut flora): Guenter *et al.* (1991) demonstrated a significant increased incidence of diarrhoea when entrally fed patients were being treated with antibiotics (41% versus 3%);
■ excessive fluid (colonic absorption is limited to about 4.5 litres each day);
■ reduced water reabsorption from hypoalbuminaemia or hypoperfusion (both common in ICU);
■ sorbitol (used in some elixirs, such as paracetamol suspension): exerts higher osmotic gradients than plasma, drawing fluid into the bowel (McClave *et al.*, 2016).

Likely causes of diarrhoea should be identified and where reasonably possible treated. If treatment is not reasonably possible, nurses should attempt to alleviate problems and risks. Enteral feeds seldom cause diarrhoea, so should not usually be stopped if diarrhoea occurs (Blaser *et al.*, 2017).

Diarrhoea can be a homeostatic way to remove pathological bowel bacteria, so reducing motility may cause/prolong infection. The most important pathogenic cause of healthcare-associated diarrhoea is *Clostridium difficile* (Weston, 2013). Pathogen removal should not be inhibited, but samples should be sent for culture and appropriate antibiotics prescribed. Tirlapur *et al.* (2016) suggest that diarrhoea in ICU patients is unlikely to be caused by pathogens.

Diarrhoea not caused by pathogens may be managed by:

- reducing gut motility – e.g. codeine phosphate, loperamide;
- changing to fibre feeds;
- probiotics, such as *Saccharomyces boulardii* (Allen *et al.*, 2010), although current evidence does not support their use in critically ill patients (Jack *et al.*, 2010).

Bowel contents are normally rich in electrolytes, including potassium and bicarbonate (Yassin and Wyncoll, 2005), so diarrhoea may cause hypokalaemia and metabolic acidosis.

Some ICU patients experience cramp pains when the gut recommences function or is overactive. This typically causes spasmodic pain (many patients will move their hands towards their abdomen) and irritability. Antispasmodic drugs, such as hyoscine nutybromide (Buscopan) can provide symptom relief.

Diarrhoea is distressing and socially embarrassing for patients (and visitors) and may excoriate skin and spread bacteria into wounds, lines or urinary catheters. Patients should therefore be reassured, washed and given clean linen. Faecal collections systems may reduce psychological distress and physiological risks such as infection (Echols *et al.*, 2004; Yassin and Wyncoll, 2005) and skin breakdown.

Constipation

Bowel habits can vary greatly between individuals, so defining constipation is problematic, but Lindberg *et al.*'s (2011) suggestion of bowel motions every three to four days or less is typical of most definitions. Constipation may be due to problems with:

- transit or
- evacuation.

(Lindberg *et al.*, 2011)

Unless the patient has pre-existing problems with evacuation, reduced transit is likely to be the problem in ICU, often caused or compounded by:

- dehydration;
- immobility;
- drugs reducing gut motility (e.g. opioids);
- gut damage from hypotension and hypoxaemia (Gacouin *et al.*, 2010).

Constipation can cause:

- discomfort
- agitation

- delayed weaning (Gacouin *et al.*, 2010)
- and other problems.

Bowel management should include assessment of possible constipation through:

- identifying when bowels were last opened, and type of stool passed;
- observing and palpating for abdominal distension;
- possibly, digital rectal examination ("PR");
- if hard stools are present in the rectum, giving stool softeners, enemas or (sometimes) manual evacuation of faeces.

R.C.N. guidelines (2008) list contraindications and cautions to digital rectal examination.

There are various types of laxatives; those used in ICU are usually:

- bulk-forming, stimulating peristalsis (e.g. fibre in feeds);
- peristaltic stimulants (e.g. senna);
- stool softeners (e.g. lactulose).

(Collins and O'Brien, 2015)

Osmotic laxatives should be avoided in hypovolaemic patients or patients with poor gut perfusion. If oral/nasogastric laxatives fail, glycerol suppositories may be useful, but these often necessitate help to position the patient.

Colostomies

Major bowel surgery often necessitates colostomy formation. Colostomy care is the same in ICU as elsewhere, except that ICU patients can seldom care for their own colostomies. Colour and perfusion of stomas should be checked at least once every shift and any concerns reported. Most trusts employ stoma nurses, who should be actively involved.

Implications for practice

- early and adequate nutrition hastens recovery and reduces endogenous infection;
- while multidisciplinary expertise is useful, nurses should both assess their patients' nutritional needs and co-ordinate care to ensure patients are adequately nourished;
- if the gut works, use it – enteral feeding is *usually* preferable;
- nurses may need to initiate standard protocol feed regimes, but dieticians should individually assess patients as soon as reasonably possible;
- success in establishing feeds should be assessed through;

  - gastric aspirates;
  - bowel function;

- most UK ICUs use gastric residual volumes to assess absorption, volumes exceeding 200 ml in four hours often indicating need for prokinetics;
- if nasogastric feeding fails, other options include jejunal tubes;
- diarrhoea is rarely caused by nasogastric feeding, so is not an indication to stop feeds;
- bowel function should be assessed on admission, reviewed each shift. Frequency, type and amount of stool should be recorded;
- the Bristol Stool Form assessment provides a useful way to quantify bowel evacuations;
- senna is usually the best laxative for ICU use, and is usually best given at night;
- overactive bowels can be slowed with drugs such as codeine phosphate or loperamide;
- bowel spasm distress may be relieved by antispasmodics (e.g. Buscopan);
- faecal collection systems can reduce distress to patients from frequent diarrhoea and subsequent washes and changes, and reduce infection risks to others;
- Stoma nurse specialist should be involved in care of all patients with newly formed stomas.

Summary

Malnutrition causes much ill health, delays recovery and increases mortality. Early and appropriate nutrition, preferably enteral, is fundamental to care. Protecting the gut may prevent sepsis. Nurses therefore should assess nutritional needs.

Many ICU patients are unable to identify need to defecate or report constipation, yet are prone to bowel dysfunction. Nurses should therefore monitor bowel function. Diarrhoea frequently occurs in ICU patients, usually being caused by disease or treatments.

Further reading

Most ICU texts include substantial chapters on nutrition, and articles on nutrition frequently appear in medical and nursing journals. Major guidelines and reports include Singer *et al.* (2009), McClave *et al.* (2016), Blaser *et al.* (2017) and N.C.E.P.O.D. (2010a). Gandy (2014) is the key (dieticians) text. Websites such as that of the British Association of Parenteral and Enteral Nutrition (BAPEN) and European Society for Clinical Nutrition and Metabolism (ESPEN) contain current material and guidelines. Preiser *et al.* (2015) and Sertaridou *et al.* (2015) provide useful reviews. The R.C.N. (2008) provides guidelines on bowel care.

Clinical scenarios

Richard Lewis is 71 years old and weighs approximately 70 kg, with arm span of 1.88 metres. He was admitted to ICU 15 days ago following emergency surgery for a perforated appendix. He is a smoker and has a tracheostomy to facilitate weaning from mechanical ventilation. His glycaemic control maintains his blood sugar at 8.7 mmol/litre with intravenous insulin infusion of 0.5 units/hour.

Richard is fed via a nasojejunal (NJ) tube in his right nostril. He receives 65 ml/hour of Nutrison Protein Plus (1.25 kcal/ml). He has diarrhoea > 800 ml/day, which is infected with *Clostridium difficile* and treated with continuous vancomycin infusion.

Q1. Calculate Richard's body mass index (BMI). Prior to dietetic assessment, what type of feed and target volume would your unit use? Identify other information needed to complete assessment.

Q2. Analyse Richard's feeding regime including total daily calories, the potential benefits and risks of feeding approach and type of enteral feed.

Q3. Consider strategies to manage Richard's diarrhoea and prevent cross-infection. What faecal management systems are available in your clinical area and what are criteria for their use? What other resources are used to manage patients' diarrhoea?

Mouthcare

Contents

Fundamental knowledge

Oral anatomy
Composition of dental plaque

Introduction

Hygiene is a fundamental activity of living. Poor oral care in ICU contributes to ventilator-associated pneumonia (VAP), so most recent studies, such as Grap *et al.* (2011), focus on how improved care can reduce VAP. Other evidence is sparse and weak (El-Rabbany *et al.*, 2015), with less interest in wider aspects of oral care in ICU, such as reducing long-term dental decay (O'Reilly, 2003).

Oral hygiene provides psychological comfort (O'Reilly, 2003). The mouth is used for communication – lip-reading is possible despite intubation, while following extubation oral discomfort may make speech difficult. The mouth is also associated with intimate emotions (smiling, kissing). Patients with, or thinking they have, dirty mouths or halitosis may feel (psychologically) isolated.

Providing oral hygiene merely replaces activities ICU patients would perform for themselves, if able. Mouthcare should therefore:

- maintain hygiene;
- keep the oral cavity moist;
- promote comfort;
- protect from infection;
- prevent trauma;
- prevent dental decay.

Anatomy

Saliva is released from glands (see Figure 10.1). Secretion increases with:

- oral pressoceptor stimulation (from anything in the mouth, including endotracheal tubes);
- oral chemoreceptor stimulation (especially acids);

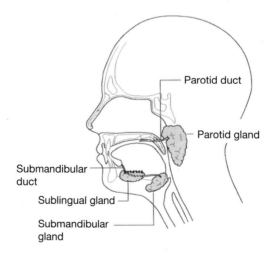

Figure 10.1 Oral (buccal) cavity

- thoughts of food;
- smelling food (in environment, on clothing);
- lower gut irritation.

However, ICU patients may develop dry mouths (xerostomia) from:

- absence of oral intake;
- reduced saliva from drugs (e.g. morphine, diuretics) and sympathetic nervous system stimulation;
- drying (convection) from mouths wedged open by oral endotracheal tubes.

So saliva secretion may be excessive or diminished. Saliva contains many chemicals, including immune defences, so excess or deficits can cause colonisation/infection and ulceration. While it is normally slightly acidic (pH 6.75–7.0 (Marieb and Hoehn, 2016)), Treloar (1995) found mean salivary pH of 5.3 in ICU patients, which is more likely to cause tooth decay.

Saliva may be serous (containing ptyalin, which digests starches) or mucous (containing mucin, a lubricant). Sympathetic vasoconstriction and dehydration reduce salivary gland perfusion, making saliva viscous and mucin-rich – dry mouths are familiar from "fight or flight" responses. Endogenous sympathetic stimulation from stress may be compounded by exogenous catecholamines (adrenaline/noradrenaline). Saliva production also decreases with age – most ICU patients are old.

Plaque

Plaque (sugar, bacteria and other debris) metabolises to acids, especially lactic acid. Plaque can contain 10^8–10^{11} bacteria per gram (Murray et al., 2009). Accumulated plaque calcifies into calculus or tartar, disrupting seals between gingivae and teeth. Gingivitis (sore, red and bleeding gums) occurs within 10 days of plaque formation (Kite and Pearson, 1995).

Plaque is not water-soluble, so mouthwash solutions are not a substitute for brushing. Oral neglect enables bacteria to multiply around teeth and dissolve bone (periotonitis/periodontal disease). Periodontitis is the main cause of adult tooth loss, so neglect in ICU can have rapid and enduring effects.

Infection

Micro-organisms grow readily in ICU patients' mouths because:

- mouths are warm, moist and static;
- saliva accumulates at the back of throats, especially if gag/swallowing reflexes are impaired;
- blood and plaque provide protein for bacterial growth (O'Reilly, 2003);
- normal flora is often destroyed by antibiotics;
- immunosuppression facilitates growth.

Infection is usually bacterial, but *Candida*, the most common fungal infection, can be recognised by white spots (Clarke, 1993) and, like most oral fungi, is usually susceptible to nystatin.

Excessive or purulent secretions should be removed with suction. Yankauer catheters are often best for the front of the cavity, but deep oral suction is often easier with a soft catheter. Removal of tenacious secretions may necessitate lubricating the mouth with clean water from a 5 ml syringe, usually best directed at the side of the mouth. Frequency of moistening or removing secretions should be assessed individually for each patient.

Assessment

Oral assessment should include each aspect of the cavity:

- lips
- gums
- teeth
- tongue
- hard palette
- soft tissue
- salivary production
- evidence of any infection
- evidence of any cuts/purpura/blood.

These should be assessed against risk factors from:

- overall condition;
- underlying pathology;
- treatments (including effects of drugs);
- viewing the oral cavity requires a good light (e.g. pentorch).

Many assessment tools have been developed, most being checklists. While these can provide a useful structure, assessment should be individualised to each patient, and there is little evidence of either sustained effectiveness from (Kelly *et al.*, 2010) or validity of (Berry *et al.*, 2007) any tool. Many are relatively lengthy and risk becoming one more time-consuming "tick-box exercise" that fails to be translated into nursing care.

Replacing saliva

Many mouthcare solutions and other aids have been marketed, but few remove or prevent plaque. There are artificial saliva solutions, but these are seldom used in ICU. *Sterile water*, which can be instilled using a small syringe, can provide moisture but has no cleansing properties, so is an adjunct rather than a replacement for other care.

Foam sticks are useful for moistening the mouth between cleaning (O'Reilly, 2003) but do not remove debris from surfaces or between teeth, so plaque accumulation progresses (Grap *et al.*, 2003). Frequency of moistening mouths should be individualised to patients.

Excess fluid, whether patients' own saliva or instilled water/mouthwashes, should be removed, which usually necessitates suction.

Oral decontamination

Ventilator-associated pneumonia (VAP) is a major cause or morbidity and mortality in ICUs. Most organisms infecting the lungs originate from oropharyngeal colonies, so reducing oral colonisation should logically reduce VAP.

Some mouthwashes are antibacterial: in the past many studies (such as Grap *et al.*, 2011; El-Rabbany *et al.*, 2015), found *chlorhexidine* prevented bacterial and fungal growth, so reducing VAP. However, more recent studies have found limited or no benefit, and even non-significant increased mortality from chlorhexidine (Kusahara *et al.*, 2012; Klompas *et al.*, 2014; Price *et al.*, 2014; Wong, Schlichting *et al.*, 2016), and the I.C.S. (2015) recommends not using chlorhexidine except for cardiac surgery patients. Chlorhexidine mouthwash is usually either 1% or 2%, but other strengths are available, which reduces the comparability of different studies. Logically, stronger antiseptics will kill more micro-organisms, but stronger chemicals may cause more tissue damage.

Teeth

Teeth should be brushed at least twice daily to reduce caries (de Oliveira *et al.*, 2010). However, toothbrushing does not reduce VAP (Munro *et al.*, 2009). Between brushing, additional comfort cleaning/refreshing will usually be needed. Toothbrushes (with or without toothpaste) remain the best way to clean patients' teeth (Rello *et al.*, 2007; Kelly *et al.*, 2010), loosening debris trapped between teeth and removing plaque. Technique should reflect brushing one's own teeth: brush away from gums to remove, rather than impact, plaque from gingival crevices. Manipulating toothbrushes in others' mouths, especially when orally intubated, can be difficult, so small-headed ("paediatric") toothbrushes are often most effective for brushing others' teeth (Jones, 2004). Brushing is most effective if toothbrushes are angled at 45° to gingival margins; using small, scrubbing movements for two minutes, collects and removes plaque (Dougherty and Lister, 2015). Toothbrushes can clean heavily coated tongues, and gums and tongue of endentitious patients (O'Reilly, 2003).

Fluoride toothpaste is preferable (Rattenbury *et al.*, 1999), although patients may find the taste of their usual brand comforting. Most toothpastes dry the mouth (Jones, 2004), so should be rinsed out thoroughly – sterile water from a 5 ml syringe, and continuous suction, are usually the best way to achieve this. Yankauer catheters can stimulate cough/gag reflexes, so should be used sparingly; soft catheters are usually more effective for mouthcare.

Vigorous brushing may cause bleeding, especially if patients have coagulopathies; oral care should therefore be planned holistically. If nystatin is prescribed, this should be administered following mouthcare.

Lips

Lips are highly vascular, with sensitive nerve endings. Mucosa being exposed, it can dry quickly. Lips are even more closely associated with communication (e.g. lip-reading) and intimacy (e.g. kissing) than the mouth. Lipcare can therefore prevent drying/cracking, while providing psychological comfort. Lip balm, white petroleum jelly or yellow soft paraffin is often used to keep lips moist (Bowsher *et al.*, 1999). Contrary to circulating myths, petroleum jelly neither explodes nor burns (Winslow and Jacobson, 1998).

Pressure sores

Any body surface area may develop pressure sores (see Chapter 12). Treloar's (1995) small study found multiple lip, tongue and mucosal lesions, as well as very dry mouths, in ICU patients. Endotracheal tubes and many securing devices place pressure on various tissues, including the mouth. Gingival surfaces are more susceptible to sores than teeth (Liwu, 1990), and tube tapes can lacerate lip.

Dentures

About half of older people do not have their own teeth (Watson, 2001). Intubation and impaired consciousness normally necessitates removal of any dentures, but property should be checked on admission so that dentures are not lost. Nursing records should include whether patients normally wear partial or complete dentures, and relevant care.

Dentures may easily be damaged or warp, especially if left dry or cleaned in hot water (Clarke, 1993). Dentures should usually be left soaking overnight in cold water (Xavier, 2000; Clay, 2002; O'Reilly, 2003). Toothpaste should not be used on dentures, as it can damage their surfaces (Clarke, 1993). Patients, or their family, may be able to supply their normal cleaning agents, which, if available, should be used (Xavier, 2000).

Implications for practice

- mouthcare should be individually assessed, rather than following routine/ rituals;
- toothbrushes (with or without toothpaste) are the best means for providing mouthcare;
- teeth should (usually) be brushed with toothpaste twice daily, with additional comfort cleaning between, according to individual assessment;

- fluoride toothpaste helps prevent decay;
- rinse toothpaste out thoroughly, using sterile water and suction;
- mouthwashes or moist swabs moisten the mouth but do not remove plaque;
- if pharmaceutical agents are needed, consult pharmacists;
- if patients wear dentures, maintain their normal care if possible, and record where they are stored;
- white petroleum jelly or yellow soft paraffin protects lips from cracking.

Summary

Mouthcare is too easily forgotten in the physiological crises of critical illness, but problems developing from their time in ICU can cause long-term or permanent oral/dental disease. The current paucity of material on mouthcare in ICU makes evidence-based practice difficult.

Further reading

Other than debates surrounding chlorhexidine, there has been no significant ICU literature about mouthcare for a decade, making Berry *et al.* (2007) and Rello *et al.* (2007) the most recent useful resources.

Clinical scenarios

Michael Dodd is a 22-year-old gentleman who has a past medical history of poorly controlled asthma. He presents with left lower lobe pneumonia. This is his third admission to ICU for respiratory support. He weighs 90 kg, is receiving enteral nutrition at 65 ml/hr and has been invasively ventilated for seven days. Michael's oral endotracheal tube length is 23 cm at lips, positioned on the right side of his mouth and balancing on his teeth. He has visible dental decay at gum margins with white spots on his tongue and hard palate.

Michael's intravenous drug therapy includes propofol, tazobactam and rifampicin and hydrocortisone. He has a temperature of 38.5°C, Hb 104 grams/litre, WCC 9.3 x10⁹/litre, CRP 207 mg/litre.

Q1. List equipment needed to inspect and assess Michael's oral status to include gums, tongue, salivary glands, teeth, palate, lips and jaw.
Q2. Identify Michael's risk factors for developing oral complications. Use your unit's oral assessment tool to calculate and interpret Michael's oral assessment score.
Q3. Develop a plan for Michael's mouthcare including frequency of interventions, method of brushing teeth and tongue, lip lubrication and use of any topical lotions or creams.

Chapter 11

Eyecare

Contents

Fundamental knowledge

Eye anatomy – cornea, lens, tear production, blink reflex

104

Introduction

Patients are seldom admitted to ICU for ocular pathologies, but critically ill patients can suffer eye surface disease (Dawson, 2005), especially dryness, redness and discharge (Oh *et al.*, 2009). In health, blink reflexes both moisten and protect the eye surface. But loss of blink reflexes, such as from deep sedation and paralysis, expose eye surfaces to risks of:

- infection (keratitis), especially from *Pseudomonas aeruginosa, Acinetobacter spp, Staphylococcus epidermis* (Mela *et al.*, 2010);
- exposure keratopathy (Alansari *et al.*, 2015);
- trauma and abrasion from bedding, endotracheal tube tapes and other equipment.

Positive pressure ventilation increases intraocular pressure, so causing potential "ventilator eye". This chapter does not discuss specialist ocular pathophysiologies, but reasons for and types of eyecare needed by ICU patients.

In health, eyelids protect eye surfaces. Tear production and frequent blinking maintains health and moistens eye surfaces. While many ICU patients can maintain their own ocular health, some may develop complications. Problems are more likely with:

- increased intraoccular pressure or periorbital oedema (especially prone positioning);
- impaired blink reflex, such as from paralysis (disease or chemical);
- decreased tear production;
- patient being unable to move their head;
- eye infection.

If patients are unable to maintain their own ocular health, nurses should meet this need for them. It is therefore important to assess all patients, and to provide eyecare where problems exist.

People may feel squeamish about touching eyes, but eyecare maintains physiological and psychological health. Ocular abnormalities often make patients and relatives anxious. For most people, vision is the most used sense, eye contact helping communication. So visual deficits contribute significantly to sensory imbalance. ICU nurses should therefore evaluate:

- visual appearance;
- eyecare performed;
- how care is described.

Eyecare in ICU varies greatly, with limited supporting evidence (Dawson, 2005; Leadingham, 2014; Câmara *et al.*, 2016). Evidence from other specialities (such as theatres), dated evidence, or evidence from countries where sedation practices may differ should be applied with caution. Substantive research being needed, suggestions here necessarily remain tentative.

Ocular damage

The cornea, the eye's outer surface, has no direct blood supply, otherwise sight would be impaired. It is therefore vulnerable to drying, trauma and lacerations (e.g. from pillows, endotracheal tapes, dust and particles). Blink reflexes and tear production, which normally protect and irrigate corneal surfaces, may be absent/weak. Drugs (e.g. atropine, antihistamines, paralysing agents) also inhibit tear production. If blink reflexes are absent, eyelids should be closed or corneas protected with a cover (Alansari *et al.*, 2015).

Bacteria can cause blepharitis, inflammation of eyelash follicles and sebaceous glands, resulting in redness, swelling and crusts of dried mucus collecting on the lids. Crusts may cause corneal trauma on eyelid closure with blinking. If ocular infection is suspected, it should be reported and recorded; swabs may need to be taken and topical antibiotics prescribed.

Incomplete eyelid closure or loss of blink reflexes causes corneal drying (exposure keratopathy) and can cause infection (keratitis) or corneal ulceration (Dawson, 2005; Demirel *et al.*, 2014). The cornea is the most densely innervated structure in the human body (Shaheen *et al.*, 2014), making lacerations very painful. Corneal damage exposes deeper layers to infection, while the avascularity of the cornea delays healing, often leaving opaque scar tissue. Ocular trauma may remain unrecognised until patients regain consciousness, finding their vision permanently impaired.

Normal intraocular pressure is 12–20 mmHg (average 15 mmHg). Drainage of aqueous humour, and so intraocular hypertension, subconjunctival haemorrhage and other damage, may be caused by positive intrathoracic pressure (positive pressure ventilation), tight ETT tapes, oedema, poor head alignment or prone positioning. ICU patients are therefore at high risk of intraocular hypertension. Head elevation (e.g. 30°) assists venous drainage.

Contact lenses are removed pre-operatively, but with emergency admissions may still be in place. Contact lenses or glasses, if removed, should be stored safely, and recorded in nursing notes in case of loss.

Assessment

Structured eye assessment tools are not generally used in ICUs, and with the proliferation of paper assessment tools might prove counterproductive if introduced. Nurses should assess the condition of their patients' eyes through:

- existing documentation;
- visual observation of patients;
- knowledge of normal ocular anatomy;
- verbal questions (to patients or family).

Cues to consider include:

- contact lenses/glasses;
- abnormalities (e.g. eyelids, lashes, exophthalmus); are abnormalities unilateral/bilateral?

- periorbital oedema;
- patient positioning, venous drainage;
- muscle weakness ("droopy eye");
- eye closure – do lids cover cornea completely?
- do eyes look infected/inflamed?
- do eyes look sore ("redeye" – often a sign of acute bacterial conjunctivitis)?
- tear production (excessive/impaired) – moist/dry eyes;
- blink reflex (absent, impaired, slow);
- eye pain (flinching during eye care/interventions);
- visual impairment (double, cloudy, difficulty focusing);
- how does the patient feel (e.g. are eyelids heavy)?

Closed questions are often easier for intubated patients to answer.

Unless patients have specific ocular disease, eyecare should:

- maintain ocular health;
- replace lost functions;
- ensure comfort;
- protect from trauma/infection.

Eye care is easiest to perform if the patient is positioned either supine or with head tilted backwards – this helps nurses see what they are doing and keeps solutions in the eye (Dougherty and Lister, 2015). Frequency of eyecare should be individualised to needs.

While assessing and caring for patients' eyes, nurses can also make neurological assessment of:

- pupil size and reaction;
- accommodation for near and long vision: place a finger near the patient's nose; when moved away, pupils should diverge.

Ocular damage may invalidate any or all of these tests.

Interventions

Dry eyes should be lubricated, although optimal solution or frequency remains unclear (Dawson, 2005). *Artificial tears* seem a logical replacement if tear production is inadequate. *Chloramphenicol* eye drops are often used to treat acute bacterial conjunctivitis (Sheikh *et al.*, 2012). Eye drops should be instilled into the outer side of the lower fornix (see Figure 11.1), which is less sensitive than the cornea. Over-vigorous use of eye drops on corneas resembles water torture. To minimise infection risk, solutions should be stored in a clean area. If reusable, they should be labelled with date and time of opening. Labelling or local hospital policies will identify how long solutions can be used for after opening.

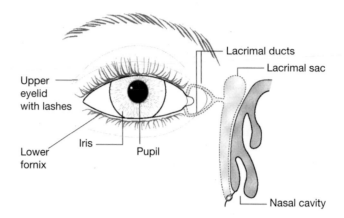

■ *Figure 11.1* **External structure of the eye**

If eyelid *closure* is incomplete, and patients cannot blink, corneal surfaces should be kept moist and covered. Some authors, such as Alansari *et al.* (2015), suggest that saline can damage the corneal surface, so recommend sterile water or commercial eye drops/lubricants. As tears are dilute saline, this seems illogical. Excess moisture should be removed delicately with soft, non-woven swabs. Many people are especially squeamish about eyes, so relatives may become especially anxious when eyes are covered.

Implications for practice

- ICU patients may suffer "ventilator eye";
- care for each patient should be individually assessed;
- if patients are unable to maintain their own ocular health, eyecare should keep eyes clean, moist and covered;
- nursing semi-recumbent helps venous drainage;
- prone positioning can damage eyes; elevating bedhead by as little as 10° and careful head alignment can reduce complications;
- eyecare solutions are potential media for infection, so should be changed regularly. In addition to expiry dates, most commercial preparations have facilities for dating time of opening. Any fluids open to the atmosphere should be discarded after each intervention;
- exposed corneas are vulnerable to trauma, so keep pillow edges, endo-tracheal tape and other equipment away from eyes.

Summary

Although patients are seldom admitted for ocular conditions, diseases and treatments can expose ICU patients to ocular damage. Yet, eyecare in ICU is often given low priority, and there is little reliable and substantiated literature to guide interventions. Preventative eyecare should be commenced on admission

(Oh *et al.*, 2009). Care inevitably relies heavily on custom, practice, rituals and anecdotal support. As part of their fundamental patient care, nurses should support/provide what their patients need. Nurses should therefore assess their patients' ocular health and risks, planning individualised care accordingly.

Further reading

Eyecare in ICU is much under-researched, and little other specialist literature exists that is directly relevant to ICU practice. Despite their relative age, Dawson (2005) and Oh *et al.* (2009) provide the most useful reviews for UK ICUs. Most more recent studies originate from countries where deep sedation and chemical paralysis are more widespread, limiting their applicability to the UK. The Marsden Manual (Dougherty and Lister, 2015) contains a useful section on eyecare, but this is not ICU-specific.

Clinical scenarios

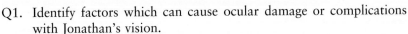

Mr Jonathan Hopkins is 48 years old and works as a computer programmer. Jonathan wears non-gas-permeable contact lenses and has a severe stigmatism in one eye. He recently required treatment for recurrent conjunctivitis. Jonathan was admitted with community-acquired pneumonia. In the first 24 hours he received respiratory support with high-flow nasal oxygen, 60 litres flow and FiO_2 of 0.5.

Q1. Identify factors which can cause ocular damage or complications with Jonathan's vision.

Q2. Jonathan developed bacterial keratitis and corneal ulceration from corneal exposure. Consider how this affected his recovery in relation to his perceptions, vision, communication interactions and pain. Reflect on the legal, ethical and professional responsibilities towards Jonathan. Has substandard practice or negligence occurred? If yes, who might be responsible?

Q3. Review eye care in your own clinical area. Is ocular assessment and eyecare:

- systematic (in both approach and documentation);
- based on a local or published guideline;
- knowledge- and/or evidence-based;
- effective at identifying patients at risk before complications occur?

Chapter 12

Tissue viability

Contents

Fundamental knowledge

Structure and anatomy of skin
Functions of skin
Pressure sore (decubitus ulcer) formation
Stages of wound healing

Introduction

Maintaining skin integrity is fundamental to care, although potentially difficult to achieve with high-risk hypotensive and immobile patients, especially if turning risks compromising vital organ function. Pressure sores are problematic in most inpatient settings, but incidence is highest in ICU – patient safety incident reports identify pressure sores as the most common cause of harm in ICU (Thomas and Taylor, 2012), although this may reflect better reporting. Approximately 10% of ICU patients develop ulcers (VanGilder et al., 2009), although statistics vary greatly – Elliott et al. (2008) found that they occurred in up to half of ICU patients, whereas Shahina et al. (2009) measured only 3.3%. Increased awareness together with significant practice changes such as reduced sedation and earlier rehabilitation should reduce this incidence. The single largest group of litigation claims in UK ICUs between 1995–2012 was positioning, skin care and nursing standards (Pascall et al., 2015). External pressures such as litigation and financial penalties could also drive change, although challenges with staffing levels could exacerbate problems.

Pressure sores increase:

- morbidity (human costs);
- mortality;
- financial costs (prolonged stay, additional treatments).

(Tayyib and Coyer, 2016)

The epidermis regenerates itself every four to six weeks (Baranoski et al., 2012), so healing is slow, exposing deeper tissues to potential infection.

ICU patients are at "high risk" for developing pressure sore because of:

- severity of illness;
- patient responses to critical illness.

(Tayyib and Coyer, 2016)

Other risk factors include:

- prolonged peripheral hypoperfusion;
- age (Terekeci et al., 2009; Kottner et al., 2013; Tayyib and Coyer, 2016);
- length of stay (Terekeci et al., 2009; Tayyib and Coyer, 2016);
- prolonged immobility (Tayyib and Coyer, 2016; Chen et al., 2017);
- cardiovascular disease (Nijs et al., 2009; Terekeci et al., 2009; Tayyib and Coyer, 2016);
- inotropes (Nijs et al., 2009; Tayyib and Coyer, 2016);
- renal replacement therapy (Nijs et al., 2009);
- mechanical ventilation (Nijs et al., 2009);
- sedatives (Nijs et al., 2009);
- body temperature > 38.5°C (Nijs et al., 2009);
- malnutrition (Terekeci et al., 2009);
- hypoalbuminaemia (Terekeci et al., 2009).

Contrary to some scoring systems, such as Waterlow (1985), Terekeci *et al.* (2009) suggest body mass index is not a risk factor.

This chapter revises pressure sore development, identifies some assessment systems available, and describes some ways of preventing pressure sores. Wound dressings are not discussed, as rapid changes in practice and availability make inclusion in this book impractical. Necrotising fasciitis, a potentially fatal dermatological pathology, is also discussed. Some evidence originates, or is sponsored/promoted by, people and commercial companies with vested interests, so should be treated cautiously.

Pressure sores

When external pressure exceeds capillary pressure, perfusion fails, leading to necrosis. *Capillary occlusion pressure*, the amount of pressure required to occlude capillaries, is often cited at 30–32 mmHg. This originates from Landis's 1930 study, which measured 21–48 mmHg in normotensive volunteers (mean 32 mmHg). ICU patients are not volunteers and are seldom normotensive. So 20–25 mmHg is generally a safer upper limit for unrelieved pressure on any tissue. Visible signs of pressure sores may appear on skin surfaces, but compression of tissue between surfaces and bony prominences can cause deeper damage (de Carvalho *et al.*, 2016) – elbow, heels, sacrum are often most at risk, but other possible sites for sores include:

- head (especially the back);
- ears;
- lips/mouth (around ETTs);
- beneath invasive equipment (e.g. hubs of arterial lines);
- skinfolds (e.g. breasts, groin, abdomen);
- chest and face if prone positioned;
- coccyx, from semi-recumbent positioning (Bell, 2008).

Hair may hide sores on backs of heads, until blood is found on pillows. Nurses should therefore proactively assess all risk areas.

Excessive moisture or dryness hastens skin breakdown. Urine is acidic, so leaks around urinary catheters excoriate skin. Perspiration makes skin excessively moist and contains urea. Faeces also contain acids. Diarrhoea, inability to alert nurses of the need for bedpans, and gathering sufficient staff to turn patients can result in anal areas being exposed to evacuated faeces, causing excoriation. Prompt hygiene and "comfort" washes reduce risks, and lubricating dry skin (e.g. with aqueous cream) can prevent breakdown. Barrier creams can reduce risks of breakdown (Kottner *et al.*, 2013), so are useful adjuncts to, but not substitutes for, nursing care.

Falls

Although falls are less common in critical care than most inpatient areas (Richardson and Carter, 2017), damage can occur from falls. Falls are more common when patients have neurological conditions or are admitted with trauma, and surprisingly are most common among patients aged 35–64 (Richardson and Carter, 2017). Falls are a national priority, so risk assessment is now standard in most UK hospitals, including in critical care.

Assessment

Pressure areas should be regularly assessed (at least once each shift), and assessment tools can provide useful cues, but become counterproductive if they are viewed as just another paper exercise. Many assessment tools have been developed, but many are complex and no more effective than clinical judgement (Anthony et al., 2010); Braden (2012) acknowledges the value of using clinical judgement together with assessment tools. The Braden tool (Bergstrom et al., 1987) remains internationally the most widely used pressure risk assessment (Chen et al., 2017; Ayello and Braden, 2002).

The most widely used tool in the UK is Waterlow (1985, updated 2005). Most UK nurses are familiar with it, and Sayar et al. (2009) concluded that it reliably predicts risk of pressure sore development in ICU. Most ICU patients predictably score "high risk", which potentially negates its value; Pender and Frazier (2005) found it unreliable for ICU, while Sanada et al. (2006) found it had high sensitivity (identified patients at risk) but low specificity (many false positives). Moore and Cowman's (2014) review of assessment tools found limited evidence, but that pressure ulcer incidence was not reduced by using assessment tools.

Prevention

Pressure ulcers have traditionally been viewed as a sign of poor care; pressure ulcers are potentially avoidable, and so require reporting. The D.O.H. (2009a) set a target of eliminating avoidable pressure sores; in 2016 the D.O.H. claimed that NHS awareness of pressure ulcers had increased and incidence had decreased. Pressure ulceration continues to be a significant cause of morbidity. Pressure on skin can be decreased either by changing position or increasing the surface area over which pressure is spread. Two-hourly pressure area care owes more to ritual than logic (Siddiqui et al., 2013) and is probably seldom practised in many clinical areas – Goldhill et al. (2008) found average time between turns in UK ICUs is 4.85 hours, frequency not being related to staffing numbers (Badacsony et al., 2007). Anecdotally, it would be surprising if frequency of turning has increased since 2008.

Support surfaces and alternating pressure mattresses can reduce tissue breakdown (Shahina et al., 2009); almost all ICUs use either *low air loss mattresses* or *tilting/kinetic beds*. Choice of *mattress* or other aids may be restricted by:

- weight limits for equipment (including hoists);
- pathology – e.g. head or spinal injury patients require a firm mattress to maintain spinal alignment;
- availability and cost, if equipment needs to be hired.

Bony prominences, such as heels, being high-risk areas for ulcer development, prophylactic heel protectors (Rajpaul and Acton, 2016) or heel pressure off-loading by supporting legs on a pillow can prevent many avoidable pressure sores. Tayyib and Coyer (2016) recommend silicone foam dressings to prevent sacral and heel pressure sores. Siddiqui *et al.* (2013) recommend continuous bedside pressure mapping, using a pressure-sensing mat to display real-time digital imaging of pressure areas.

Other "general" aspects of ICU care can reduce risk factors, such as early mobility and early enteral nutrition (Coleman *et al.*, 2013), both important interventions for various reasons and discussed elsewhere in this book.

Most hospitals employ tissue viability nurses, who are a valuable source for advice and resources, but it is also valuable for ICUs to have a tissue viability link nurse to:

- disseminate information and provide an immediate resource for staff;
- apply information to special needs and problems of ICU patients;
- audit skincare.

Necrotising fasciitis

This rare condition occurs when pathogens, often streptococcal and/or clostridium (Stevens and Bryant, 2017) infects and spreads rapidly through deep fascia (Khamnuan *et al.*, 2015), often provoking inflammation and septic shock.

Necrotising fasciitis should be treated with urgent surgical debridement and intravenous antibiotics (Khamnuan *et al.*, 2015). Evidence for benefits from hyperbaric oxygen therapy are controversial (Hunter *et al.*, 2011), there being insufficient evidence either to support or refute its use (Levett *et al.*, 2015) and it is unavailable in most hospitals.

Gross oedematous swelling of flesh may make patients almost unrecognisable, so visitors should be warned to expect distressing appearances.

Implications for practice

- ICU patients are "high risk" for pressure sore development;
- ICU patients can develop sores in many places, including backs of heads;
- pressure areas should be checked at least every shift;
- no ideal assessment tool exists for ICU, but whatever is used should be familiar to all staff;
- sores develop if external pressure exceeds capillary occlusion pressure; 20–25 mmHg is usually a safe upper limit for sustained pressure;
- hospital tissue viability nurses, and unit link nurses for tissue viability, can be a valuable resource;
- necrotising fasciitis is a rare, but potentially devastating, infection that progresses rapidly and should be treated aggressively (antibiotics and debridement).

Summary

Skin has many functions, but most importantly it forms a selective barrier which protects the body. Cost of skin breakdown can be measured in mortality, morbidity, increased length of stay in ICU, increased financial costs and litigation.

Various scoring systems have been designed to assess skin integrity and pressure sore risk, but none are ideal for ICU, and whether quantifying risk is beneficial remains unclear. Anthony *et al.* (2008) suggest that nurses may be wasting time conducting risk assessment scoring. Pressure sores continue to occur in ICU. A culture of guilt surrounding pressure sores is counterproductive; despite good nursing, sores will occur, so nurses should assess and minimise risk factors to reduce the incidence.

Further reading

Most anatomy texts include detailed chapters on skin. Surprisingly little has appeared in specialist nursing journals since the last edition of this book, but de Carvalho *et al.* (2016) and Tayyib and Coyer (2016) are among the most useful ICU-focused articles. Moore and Cowman (2014) review risk assessment tools. There are a number of wound care and tissue viability books, such as Baronoski and Ayello (2012) and journals, such as the *Journal of Wound Care.*

Websites

Braden Scale: www.bradenscale.com/braden.pdf.
Waterlow: www.judy-waterlow.co.uk/waterlow_score.htm.

Clinical scenarios

Norman Robinson is a 60-year-old gentleman who tripped on an uneven paving stone and sustained a superficial abrasion to the lateral aspect of his left knee. Within 24 hours, his leg was increasingly painful and oedematous, making him unable to extend his knee or weight bear. Two days following this fall, Mr Robinson was diagnosed with necrotising fasciitis and had aggressive surgical debridement, with application of skin grafts from his right leg. He was admitted to the ICU following surgery for mechanical ventilation and organ support. Mr Robinson is increasingly oedematous, with extensive (offensive-smelling) wound exudate from both legs and constant diarrhoea. He weighs 93 kg and is 1.68 m tall.

Vital signs include pyrexia 38.5°C, tachycardia 115 beats/minute, MAP 73 mmHg, and urine output over 60 ml/hour for the last four hours. Blood investigation reveal creatinine 218 micromol/litre, urea

18.4 mmol/litre, albumin 17 grams/litre, platelets 61×10^9/litre, Hb 85 grams/litre, WCC 14×10^9/litre. Microbiological examination of tissue from left leg shows large presence of *Staphylococcus aureus* and beta haemolytic group A *Streptococci*. Appropriate antibiotics have been prescribed.

Q1. Identify Mr Robinson's risk factors for developing further skin breakdown.

Q2. Consider the range of pressure relieving equipment in your clinical area, select appropriate mattress type, aids and other interventions to optimise skin integrity.

Q3. Review wound assessment and documentation for Mr Robinson. How should his exudative wounds and skin grafts be managed to minimise other complications and promote wound healing?

Chapter 13

Children in adult ICUs

Contents

Fundamental knowledge

Local policies about consent and child protection
Location and contents of paediatric equipment and
    resources in the workplace

Introduction

In the UK, as in most European countries (EfCCNa, 2017), children are usually nursed in dedicated paediatric intensive care units (PICUs), as this improves survival (Cogo *et al.*, 2010; Ramnarayan *et al.*, 2010). PICUs in the UK are in regional centres, and when children initially become critically ill they are often in, or admitted to, their local hospital (Lampariello *et al.*, 2010). Hospitals accepting children with trauma should have either a Level 1 (basic critical care, similar to acute wards for adults) or Level 2 (intermediate critical care, e.g. able to manage airways such as tracheostomies, and non-invasive ventilation) paediatric critical care unit (P.I.C.S., 2015a), where deteriorating children are usually managed, but they may need to be admitted to general (adult) ICUs (P.I.C.S., 2015a) if additional needs, or inadequate resources, necessitate admission. Time in adult ICUs is usually brief, until retrieval teams from paediatric ICUs (PICUs) arrive to transport patients to specialist centres (D.O.H., 1997; P.I.C.S., 2015b). The occasional emergency paediatric admission creates two main challenges for staff in general (adult) ICUs:

- when children are admitted, their condition is usually at its most critical/unstable;
- admission is so infrequent that most staff in general ICUs have little or no experience of paediatric critical care.

This chapter therefore focuses on initial management and stabilisation of critically ill children, using the ABCDE format likely to be used when stabilising children for transfer. Pandemic influenza planning in 2009 anticipated significant numbers of children being cared for on general ICUs (see Chapter 16). In a position statement, the N.M.C. (2009) acknowledged that nurses might have to care for people in unfamiliar settings or areas of practice, requiring that nurses act "responsibly and reasonably". This chapter will not discuss neonates, who would be admitted to a special care baby unit (SCBU) or neonatal ICU (NICU). Meningitis, which can also occur in adult patients, is discussed.

Children, especially young children, are still developing. Physical growth necessitates higher metabolic rates, increasing oxygen and nutritional demands, while increasing physiological waste. Many vital signs, such as heart rate, are therefore higher than with adults, with different "normal" ranges for different ages. But crises necessitating ICU admission are also likely to make many vital signs abnormal. Unless familiar with paediatric ranges, nurses need to assess which signs are significant, and often need to rely on trends. Weight-relating drug dosages and fluid volumes is usually necessary, but there can be other significant differences. Most ICUs have a paediatric trolley with standard equipment and guidance. Readers should familiarise themselves with resources available where they work – when children are admitted, time is precious.

P.I.C.S. (2015a) requires a consultant and lead nurse to be responsible for ICU policies, procedures and training relating to children, and that there should be an appropriately designed and equipped area for providing paediatric critical care for children. When children are admitted, a registered children's nurse should support the care of the child and review the child at least every 12 hours (P.I.C.S., 2015a). In practice, an RSCN often accompanies the child at admission, and often remains until the transfer team arrive.

Depending on needs, adolescents needing intensive care might remain on adult ICUs.

A: Airway

Proportionally increased oxygen demand and smaller airways make children prone to rapid desaturation (Holm-Knudsen and Rasmussen, 2009). Relatively minor inflammatory responses, or mucous, can obstruct airways, so intubation is likely to be an early priority. Paediatric endotracheal tubes and suction equipment are necessarily smaller than adult ones, making tubes more prone to obstruction by mucous and removal more difficult owing to smaller and more flimsy catheters. Being especially prone to hypoxia, children should always be preoxygenated before suction.

Traditionally, uncuffed tubes were used for younger children (Spitzer and Sims, 2016), cuffed tubes usually being a half-size smaller, and so increasing cricoid oedema and subglottic stenosis. Weiss *et al.* (2009) recommend using cuffed tubes for all children. Initially, oral tubes are usual but, once stabilised, tubes are usually changed to nasal (James and Hanna, 2014), which are more comfortable and less likely to be displaced. Nasal tubes can cause nasal sores, so skin should be inspected regularly.

B: Breathing

Children have little physiological reserve, small respiratory systems and high metabolic rates, making them very susceptible to hypoxia. Oxygen should therefore be given quickly to any hypoxic child. Gasper *et al.* (2016) suggest that normal respiratory rates (breaths/minute) are:

Newborn	30–60
6 months	30–45
1–2 years	25–35
3–6 years	20–30
7–12 years	20–25

These rates will usually be mimicked on ventilator setting. Otherwise, paediatric and adult ventilation are similar, with proportionally smaller volumes. Saturation and arterial blood gas values are similar to those of adults.

C: Circulation

Unless born with congenital abnormalities, children usually have healthy cardiovascular systems, so blood pressure monitoring is often less valuable than with adults. Cardiovascular changes often indicate respiratory dysfunction, such as hypoxia. Normal cardiovascular vital signs are:

Age	Heart rate (bpm)	Systolic BP	Diastolic BP	Mean arterial pressure
Newborn	100–180	60–850	25–24	40–60
Infant	100–160	85–105	55–65	50–90
Toddler	80–110	95–105	55–65	50–100
Preschool	70–110	95–110	55–65	50–100
School age	65–110	95–110	55–70	60–90
Adolescent	60–90	110–130	65–80	65–95

(Cockett, 2010)

Fluid resuscitation, like drugs, should be weight-related; Lampariello *et al.* (2010) define paediatric fluid resuscitation as > 20 ml/kg. If not already established, vascular access will therefore be a priority. Paediatric resuscitation algorithms differ slightly from adult ones, so should be displayed prominently in bed areas where children are nursed. Fluid balance assessment should include any nappies, dressings or other losses.

D: Disability (neurological)

As with adults, Glasgow Coma Scale (GCS) of 8 or below is an indication for intubation (R.C.P.C.H., 2015). Immature vital centres, and other brain functions, make children prone to exaggerated responses, such as fitting (Stokes *et al.*, 2004). Among other causes, fitting may be due to hypoxia, so stabilising vital signs reduces such complications, Neck muscles of young children are weak, and their head is disproportionately large, so children are prone to spinal cord injury. Children are especially susceptible to meningitis (below).

High metabolic rates make children especially susceptible to hypoglycaemia, and critically ill children may not have eaten for some time. Blood glucose should therefore be assessed.

Children are prone to extremes of temperature owing to:

- high metabolic rate;
- proportionally large surface area to body mass compared with adults (more heat lost);
- proportionally more brown fat than adults (insulation).

Children usually become pyrexial owing to infection; antipyretics do not prevent convulsions, so should only be given if the child is distressed (National Collaborating Centre for Women's and Children's Health, 2013).

Analgesics and sedatives used are likely to be similar to those used for adults, with smaller (weight-related) doses. In PICUs, midazolam remains the most frequently used sedative, while fentanyl and morphine remain the most frequently used analgesics (Kudchadkar *et al.*, 2014), although there is con-siderable variance. Traditionally propofol has often been avoided, because of concerns about "propofol syndrome" (metabolic acidosis, lipidaemia, cardiac failure, dysrhythmias, death), although propofol syndrome rarely occurs (Jenkins *et al.*, 2007) – a recent study of 174 children sedated with propofol found that none suffered "propofol syndrome" (Svennson and Lindberg, 2012). Nevertheless, few PICUs use propofol (Kudchadkar *et al.*, 2014). Propofol is only licensed for adult (over 18 years of age) use (B.N.F., 2017). The nature of crisis admis-sion prior to impending retrieval means that relatively deep sedation will be targeted.

If raised intracranial pressure is suspected, the child should be nursed at 20° to optimise cerebral drainage and reduce risk of coning (R.C.P.C.H., 2015).

Parents usually help provide children with comfort and reassurance, but the admission is usually emotionally traumatic for parents (Stremler *et al.*, 2017), and crises surrounding admission often necessitate medical interventions over family involvement. Parents often experience guilt and anger, however illogical both may be. Even more than relatives of adult patients, they need information and emotional support. Parents should have 24-hour access to visit their child (P.I.C.S., 2015a).

E: Exposure

Like all patients, children should be thoroughly examined ("exposed") for any other signs of injury; in children this may include non-accidental injury (see below).

For transfer, children should be "mummy wrapped" in insulating blankets, with woollen hats and gloves. As well as retaining heat, this also protects vascular access and makes them easier to handle during transfer.

Drugs

Unlike most adult doses, paediatric drugs dosages are usually prescribed according to patients' weight or body surface area. Weight will usually have been recorded on admission. If children have not been weighed recently, parents may know or have some health records. If no other source is available, weight can be estimated in children over one year of age by adding four to their age, and doubling the sum:

$$\text{weight} = (\text{age} + 4) \times 2$$

Until one year of age, 10 kg is usually a fair estimate of likely weight. Most units keep paediatric formularies and quick reference guides with paediatric equipment.

Drugs are sometimes given intraosseously, but nurses should only use this route if competent to do so.

Transfer

Early transfer will normally be planned and be managed by retrieval teams. Prior to their arrival, their centres will usually have offered advice. Otherwise, preparation for transfer is similar to adults (see Chapter 47).

Legal aspects

Children have potentially different status in law to adults. Following the *Gillick* case and the 1989 Children Act, concepts of legal "minors" have changed from age-related to competence-related (Dimond, 2015). Actions are often undertaken in patients' "best interests" (see Chapter 48), but this is even more problematic with children than with adults (Birchley *et al.*, 2017). Nurses should clarify what rights children and others do, and do not, have. If in any doubt, advice should be sought from their trust's legal department, or out-of-hours escalated to senior management.

Each year 2–3% of children in the UK are abused, one in every thousand of these resulting in serious injury (Russell and McAuley, 2009). Vague history, or bruising that is not adequately accounted for, may indicate non-accidental injury. Head injury, and especially subdural haemorrhages in infants, are the most common reason for abused children to need intensive care (Russell and McAuley, 2009). Suspected abuse should be reported, but is emotionally, legally and politically contentious, so should be referred to senior staff. Written records and verbal reports should remain factual.

Meningitis

Infection can cause inflammation of the meninges, or subarachnoid space. Viral meningitis is more common and less serious than bacterial meningitis. Bacteria usually responsible for childhood meningitis are:

- *Streptococcus pneumoniae*;
- *Neisseria meningitides*;
- *Haemophilus influenza* type b (Hib).

(McIntyre *et al.*, 2012)

Incidence peaks under one year of age, before immunity matures, with a lesser peak in those aged 15–19 (Wilcox, 2012). Meningitis can progress rapidly, death following within hours of mild non-specific febrile symptoms. Neck stiffness is often the earliest specific symptom. Meningitis can cause long-term health complications, especially hearing loss, so survivors should be followed up by paediatric services. Prompt and appropriate treatment is therefore vital.

Meningitis is usually diagnosed by lumbar puncture – infected cerebrospinal fluid (CSF) contains protein and leukocytes. N.I.C.E. (2010c) lists contraindications to lumbar puncture, especially suspected raised intracranial pressure, as the procedure could cause *tentorial herniation* ("coning"). Treatment is mainly intravenous antibiotics, with aggressive system support. Meningitis usually causes photophobia, so children should be nursed in a dark room.

Meningitis is a notifiable disease (N.I.C.E., 2010c), so all contacts should be traced. Antibiotics are usually given to everyone who had prolonged contact with bacterial meningitis during the previous week.

Implications for practice

- children are rarely admitted to adult ICUs, but when they are, are usually in crisis, awaiting transfer to regional PICUs. An ABCDE approach is useful to stabilise the child prior to transfer;
- respiratory failure is the most common cause for ICU admission;
- primary cardiovascular disease is rare; cardiovascular failure is usually secondary to hypoxia;
- pyrexia is usually a symptom of disease, which should be the focus of treatment; antipyretics should only be given if the child is distressed;
- most units have a trolley with readily accessible paediatric equipment, including:

  - paediatric drug formularies;
  - paediatric resuscitation guidelines;
  - regional PICU protocols;

- staff should familiarise themselves with local paediatric equipment;
- paediatric drug doses are almost always far smaller, usually varying with size/age. Before giving any drugs, nurses should carefully check prescriptions and amounts, seeking further advice if concerned about anything;
- paediatric nurses usually accompany children admitted to adult ICUs, and are a useful resource for any aspects staff are unsure about;
- parents usually suffer guilt and anxiety, so need information and support, and whenever possible should be actively included in the child's care;
- waiting rooms should cater for siblings – toys, small chairs and information booklets;
- if unsure of children's legal status, or concerned about non-accidental injury, seek advice from senior staff;
- meningitis usually begins with non-specific fever-like symptoms, but bacterial meningitis can be rapidly fatal. Neck stiffness is usually the earliest specific symptom;
- meningitis is a notifiable disease; anyone having prolonged contact with bacterial meningitis during the previous week should be given prophylactic antibiotics.

Summary

Paediatric admissions to adult ICUs are rare, but when they occur are usually brief, with the aim of stabilising for transfer. This is challenging and stressful for staff with little or no familiarity of paediatric nursing. Principles of nursing critically ill children are largely similar to nursing adults, with proportionally smaller volumes and sizes. Adult ICU nurses are usually unfamiliar with these sizes, so should carefully check all prescriptions and calculations, seeking advice if they have any concerns.

Parents and siblings usually experience extreme psychological crises, needing information and support. Family should be prepared and involved in care as much as possible.

Further reading

One of the more useful books about children for general ICU nurses is Cockett and Day (2010). Murphy *et al.* (2009) provide useful case studies. There are a number of handbooks, such as Gasper *et al.* (2016), which provide easily accessibly information; many adult ICUs have handbooks and other material for emergency paediatric guidance. N.I.C.E. (2010c) provides guidelines about meningitis.

Regional PICUs often provide open websites which usually include useful general information, and specific guidance for ICUs needing to transfer children. The Paediatric Intensive Care Society also has an informative website, which includes the standards (currently 2015) for paediatric critical care, aspects of which apply to general (adult) ICUs admitting children.

Support groups

Childline: 020 7825 2505;
Meningitis Research Foundation 0808 800 3344 (England; for other countries, check with website);
National Meningitis Trust helpline 0808 801 0388;
NSPCC Child Protection helpline 0808 800 5000;

Clinical scenarios

Annabel White is a healthy 15-year-old who ingested an unknown amount of alcohol at a local nightclub. On admission to the adult ICU, Annabel is conscious but disorientated, with a self-ventilating respiratory rate of 39 breaths per minute, tachycardia (164 beats per minute) with hypotension (80/40 mmHg). Blood investigations reveal metabolic acidosis and hypoglycaemia. Annabel's parents are aware of her admission but not yet present.

Q1. Review local hospital policies on paediatric admissions to ICU. What documentation is needed and who should be informed about Annabel's admission?

Q2. Annabel is non-compliant with interventions, for example oxygen therapy, positioning and assessment. Consider issues regarding her autonomy, legal age of competence and consent. Can Annabel refuse treatment? Who should advocate for Annabel and give consent on her behalf?

Q3. Consider the impact of the ICU environment on Annabel and the impact of her presence on other ICU patients and staff. Outline nursing strategies which may be used to promote compliance and stabilise her condition.

Chapter 14

Older patients in ICU

Contents

Introduction

Like most countries, the UK has an ageing population (Guzman-Castello *et al.*, 2017), so unsurprisingly increasing numbers of older people are admitted to hospitals (C.Q.C., 2012); they are the most acutely ill in hospital (Hayes and Ball, 2012) and form the majority of ICU admissions (Pisani, 2009; Ehlenbach *et al.*, 2010). Healthcare should be provided according to clinical need, regardless of age (D.O.H., 2001; International Council of Nurses, 2006). Yet, limited material appears about older people in specialist literature, making them a potentially neglected majority.

Age is not a disease, and diseases suffered by older people are not unique to their cohorts. Physiological ageing, multiple pathology and polypharmacy often complicate their physical needs, while negative attitudes by society, hospitals and staff may limit access to services or mar their psychological care (D.O.H., 2001). Admission of older people to ICU raises ethical questions:

- should there be age-limits for ICU admission?
- with limited resources, should resources be allocated between different groups?
- should age be a factor in resource allocation?
- is there a need for specialist input from healthcare of older people (HCOOP) teams?
- if only one bed were available but two patients needed ICU admission, how would readers react to that bed being given to the older patient?

Most older people are healthy, but healthy people are not admitted to ICU. This chapter outlines effects physiological ageing can have on major body systems before focusing on wider social and attitudinal issues.

Ageing

Ageing can be:

- chronological (number of years lived);
- sociological (role in society, e.g. retirement);
- physiological (physical function).

de Beauvoir (1970)

Chronological ageing, often over 65, is statistically simple and clear, so adopted by much medical literature, especially quantitative research, and (with qualification) by the D.O.H. (2001), but is usually medically arbitrary, failing to recognise each person's uniqueness and individuality. While used here for convenience, increased life expectancy and (often) increased function (Newton *et al.*, 2015) into later years makes whether 65 is "old" questionable. Nurses should approach each person as an individual, rather than chronological stereotype, making inclusion of age during handover of dubious value.

Ageing almost inevitably brings decline in most physiological functions, although rates of decline vary between systems and individuals. *Reserve function* – the difference between actual level of function and minimum function needed for homeostasis – provides a barrier against disease. Progressive decline in reserve function increases likelihood of chronic and multiple disease in later years, such as diabetes mellitus.

Physiological effects

Hypertension, reduced stroke volume and cardiac output and other chronic *cardiovascular* changes are partly age-related (Vanhoutte, 2002; Richardson *et al.*, 2004), but mainly from acquired damage, especially from smoking (Fogarty and Lingford-Hughes, 2004). Older people may suffer various cardiovascular diseases, including:

■ dysrhythmias, especially atrial fibrillation (see Chapter 22);
■ coronary artery disease;
■ heart valve disease;
■ atherosclerosis;
■ peripheral vascular disease.

Poor perfusion affects all other body systems.

Nearly all aspects of *respiratory* function significantly decline with age (Mick and Ackerman, 2004; Richardson *et al.*, 2004), making acute respiratory failure more likely (Behrendt, 2000).

Central nervous system degeneration progresses throughout life. Neurophysiological changes are complex, but older people are at greater risk from the three Ds:

■ dementia
■ delirium
■ depression.

Incidence of depression is greater in older people in hospital than those in the community (Dennis *et al.*, 2012). Critical illness often precipitates cognitive decline (Ehlenbach *et al.*, 2010), making this group of patients at especially high risk of delirium. Reality orientation can be useful but may provoke aggression (see Chapter 3); alternative approaches, such as validation therapy (Feil, 1993), seek to empower rather than control people. But most approaches rely on verbal responses, limiting their value for intubated, sedated patients. Communication can be problematic with all ICU patients, but acute limitation may be compounded by dysphasia, hearing loss, impaired vision or impaired memory (Happ *et al.*, 2010). Communication needs should therefore be individually assessed – relatives may be a valuable source for information or achieving communication. Happ *et al.* (2010) recommended communication rounds and communication case conferences, using such resources as speech and language therapists.

Kidney function declines with age (Tonelli and Riella, 2014), potentially causing abnormal biochemistry, such as elevated serum creatinine, but like most other critically ill patients acute kidney injury is usually caused by hypovolaemia. Drug clearance is reduced (Richardson *et al.*, 2004), making older people potentially more sensitive to effects of many drugs. Although older people are more likely to have pre-existing problems such as incontinence and prostatic obstruction, these are alleviated by catheterisation.

With advancing age, *skin* becomes thinner, fragile and poorly perfused, making it prone to sheering pressure sores, with wounds that take longer to heal (Richardson *et al.*, 2004). Most pressure sores occur in older people, hence the weighting for age on the Waterlow (1985) and other assessment scales, although these arguably reinforce negative stereotype of (chronological) age. Pressure area aids can reduce incidence of pressure sores, but optimising endogenous factors (nutrition, perfusion) reduces risks. Reduced capillary perfusion may impair cutaneous drug absorption (e.g. GTN/fentanyl patches) and removal of metabolic waste, although whether this is clinically significant is questionable.

Gastrointestinal function declines with age (Eliopoulos, 2013), but the gut's large functional reserve normally sustains adequate function (Firth and Prather, 2002), although gastric emptying may be slower (Richardson *et al.*, 2004).

Liver dysfunction is mainly pathological rather than chronological (Eliopoulos, 2013). Reduced ability to metabolise drugs may necessitate reduced doses and more careful monitoring of plasma drug levels.

Older people are more frequently *malnourished* than younger people (Devlin, 2000) owing to factors such as poverty, poor mobility, maldentition, reduced gut motility, digestive problems, lack of facilities or chronic bowel dysfunction. Malnourishment may delay recovery, weaning and rehabilitation.

As *muscles* and bone atrophy, they are replaced by fat. Fat repels water, one of many factors making older people more prone to dehydration. As calcium metabolism declines, less is absorbed, while stored (skeletal) calcium is leached, reducing bone density, so making bones more brittle and liable to fracture. Muscle weakness contributes to delayed weaning from ventilation and prolongs rehabilitation.

Outcome

Most studies about older ICU patients measure mortality, increasingly to hospital discharge or later. For example, Ford *et al.*'s (2007) study of post-operative octogenarians found that one fifth died in ICU and one third died in hospital, but mortality was higher if vasoactive drugs were needed. Some other studies show more favourable outcomes; for example, Yaran (2012) found that very old ICU patients had fewer acute illnesses and co-morbidities than relatively younger patients, but this may reflect covert ageism: numbers of very old patients admitted to intensive care was lower than numbers of relatively younger patients. Aggarwal *et al.* (2017) suggest older people have similar ICU outcomes to younger patients. Lerolle *et al.* (2010) found that survival had increased among older ICU patients. Thomas *et al.* (2014) found that a significant proportion of over 85s were discharged home. Flaatten *et al.* (2017) suggest that frailty, rather than chronological age, influences survival in the very old (>80), measuring ICU and 30-day mortality as 22.1% and 32.6%, respectively. The diversity of findings probably reflects diversity of practice towards older people. But it also illustrates the relative futility of judging by chronological age rather than physiological condition. Decisions to admit, or ration care, should be based on health needs and benefits rather than years lived (Nates *et al.*, 2016).

If patients do not require ventilation, age has no effect on ICU survival (Farfel *et al.*, 2009). So, outcomes are broadly similar to other groups of patients (see Chapter 50). Underlying physiological function does affect outcome (Boumendil *et al.*, 2004), so physiological rather than chronological age-related criteria for ICU admission may be justified. Morbidity is less often studied, although acute hospitalisation often precipitates cognitive and functional decline (Courtney *et al.*, 2011), and critically ill older people are more likely to develop post-traumatic stress disorder (Wallen *et al.*, 2008) and dementia (Ehlenbach *et al.*, 2010), which raises the challenge of whether, and if so how, morbidity can be reduced.

N.C.E.P.O.D. (2010b) suggests that older people arguably have specialist needs which benefit by input from teams specialising in healthcare of older people (HCOOP), although evidence is drawn from other specialities. Their findings suggest that older people receive good care in ICU, even though anecdotal evidence suggests that HCOOP teams generally have little input into ICU care.

Ageism

"Ageism", the "notion that people cease to be people ... by virtue of having lived a specific number of years" (Comfort, 1977, p35), may be overt (e.g. refusing services to people over a certain age) or covert (e.g. attitudes).

Overt chronological age criteria for critical care admission are now rare (D.O.H. 2001; N.C.E.P.O.D., 2010b) and unacceptable (Preston *et al.*, 2008). Hubbard *et al.* (2003) suggest that people are not denied access to critical care because of age. Although not repeated in later documents, the W.H.O. (2007) response to fears of global influenza pandemic acknowledged the "fair innings" arguments for prioritising services towards younger people, instructing that age-based rationing should only be adopted after widespread public consultation, while O'Brien *et al.* (2009) found that older patients with sepsis were more likely to have ceilings of treatment, even if prognosis was similar to that of younger patients.

Predictive scoring (e.g. APACHE (Knaus *et al.*, 1985)) can create covert ageism – APACHE II scores chronological age to account for physiological ageing, as well as scoring pathophysiologies. APACHE scores of older people are therefore disproportionately increased and do not reflect length of stay or severity of disease (Laskou *et al.*, 2008). N.C.E.P.O.D. (2010b) found low admission rates among older people, which suggests that covert (subjective) criteria may remain, making healthcare for critically ill older adults a lottery.

Older people may have sensory or expressive communication difficulties. While staff should optimise communication, they should beware of insidious prejudice, stereotyping or other negative attitudes, such as speaking loudly to all older people, rather than assessing whether they have any deficit and if so how to compensate for it.

Many older people were born before the National Health Service existed, when society and social values were very different; doctors (and nurses) were presumed to always know best. Their beliefs and values may therefore differ significantly from those of nurses caring for them; different generational values may cause misunderstandings. Nurses should empower choices, which with older people may take more encouragement.

Bereavement, social mobility and physical immobility may leave older people isolated, deprived of social supports (families, friends). Friends/family may treat the older person as a burden. Psychological isolation can become self-fulfilling, encouraging older people to adopt childlike, dependent behaviour and/or appear confused. Stereotypes may be widespread, and insidious in their effect, but nursing care should be individualised to each person (Meyer and Sturdy, 2004). Deeny (2005 p325) suggests that the "care of critically ill older people . . . may cause us to modify physical environments, reflect on professional attitudes, revise education and training and be more collaborative with older people advocacy groups and experts from outside critical care".

Implications for practice

- older patients already form about half of UK ICU admissions; numbers will probably increase, so ICU nurses should actively consider needs and quality of care;
- function of all body systems declines with age, but most older people are healthy. When acute ill health necessitates ICU admission, care should anticipate recovery;
- reduced function, and possible multipathology, necessitates individualised, holistic care;
- confusion should be treated as acute and reversible, until proven otherwise;
- sensory or expressive communication limitations may be acute or chronic, so should be individually assessed, and individualised strategies planned to overcome limitations;
- in-service and post-registration education should include significant focus on nursing older people in ICU;
- ageism, insidious throughout society, can easily, and insidiously, influence care; reflecting on and evaluating nursing care (individually and in groups) helps identify areas for development.

Summary

Definitions of "old" are arbitrary. Chronological ageing is widely used, but arguably a poor indicator of healthcare needs. If old is over 65, many ICU patients are "old" and appear to have similar mortality rates to younger patients. Morbidity, and needs, are less often studied, making older people a potentially neglected majority. Paucity of literature on older patients in ICU makes this one of the most neglected aspects on ICU nursing.

Pathologies experienced by older people are largely those suffered by younger patients. Multiple pathologies, system dysfunction and slower metabolism make physiological needs of older patients complex. ICU admission can also threaten psychological and social health. Nurses can humanise potentially threatening and ageist ICU environments to meet the needs of older patients.

Further reading

de Beauvoir (1970) provides highly readable, challenging sociological perspectives. Medical studies of age-related outcome frequently appear, but otherwise literature on older people in ICU is infrequent. Eliopoulos (2013) is one of the best textbooks about nursing older people. N.C.E.P.O.D. (2010b) reviews ongoing problems of discrimination faced by older people in healthcare. Yaran (2012) is one of the few recent studies focusing on older people in ICU.

Clinical scenarios

Albert Rose is an active and independent 89-year-old who was admitted to the ICU following emergency laparotomy for a perforated bowel. He has an ileostomy and two abdominal drains, from which he has lost two litres of blood within the first four hours. He is mechanically ventilated with an Hb of 76 grams/litre and haematocrit (Hct) of 27%.

Q1. What are the main age-related physiological changes and expected normal values for an 89-year-old in ICU? What are the implications of these changes in managing Mr Rose's treatments?

Q2. What is the significance of Mr Rose's Hb for his recovery? List possible reasons for and against blood transfusion for Mr Rose, and decide whether you think blood should be transfused.

Q3. Remembering possible outcomes for Mr Rose following discharge from hospital, develop a plan to promote his physical and mental recovery.

Chapter 15

Infection prevention and control

Contents

Fundamental knowledge

Standard precautions
Asepsis
Immunity (see Chapter 25)
Common healthcare-associated infections
Local infection control guidelines

Introduction

More than a quarter of patients admitted to ICU have infections, nearly half of which are healthcare-associated (Dhillon and Clark, 2009). Infection can also occur following admission – one quarter of all hospital infections occur in the ICU (Allen, 2005). Infection increases morbidity and mortality. Critical illness causes immunosuppression (Hunter, 2012), making patients more susceptible to opportunistic infection that healthy people, such as staff and visitors, would resist. Preventing and controlling infection has always been challenging, but increasing mutation of organisms into multiresistant strains has created additional problems (Larson *et al.*, 2010; C.D.C., 2013); evolution of extended spectrum beta-lactamase (ESBL), an intracellular enzyme, has enabled cross-resistance between different species of bacteria. Too often, solutions remain elusive.

Microbiology is a huge topic; this chapter summarises problems caused by infection, briefly describes some problem organisms, and suggests key strategies that can help reduce incidence of infection.

Organisms typically take 48 hours to cause infection, so healthcare-associated infection (HCAI) is defined as occurring more than 48 hours after admission, and ventilator-associated pneumonia (VAP) as occurring more than 48 hours after intubation.

Sources

For each human body cell, we carry more than 10 bacterial cells (Maczulak, 2010). Every 40 minutes we shed up to one million dead skin cells (Gould, 2012), which leave skin-surface bacteria in the environment. Closed circuits prevent environmental contaminants accessing patients' internal environments, so should only be broken if essential. Having micro-organisms in and on the body is normal; as long as they do not cause harm, they are colonising the body. But when they cause a pathological response (disease), infection occurs. Destroying commensals (non-harmful organisms) with antibiotics enables opportunist infection from resistant organisms.

Infection can be:

- endogenous or
- exogenous.

Endogenous infection, from organisms already harboured by patients, in ICU usually occurs through the:

- respiratory tract (e.g. ventilator-associated pneumonia)

but can also occur through:

- skin, especially though central venous lines (Loveday *et al.*, 2014)
- the gut (Hall and Horsley, 2007).

Exogenous infection is usually through:

■ contact (staff, procedures, equipment)

but can also be:

■ airborne.

Exogenous cross-infection causes up to one third of HCAIs, at least half of which are preventable (Harbath *et al.*, 2003).

Organisms

Bacteria remain the most common cause of infections, so form the focus of organisms discussed in this chapter. Significant viral and fungal infections in ICU are increasingly common, so fungi are mentioned. Viruses are not discussed here but are in other chapters (see index for specific organisms). Other types of organisms, such as prions (the cause of Creutzfeldt–Jakob disease), are seldom significant in ICU, so are not discussed in this book.

Bacteria are classified as gram "positive" or "negative" (Pitt, 2007), depending on response to laboratory staining. Gram-positive bacteria generally reside on skin, in air or the environment, whereas gram-negative bacteria generally originate from the bowels, soil or water (Pitt, 2007). Gram-positive organisms include:

■ *Staphylococci*
■ *Clostridium*
■ *Enterococci*
■ *Streptococci*
■ *Tuberculosis bacillus.*

Gram-negative organisms include:

■ *Acinetobacter*
■ *Enterobacter*
■ *Escherichia coli*
■ *Helicobacter pylori*
■ *Klebsiellae*
■ *Proteus*
■ *Pseudomonas*
■ *Serratia.*

Gram-negative organisms have thinner cell membranes, so produce endotoxins for protection. Endotoxin stimulates inflammatory responses. There are many strains of each species, resistance often varying between different strains, and so recommended antibiotics may differ.

Bacteria

Most strains of *Staphylococci aureus* remain meticillin-sensitive (*MSSa*), but *meticillin-resistant Staphylococcus aureus* (*MRSa*) has become problematic. Between one third and half the population are colonised with *S. aureus* (Lim and Webb, 2005), creating a large reservoir for potential infection. Although *MRSa* may be acquired in ICU, transmission from either staff or the environment is unlikely (Price *et al.*, 2017).

Whether patients with *MRSa* should be isolated remains controversial (Cepeda *et al.*, 2005; Garvey and Belligan, 2009); current guidelines suggest isolation should be considered, depending on facilities and risk (Coia *et al.*, 2006). Together with *pseudomonas*, *Staphylococcus aureus* remains the main cause of ventilator-associated pneumonia (Rello *et al.*, 2014).

Pseudomonas is one of the commonest causes of ventilator-associated pneumonia (Caserta *et al.*, 2012; McCarthy, 2015; Dasgupta *et al.*, 2015; Fernández-Barat *et al.*, 2017). It especially colonises moist environments, such as washbasins (Cholley *et al.*, 2008), and is a common cause of pneumonia, bloodstream infections, urinary tract infections, and surgical site infections (C.D.C., 2013). Resistance among pseudomonads is increasing (Tumbarello *et al.*, 2013; Fernández-Barat *et al.*, 2017).

Enterococci are normal gut flora, but the third most common cause of healthcare-associated infection (Gould, 2008), especially urinary tract infections (Heintz *et al.*, 2010). *Enterococci* are hardy organisms, surviving more than one week in the environment (Zirakzadeh and Patel, 2006). *Glycopeptide-resistant Enterococci* (*GRE* – still often called by its former name of *Vancomycin-Resistant Enterococci* – *VRE*) usually inhabit the gut but may colonise other parts of the body. Although pathogenicity is relatively low, it is resistant to most antibiotics and can transfer resistance to *MRSa*, so co-infection is fairly common (Zirakzadeh and Patel, 2006), making it a major threat to already critically ill patients. VRE infections are usually managed by barrier nursing, although barrier nursing does not appear to reduce transmission rates (Huskins *et al.*, 2011). Once identified, screening is pursued through weekly rectal/stoma swabs.

Clostridium difficile infection is the most common cause of both diarrhoea (Freedberg *et al.*, 2016) and infections (Magill *et al.*, 2014) in hospitals, especially among older people (Freedberg *et al.*, 2016). First identified in 1935, the organism remained relatively unproblematic until 2001, when the 027 strain mutated (Pépin *et al.*, 2005; Kelly and LaMont, 2008). *C. difficile* is resistant to most broad-spectrum antibiotics, infection typically occurring as opportunistic infection when other gut flora are destroyed by antibiotics (Shannon-Lowe *et al.*, 2010; Sourial *et al.*, 2014).

Infection typically causes explosive diarrhoea, spreading spores into the environment, where they can survive for months (Freedberg *et al.*, 2016). Alcohol handrubs are ineffective (Wren, 2009).

Acinentobacter is normally found in water and soil, but *Acinitobacter baumannii* (*Acb*) is a common skin-surface organism (Grice and Segre, 2011).

Infection is usually from multiresistant strains (Munoz-Price and Weinstein, 2008).

Tuberculosis bacilli (TB), once thought largely a disease of the past in Western countries, has made a resurgence in recent decades, although this decade UK incidence has started to decrease (Public Health England, 2016a). It primarily occurs in large urban areas (Public Health England, 2016a), especially in association with HIV (Lawn and Zumla, 2011; W.H.O., 2014a). TB has always been a challenging organism to treat, necessitating prolonged courses of antibiotics, but recent emergence of drug-resistant strains (Dheda *et al.*, 2014) creates additional problems.

Carbapenem-resistant enterobacteriaceae (CRE, alias *New Delhi Metallo Beta-Lactamase – NDM-1*, sometimes called carbapenemase-producing *entero-bacteriacae – CPE*), the most recent "super-threat", is increasingly prevalent (C.D.C., 2013; W.H.O., 2014b), especially in ICUs (Dautzenberg *et al.*, 2015). As carbapenems, such as meropenem, are the "last resort" antibiotic (W.H.O., 2014b), treating CRE is difficult. Most trusts therefore screen on admission, asking questions about travel.

Fungi

Fungal infection and mortality among critically ill patients are rising (Paiva *et al.*, 2016). The most common fungal infection in ICU is from *Candida*. Although *Candida albicans* remains the most prominent species, both *Candida glabrata* and *Candida parapsilosis* cause significant incidences of infection in ICUs (Paiva *et al.*, 2016). Traditionally, fluconazole, and other azoles, have been the main antifungal treating, but resistant *Candida* species are increasingly problematic (C.D.C., 2013). ICU patients are especially susceptible to oral and skinfold fungal colonisation/infection, which can be sources for bloodstream infections (C.D.C., 2013; W.H.O., 2014b), so these areas should be inspected carefully, and maintaining hygiene contributes to reducing infection. Oral *Candida*, often diagnosed by a white coating of the tongue, is usually susceptible to nystatin.

Ventilator-associated pneumonia

Ventilator-associated pneumonia (VAP) is the most common HCAI in ICU, occurring in up to one quarter of patients (Blot *et al.*, 2011) and increasing mortality risk by 14% (Sedwick *et al.*, 2012). Hunter (2012) suggests the most common sources are micro-aspiration of oropharyngeal secretions and microbial biofilm on endotracheal tubes, although improved technology, such as silver-coating of tubes, make applicability of older research and statistics questionable. VAP mortality is estimated at 9% (Hunter, 2012). Reducing VAP risks is problematic, but many interventions identified elsewhere in this chapter can contribute to reducing incidence. Drakulovic *et al.*'s (1999) classic 1998 study recommended nursing patients at 45°, to reduce aspiration and VAP, but, as this has proved largely unachievable, most units aim for angles of 30° (Hellyer *et al.*, 2016).

Laboratory screening

Nurses collect most specimens sent for microscopy, culture and sensitivity (MC+S). Records of when specimens were sent should be kept – a pathology flow sheet – is useful. Each shift, nurses should review what has been sent, request any outstanding results, and alert medical staff to any concerns.

Preliminary reports from blood cultures may be available after 24 hours, as some organisms can be visually identified after this time. Confirmed, detailed reports are normally available after 48 hours, with sensitivity (recommended antibiotic) usually following 72 hours. Debate persists about indications for blood cultures, many units taking cultures if patients' temperatures exceed an identified limit – often 38–38.3°C. Such figures reflect greater likelihood of infective rather than metabolic pyrexia (see Chapter 8) but are not always reliable.

With increasing global antibiotic resistance (NHS England, 2016), antibiotic governance/stewardship encourages restricting use, and therefore microbial exposure, to where they will be effective. The biomarker procalcitonin indicates whether antibiotic therapy is effective (de Jong et al., 2016; Schuetz and Müeller, 2016), enabling earlier discontinuation of ineffective therapy.

Controlling infection

Unfortunately, compliance with infection control measures remains suboptimal (Gammon et al., 2008). *Antibiotics* generally remain the best way of treating existing infections, although prevention is better than cure. Appropriate antibiotics should be prescribed by medical staff, usually with advice from microbiology. Duration of treatment with antibiotics should be identified and clearly recorded, usually on drug charts. Nurses should inform medical staff if prescriptions are due for review. Some antibiotics have narrow therapeutic ranges (e.g. gentamycin, vancomycin), necessitating blood tests to check serum levels; staff should check local protocols, and clarify the appropriate time before and/or after antibiotic dose. Increasingly, some antibiotics, such as vancomycin, are being administered through continuous infusion to achieve more effective therapy (Bassetti et al., 2016).

Invasive cannulae cause one third of healthcare-associated infections, with central lines remaining the single main cause of nosocomial septicaemia (Loveday et al., 2014). Vascular access and other invasive devices are necessary with sicker patients, but unneeded devices should be removed. Routine replacement of both peripheral and central lines is no longer recommended (Loveday et al., 2014). Infection risks increase when dressings or lines are changed, so unless there is a specific contraindication, clean and intact line dressings should remain in place for seven days (Loveday et al., 2014), and administration sets used for 96 hours (Loveday et al., 2014). Insertion dates of all invasive equipment should be clearly recorded.

Moving *equipment* between patients can spread infection. Where dedicated equipment is not practical (e.g. portable X-ray, 12-lead ECG), it should be cleaned after use (Loveday et al., 2014).

Airborne bacteria may be transmitted through:

- dust
- skin scales
- droplets.

Airborne infection is significantly reduced by use of in-line suction catheters (see Chapter 5). Other ways to reduce airborne infection on ICU include:

- planning higher-risk procedures at times of least disturbance;
- careful disposal of linen (e.g. bringing linen skips/bags to bedsides, carefully rolling linen inwards to trap skin scales);
- airflow systems.

Hand hygiene remains the simplest, easiest, cheapest and most important way to reduce transient colonisation (Loveday *et al.*, 2014). Healthcare-associated infections are mainly transmitted by hand, yet compliance with recommendations is usually low (Allegranzi *et al.*, 2013). Hand hygiene should be performed before each patient care episode (Loveday *et al.*, 2014), which the World Health Organization (W.H.O., 2005) summarised as the five moments for hand hygiene:

1. before touching a patient;
2. before clean/aseptic procedure;
3. after body fluid exposure risk;
4. after touching a patient;
5. after touching patient surroundings.

Alcohol rubs should be used for decontaminating hands, except where:

- hands are visibly soiled;
- hands are potentially contaminated with body fluids;
- when caring for patients with vomiting or diarrhoea.

(Loveday *et al.*, 2014)

The third exclusion is because some organisms, such as *C. difficile* and *Norovirus*, may survive alcohol rubs. Sufficient amounts should be dispensed (this varies between products), spread fully over hands, and allowed to dry. Local infection control departments can advise amount and time for products used.

Hand hygiene should cover all areas of the hand, including thumbs, fingertips and backs of hands. Hands should be dried thoroughly after washing as moisture, including wet alcohol, facilitates bacterial growth. Patients and relatives have been encouraged to challenge staff about hand hygiene (N.P.S.A., 2004a); staff have a professional duty to challenge anyone about to touch patients without performing adequate hand hygiene. Anyone (staff or family) visiting any patient on ICU should clean their hands before entering the unit. Alcohol rubs should be placed by each entrance to the unit, with prominent signs informing people to prevent infection by cleaning their hands.

Personal protective equipment (PPE – aprons, gloves) reduce colonisation/infection from patients to staff. Aprons also reduce transmission of bacteria from clothing, so should be worn by anyone having patient contact. Colour-coded aprons for each bed-space encourages staff to change aprons when moving between patients. Gloves significantly reduce cross-infection (Loveday *et al.*, 2014), so should be worn whenever manipulating invasive devices, preparing intravenous drugs, or nasogastric/jejunal feeds, drugs or fluids.

Documentation helps identify when actions are required. Useful documentation includes charts for:

■ equipment changes
■ specimens sent and results.

Inadequate staffing (quantity and skill mix) increases cross-infection (Knoll *et al.*, 2010; Aiken *et al.*, 2016).

Pneumonia in ICU patients usually originates from nasal, oropharyngeal or gastric flora (Torres *et al.*, 2009). *Selective oral/digestive decontamination* (SOD/SDD) can prevent pathogen colonisation, and so can VAP (Price *et al.*, 2014). Concerns that SDD/SOD may increase bacterial resistance (Oostdijk *et al.*, 2010) are unfounded (Daneman *et al.*, 2013), but it is not commonly practised in the UK (Hunter, 2012; Sertaridou *et al.*, 2015), remains under-researched (Daneman *et al.*, 2013), and might be consigned to a similar fate as chlorhexidine mouthwashes.

Implications for practice

■ ICUs often provide high-tech and expensive treatments for patients, but too often microbes can undermine efforts, increasing mortality and morbidity;

■ infection prevention and control are important in all clinical areas, but the physiological vulnerability of critical illness places ICU patients at especially high risk of, and from, infection;

■ hand hygiene should be carried out before and after each aspect of care, and before approaching and after leaving each bed area;

■ alcohol handrubs should be available at each bed area, and be used before and after any patient contact. Staff should know how much to use, and how long it takes to dry;

■ some infections, such as *C. difficile* and *Norovirus*, are resistant to most alcohol handrubs (although, depending on products available, some suitable handrubs might be supplied by the infection prevention and control team), necessitating handwashing; with these infections, remove handrubs from the bed area to remind staff to use soap and water;

- nursing/medical documentation should include easily accessible flow sheets of specimens sent, and results. Each entry should be dated and signed;
- equipment (e.g. heat moisture exchangers) should be changed according to manufacturer's instructions; catheter mounts should be changed at the same time as humidifiers. Generally, respiratory equipment should be changed at least daily;
- maintaining closed circuits, and minimising disconnection, reduces opportunities for environmental organisms to colonise/infect patients;
- invasive techniques and disconnection of intravenous lines should, when possible, avoid times of dust disturbance (e.g. floor cleaning, damp dusting);
- strict asepsis must be observed when breaking/bypassing normal non-specific immune defences, such as when handling intravenous circuit, treating open wounds, or procedures involving the trachea, stomach or jejunum;
- colour coding bed areas (aprons, equipment) discourages inappropriate movement between bed-spaces.

Summary

We do not live in a sterile world, and our bodies are not sterile. Preventing infection is not always possible, but infections incur high mortality and morbidity. While antimicrobial agents may be able to treat infections, prevention is humanly (and financially) preferable.

Hand hygiene remains the most important way to prevent infection. Hygiene is helped by adequate and appropriate facilities, including accessible alcohol handrubs, aprons and unit guidelines/protocols. All multidisciplinary team members should be actively involved in making decisions, nurses having an especially valuable role in co-ordinating and controlling each patient's environment, and challenging anyone who exposes their patient to unreasonable risk of infection.

Further reading

Much has been written about infection prevention and control, which makes many articles date quickly. As well as specialist journals, such as the *Journal of Hospital Infections*, most journals frequently publish articles on the topic. Loveday *et al.* (2014) is the national guideline for infection control, while the Department of Health, NHS England, NHS Scotland and other national bodies provide UK guidance. C.D.C. publications (e.g. 2013) provide American perspectives, while the W.H.O. provide international reports and guidelines (e.g. 2014b), many of which apply or are transferable to the UK. Weston (2013) provides nursing perspectives. Staff should be familiar with local policies.

Clinical scenarios

Nadeen Persad, a 32-year-old with chronic kidney disease, was successfully resuscitated following cardiopulmonary arrest. She is admitted to ICU for monitoring. An ICU doctor and Outreach nurse (who is four months pregnant) go with appropriate transfer equipment to retrieve the patient while an ICU bed is prepared for the admission. On arrival to ward, the ICU doctor and nurse are informed that Nadeen has active pulmonary *Tuberculosis* and *Acinetobacter* in her diarrhoea.

Q1. Consider the common transmission modes and pathogenicity of *Tuberculosis* and *Acinetobacter*. Specify the infection control precautions to be followed in order to minimise potential cross-transmission of the micro-organisms to other patients and staff when transferring and admitting Nadeen to the ICU.

Q2. In addition to the prepared bed area, the ICU has two protective isolation rooms available where airflow in one room is under positive pressure and the other room is under negative pressure. Which side room is more appropriate for Nadeen, and why?

Q3. Management of Nadeen's infections focused on three main areas:

- containment (e.g. screening of staff and visitors);
- prevention of cross-transmission (exogenous – to other patients; endogenous – to other sites within Nadeen);
- eradication (antibiotics).

Design an evidence-based nursing care plan for Nadeen while on ICU. Include a holistic nursing approach, integrating professional, psychosocial, psychological and physical aspects.

Chapter 16

Pandemic planning

Contents

Fundamental knowledge

Community-acquired infections and their transmission
Pathology of pneumonia
Source isolation precautions

Introduction

Throughout history there have been epidemics, many causing high mortality. These epidemics have almost invariably been caused by viruses, usually influenza, which have mutated often from other species to become highly contagious and pathogenic. Over half the known human pathogens have originated in other species (Stein, 2009). Recent epidemics have prompted historical analysis, suggesting semi-predictable patterns. Epidemics/pandemics were anticipated during the first decade of this century, for which extensive preparations were made. Arguably, preparations have so far exceeded effects of the disease, at least in the UK, creating dangers of complacency towards future outbreaks. Influenza pandemic remains the top risk in the UK Cabinet Office National Risk Register of Civil Emergencies (2016) (NHS England, 2016). This chapter reviews the historical evidence, what has been learned from recent preparations and outbreaks, and suggests likely implications for future practice.

Twentieth-century pandemics

Since the sixteenth century there have been an average of three pandemics each century, at intervals of 10–40 years (Saidi and Brett, 2009). Records and evidence from the twentieth century are considerably larger than from previous centuries. The worst pandemic of the twentieth century was "Spanish 'flu" (H1N1), which began in 1918, killing about 50 million people, 3% of the world's population (Morens *et al.*, 2010). Although populations were vulnerable owing to generally poorer health, debilitation in the aftermath of the First World War, and lack of knowledge about the virus, the virus seems to have been an especially lethal strain – emerging from birds into humans and swine simultaneously (Zimmer and Burke, 2009). Infections persisted for years, with often devastating long-term effects, such as the encephalitis lethargica of 1917–1923 described by Sacks (1990). Survival was highest among socially isolated populations (Stein, 2009), although mortality among doctors and nurses treating influenza victims was also surprisingly low (Shanks *et al.*, 2011). Partly owing to the extent, and partly because of survivor, evidence and records being available once microbiological research could seek answers, this outbreak has become the benchmark against which modern pandemics are assessed (Saidi and Brett, 2009).

Further influenza pandemics occurred in 1957 (H2N2; "Asian 'flu") and 1968 (H3N3 "Hong Kong"), each killing about one million people. Like the 1918 outbreak, mortality was highest among young adults aged 15–34 (Saidi and Brett, 2009). Both outbreaks brought a second wave, the one from the 1968 virus occurring 16 months after the first UK cases (D.O.H., 2009b). As the last major pandemic was in 1968, another pandemic is overdue.

This century, most outbreaks have occurred in East Asia, mutating from animal viruses (Wen and Klen, 2013), but outbreaks have occurred else-where, often resulting from international travel by carriers. Avian viruses do not replicate efficiently in humans, but swine ones do (Stein, 2009). Severity inevitably varies between viruses, although H1N1 outbreaks in both 2001 and 2009 might have become more devastating with less knowledge and preparedness.

Influenza

Influenza A develops new strains every two to three years (Saidi and Brett, 2009). Most infections cause mild respiratory disease, although each year people do die from influenza, usually among the more vulnerable groups, such as older people (Public Health England, 2017). Influenza vaccinations for vulnerable groups, and healthcare workers, are now standard practice. All medicines, including vaccinations, have risks, making some people reluctant to receive vaccination. For example, there were (unsubstantiated) claims that H1N1 vaccines caused Guillain-Barré Syndrome (Nachamkin *et al.*, 2008). Influenza vaccines no longer contain live viruses but are suspended in egg; current guidelines (Greenhawt *et al.*, 2018) suggest that people with egg allergies can safely receive vaccines.

Incubation times vary for viruses but, based on previous experiences, W.H.O. (2017) presumes one to three days is likely, followed by a 0.5- to two-day latent period. Preventing spread and tracing contacts will therefore be difficult (W.H.O., 2017).

Some immunity develops following exposure, but whether it is lasting is questionable. Pandemics have appeared approximately one generation apart, infection being highest in children (Miller *et al.*, 2010) and younger adults, possibly because they lack immunity from exposure during previous pandemics (Chowell *et al.*, 2009; Miller *et al.*, 2010). Unlike most ICU patients, victims are therefore:

- young and
- suffering single or dual organ failure (lungs, often complicated by cardio-vascular),

although kidney injury often occurred, more than one fifth of patients needing renal replacement therapy (Brauser, 2010). With the 2009 outbreak, most deaths occurred in people with pre-existing chronic disease (Fajardo-Dolci *et al.*, 2010), although acute kidney injury increased both length of stay and mortality (Brauser, 2010). The 2003 outbreaks caused infections and deaths among healthcare workers, in many cases probably from occupational exposure (Manocha *et al.*, 2003; Lapinsky and Granton, 2004). The 2008 epidemic caused no secondary infections among healthcare workers in Mexico (Perez-Padilla *et al.*, 2009).

Rationing

Recent outbreaks have caused severe respiratory failure and ARDS, mainly in young adults and children (Perez-Padilla *et al.*, 2009). Pandemic influenza is likely to cause overwhelming need for invasive ventilation, exceeding availability of ICU and PICU beds. Utility ethics, "saving most lives" (W.H.O., 2017), is likely to guide local, national and international practice. Contingency planning for recent threatened pandemics included:

- creating beds for invasive ventilation in areas such as operating theatres;
- using staff from other wards/departments, who have transferable skills.

Although contingency planning should enable some increase in resources, it is unlikely to prove sufficient (Saidi and Brett, 2009; Sprung *et al.*, 2010), making rationing of resources inevitable. Non-emergency operations and other treatments are likely to be suspended. If demand continues to exceed supply, triaging admissions to exclude those:

- too well;
- too sick to benefit; or
- with co-morbidities likely to limit short-term survival

is almost inevitable (Bailey *et al.*, 2008), which will raise ethical questions of who should be denied resources (W.H.O., 2017). National, professional and local guidance is likely to be issued, but these inevitably deal with generalisations and cannot always solve specific dilemmas faced by nurses "at the bedside".

While contingency planning is laudable, creating temporary "ICUs" will almost inevitably mean less than ideal environments. Staff drafted from elsewhere are likely to feel stressed/frustrated. New ways of working may be necessary; for example, experienced ICU nurses may have to oversee relatively large numbers of patients, prescribing care for staff with transferable skills who are not experienced or confident in ICU nursing. Similarly, medical staff and professions allied to medicine may be drafted in, and face similar stressors. Coupled with risks of occupational exposure to a potentially fatal and highly virulent virus, staff may be sick or opt not to work. Rankin's (2006) survey of the 2003 Toronto outbreak found:

- two of the 44 victims were nurses exposed through their work;
- at least 79 nurses missed 15 days or more owing to sickness;
- nurses worked long hours, sometimes 14.5 hours a day;
- nurses became "social lepers";
- the worst aspect for nurses was fear of the unknown.

In Taiwan in 2003, nearly three quarters of the nursing workforce felt that their job put them at risk, although only a minority wanted to leave their jobs (Shiao *et al.*, 2007); UK cultural differences might draw different responses – Saidi and Brett (2009) estimate that up to half of staff may be absent.

Problems will be compounded by reduction of normal sources of supply. Both inside and beyond hospitals, workforces will be depleted. What this will affect most is unpredictable, but shortages of drugs, oxygen, equipment, linen or transport could occur, necessitating further local rationing, potentially encouraging less than ideal practices. Social isolation improves survival from epidemics (Stein, 2009), so curfews and restrictions on mobility may be imposed. A pandemic is therefore likely to prove difficult, for many reasons, but adequate contingency planning can reduce some of the stresses and burdens.

Some experience of implementing disaster planning has been gained through major terrorist attacks, such as 9/11 (2001, New York) and 7/7 (2005, London), but these attacks were of limited duration, affecting finite numbers of victims in small geographical areas. When pandemics surface, initial and secondary waves are expected, but duration and effects remain largely speculative.

Treating victims

Austerity necessitates prioritisation, so adopting an ABCD approach to assessment, treatment and care is helpful.

Airway. Respiratory failure usually necessitates intubation and invasive ventilation. While such airway management is familiar to ICU nurses, many victims are likely to be young children. Need will probably exceed PICU resources, so adult ICUs are likely to care for significant numbers. Nurses and other staff in adult ICUs usually have very limited experience of caring for children (see Chapter 13). During recent pandemics, many deaths (30–90%) have occurred from bacterial co-infections (Mina and Klugman, 2014).

Breathing. Conventional artificial ventilation is likely to be needed. Modes will probably largely follow those familiar to the unit staff, although Liu *et al.* (2010) recommends lung recruitment manoeuvres (low TV and high PEEP with breaks e.g. ARPV). Liu *et al.* (2010) also suggest inhaled nitric oxide (vasodilator) and inhaled aerolised prostacyclin, Non-invasive ventilation is unlikely to be effective. Aerolised viruses place staff and visitors at risk, so closed circuits should be maintained as far as possible, with filters to minimise risks. Aggressive weaning and transfer to lower-dependency areas should be possible after a very few days.

Cardiovascular. Shock commonly complicates severe respiratory failure from influenza, and myocarditis may occur. Steroids should be avoided, as they may cause shedding of virus particles. Experience from the 2009 outbreak suggests that fluid resuscitation is seldom needed.

Disability. Severe disease usually necessitates sedation, and occasionally paralysis. Drugs used are unlikely to differ from standard practice, remembering that paediatric doses of nearly all drugs are smaller than adult ones, and usually weight-related. Glucose supplements and early enteral feeding are likely to be beneficial.

Prevention

Virulence of epidemic influenza will necessitate precautions to minimise risks to staff and family. Although specific precautions are likely to be suggested for each threatened epidemic, other patients, staff and visitors should be protected by source isolation, including isolation rooms, preferably with negative pressure, and personal protective equipment. Current guidance is provided by Public Health England (2017), but guidance is likely to be updated and replaced frequently, especially should outbreaks occur – employers are likely to disseminate updates during pandemics.

Implications for practice

- historical evidence suggests pandemic influenza is overdue;
- pandemic influenza is likely to affect much of the population;
- disease is likely to cause life-threatening respiratory failure in large numbers of young adults and children;
- shortage of beds, staff, equipment and other supplies may necessitate rationing and triage that staff may find ethically uncomfortable;
- social pressures outside hospitals are likely to impact on health services;
- pandemic planning aims to minimise avoidable mortality and morbidity;
- risk of transmission to staff is high, so infection control and occupational health departments should be involved to provide advice and monitoring.

Summary

Despite extensive research particularly during the twenty-first century, much clearly remains unknown and unpredictable about influenza pandemics. Mild outbreaks of influenza are an annual occurrence. The influenza virus frequently mutates, making prediction of strains, and therefore vaccination, problematic. In the twentieth century, pandemics generally occurred once per generation, the last major pandemic occurring in 1968. A pandemic within the next few years therefore seems likely. In 2003 and 2009, outbreaks occurred which failed to become the threatened pandemic. These, and historical analysis, have provided some experience of likely problems and solutions, but have also encouraged some public scepticism and complacency. A full pandemic is likely to overwhelm healthcare resources, necessitating rationing, triage and uncomfortable ethical choices. Planning aims to limit the impact of the looming disaster.

All trusts have disaster plans, but on the rare occasions these have been needed they have generally been used for brief occurrences. Pandemics persist, without certainty of their geographical or chronological limitations. Pandemic planning has become part of healthcare, in the hope that when the next major outbreak occurs mortality and morbidity can be minimalised.

Further reading

A flurry or reports and analyses has followed recent outbreaks. At the time of writing, the last significant outbreak was 2009, making evidence dated. Zimmer and Burke (2009) provide a historical review, but guidelines are likely to change with each threatened pandemic, so the most appropriate reading will be currently available evidence. Readers should check websites such as:

- Department of Health and the national public health bodies;
- the World Health Organization;
- professional organisations such as the N.M.C. and G.M.C.;
- bodies such as the R.C.N. and B.M.A.;
- local trust intranet.

Sprung *et al.* (2010) provide ICU-specific guidelines for epidemic or mass disaster, although many aspects may be outdated when another outbreak occurs.

Clinical questions

Q1. Find out and read the current contingency plans for your trust and ICU.

Q2. Identify what resources, including equipment, are available in your unit to cope with pandemic influenza.

Q3. List at least six significant effects that activation of these plans would be likely to have on your own current daily work.

Part III

Monitoring

Chapter 17

Respiratory monitoring

Contents

Fundamental knowledge

Respiratory anatomy and physiology
Normal mechanics of breathing – muscles, negative pressure
Haemoglobin carriage of oxygen (see Chapter 18)
Cough reflex and physiology

Introduction

There are many ways to assess and monitor breathing. As with all patients, respiratory rate and depth remain important, but artificial ventilation necessitates additional monitoring. This chapter includes:

■ auscultation
■ ventilator observations, including waveform analysis.

Assessments primarily used by other professions, such as chest X-rays and bronchoscopy, are not discussed. As with all observations, trends should be assessed, and interpreted holistically, in the context of individual patients.

Visual

Respiratory history is usually gained from individual handover and interdisciplinary notes – medical, nursing, physiotherapy. Additional valuable fundamental information can be gained visually:

■ skin colour and texture (and any clamminess) indicates perfusion – especially lips and tongue;
■ finger clubbing or "nicotine stains" on fingers, indicating smokers; abnormal chest shape ("barrel", "pigeon") indicate chronic respiratory disease;
■ for self-ventilating patients, accessory muscle use and intercostal recession indicate respiratory distress;
■ shallow breathing may reflect reduced demand, but with tachypnoea indicates other problems – possibilities include pain or limited airflow;
■ unequal chest wall movement – causes should be investigated, but could include pneumothorax.

Other signs of respiratory problems include:

■ inability to complete sentences without pausing for breath;
■ sudden confusion – more often caused by hypoxia than nonrespiratory factors;
■ cyanosis – a late sign, appearing only with desaturation < 85–90%, and not appearing with severe anaemia (< 30–50 grams/litre (Lumb 2017)).

Sputum should be observed for:

■ volume
■ colour (see Table 17.1)
■ consistency (e.g. frothy, tenacious, watery)
■ purulence
■ haemoptysis.

Type and amounts of sputum, and frequency of suctioning, should be recorded.

Table 17.1 Sputum colour – possible causes

Colour	Possible cause
Black	Tar (cigarette smoking) Old blood Coal (in ex-miners) Smoke inhalation (rescued from fires) Saliva staining (e.g. iron therapy)
Pink	Fresh blood (frothy pink sputum often indicates pulmonary oedema)
Cream, green	Infection (green = probable *pseudomonas*)
Rusty	Probable pneumoccal pneumonia
Yellow	Infection Allergy (e.g. asthma)

Tactile

Movement of sputum in larger airways can create vibration on the chest wall, which may be felt by placing a flat hand palm-down across the sternum ("fremitus", "tactile crepitations"). Although not as reliable as auscultation, this can quickly identify need for, or effectiveness of, suction.

Auscultation

Breath sounds are created by air turbulence, and are useful to assess:

- intubation (bilateral air entry);
- bronchial patency/bronchospasm;
- secretions;
- effect of suction (before and after).

Breath sounds should be assessed at the start of each shift. Most stethoscopes have two sides: the *bell* (useful for focused sounds, like the heart) and the larger diaphragm (useful for more diffuse sounds, such as lungs). Stethoscopes are usually best placed over:

- right and left main bronchi, then
- mid lobe (usually just to the side of the nipple), then
- bases of lungs (front, side or back),

comparing sounds from both lungs (see Figure 17.1). All sounds are created in bronchioles, but transmitted, and dulled, through lower airways. Chest (and abdominal) sounds can be deceptive, so should not be absolutely relied upon.

Sounds may be normal, abnormal, diminished or absent. Abnormal sounds may be heard on inspiration, expiration, or on both phases, so, having identified abnormal sounds, nurses should listen to further breaths to identify on which

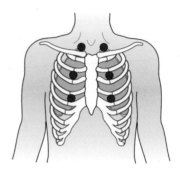

Figure 17.1 Auscultation sites for breath sounds (anterior chest wall)

phases sounds occur. Names of sounds vary between texts, but normal sounds are often called:

- bronchial: high-pitched, loud, air blowing through a tube (the trachea);
- bronchovesicular: medium pitch, heard at lung apices;
- vesicular: low pitch and volume, like rustling wind, heard in most parts of lungs.

Abnormal sounds include:

- stridor: monophonic inspiratory wheezes from severe laryngeal or tracheal obstruction;
- wheeze (rhonchi): obstruction of lower airways;
- crackle (rales, crepitations): on inspiration only, this indicates atelectasis, usually from a problem outside alveoli; if present on both inspiration and expiration, this usually indicates sputum;
- pleural rub: grating sound caused by friction between inflamed pleural surfaces from pleural disease (e.g. pneumonia, pleurisy).

Absent sound may indicate absent airflow:

- obstruction (sputum plug);
- atelectasis;
- pneumothorax/pleural effusion;
- emphysema;
- or lack of transmission to the chest wall (e.g. obesity, small tidal volume).

Artefactual sounds include:

- heartbeat;
- gut movement;
- clothing;

■ friction of stethoscope against equipment (e.g. cotsides);
■ chest hair (crackles).

Interpreting breath sounds is a skill. Listening to healthy lungs (your own) is an essential baseline. Readers unfamiliar with listening to abnormal breath sounds should ask a respiratory physiotherapist or other expert to auscultate with them. Recordings of breath sounds (see further reading) are also valuable.

Waveform analysis

Each breath has three active phases:

■ inspiration
■ inspiratory hold (or "pause" or "plateau")
■ expiration.

See Figure 17.2.
A fourth phase is passive:

■ expiratory hold.

Inspiration affects, and is affected by, bronchial muscle stretch, so patients with chronic obstructive pulmonary disease cannot fully dilate bronchi during short inspiratory time. Most gas exchange occurs during plateau (peak inflation pressure). Expiration is passive recoil; short expiration time of muscle spasm (asthma) causes gas trapping (and distress).
Most ventilators can display three waveforms:

■ pressure
■ flow
■ volume,

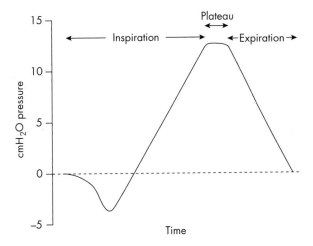

■ *Figure 17.2 Breath waveform*

157

all plotted against time. From these, two loops are usually available:

- pressure/volume
- flow/volume.

Waveform indicates effectiveness of modes and settings (Branson, 2005). Although each option is described separately below, similar information is often transferable between displays. Most discussion below is given for the pressure/volume loop, which in the author's view is the most immediately valuable of all.

Pressure (Figure 17.3) graphs indicate compliance. The slope should be linear. Increased slope near the end of inspiration indicates reduced compliance (hyperinflation). If the slope reduces during inspiration, compliance is increasing, indicating lung recruitment (Macnaughton, 2006). High pressure can cause barotrauma (see Chapter 4), so settings usually aim to maximise volume while minimising pressure. Ventilators include pressure limits and alarms, but pressure graphs provide detailed visual information about pressure.

Flow (Figure 17.4) graphs are useful for assessing triggered (patient-initiated) breaths. Triggering is shown below the baseline and should be followed by rising inspiratory flow (above the baseline). Triggers without inspiratory flow indicate wasted work of breathing, so sensitivity should be reduced. Expiratory flow normally returns below the baseline; if it fails to return to the baseline, gas trapping (auto-PEEP; bronchospasm) is occurring.

Reducing settings (respiratory rate, tidal volume, pressure support) reduces flow. Flow may also be improved (smaller waveform) by bronchodilators.

Volume graphs (Figure 17.5) are possibly the least useful waveform, as tidal and minute volumes are measured elsewhere on ventilators, but loss of volume indicates air leaks.

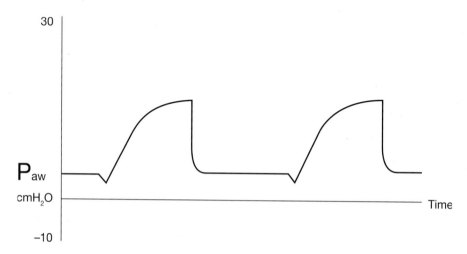

Figure 17.3 Pressure waveform

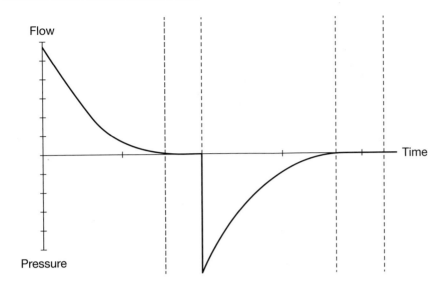

Figure 17.4 Flow waveform

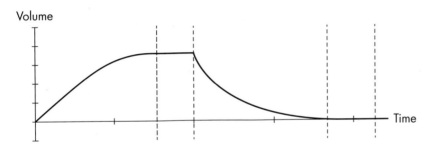

Figure 17.5 Volume waveform

Pressure/volume (Figure 17.6) loops indicate compliance, and are probably the most valuable visualisation of ventilation. At the start of inspiration, alveolar (and so lung) compliance is poor, causing significant increase in pressure with little increase in volume. After a critical point, alveoli inflate easily, causing volume to rise significantly, with little further increase in pressure. A reversed picture on expiration gives normal pressure/volume loops a rhomboid shape. Although pressure and volume measured are throughout the lung fields, it may be helpful to think of the loop display as a single alveolus. Abnormal shapes include:

■ jagged ("sawtooth") lines on inflation and deflation indicate fluid (Sole *et al.*, 2015; Paratz and Ntoumenopoulos, 2014), usually mucus; if water humidifiers are used, water in tubing can cause the same effect;

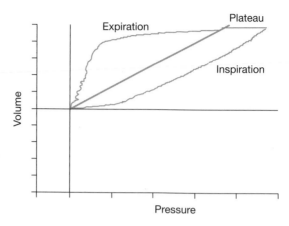

Figure 17.6 Pressure/volume loop

- "beaking" (extending far to the right at the end of inspiration) indicates over-distension, usually resolved by reducing pressures (e.g. PEEP, pressure support, tidal volume);
- wide loops indicate excessive ventilation, usually resolved by reducing tidal/minute volume;
- flattening (increased tilting to the right) indicates worsening compliance (Pipbeam, 2006), while increasing tilts to the left indicate improving compliance;
- incomplete loops indicate either air leaks or gas trapping – the flow waveform should be checked to confirm there is a problem.

Changing settings to adjust the shape (width) of the loop can maximise volume while minimising peak pressure. In pressure-driven modes, this loop may not show abnormalities as ventilation will be reduced to maintain preset pressures.

Flow/volume (Figure 17.7) indicate air trapping (auto-PEEP) and air leaks (Pipbeam, 2006):

- bronchoconstriction/dilatation (changes in flow);
- loss of volume if expiratory wave fails to return to the start of inspiration on the horizontal axis (= leak);
- loss of flow if expiratory wave fails to return to the start of inspiration on the vertical axis (= gas trapping);
- sawtooth (jagged) lines indicate fluid (usually mucus) (Sole *et al.*, 2015).

Manufacturers' booklets often provide usefully illustrated guides to what is available, and readers not familiar with observing waveforms should set up a ventilator circuit with a test lung, viewing various modes and manipulating the test lung to mimic coughs, a triggered breath and resistance.

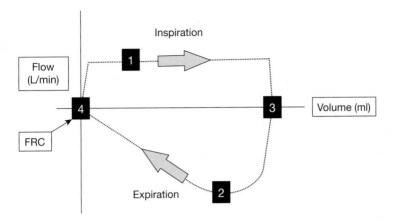

Figure 17.7 Flow/volume loop

Indexed measurements

Attempts to rationalise and weaning have encouraged quantification of respiratory function, usually indexed to patient size. Two examples are oxygen index (OI):

$$= \frac{FiO_2 \times MAP \times 100}{PaO_2}$$

and rapid shallow breathing index (RSBi):

$$= \frac{\text{respiratory rate } (f)}{\text{tidal volume } (V_t) \text{ in litres}} .$$

Advocates claim that oxygen index above 26 or RSBi below 100 indicates likely successful weaning, but reliability of either measurement remains unclear; Monaco *et al.* (2010) suggest that RSBi is not clinically useful to predict weaning. Trachsel *et al.*'s (2005) paediatric study found that oxygen index predicted outcome.

Pulse oximetry

Pulse oximetry is non-invasive and continuous, so is a useful means to monitor oxygenation. Most authors suggest saturation measured by oximeters is within 2% of measurement using arterial blood gas (Jubran, 2015), although Nitzan *et al.* (2014) suggest a 3–4% error range. Oximetry measures saturation of haemoglobin – the oxygen stored in the haemoglobin "bank".

Limitations of oximetry include:

- *Poor perfusion.* Pulse oximetry calculates saturation by measuring light absorption through a finger or other tissue. Only 2% of total light absorption is by blood, so poor blood flow causes unreliable signals ("noisy signal"). Most oximeters in ICU show capillary pulse waveforms (*plethysmograph* or "pleth"), which should reflect arterial pulses. Poor waveforms indicate insufficient signal (blood supply), probably making low readings spurious. Repositioning probes, or warming peripheries, may improve accuracy. Some oximeters display a perfusion index or bar graph, indicating blood flow sensed by the probe.
- *Anaemia.* Oximetry measures percentage saturation of haemoglobin, not quantity of haemoglobin, or oxygen, available. Saturation should be interpreted in relation to haemoglobin levels.
- *Dark colours* either on the skin/nail surface or in blood (e.g. bilirubinaemia) absorb more red light, causing potential under-readings. In the past, significant under-readings have been measured with darker nail varnishes – Coté et al. (1988) measured 10% differences. Perhaps owing to technological advances, more recent studies measure non-significant differences (Rodden et al., 2007; Hinkelbein and Genzwuerker, 2008; Sharma et al., 2015), There is probably no advantage to removing nail varnish for pulse oximetry.
- *Oxygen dissociation.* Pulse oximetry measures the saturation of haemoglobin by oxygen, not the partial pressure is plasma (PaO_2 measured by ABGs), which will determine oxygen delivery to cells (see Chapter 18)

Capnography

Capnography (end-tidal carbon dioxide; $etCO_2$) enables continuous non-invasive breath-by-breath monitoring of expired concentrations and should be used on all intubated ventilated patients (I.C.S., 2011a; Checketts et al., 2015). End-tidal carbon dioxide usually differs slightly from arterial blood gas measurement; often the difference is less than 1 kPa but it can vary considerably between patients, especially with V/Q mismatch (e.g. COPD, ARDS). End-tidal CO_2 remains reasonably consistent within individual patients, so displayed figures provide a useful trend rather than an absolute (actual) level – if end-tidal values change, they reflect similar changes in arterial levels. Differences are increased with dead space, so attachments should be placed as close to the endotracheal tube as possible.

As well as measuring end-tidal carbon dioxide and respiratory rate, capnogram waveforms may indicate problems. Normal flow creates a slightly rising plateau, but airway obstruction creates "shark's fin" waveforms (see Figure 17.8).

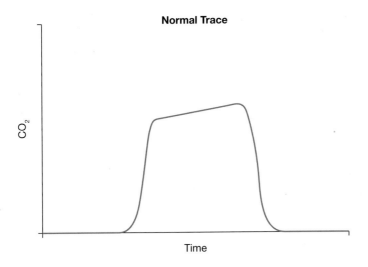

Normal Trace

CO$_2$

Time

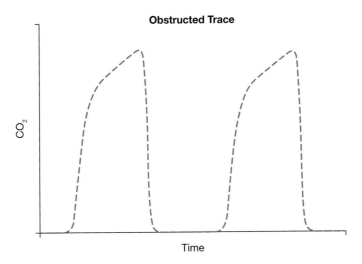

Obstructed Trace

CO$_2$

Time

Figure 17.8 Capnograms

Implications for practice

■ information should be interpreted holistically – in the context of other relevant observations, underlying disease, and treatments;

■ ICU nurses should undertake and document visual, tactile and auscultatory respiratory assessment on all patients;

■ pulse oximetry provides a continuous guide of oxygenation, but is limited by the amount of haemoglobin to carry oxygen and factors that affect oxyhaemoglobin dissociation;

- capnography provides a useful trend of carbon dioxide removal and should be used with all invasive ventilators;
- ventilator waveform display indicates airway response to ventilation, enabling optimal adjustment of settings; pressure/volume loops indicate compliance, so are usually the most useful single display.

Summary

Respiratory monitoring is fundamental to intensive care. Much can be assessed noninvasively, by listening and looking. Ventilators provide much information, especially through waveforms display. Readers should take early opportunities to become familiar with available means of respiratory monitoring on their units. Whatever means is used, observations can only be as reliable as those making and interpreting the observations. ICU nurses therefore should understand the physiology and mechanics of lung function and pathophysiology. Respiratory monitoring is therefore fundamental to care underlying many of the pathologies discussed in the third section of this book.

Further reading

Most texts describe widely used methods of monitoring. Classic texts include Lumb's (2017) respiratory physiology. For staff wishing to develop skills of X-ray interpretation, Corne and Kumaran (2016) is a useful resource. Lung sounds are easiest to understand if heard, with accompanying description; websites include:

www.easyauscultation.com/lung-sounds.
www.practicalclinicalskills.com/lung-sounds.
www.practicalclinicalskills.com/breath-sounds-reference-guide.

Acknowledgement

The section on waveform analysis is based largely on a workshop by Jane Roe and Rosie Maundrill presented at the B.A.C.C.N. 2008 National Conference.

Clinical scenarios

Kathleen Fogarty is a 58-year-old lady who was admitted to ICU for mechanical ventilation to support deteriorating respiratory function. The cause of her recent deterioration is unknown, but possible diagnoses include bronchospasm, basal pneumonia, and aspiration of upper airway secretions.

Kathleen has a visible and widespread drug-related erythematous rash, worse at extremities, and extensive oral ulcerations. Kathleen's sputum is thick, mucopurulent, yellow-green and copious. On auscultation, she has expiratory phase and late expiratory wheeze, vesicular breath sounds are diminished in apices, and crackles in right base. Kathleen's E_TCO_2 is 6.5 kPa and SpO_2: 94%.

Q1. Identify and interpret Kathleen's abnormal lung sounds; explain their relevance to other results and her recent deterioration.

Q2. What additional investigations or monitoring would help assess Kathleen's respiratory function? Include rationales for your choice.

Q3. How would you describe the means used in Q1 and Q2 to a student nurse with whom you are working?

Chapter 18

Gas carriage

Contents

Fundamental knowledge

Pulmonary anatomy and physiology (including vasculature)
Normal respiration (including chemical + neurological
   control and mechanics of external respiration)
Dead space
Haemoglobin – anatomy and physiology (erythropoietin,
   erythropoiesis, oxygen binding)
Types of anaemias

Introduction

Textbooks such as this necessarily focus on one aspect at a time (reductionism). But body systems function as parts of the whole body, not in isolation. Cardiovascular and respiratory functions are particularly closely interdependent: delivering oxygen and nutrients to tissues, while removing carbon dioxide and other waste. Respiration should achieve adequate tissue oxygenation, so gas movement across lung membranes forms *external respiration*, while gas movement between tissue cells and capillaries forms *internal respiration*.

This chapter focuses mainly on internal respiration, identifying factors that affect tissue perfusion and oxygenation. The structure of haemoglobin and its effect on oxygen carriage and the oxygen saturation curve are identified. Carbon dioxide carriage is also discussed. Aspects of arterial blood gas results are mentioned but developed more fully in the next chapter.

Pressure of gases

Gas transfers across semipermeable membranes (capillaries) from areas of greater to lesser pressure (concentration). Partial pressure of arterial oxygen (PaO_2) therefore indicates oxygen available for diffusion into cells.

Air is approximately 21% oxygen and 79% nitrogen, with negligible amounts of other gases – only 0.04% is carbon dioxide. Representing the whole of inspired air as 1, the faction of inspired oxygen (FiO_2) in air is 0.21. The common practice of recording FiO_2 as 21 for patients not receiving supplementary oxygen is technically incorrect – an FiO_2 of 21 is 2100% oxygen.

Barometric, and so alveolar, pressure at sea level is 101.3 kPa. Total atmospheric pressure includes water vapour. Pressure of water vapour is variable, but at sea level and 37°C ("normal" body temperature) in the UK is about 6.3 kPa. This leaves approximately 95 kPa for all gases. The partial pressure of oxygen in (warm) air is therefore 21% of 95 kPa (=19.95 kPa), Table 18.1 outlines typical gas pressures in airways.

Before reaching alveoli, inhaled air is diluted with "dead space" air – air remaining in airways from the last breath out. "Dead space" air is relatively carbon dioxide-rich and oxygen-poor, further diluting the partial pressure of oxygen reaching the alveoli. As long as oxygen tensions (partial pressure) are

Table 18.1 Typical partial pressures of gases at sea level (approximate)

	Concentration in air (%)	Pressure in air (kPa)	Pressure in (healthy) alveoli (kPa)
water vapour		variable	6.3
oxygen	21	21.27 in dry air	13.3
carbon dioxide	0.03	0.03 in dry air	5.3
nitrogen	79	80 in dry air	76.4

higher in alveoli than pulmonary capillaries, oxygen diffuses into blood. Similarly, higher carbon dioxide tensions in pulmonary capillaries than alveoli enable transfer into alveoli.

Physiological adult dead space is about 150 ml, with additional pathological dead space when alveoli are not perfused. Artificial ventilation dead space begins at the inspiratory limb ("Y" connector) of ventilator tubing, hence the practice of cutting endotracheal tubes. As physiological dead space remains constant, breath size affects partial pressure of oxygen reaching alveoli.

Oxygen carriage

Oxygen is carried by blood in two ways:

- plasma (1.5–3%)
- haemoglobin (97–98.5%).

Oxygen is not very soluble, so at normal (sea-level) atmospheric pressure 3 ml of oxygen dissolves in every litre of blood (Lumb, 2017), insufficient to maintain life. Haemoglobin solves this problem: its high affinity for oxygen helps it collect and transport the vast majority of oxygen in our blood. The small amount of dissolved oxygen exerts the partial pressure in blood (PO_2), which can diffuse into cells. Maintaining partial pressure of oxygen therefore in part depends on adequate dissociation of oxygen from haemoglobin.

Tissue oxygen supply is therefore affected by:

- haemoglobin level (Hb);
- oxygen saturation of haemoglobin (SO_2);
- oxygen dissociation from haemoglobin;
- partial pressure of oxygen in blood (PO_2);
- perfusion (blood) pressure.

Perfusion pressure is discussed in other chapters.

Haemoglobin

Erythrocytes are mainly haemoglobin. With average diameters of 7 micrometres (μm), erythrocytes are slightly larger than most capillaries (5–6 micrometres), necessitating them to deform (Patel and Burnard, 2009). The poor solubility of oxygen is thus overcome by placing haemoglobin, and oxygen, close to capillary walls.

Physiological normal levels for haemoglobin (Hb) are 130–180 grams/litre (male) and 110–150 (female). Haemoglobin largely determines viscosity of blood. Less viscous blood flows more easily through small vessels (capillaries), so optimum oxygen delivery to cells is a paradoxical balance between:

■ high haemoglobin (more viscous blood) carries more oxygen;
■ low haemoglobin (less viscous blood) flows more easily through capillaries.

Survival from critical illness is highest when haemoglobin is 70–90 grams/litre (Hébert *et al.*, 1999), although specific groups, such as older people, may benefit from higher levels (Norfolk, 2013), possibly 80–100 grams/litre.

SaO_2-SvO_2

While haemoglobin transports oxygen efficiently, its high affinity for oxygen limits dissociation: only 20–25% of available oxygen normally unloads, making normal venous saturations (SvO_2) 70–80% (Nitzan *et al.*, 2014). The SaO_2–SvO_2 difference therefore indicates tissue uptake (consumption) of oxygen, with low SvO_2 indicating tissue hypoxia (Wagstaff, 2014) from:

■ increased demand (Nebout and Pirracchio, 2012); or
■ reduced supply, e.g. from low cardiac index (Perner *et al.*, 2010), anaemia (Nebout and Pirracchio, 2012),

so consider increasing:

■ supply (FiO_2)
■ carriage (Hb).

Small differences indicate low uptake, which may be from:

■ low demand
■ low delivery (e.g. poor perfusion, oedema).

Oxygen dissociates readily if haemoglobin is fully or highly saturated, but lower saturations reduce dissociation. This variable relationship between SaO_2 and PaO_2 is shown in the S-shaped oxyhaemoglobin dissociation curve (see Figure 18.1).

Factors that can change ("shift") oxyhaemoglobin dissociation include:

■ temperature
■ pH
■ 2,3 DPG levels
■ some haemoglobinopathies (e.g. foetal haemoglobin – see below).

Shifts to the left reduce, while shifts to the right increase, dissociation (see Table 18.2). If dissociation is reduced, saturation (SaO_2) may remain high, despite low partial pressures (PaO_2), potentially dangerous when relying just on pulse oximetry.

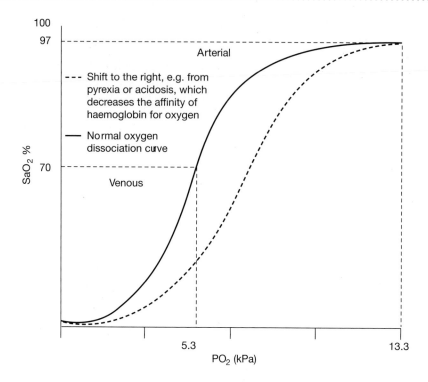

Figure 18.1 Oxygen dissociation curve

Table 18.2 Some factors affecting oxygen dissociation

curve shifts to right (increased oxygen dissociation from haemoglobin) with
    increased temperature
    acidosis (pH) – the Böhr effect
    increased 2,3 DPG (diphosphoglycerate)
    increased CO_2

curve shifts to left (decreased oxygen dissociation from haemoglobin) with
    reduced temperature
    alkalosis
    (some) haemoglobinopathies (e.g. HbF)
    decreased 2,3 DPG (diphosphoglycerate)
    carbon monoxide
    decreased CO_2

Pyrexia and acidosis increase oxygen demand, but by shifting the curve to the right also increase oxygen supply at tissue level. 2,3 DPG (2,3-diphosphoglycerate), a chemical in erythrocytes which aids oxygen dissociation from haemoglobin. If Hb is below 60 grams/litre, levels are increased (Lumb, 2017), which improves oxygen supply when carriage is reduced.

V/Q ratio

V/Q ratio is the relationship between the volumes of air (ventilation – V) and blood (perfusion – Q) reaching lungs. An average healthy 70 kg adult at rest typically breathes four litres of air each minute and has a cardiac output of five litres, making normal V/Q ratio 4:5, which can also be expressed as a percentage (80%) or decimal fraction (0.8).

Radiography (V/Q scans; CTPA) uses contrast to visualise perfusion to lungs. V/Q mismatches occur with:

- "shunting", where blood perfuses unventilated alveoli, and so does not exchange gases;
- unventilated alveoli which remain perfused – e.g. mucus plugs or atelectasis if perfusion remains, typically because of inflammation causing vasodilation ("pathological dead space").

The A-a gradient and P/F ratio, both measured with arterial blood gases (provided oxygen delivered to the patient is entered), indicate shunting (see Chapter 19).

Cell respiration

The purpose of breathing is:

- to supply tissue cells with sufficient oxygen to enable aerobic metabolism in mitochondria;
- to remove carbon dioxide, a metabolic waste product.

Measuring mitochondrial respiration is not practical, so cruder parameters (e.g. arterial gas tensions) are measured instead. However, measured parameters only partly indicate delivery of oxygen to cells and removal of carbon dioxide.

Partial pressures of oxygen progressively fall with further stages of internal respiration: normal capillary pressure of oxygen at 6.8 kPa gives tissue pressure of 2.7 kPa, and mitochondrial pressure of 0.13–1.3 kPa. Conversely, intracellular carbon dioxide tensions are higher. These pressure gradients create *internal respiration*.

Oxygen debt

In hypoxic conditions, oxygen and glycogen are withdrawn from haemoglobin and myoglobin (muscles), creating a "debt" that is normally repaid once high oxygen demand ceases. So, after completing strenuous exercise we continue to breathe deeply. Anaerobic metabolism produces lactic acid.

Prolonged critical illness can cause cumulative oxygen debt, which, with recovery, flushes toxic acids and cytokines into the circulation, causing potential reperfusion injury (see Chapter 24).

Oxygen toxicity

Metabolism of oxygen releases a few oxygen radicals – highly reactive and unstable atoms than can cause tissue damage. In health, the body has many antioxidant chemicals to protect it. But, in ill health, antioxidant defences are often depleted, while oxygen radical release is often increased, especially with hyperoxia (Knight *et al.*, 2011; Ward *et al.*, 2011), so prolonged exposure to high concentrations of oxygen can damage lung tissue. There have also been concerns that high-concentration oxygen also "washes out" nitrogen from lungs – nitrogen being an inert gas, and the majority (79%) of air, may help prevent atelectasis; increasing oxygen concentration would therefore reduce nitrogen, potentially causing atelectasis. Although identified in some literature, evidence to support concerns about "nitrogen washout" is very weak.

Although precise concentrations and times are disputed, prolonged use of high-concentration can cause oxygen toxicity, causing lung damage. Amount and duration for oxygen toxicity is unclear but Kallet and Matthay (2013) suggest that "prolonged" use of more than 50% is toxic.

Traditionally, although with little evidence, toxicity is presumed to occur with FiO_2 over 0.6 for more than 24 hours. Severe critical illness may necessitate risking oxygen toxicity to preserve cell (and so the patient's) life.

Carbon dioxide transport

Air contains virtually no carbon dioxide (0.04%). Metabolism typically produces 200 ml of carbon dioxide every minute. Carbon dioxide diffuses by concentration gradients from cells into capillary blood, and from pulmonary capillaries into alveoli. In most people, breathing is normally primarily in response to the hypercapnic drive, aiming to keep $PaCO_2$ at 5.3 kPa (Bourke and Burns, 2015). Carbon dioxide is also vasoactive, stimulating vasodilation.

Carbon dioxide carriage is relatively simple compared with oxygen carriage. It is carried in blood in three ways:

- plasma (normally about 10%);
- haemoglobin (normally about 20%);
- bicarbonate (normally about 70%).

Plasma. Carbon dioxide is approximately 20 times more soluble than oxygen, so is readily carried in solution by plasma.

Haemoglobin. Carbon dioxide is carried as carbaminoglobin. Carbon dioxide binds to globin, not haem, so (unlike carbon monoxide) does not displace oxygen.

Bicarbonate. Most carbon dioxide carriage is in plasma bicarbonate (H + CO_2 + O).

Some blood gas analysers measure total carbon dioxide carried (tCO_2), as a proportion of either volume (%/vol) or quantity (mmol/litre).

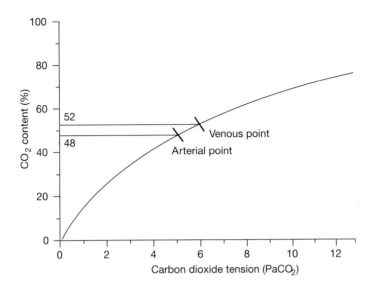

Figure 18.2 Carbon dioxide dissociation curve

Diffusion of carbon dioxide occurs through simple tension gradients, making the carbon dioxide dissociation curve virtually linear (see Figure 18.2). Like the oxygen dissociation curve, carbon dioxide dissociation can move to the right or left. Rightward shifts (lowering carbon dioxide content per unit of pCO_2) occur with raised oxygen concentrations in blood – the "Haldane effect".

Hypercapnia vasodilates, improving cardiac output and tissue perfusion (Geijer *et al.*, 2016), typically causing a flushing appearance to facial skin.

Haemoglobinopathies

Critical illness may be complicated by haemoglobinopathies. Sickle cell disease and thalassaemia, two of the more common haemoglobinopathies, are discussed in Woodrow (2016). Two rare haemoglobinopathies are outlined here. Carbon monoxide is included in the next chapter.

Methaemoglobin (MetHb) is caused by the iron in haemoglobin oxidising, changing it from a ferrous to ferric state, which reduces oxygen carriage. A few drugs can cause methaemoglobin, including nitric oxide (NO), a gas occasionally used to dilate pulmonary capillaries and so improve oxygenation. MetHb is measured by many blood gas analysers.

Foetal haemoglobin (HbF) has a higher affinity for oxygen than normal adult haemoglobin (HbA), so reducing tissue oxygenation. Conversion to adult haemoglobin normally occurs around six months of age (Robson *et al.*, 2014), but foetal haemoglobin can (abnormally) persist throughout life.

Implications for practice

- oxygen is vital for life, so adequate oxygen delivery to cells, as well as adequate oxygen carriage by haemoglobin, should be achieved;
- oxygen dissociation from haemoglobin is affected by various factors (see Table 18.2), including pH and temperature;
- PaO_2 measures plasma oxygen, whereas SaO_2 measures oxyhaemoglobin. Relationship between SaO_2 and PaO_2 is variable, so high saturations do not guarantee tissue oxygenation;
- prolonged high-concentration oxygen ($FiO_2 > 0.5$ for > 24 hours) can cause toxic lung damage, so should be avoided if possible.

Summary

Oxygen is primarily carried by haemoglobin (SO_2), but partial pressure in plasma (PO_2) creates the pressure gradient for transfer to tissues. Complex, changeable relationships between SO_2 and PO_2 are shown by the oxygen dissociation curve, which may be "shifted" to the right or left by various factors. Most oxygen is carried by haemoglobin, but, as haemoglobin also affects viscosity of blood, high haemoglobin creates the paradox of increasing oxygen carriage but reducing delivery. Carbon dioxide is carried in various ways, most often in the form of serum bicarbonate.

Further reading

Most physiology texts contain useful chapters on gas carriage, Lumb (2017) being especially useful. The British Thoracic Society (B.T.S., 2017) acute oxygen therapy guidelines are useful, even though specifically excluding applicability to ICU.

Clinical scenarios

Nina Walker is 36 years old and was admitted to the ICU with a head injury and fractured spine at C5 from falling down stairs. The first blood gas taken was from a central vein while Nina was self-ventilating via a face mask with FiO_2 0.6, in supine position wearing a hard collar. The second blood gas is arterial, taken 12 hours after intubation, with mechanical ventilation using spontaneous mode and FiO_2 0.25. Nina's respiratory rate is 16 bpm, her Hb is 98 grams/litre and core temperature at 12 hours is 35.7°C. Both gases are temperature-corrected.

Blood gas and electrolyte values on admission to ICU 12 hours later are:

	Central venous blood FiO$_2$ 0.6	Arterial blood FiO$_2$ 0.25
Temperature	35.9°C	35.7°C
pH	7.27	7.51
PaO$_2$ (kPa)	3.30	13.36
PaCO$_2$ (kPa)	6.84	3.80
HCO$_3$ (mmol/litre)	21.1	25.3
BE (mmol/litre)	-2.5	+0.3
Lactate (mmol/litre)	3.3	1.9
SO$_2$ (%)	48.5	97.9

Q1. How is the oxygen dissociation curve (Figure 18.1) affecting Nina's PO$_2$ with the arterial gas? What factors have altered the position of the dissociation curve? Repeat this using the carbon dioxide dissociation curve (Figure 18.2).

Q2. What other factors will influence Nina's oxygen and carbon dioxide exchange at alveolar and cellular (tissue) levels?

Q3. What other assessments can be used by nurses to monitor effectiveness of oxygen transport to Nina's tissues – e.g. visual observation, laboratory investigations, oximetry?

Chapter 19

Blood gas interpretation

Contents

Fundamental knowledge

Cell metabolism (oxygen consumption, ATP production, carbon dioxide production)

Introduction

Arterial blood gas analysis provides valuable information about acid–base balance and respiratory and metabolic function. Analysers also provide additional useful information about various metabolites and electrolytes. Therefore, arterial blood gas sampling and analysis is a core skill for ICU staff. Analysers and many "normal ranges" vary between units, so using sample printouts from your unit may be helpful. The UK measures gases in kilopascals (kPa) – the SI unit. The USA uses mmHg: 1 kPa is 7.5 mmHg. A similar, more ward-focused, version of this chapter is included in Woodrow (2016).

Acid/base definitions

Acids can release hydrogen ions; bases (alkali) can accept (buffer) hydrogen ions. Strong acids (e.g. hydrochloric) release many free hydrogen ions, whereas weak acids (e.g. carbonic) release few. Acid/base balance is the power of hydrogen ions (pH) measured in moles per litre ("power" in the mathematical sense). The power of hydrogen ions can be controlled (balanced) either through *buffering* or exchange. Hydrogen (H^+), a positively charged ion (cation), can be buffered by a negatively charged ion (anion), such as bicarbonate (HCO_3^-).

pH measurement

Chemically, the pH scale ranges from 0–14, making pH 7 chemically neutral. Normal arterial pH range is 7.35–7.45, making blood (in pure chemistry terms) slightly alkaline. Blood pH < 7.35 is acidotic, while pH > 7.45 is alkalotic. If arterial acid–base balance is ideal (pH 7.4), each litre of blood contains 0.00004 millimole (or 40 nanomoles, nmol) of hydrogen. Keeping this wide range of hydrogen ions that substances can release or accept within a scale of 0–14 is achieved using a negative logarithm. Unfortunately, few people think logarithmically.

A logarithm expresses numbers as a (mathematical) power:

- $10^1 = 10$,
- $10^2 = 10 \times 10 = 100$,
- $10^3 = 100 \times 10 = 1000$,
- $10^4 = 1000 \times 10 = 10,000$,

each addition to the power (log) causes a tenfold increase to the actual number. Bacteria and blood cells, being very numerous, are usually measured using the log of 10. Negative logarithms similarly represent very small divisions by subtraction from the log:

- $10^0 = 1$;
- $10^{-1} = 0.1$;
- $10^{-2} = 0.01$.

Changing pH by one represents a tenfold (logarithmic) change in hydrogen ion concentration (acidity), while changing pH by 0.3 doubles or halves concentrations:

- pH 7.7 = 20 nmol/litre H^+
- pH 7.4 = 40 nmol/litre H^+
- pH 7.1 = 80 nmol/litre H^+
- pH 6.8 = 160 nmol/litre H^+

Cell metabolism produces acids, so hydrogen moves from intracellular to extracellular fluid through concentration gradients, intracellular (where hydrogen is produced) concentrations being highest (normal intracellular pH is 7.0 (Marieb and Hoehn, 2016)). Interstitial and venous pH has traditionally been viewed as 7.35 (Marieb and Hoehn, 2016), although some recent evidence (Byrne *et al.*, 2014; McKeever *et al.*, 2016) suggests that differences between arterial and venous pH are no more than 0.03.

Transient derangement may be survivable, but sustained blood pH outside 6.8–7.8 is incompatible with life (Hennessey and Japp, 2016), pH below 6.8 usually leads to coma and death, while pH over 7.8 overstimulates the nervous system, causing convulsions and respiratory arrest.

Blood acid–base balance is the sum of:

- respiratory and
- metabolic (renal function, liver function, chemical buffers)

balance, so causes of deranged pH must be sought from other results.

Respiratory balance

Carbon dioxide dissolves in water to form carbonic acid:

$$CO_2 + H_2O \leftrightarrow H_2CO_3,$$

a weak (pH 6.4), unstable acid, the main acid in blood. Being unstable, carbonic acid usually dissociates back into water and carbon dioxide. Haemostasis of carbon dioxide is normally maintained by adapting removal through ventilation (rate and depth of breathing). As carbon dioxide forms the main acid in blood, it is considered a *potential* acid (lacking hydrogen ions, it is not actually an acid, but it can help create an acid), so:

- *respiratory acidosis* is failure to remove sufficient carbon dioxide (i.e. high $PaCO_2$);
- *respiratory alkalosis* is excessive removal of carbon dioxide (i.e. low $PaCO_2$).

Hypercapnia stimulates respiratory centres to increase ventilation (rate and depth), removing more carbon dioxide. So, although respiration cannot remove

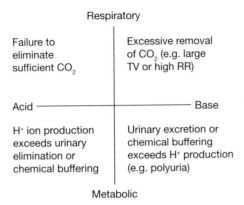

Respiratory

Failure to eliminate sufficient CO_2 | Excessive removal of CO_2 (e.g. large TV or high RR)

Acid ———————————————— Base

H^+ ion production exceeds urinary elimination or chemical buffering | Urinary excretion or chemical buffering exceeds H^+ production (e.g. polyuria)

Metabolic

■ Figure 19.1 Origin of acid/base imbalance

hydrogen ions, it can inhibit carbonic acid formation, restoring homeostasis. Respiratory acidosis is caused by hypoventilation. Respiratory alkalosis is caused by hyperventilation.

In health, respiratory response to acidosis is rapid: doubling or halving alveolar ventilation can alter pH 0.2, returning life-threatening pH of 7.0 to 7.2 or 7.3 in three to 12 minutes (Hall, 2016).

Metabolic balance

Metabolic balance is more complex. Acids are:

■ ingested (e.g. wine, many IVIs – see Chapter 33)
■ produced (metabolism)

removed through the

■ kidneys

and buffered by:

■ chemicals.

Bases (e.g. bicarbonate) are:

■ produced
■ reabsorbed (renally)
■ ingested/infused (e.g. antacids).

Hydrogen (H^+) ions, an essential component of any acid, are removal by the kidney or buffered by bases. Acidosis therefore occurs if:

■ hydrogen production exceeds removal (excessive production; kidney injury);
■ buffer production is insufficient (especially, liver failure).

Metabolic acidosis may also be caused by:

■ tissue acids (lactic or keto acids) or
■ hyperchoraemia.

Ketones are produced from fat metabolism, fat being used for metabolism if glucose is not available. Lactate is released with anaerobic metabolism, usually from perfusion failure. Ketones and lactate both form acids. Hyperchloraemia increases dissociation of hydrogen ions from body water to form hydrochloric acid. Hyperchloraemic acidosis is usually caused by excessive saline infusion (Shaw *et al.*, 2014; Zhou *et al.*, 2014).

Metabolic alkalosis is usually caused by excessive removal/buffering of hydrogen (H^+) ions or excessive production/absorption of bases due to:

■ polyuria;
■ hypokalaemia (causing excess H^+ in urine);
■ gastric acid loss (e.g. excessive nasogastric drainage, vomiting);
■ excessive buffers (e.g. increased production, colonic reabsorption from constipation).

With acute illness acidosis is usually the problem. Any alkalosis is usually compensatory, and if compensatory should not be treated.

Renal control

Other than insignificant transdermal loss, hydrogen ions are only removed from the body in urine, being actively exchanged into glomerular filtrate when other cations (mainly sodium) are reabsorbed. The extent of active hydrogen ion excretion into urine is seen on urinalysis: normal blood (from which urine is formed) pH is 7.4, while normal urinary pH is 5.0. Kidney injury therefore causes metabolic acidosis.

Kidneys usually excrete 30–70 mmol of hydrogen ions daily, but after a week or more can remove 300 mmol daily.

Chemical buffers

Chemical buffers respond rapidly, within seconds, balancing hydrogen ions by binding acids to bases. They do not eliminate acids from the body.

Bicarbonate is the main chemical buffer of extracellular fluid, responsible for half of all chemical buffering. Hydrogen ions are essential to produce bicarbonate (HCO_3). Bicarbonate can combine with hydrogen to produce carbonic acid:

$$HCO_3^- + H^+ \leftrightarrow H_2CO_3$$

Phosphate (PO_4^{3-}) is the least important buffer in blood, but the main urinary, interstitial and intracellular buffer.

Plasma and proteins. Albumin is the main plasma protein, although histidine (in haemoglobin) is also a significant buffer. Hypoalbuminaemia, common in critical illness, therefore reduces metabolic buffering.

Chemical buffers are produced in many places, but especially in the liver, therefore hepatic failure causes metabolic acidosis.

Acidosis

Acidosis (blood pH < 7.35) may be:

- respiratory = failure to excrete sufficient carbon dioxide (high pCO_2);
- metabolic = failure to excrete/buffer sufficient H^+ ions (base excess below –2; HCO_3 below 22);
- mixed (respiratory + metabolic).

Acidosis:

- increases respiratory drive;
- shifts the oxygen dissociation curve to the right, increasing oxyhaemoglobin dissociation ("Böhr" effect). Treating acidosis rather than underlying causes therefore deprives hypoxic tissues of available oxygen;
- reduces blood carriage of carbon dioxide (Cavaliere *et al.*, 2002);
- is negatively inotropic (Curley and Laffey, 2014; Khitan *et al.*, 2015), and reduces effectiveness of infused inotropes;
- impairs clotting (Engström *et al.*, 2006).

Acidosis is a symptom, not a disease, so treatment should focus on underlying pathologies. For example, permissive hypercapnia (see Chapter 27) induces respiratory acidosis but can protect lungs. Oxygen delivery to peripheries should be optimised, without increasing cell metabolism.

Sodium bicarbonate infusions have traditionally been used to reverse acidosis. As bicarbonate is the main chemical buffer in blood, this appears logical. Metabolic acidosis primarily originates from generation of hydrogen ions in cells. Bicarbonate is essentially an extracellular chemical, so increasing serum bicarbonate will not counter intracellular acidosis. Bicarbonate can dissociate into carbon dioxide (plus water), which can transfer into cells, exacerbating acidosis (Kraut and Madias, 2014; Velissaris *et al.*, 2015). Also increasing serum bicarbonate induces alkalosis, which reduces oxygen dissociation from haemoglobin (shifts the oxygen dissociation curve to left). Resuscitation Council (UK) (2015) adult guidelines do not mention bicarbonate.

Tonometry

Hypoxic tissues metabolise anaerobically, producing more hydrogen ions. The gut being highly vascular, gastric (intramucosal) pH (pHi) may indicate acidaemia. Zhang *et al.*'s (2015) meta-analysis suggests that pHi-guided therapy can reduce ICU mortality, although Mythen's (2015) editorial acknowledges lack of evidence from robust randomised controlled trials. For accuracy, feed should be aspirated before measurement (Marshall and West, 2003), which limits its clinical usefulness.

Taking samples

Blood gas samples should not be taken within 20 minutes of any changes to ventilation, or any interventions that affects respiratory function (Hennessey and Japp, 2016).

Potential sampling errors than may affect results include:

- *dilution* from saline flush, if insufficient fluid is withdrawn from the "deadspace" of arterial lines; blood should be clearly free of saline, but sampling ports are usually close to the cannula, making 0.5–1 ml usually sufficient discard;
- excessive *negative pressure* may damage cells (haemolysis), causing potassium release; if pressure is needed, it should be gentle, steady and minimal;
- *air* in samples causes falsely low readings, so should be expelled (Szaflarski, 1996). Samples should be covered immediately to prevent atmospheric gas exchange;
- *delay in analysing* causes inaccuracies, as blood cells in samples continue to metabolise: potassium and carbon dioxide levels increase, pH and oxygen fall. As ICUs usually have analysers on the unit, this rarely causes significant problems, but usually justifies interrupting routine calibrations;
- *erythrocyte sedimentation* may cause either concentrated plasma or concentrated cells to enter the analyser, affecting many results, especially haemoglobin; samples should be mixed continuously, rotating with a thumb roll, not vigorous shaking (which causes haemolysis).

When taking samples, these pitfalls should be avoided, but they should also be considered when interpreting results, especially if the sample has been obtained by someone else.

Interpreting samples

Like all skills, interpreting results improves with practice, and benefits from using a systematic approach. There are four main sections to blood gas results, each with a very few key measurements:

- pH;
- respiratory ($PaCO_2$, PaO_2, SaO_2);
- metabolic (HCO_3, SBC);
- "add-ons" (electrolytes, metabolites).

Not all results are always printed together, and there will be other (usually less valuable) results, some of which are included below.

This chapter describes key measurements, many analysers offering additional results. "Normal" ranges are listed individually, but the five key ones are also gathered in Table 19.1. Standard abbreviations used for some other measurements are listed in Table 19.2. Electrolytes and metabolites, measured by most analysers, are listed in Table 19.3; lactate is included in this chapter but others are discussed in Chapter 21. Having a printout from a patient you have recently cared for will be useful while reading through this section.

Temperature affects dissociation of gases, so PaO_2, $PaCO_2$, and therefore pH results differ with different temperatures – seen by reanalysing samples at different temperatures. Theoretically, analysing samples at the patient temperature ("pH-stat") reflects gas dissociation in the individual patient. Even if staff have confidence in both the thermometer and the measured temperature, temperature differs in different parts of the body. Analysing all samples at 37°C ("alpha-stat") provides consistency, is easier and safer (Bisson and Younker, 2006) and is recommended by the USA AARC Clinical Practice Guidelines (Davis *et al.*, 2013). Most ICUs no longer temperature-correct gases (Smith and Taylor, 2005), but consistency of all staff is more important than abstract debate.

pH

Normal: 7.35–7.45

pH measures overall acidity or alkalinity of blood; it does not differentiate between respiratory and metabolic components. (NB Ph = *pharmacopoeia* or *phenyl*)

Table 19.1 Normal ranges for arterial blood gases

pH	7.35–7.45
$PaCO_2$	4.6–6.1 kPa
PaO_2	12.0–14.6 kPa
HCO_3	22–29 mmol/litre
BE	±2 mmol/litre

Table 19.2 Some abbreviations commonly found on blood gas samples

F	=	Fractional concentration in dry gas
I	=	ideal
P	=	pressure, or partial pressure
Q	=	volume of blood
A	=	alveolar
a	=	arterial
c	=	capillary
v	=	venous

PaCO₂

Normal: 4.6–6.1 kPa (British Thoracic Society – B.T.S., 2017)

Carbon dioxide dissolves in water, forming carbonic acid (see above). High carbon dioxide tension (high $PaCO_2$) therefore indicates respiratory acidosis, while low carbon dioxide tension indicates respiratory alkalosis. Whether CO_2 from venous gases is reliable and/or useful is debated, but arguably $PvCO_2$ can indicate trends for adjusting ventilation in patients who do not have arterial lines. Ideal arterial $PaCO_2$ = 5.3 kPa (Bourke and Burns, 2015).

tCO₂ (or ctCO₂)

Normal: 21.6–22.5 mmol/litre (48–50 vols%)

Although most carbon dioxide is carried in bicarbonate, nearly one third is carried either is solution (as carbonic acid) or by haemoglobin. tCO_2 measures the total carbon dioxide in plasma. This measurement is generally of limited use.

PaO₂

Normal: 12.0–14.6 kPa (B.T.S., 2017)

PaO_2 measures partial pressure of oxygen in plasma. This is a very small amount (normally about 3%) of oxygen in blood, but as gas exchange relies on pressure gradients, partial pressure of oxygen determines tissue oxygenation. PO_2 from venous gases has little meaning and should be ignored.

Saturation

Normal: 97–98%

Arterial saturation indicates percentage saturation of haemoglobin by oxygen and is the same as SpO_2 measured by pulse oximeters (see Chapter 17). Blood gas analysers use many colours to calculate saturation; pulse oximeters use only two, so analysers are more accurate, especially if carbon monoxide is present. Venous saturation is discussed in Chapter 18.

a-A gradient

Normal: 2–3.3 kPa (depending on age)

Alveolar arterial (A-a) gradient indicates whether "*shunting*" is occurring. Measurement is only available if FiO_2 is entered into the analyser. As significant shunting is probably occurring if high concentrations of inspired oxygen are needed, the need to quantify shunting is questionable.

P/F ratio

Normal: 40 mmHg (200 if measured in mmHg)

This is the ratio between PaO_2 and FiO_2. Low P/F ratio indicates problems with gas exchange (Drahnak and Custer, 2015), arguably providing a better indication of shunting than A-a gradient. As with A-a gradient, the need to quantify shunting is questionable, although algorithms for adjusting ventilation modes such as APRV often rely on P/F ratio. Measurement is only available if FiO_2 is entered into the analyser.

FCOHb

Normal (non-smoker) < 2%

Half-life of carbon monoxide is about five hours in air, reducing to 90 minutes if breathing pure oxygen (B.T.S., 2017), so pure oxygen should be given to patients with carbon monoxide poisoning.

HCO_3^-

Normal: 22–29 mmol/litre (Pathology Harmony)

Bicarbonate is the main buffer in blood, so low bicarbonate indicates metabolic acidosis, while high levels indicate metabolic alkalosis. While most bicarbonate is produced by the metabolic system, some is also produced from carbon dioxide:

$$CO_2 + H_2O \leftrightarrow H_2CO_3 \leftrightarrow HCO_3^- + H^+$$

(carbon dioxide + water form carbonic acid, which can dissociate to bicarbonate and a hydrogen radical)

Bicarbonate production from carbon dioxide is normally negligible but becomes increasingly significant with hypercapnia. Actual bicarbonate (ABC, the amount measured) therefore includes both metabolic and respiratory production. Microchip calculation enables removal of the respiratory component by adjusting the measurement to standard conditions (temperature 37°C and $PaCO_2$ 5.3 kPa), giving a *standardised bicarbonate* (SBC, HCO_3^-std). Although a derived measurement, SBC gives more reliable indication of metabolic function than ABC (HCO_3^-). Many machines now only display standardised figures.

Base excess (BE)

Normal: ±2 mmol/litre (= milliEquivalents/litre; mEq/L)

Base excess measures metabolic acid/base balance, indicating moles of acid or base needed to restore one litre of blood to pH 7.4. Unlike pH, base excess is a linear scale, so easier to understand. Neutral is zero and positive base excess is too much base (alkaline; metabolic alkalosis), while negative base excess is insufficient base (metabolic acidosis).

Base excess is calculated from Hb and pCO_2 (Lumb, 2017), so, although viewed as a metabolic figure, carbon dioxide also affects measured base excess. Standardised base excess (SBE, BE-std) is therefore more accurate and indicates metabolic balance. Many machines now only display standardised figures.

Anion gap

Normal: 10–18

This measures the difference (gap) between measured cations and measured anions:

$$(Na^+ + K^+) - (Cl^- + HCO_3^-)$$

In health, cations and anions are balanced, but there are more anions than cations not measured by analysers, hence the gap. In sepsis, a high anion gap is often caused by lactate (Velissaris *et al.*, 2015); as lactate is usually measured by blood gas analysers, inferring it from the anion gap seems futile. Arguably, the anion gap is an archaic way of assessing acid/base balance, and it is usually unreliable in critically ill patients owing to the anion albumin almost invariably being low (Sood *et al.*, 2010).

Lactate ($C_3H_5O_3^-$)

Normal < 1 mmol/litre

Metabolism normally produces about 0.8 mmol/kg/hour of lactate (Cooper *et al.*, 2014), but anaerobic metabolism significantly increases production. Lactate is converted into lactic acid (pH 3.4), causing/increasing metabolic acidosis. Raised lactate indicates perfusion failure, with mortality increasing as lactate rises (Kraut and Madias, 2014). Much evidence for detrimental effects of lactate originates from studies with sepsis; whether lactate predicts mortality in most pathologies (Kraut and Madias, 2014) or only with cardiovascular failure (Ansen *et al.*, 2009) is disputed; lactate is useful as fuel source in sports medicine (Hall *et al.*, 2016) and neurology (Jalloh *et al.*, 2013). While lactate may pose few risks to healthy bodies, in critically ill patients it can cause life-threatening metabolic acidosis (Greaves *et al.*, 2012). The normal levels above are widely cited, including in Dellinger *et al.*, 2013, but not the 2017 international sepsis guidelines; it also conflicts with Pathology Harmony (the national UK reference range for biochemistry), which suggests that normal ranges are 0.6–2.2 mmol/litre.

Compensation

Homeostasis aims to keep blood pH 7.4. Overall pH of blood is the balance of both respiratory with metabolic function (see Figure 19.1). If able, the body compensates for a problem with one by an equal and opposite reaction with the other:

When analysing acid/base balance, identify:

- whether pH is normal (7.35–7.45);
- respiratory acid/base balance (pCO_2);
- metabolic acid/base balance (bicarbonate, base excess).

Table 19.3 Main electrolyte + metabolite results measured by most blood gas analysers

electrolyte/metabolite	normal range
sodium (Na$^+$)	133–146 mmol/litre
potassium (K$^+$)	3.5–5.3 mmol/litre
calcium (Ca^{++}, also written Ca^{2+})*	1.1–1.3 mmol/litre
chloride (Cl$^-$)	95–108 mmol/litre
glucose	3.5–8 mmol/litre (adult, non-diabetic (Diabetes UK, 2017))
lactate	< 1 mmol/litre

* NB blood gas analysers measure ionised calcium, not total calcium; biochemistry laboratories measure total calcium. See Chapter 21.

If pH is normal but respiratory and metabolic balances are abnormal and opposite, compensation is successful. If pH is abnormal, compensation is incomplete (if metabolic and respiratory balances are opposite) or absent (if metabolic and respiratory balances are not opposite).

Critical illness often causes acidosis – respiratory (respiratory failure) or metabolic (e.g. kidney or liver failure). Alkaloses are usually compensatory. Respiratory compensation occurs quickly (within minutes) but metabolic compensation takes hours or days to be fully effective (and to fully reverse) (Bourke and Burns, 2015). So metabolic compensation only occurs in response to prolonged respiratory complications. Metabolic "overshoot" may be seen in ICU where artificial ventilation resolves a primary respiratory acidosis, but metabolic compensation persists after the primary problem has been removed/resolved.

Five steps

From the four sections identified at the start of this section, core blood gas analysis can be achieved in five steps:

- pH – is it normal? If not, is acidosis or alkalosis present?
- respiratory (PaCO$_2$ = ventilation + respiratory acid/base balance; PaO$_2$ + SaO$_2$ = oxygenation);
- metabolic acid/base balance (HCO$_3$, SBC);
- is compensation occurring? If so, which way? Is it fully or partly successful (short cut: acidosis is usually the problem; alkalosis is usually compensation)?
- "add-ons" (electrolytes, metabolites).

Most normal ranges for venous blood gases are similar to arterial, except for PO_2 (Treger *et al.*, 2010), and arguably pCO_2 (Byrne *et al.*, 2014; McKeever *et al.*, 2016). Venous gases may prevent the need for arterial stabs when patients do not have arterial lines. Being more useful in clinical areas outside ICU, they are discussed further in Woodrow (2016).

Implications for practice

- acidosis is usually caused by disease, alkalosis usually by compensation;
- survival is only possible within a very narrow range of blood pH;
- analyse blood gases systemically, using the five-step approach;
- standardised bicarbonate and base excess levels should be used rather than actual HCO_3^- and BE (many analysers now only display standardised figures);
- gases should not be temperature-corrected unless there is an exceptional reason;
- most results from venous gases are comparable to arterial. PvO_2 is not useful, $PvCO_2$ may be discrepant, but can suggest trends. SvO_2 (when compared with SaO_2) indicates oxygen uptake.

Summary

Blood gas analysis remains one of the most valuable means of monitoring respiratory and metabolic function. ICU nurses both take and interpret arterial blood gas samples, so need to know potential sources of error (sampling, transporting), standard unit practices (e.g. whether or not to enter patients' temperature) and how to interpret results, in a logical sequence, in the context of their patient. "Normal" figures may vary slightly but principles remain applicable.

Further reading

Chapters on acid–base balance are included in many physiology, ICU and clinical chemistry/biochemistry texts. Hennessey and Japp (2016) and Foxall (2008) provide useful handbooks, with many scenarios for practice. Articles periodically appear in journals. Kraut and Madias (2014) provide a useful review of lactic acidosis.

Clinical scenarios

Arterial blood gas analysis on admission to ICU:

Patient 1: 36-year-old female who is unconscious from taking aspirin overdose.

Patient 2: 45-year-old male, known alcoholic with history of vomiting, had developed difficulty breathing.

Patient 3: 62-year-old male with a history of congestive cardiac failure with 15% ejection fraction, developed pneumonia and bilateral pleural effusions.

Patient 4: 75-year-old female, had a dynamic hip replacement, developed a chest infection, reduced respiratory function and possible pulmonary embolism.

	Patient 1	Patient 2	Patient 3	Patient 4
FiO_2	0.6	0.35	0.28	0.4
pH	7.25	7.55	7.48	7.29
PaO_2 (kPa)	9.32	11.9	12.6	7.49
$PaCO_2$ (kPa)	8.10	4.6	3.05	11.05
HCO_3 (mmol/litre)	21.2	34.4	20.1	33.7
BE (mmol/litre)	1.9	6	-6.3	12.4
Lactate (mmol/litre)	1.5	0.7	0.8	0.5

Q.1 Identify acid–base status of the four blood gases (acidosis, alkalosis, respiratory, metabolic, compensated or uncompensated).

Q2. Analyse likely causes of acid–base imbalances. How might abnormalities affect organs/systems, and how can ICU nurses anticipate and minimise adverse effects?

Q3. List potential sources of error, and how these might affect results.

Chapter 20

Haemodynamic monitoring

Contents

Fundamental knowledge

Experience of using invasive monitoring (including "zeroing")
Cardiac physiology – atria, ventricles, valves
Cardiac cycle: systole, diastole
Relationship between cardiac electrical activity (ECG) and
    output (pulse, blood pressure)
How breathing affects venous return
V/Q mismatch
Oxygen dissociation (see Chapter 18)

Introduction

The purpose of the cardiovascular system is perfusion, supplying cells with oxygen and glucose needed for normal aerobic metabolism (energy) and removing metabolic waste (carbon dioxide, metabolic acids, water). Without perfusion, cells die. Haemodynamic monitoring therefore aims to indicate perfusion.

The quest to monitor and manage the cardiovascular systems of critically ill patients has resulted in a plethora of technologies, many of which have largely been consigned to history. As the PAC-Man study illustrated (Harvey *et al.*, 2005), there is limited, and questionable, evidence that technology provides superior results to empirical treatment. More invasive (e.g. cardiac output monitoring) modes generally provide more information, but create more problems/risks, and how much that quantitative information adds over clinical acumen will probably continue to be debated. Options chosen therefore depend on balancing benefits against burdens. Monitoring equipment is diagnostic, not therapeutic, so once risks outweigh benefits, or maximum time limits are reached, it should be removed.

"Normal" figures are cited here as a guide, but many assume "average" 70 kg patients, and individuals can have wide healthy variations, so trends are more important than isolated measurements.

Visual

Pale, discoloured, cyanosed or clammy skin indicates poor perfusion – whether from hypovolaemia, vascular disease or excessive vasoconstriction. Although non-invasive and easily visible, skin discolouration may be acute or chronic, and has limited value in critical illness. Peripheral warmth and pulses indicate perfusion and are especially important to assess after vascular surgery. Excessively warm and flushed peripheries indicate excessive vasodilatation (e.g. sepsis). Poor perfusion could be volumetric (hypovolaemia) or cardiovascular (heart failure, vascular disease).

Capillary refill measures peripheral perfusion. Capillary refill is assessed by pressing on skin for five seconds. On releasing pressure, initial blanching should vanish within two seconds (Jevon and Ewens, 2012). Delayed capillary refill indicates peripheral perfusion failure, from hypotension, hypovolaemia or excessive peripheral vascular resistance, but does not indicate central perfusion.

Arterial blood pressure

This is the pressure exerted on arterial walls. Pressure is determined by flow and resistance. Flow is affected by driving force (cardiac output or left ventricular ejection) and viscosity. Resistance (afterload) is both vascular (constriction, atherosclerosis) and interstitial (e.g. oedema). Capillary blood flow ("microcirculation") is reduced if blood viscosity increases (see Chapter 21).

Systolic pressure indicates perfusion, although mean arterial pressure (MAP) is a better measure of this, being the average pressure across the pulse cycle, whereas systolic is the transient peak. Vascular resistance causes systolic pressure to increase towards peripheries, so pedal arterial lines usually measure higher systolic pressures than radial ones.

Diastolic pressure is the pressure exerted on arterial walls between pulses. Abnormally low diastolic pressure (< 80 mmHg) usually indicates vasodilatation. Once circulating volume is optimised with fluids, vasopressors (e.g. noradrenaline) may be needed.

Of the three pressures, MAP is usually the most valuable pressure, as it indicates whether pressure is adequate to perfuse tissues. "Normal" MAP is about 90–105 mmHg. Organ perfusion needs a MAP of at least 65 mmHg (Rhodes et al., 2017); a minimum of 70 mmHg is frequently used to guide inotropic therapy. Traditional beliefs that hypertensive patients may need higher pressures to perfuse organs was not supported by Asfar et al.'s (2014) study, although Joannidis et al. (2017) recommend a target MAP of 80–85 mmHg for renal protection in septic shock.

Pulse pressure, the pressure created by each pulse (systolic minus diastolic), indicates vessel response to pulse. Stereotypical normal pulse pressure is:

120 – 80 = 40 mmHg

High (wide) pulse pressures usually indicate vascular disease, such as atherosclerosis (Task Force, 2013), while low (narrow) pulse pressures usually indicate arterial hypovolaemia, which may be caused by:

- systemic hypovolaemia
- poor cardiac output
- excessive vasodilatation.

Other haemodynamic monitoring (e.g. stroke volume variation) may indicate likely causes.

Non-invasive blood pressure measurement

Cuff pressure monitoring provides adequate information for most hospitalised patients, but greater frequency and accuracy is usually needed in ICU. Incorrect-sized cuffs give erroneous readings: smaller cuffs over-read, while larger cuffs under-read. Compared with intra-arterial measurement, "dampening" of measurement between arteries and skin surface cause lower systolic and higher diastolic measurements with non-invasive blood pressure – Picone et al. (2017) measured differences in single figures, whereas Ilies et al.'s (2012) study comparing fingertip devices and intra-arterial measurement supported the traditionally cited differences of 15–20 mmHg between systolic pressures.

Intra-arterial measurement

Direct (invasive) arterial pressure monitoring provides:

- continuous measurement;
- visual display;
- access for arterial blood for sampling.

Pulse waveform (see Figure 20.1) indicates cardiac function:

- the area beneath the wave indicates pulse volume;
- the upstroke indicates myocardial contractility; normally it should be almost vertical; shallower upstrokes indicate poor flow; changes in shape can indicate response to inotropes (Easby and Dalrymple, 2009);
- downstrokes are normally almost vertical, like the upstroke; more gentle downslopes occur with vasoconstriction (Easby and Dalrymple, 2009);
- the dicrotic notch (closure of the aortic valve) normally occurs about one quarter to one third of the way down the downstroke; its position indicates peripheral vascular resistance (high dicrotic notch = vasoconstriction, low = vasodilatation (Easby and Dalrymple, 2009)); poorly defined or absent dicrotic notches indicate aortic valve incompetence;
- extensive systemic vasodilatation and low systemic vascular resistance (e.g. sepsis) can cause an anacrotic notch on upstrokes, with widening of the dicrotic notch.

Stroke volume is affected by intrathoracic pressure, so breathing causes "arterial swing" – variance in height between different arterial waveforms. Provided cardiac rhythm is regular, this is normally slight, but significant arterial swing usually indicates hypovolaemia (Perel *et al.*, 2014). Irregular

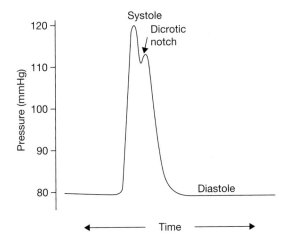

Figure 20.1 Arterial trace

rhythms, such as atrial fibrillation, cause variable stroke volumes, so no notice should be taken or arterial swing, pulse pressure variation or stroke volume variation with irregular rhythms. Many monitors can display pulse pressure variation (PPV – discussed in cardiac studies, below). Rises in late inspiration can also be caused by cardiac overload.

Disconnection, or significant oozing around arterial cannulae, can cause rapid blood loss, so security of connections should be checked, sites covered by transparent bio-occlusive dressings, and (if possible) placed where easily observed. Waveform display should be continuously monitored, with alarms set to give early warning of problems such as hypertension, hypotension and disconnection. Although rare, arterial lines can occlude arteries, so care should include checking colour, warmth and capillary refill of extremities beyond cannulae.

Transducers should be "zeroed" at midaxillary level – open the port from the monitor to air, and press calibration ("zero").

Errors can be caused by:

■ transducer level – should be at heart level; small changes in height cause large errors in measurement;
■ occlusion – patency should be maintained with continuous infusion (normally at 300 mmHg) with 0.9% saline, with or without heparin (Woodcock *et al.*, 2014);
■ drugs – no drug should be given through arterial lines (bolus concentrations can be toxic), so lines should be colour-coded red (N.P.S.A., 2010).

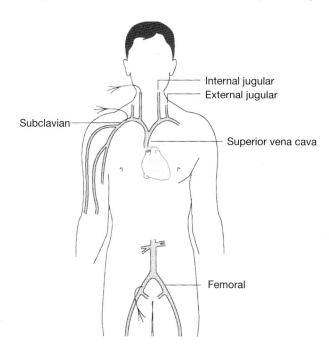

Internal jugular
External jugular
Subclavian
Superior vena cava
Femoral

■ *Figure 20.2 Main central venous cannulation sites*

Central venous catheters (CVCs)

Traditionally, central venous pressure (CVP), the pressure of blood returning to the right atrium, was viewed as indicating preload, and so blood volume, but CVP is a poor predictor of haemodynamic responsiveness (Marik and Cavallazzi, 2013; Marik and Bellomo, 2016).

Normal CVP for self-ventilating patients is 0 to +8 mmHg (mean +4 mmHg). Positive intrathoracic pressure increases this slightly, so PEEP/CPAP should be deducted from pressure measured. Very high pressures (> 18 mmHg) may indicate pulmonary oedema. Ideally, pressure measured should be as close to the right atrium as possible, the distal (brown) lumen of central venous catheters (CVCs). While CVP is of dubious value, waveform display does confirm patency of the catheter. Figure 20.3 shows components of the normal CVP waveform.

Dangers

Inserting central lines can puncture any surrounding tissue (lung puncture = pneumothorax, arteries, myocardium). Insertion may also accidently be retrograde (e.g. passing up, rather than down, the internal jugular vein (Goulding, 2014)). Nurses assisting during insertion should observe patients and monitors (ECG, airway pressures), reporting any concerns. Once inserted, lines should be secured (stitches or securing device) and position confirmed before use for any drugs or infusions. Position is usually confirmed through a chest X-ray but may also be confirmed using real-time fluoroscopy and ECG guidance (Bodenham *et al.*, 2016).

Once inserted, problems include:

- infection
- dysrhythmias
- air emboli.

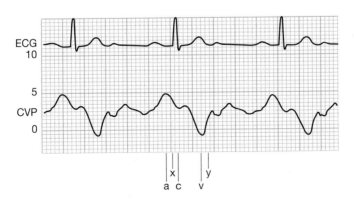

Figure 20.3 CVP waveform

Infection. The D.O.H. (2007) suggest that CVCs are responsible for more than two fifths of sepsis, although evidence for such statements is often very old. Loveday *et al.* (2014) do not cite infection rates but extensively discuss CVC and infection. Traditionally, femoral lines have been associated with greatest infection risk, although Parienti *et al.* (2015) found similar infection rates for femoral and internal jugular lines. All invasive devices are infection risks, but it is wise to view CVCs as potentially the most risky.

Dysrhythmias can be precipitated by many causes, including mechanical irritation from catheters advancing into the heart. ECG should be continuously monitored and any unexplained dysrhythmias reported and recorded.

Air emboli. Small bubbles, often seen in intravenous lines, are usually safely absorbed, but (self-ventilating) negative intrathoracic pressure of 4 cmH_2O could draw 90 ml of air in one second through an 18-gauge needle (Polderman and Girbes, 2002). Central lines should, whenever possible, be easily visible and checked regularly, especially with self-ventilating patients. Nurses should regularly check all connections are secure. If significant air embolus is suspected, the patient should be placed head-down and left lateral tilt, which may enable aspiration of air from the line (Bodenham *et al.*, 2016).

Removal

During removal of internal jugular or subclavian CVCs, negative pressure inspiration could entrain an air embolus between the time the catheter is removed and the site closes. CVCs should therefore be removed with the patient either supine or in the Trendelenburg position (bedhead angled downwards) (R.C.N., 2016), placing the exit site below heart level (Bodenham *et al.*, 2016). As the Valsalva manoeuvre (forced expiration with closed mouth, like straining at stool) is rarely practical for ICU patients, self-ventilating patients should breathe out and hold their breath (out) during removal, so intrathoracic pressure equals atmospheric pressure. With positive pressure ventilation, the positive intrathoracic pressure should prevent air entry. Once bleeding has stopped, an occlusive dressing should be placed over the site (Bodenham *et al.*, 2016).

PICCs

Peripherally inserted central cannulae (PICCs) have a lower infection risk than CVCs. Most are double-lumen, so will often not provide sufficient access for ICU needs. Woodrow (2016) discusses options for vascular access in more detail.

Cardiac output monitoring

Also called flow monitoring, this provides more information about both cardiac and vascular function, giving both direct and derived measurements. Derived measurements rely on information given by staff, such as:

■ body mass index (or ideal body weight) derived from height and weight;
■ haemoglobin;
■ central venous pressure.

There are various technologies, not all of which provide the same measurements. Indexed measurements are derived from input information of patient size and are usually used as normal ranges and remain the same for all patients. Common measurements, derivations and abbreviations are described below, with normal ranges summarised in Table 20.1. All systems are less reliable with irregular rhythms (e.g. atrial fibrillation), but many of the measurements can be taken over a longer time (e.g. 30 seconds), which usually provides sufficiently reliable results for treatment.

Pulmonary artery catheters (PACs; also called pulmonary artery floatation catheters – PAFCs – and "Swan Ganz") have largely been replaced by less invasive alternatives. Any readers encountering one should only use it if competent to do so; many older ICU texts describe PAFCs. Some measurements below are only available with PAFCs; these have been retained in the list, for benefits of staff using this technology.

Less invasive options include:

■ PiCCO – pulse indicator contour cardiac output;
■ LidCo – lithium derived cardiac output;
■ transoesphageal Doppler.

All three analyse arterial pulse waveform (contour) to derive measurements. Comparability and reliability of all technologies have been much studied and disputed, but most measurements are reliable (Lamia *et al.*, 2008).

Non-invasive means include:

■ thoracic electrical bioimpedance;
■ radial pulse applanation tonometry.

Truijen *et al.* (2012) suggest that non-invasive modes correlate well with invasive methods, but noticeably exclude ICUs from clinical areas discussed.

Thoracic electrical bioimpedance (TEB) uses ECG-like electrodes, measuring differences in thoracic resistance (bioimpedance) to high-frequency, very low-magnitude electrical currents. Aortic flow supplies less than 1% of thoracic bioimpedance, so high signal-to-noise ratio may cause significant inaccuracies. Whole-body electrical bioimpedance is accurate (Cotter *et al.*, 2004), but TEB less so (Chaney and Derdak, 2002) and it has not been widely adopted in UK ICUs.

Radial pulse applanation tonometry. Various peripheral devices have been developed. Saugel *et al.*'s (2014) "clinically acceptable agreement" margin of 23% with more conventional modes suggests this is not currently useful for ICU, but future technology may improve accuracy.

Measures and meanings

Normal ranges below are those of healthy resting adults. Figures that are not indexed are usually based on 70 kg adults. The sequence below, and many of the normal ranges, are from Pulsion Medical Systems (2008).

1. Oxygenation

Central venous oxygenation (SvO$_2$) (see Chapter 18)

Delivery of oxygen (DO$_2$)
Normal: DO$_2$ 950–1150 litres/minute

Delivery of oxygen index (DO$_2$I)
DO$_2$I 400–650 ml/minute/m^2
This indicates whether oxygen reached its target – the tissues.

Consumption of oxygen (VO$_2$)
Normal: VO$_2$ 200–290 litres/minute

Consumption of oxygen index (VO$_2$I)
VO$_2$I 125–175 ml/minute/m^2

Oxygen is needed by all cells, so delivery has little value unless tissues extract it.

2. Flow

Cardiac output (CO)
Normal: 4–8 litres/minute

Cardiac index (CI) sometimes called pulse contour cardiac index (PCCI)
Normal: 3.0–5.0 litres/minute/m^2
Cardiac output is the volume of blood ejected over one minute. If able, hearts compensate for problems, such as critical illness, by increasing cardiac index. Inotropes (e.g. adrenaline, dobutamine) are used to increase cardiac index. Low cardiac index indicates myocardial dysfunction.

Stroke volume (SV)
Normal: 60–130 ml

Stroke volume index (SVI)
Normal: 40–60 ml/m^2
Stroke volume is the amount of blood ejected with each contraction of the heart, so HR $\times$ SV = CO. Stroke volume relies on adequate preload and muscle contractility; if stroke volume is poor, preload should be optimised with fluids before using inotropes.

3. Preload

Global end-diastolic volume index (GEDI)
Normal: 680–800 ml/m^2
 Preload is the volume of blood returning to the right side of the heart, the "filling pressure". Traditionally, preload was assessed through CVP, but, as identified above, pressure and volume having poor correlation, making CVP a poor indicator of fluid status (preload). GEDI measures volume, so is a better indicator of preload.

Intrathoracic blood index (ITBI)
Normal: 850–1000 ml/m^2
 Blood volume in lungs determines perfusion, but (without other factors) also influences oedema. Per se, ITBI is of limited use, but other measures below are derived from it.

4. Volume Responsiveness

Stroke volume variation (SVV)
Normal: < 10%
 Stroke volume varies with changes in intrathoracic pressure (breathing). In health, provided heart rhythm is regular, variations are small, but hypovolaemia increases variations. SVV > 10% indicates need for fluids, provided the chest is not open (Wyffels *et al.*, 2010). Hypotension with SVV < 10% is usually an indication for inotropic support.

Pulse pressure variation (PPV)
Normal: < 10%
 Accessible through many bedside monitors, PPV is similar to SVV; PPV more than 13–15% indicates hypovolaemia (Pinsky, 2014). PPV and SVV quantify "arterial swing". Spontaneous breathing and irregular rhythms, especially atrial fibrillation, cause variable ventricular filling times and stroke volumes, largely invalidating use of SVV and PPV (Pinsky, 2014), although arguably they can indicate useful trends.

5. Afterload

Systemic vascular resistance (SVR)
Normal SVR: 800–1200 dynes/second/cm^5

Systemic vascular resistance index (SVRI)
SVRI: 1700 – 2400 dynes/second/cm^5/m^2
 Systemic vascular resistance ("afterload") is the resistance met by cardiac output from blood vessels. Blood pressure is the sum of HR × SV × SVR. Excessive vasodilatation (distributive shock, such as sepsis) reduces SVR. SVR monitoring is therefore useful for inotrope/vasopressor therapy.

6. Contractility

Cardiac function index (CFI)
Normal: 4.5–6.5 litres/minute
This is the fraction of preload pumped out by ventricles in one minute, so indicates cardiac contractility. Contractility can be increased with positive inotropes, such as dobutamine.

Left cardiac work (LCW)
Left cardiac work index (LCWI)
Normal LCWI: 3.4–4.2 km⁻m/m²

Normal LCWI: 3.4–4.2 km m/m²

Left ventricular stroke work (LVSW)
Left ventricular stroke work index (LVSWI)
Normal LVSWI: 50–60 gm m/m²
Managing severe left ventricular failure is a delicate balance between maintaining adequate cardiac output and myocardial oxygenation. Insufficient work deprives the brain of oxygen; excessive work deprives the myocardium of oxygen.

Right cardiac work (RCW)
Right cardiac work index (RCWI)
Right ventricular stroke work (RVSW)
Right ventricular stroke work index (RVSWI)
Normal RCW: 0.54–0.66 km m/m²
RVSWI: 7.9–9.7 gm m/m²
Measuring right ventricular function assists management with right heart failure.

Global ejection fraction (GEF)
Normal: > 50% (Task Force, 2016a); 25–35% (Pulsion, 2008)
More often calculated from echocardiograms (see below), ejection fraction is the fraction of blood ejected from ventricles in relation to the volume they contain, so indication of myocardial health.

Cardiac power index (CPI)
Normal: 0.5–0.7 watts per square metre (W/m²)
This indicates cardiac performance, so may be useful with cardiogenic shock.

7. Pulmonary Oedema

Extravascular lung water index (EVLWI)
Normal: 3–7 ml/kg
Interstitial fluid volume is considerably larger than blood volume. But, as oxygen is not very soluble, excess interstitial fluid creates a barrier to oxygen transfer exchange. Extravascular lung water is increased with either:

■ increased pulmonary vascular permeability (inflammation) or
■ increased hydrostatic pressure (heart failure).

(Zhang *et al.*, 2012)

Conditions such as heart failure and inflammatory responses from sepsis or acute respiratory distress syndrome (ARDS) increase extravascular lung water. EVLWI measurement has proven especially valuable for diagnosing and treating ARDS (Kushimoto *et al.*, 2012). EVLWI will not identify a pleural effusion, which being in the pleura is outside interstitial lung tissue.

Pulmonary vascular permeability index (PVPI)

■ 1.0–3.0 = cardiogenic (hydrostatic) oedema (heart failure);
■ > 3.0 = permeability oedema (inflammation).

PVPI differentiates causes of pulmonary oedema and is derived from the ratio between EVLW and intrathoracic blood volume (ITBV), based on pulmonary blood volume invariably being one fifth of intrathoracic blood volume. Measurements through femoral cannulation under-read (Berbara *et al.*, 2014), so should either be adjusted or treated cautiously.

Pulmonary artery pressure (PAP)

Normal: $\dfrac{8–15}{15–25}$ mmHg

Pulmonary vascular resistance index (PVRI)
Normal: PVR < 250 dynes/second/cm^5
 PVRI 255–285 dynes/second/cm^5/cm^2
Pulmonary hypertension creates the afterload for the right side of the heart and is increased with lung disease, and decreased with either right-sided heart disease or low preload.

Pulmonary capillary wedge pressure (PCWP)
Normal 6–15 mmHg
This is only available with PAFCs and indicates left atrial filling pressure.

Echocardiogram

Ultrasound echocardiogram enables visualisation and measurement of the heart and blood flow through central vessels, so is valuable for medical diagnosis. Among the most frequent measurements from echocardiography (cardiac ultrasound) is left ventricular *ejection fraction*. The average healthy adult left ventricle can hold about 130 ml of blood but only ejects 70–90 ml, in health increasing to meet oxygen demand. The volume ejected can therefore be expressed as a fraction, or more often percentage, of total ventricular volume. Normal healthy ejection fraction is > 50% (Task Force, 2016a). Smaller ejection

Table 20.1 **Normal cardiac output study parameters (not all parameters are available on all technologies)**

CFI	4.5–6.5 litres/minute
CI/PCCI	3–5 litres/minute/m^2
CO	4–8 litres/minute
CPI	normal: 0.5–0.7 W/m^2
CVP (self-ventilating)	0 to +8 mmHg (right atrial level); with artificial ventilation, subtract PEEP from measured CVP
DO$_2$	900–1100 litres/minute
DO$_2$I	400–650 ml/minute/m^2
EVLWI	3–7 ml/kg
GEDI	680–800 ml/m^2
GEF	25–35%
ITBI	850–1000 ml/m^2
LCWI	3.4–4.2 kg/m/m^2
LVSWI	50–60 gm/m/m^2
PAP	10–20 mmHg
PPV	< 10%
PVPI	1.0–3.0 = cardiogenic oedema; > 3.0 = permeability oedema
PVR	< 250 dynes/second/cm^5
PVRI	255–285 dynes/second/cm^5/cm^2
RCW	0.54–0.66 km/m/m/m^2
RVSWI	7.9–9.7 gm/m/m/m^2
SSV	< 10%
SV	60–130 ml
SVI	40–60 ml/m^2
SvO$_2$	75%
SVR	800–1200 dynes/second/cm^5
SVRI	1700–2400 dynes/second/cm^5/m^2
VO$_2$	200–290 litres/minute
VO$_2$I	125–175 ml/minute/m^2

fractions usually indicate extensive left ventricular damage, usually from myocardial infarction.

Implications for practice

- skin colour, warmth and capillary refill time indicate peripheral perfusion;
- diastolic blood pressure and pulse pressure indicate systemic vascular resistance;
- mean arterial pressure (MAP) indicates perfusion pressure;
- intra-arterial blood pressure monitoring is usually more accurate, and slightly higher, than non-invasive measurement, provided arterial traces do not look dampened;
- cardiac output studies enable titration of fluids, inotropes and vasopressors to optimise haemodynamic status in critical illness;
- with cardiac output studies, indexed measurements are adjusted to body surface area (m^2), so are usually used;
- each shift, identify target parameters for your patient.

Summary

Haemodynamic monitoring necessarily forms a major aspect of intensive care nursing, which has prompted a plethora of technologies to measure various aspects. Evidence can be found to support, and often confute, most options. Quantification provides reassurance about effectiveness of therapies; whether risks and costs involved are justified by reduced mortality and morbidity is often less clear. Nurses should actively assess and, where possible, initiate appropriate monitoring. Equipment should only be used by staff competent to do so, and within manufacturers' guidelines and time limits.

Further reading

Readers should access instruction manuals and websites of equipment used on their units. Pinsky (2014) provides an overview of many currently available technologies. The R.C.N. (2016) and Bodenham *et al.* (2016) provide guidance for different types of vascular access devices.

Clinical scenarios

Mrs Ellen Harrison, 62 years old, is admitted to the ICU with community-acquired pneumonia and sepsis. She is sedated, mechanically ventilated with intravenous infusions of noradrenaline at 0.4 mcg/kg/min and dobutamine at 0.5 mcg/kg/min. Mrs Harrison is 1.75 m tall and weighs 75 kg (body surface area of 1.90 m²). Cardiac output measurements are commenced to guide inotropic therapy.

Her haemodynamic profile reveals:

BP	140/50 mmHg (MAP 80 mmHg)
HR	112 beats/minute
Rhythm	Sinus tachycardia with self-terminating runs of unifocal ventricular ectopics
CI	2.9 litres/minute/m²
SVI	32 ml/beat/m²
SVRI	1416 dynes/second/cm⁵/m²
GEDI	920 ml/m²
EVLWI	6 ml/kg
SvO₂	81%

Q1. Evaluate risks and benefits of cardiac output monitoring mode(s) used on your unit with other options described in this chapter. Discuss your findings with colleagues who have experience of using other modalities.

Q2. What are the likely cause and implications of Mrs Harrison's results? Is she adequately perfused and delivering sufficient oxygen to tissues? Will she be warm, cool, dilated or constricted?

Q3. How might you adjust Mrs Harrison's vasoactive drugs to optimise her status? Devise a plan of care to include rationales for choice of prescribed drugs and/or fluid therapies and haemodynamic goals.

Blood results

Contents

Introduction

Blood is a transport mechanism, so its contents reflect body activity. Recognising abnormal values and knowing what to do about them enables early and appropriate interventions. This chapter outlines main haematology and biochemistry results. Liver function tests are outlined in Chapter 41 and cardiac markers (e.g. troponin) are included in Chapter 29.

Although results are discussed individually below, low levels may be caused by:

- dilution
- loss
- failure of supply or production,

while high levels may be from:

- dehydration (haemoconcentration);
- excessive intake/production;
- failure to metabolise or remove (e.g. hepatic or renal dysfunction).

Dilution (from large-volume intravenous infusion) and haemoconcentration (from excessive drainage or fluid shifts) are not identified specifically below but should always be considered as possible causes of abnormal results.

When analysing results, consider whether abnormalities are a:

- symptom (of a problem)
- problem
- symptom and a problem.

Treat problems, not symptoms.

Erroneous results may be caused by sampling errors, such as venepuncturing limbs where IVIs are running, or withdrawing insufficient fluid from deadspace of arterial lines. Any results appearing inconsistent with patients' clinical state should be rechecked.

Many treatments for acute abnormalities are identified, but other treatments are possible. Treatments identified are those normally used on ICU, so are not necessarily appropriate/safe in other settings. Management of chronic disorders may be very different and are not discussed in this book. Ranges cited are normally for venous blood. Most ICUs send arterial samples, which for practical purposes probably correlate with venous levels. In the UK, biochemistry laboratories use the national reference range (Pathology Harmony). Readers outside the UK should check local reference ranges.

Most samples in ICU are obtained from lines rather than venous stabs. Obvious deadspace of lines should be cleared to avoid diluting sample. Excessive clearance can cause significant cumulative blood loss, causing anaemia and necessitating transfusion (Gallando García et al., 2012). Villata-Garcia et al.

(2017) found that discarding 2 ml before taking samples from CVCs correlates with levels from venous stab. For most lines (arterial or venous), 2 ml is often a reasonable amount, but this depends on deadspace before the aspiration port.

Haematology

Blood has three types of cells:

- erythrocytes (red blood cells – RBCs);
- leukocytes (white cells);
- platelets,

so a full blood count includes:

- haemoglobin (oxygen carriage);
- white cell count (WCC – immunity), with specific types of white cells also measured;
- platelets and other clotting measurements.

Albumin, total (plasma) protein and clotting are also discussed. All blood cells are produced by bone marrow, so diseases or treatments causing bone marrow suppression affect counts of all cells. The main erythrocytes tests are summarised in Table 21.1.

Haemoglobin (Hb)

Normal: 130–180 grams/litre (men) 115–165 (women)

Polycythaemia (raised levels), usually an adaptive response to chronic hypoxia, can be caused by living at high altitudes, but in the UK is usually caused by chronic lung, or sometimes cardiac, disease.

Critical illness usually causes low levels from:

- blood loss;
- dilution;
- reduced erythropoiesis;
- premature haemolysis from disease (e.g. sepsis) and haemofiltration;
- and sometimes anaemia or other causes, including iatrongenic.

Table 21.1 Haematology normal ranges – red cells

Hb	males	130–180 grams/litre
	females	115 – 165 grams/litre
PCV /Hct	males	40 – 52%
	females	36 – 48%

Haemoglobin transports nearly all oxygen in arterial blood, so low haemo-globin reduces oxygen-carrying capacity. Oxygen delivery to cells is a paradox between oxygen carriage (erythrocytes) with oxygen delivery (plasma). Blood is plasma and cells; plasma is mainly (90–95%) water, and most blood cells (99%) are erythrocytes. Higher haemoglobin concentrations therefore make blood thicker, while lower levels make it more dilute. Dilute blood flows more easily through capillaries, increasing oxygen delivery to tissue cells (Lumb, 2017). So dilute blood carries less oxygen but delivers it more effectively. Moderate anaemia improves survival from critical illness, survival being highest with Hb 70–90 grams/litre (Hébert *et al.*, 1999; Retter *et al.*, 2012), although some authors, such as Goodnough and Schrier (2014), suggest that older people may need slightly higher levels.

Because most blood cells are erythrocytes, packed cell volume (PCV), or haematocrit (Hct), also indicates erythrocytes, as a percentage of total volume.

Treatment. Acutely low Hb may be treated by blood transfusion, although, as identified in Chapter 18, unless there are other indications, blood should not be transfused if Hb is above 80 grams/litre (Norfolk, 2013); Hébert *et al.*'s (1999) threshold of 70 grams/litre is used in US guidelines (Carson *et al.*, 2016) and is probably a more appropriate transfusion threshold for most ICU patients.

White cell count (WCC)

Normal: $4{-}11 \times 10^9$/litre

Although often called white blood cells (WBC), most white cells live outside the bloodstream. For example, only 2–3% of neutrophils (by far the most numerous type of white cell) are in the bloodstream (Storey and Jordan, 2008). White cells use blood to move about; inflammation attracts white cells back into blood so they can move to infected areas. Hence, new infections cause rapid rises in WCC, especially neutrophils.

Increases may be caused by non-infective triggering of immunity, while immunodeficiency can cause a lack of response to infection. Severe/prolonged infection may deplete reserves, hence low counts (< 4) may indicate severe sepsis. Infection cannot therefore be excluded if counts are normal or low.

There are two main groups of leukocytes:

- granulocytes
- agranulocytes,

identified by whether or not cell membranes contain granules. Granoclytes tackle acute infections, whereas agranulocytes provide longer-term defences. Both main groups have further subtypes of cells. Normal counts are identified in Table 21.2.

Treatment. Usually, underlying causes are treated – e.g. infection with antibiotics. Low neutrophil count may be an indication for protective isolation (reverse barrier nursing). Low counts (leukopaenia) can be treated with granulocyte colony stimulating factor (G-CSF), but this takes some days to work so, although useful for oncology, it has little value in critical illness.

Granulocytes

There are three types of granulocytes:

- neutrophils (polymorphoneuclear, so "polymorphs");
- basophils;
- eosinophils;
- identified by laboratory staining.

Most leukocytes (50–70%) are neutrophils. Neutrophils are the first and main defence against infection, destroying bacteria by phagocytosis, resulting in pus. With infection, neutrophil count rises before other types of leukocytes.

Basophils and eosinophils are not usually significant in critical illness but both may indicate allergic reactions (Storey and Jordan, 2008).

Agranulocytes

There are two types of agranulocytes:

- lymphocytes – T and B cells
- monocytes.

Agranulocytes are an important part of immunity, lymphocytes recognising and tackling antigens, and monocytes migrating into tissues. They have limited value for critical illness, but excessive/inappropriate lymphocyte reactions can cause anaphylaxis.

Platelets (thrombocytes)

Normal levels: 150–400 × 10⁹/litre

Platelets, which are cell fragments, circulate for about 10 days. Normally kept inactive by endovascular chemicals (e.g. prostacyclin, nitric oxide), they

Table 21.2 Haematology normal ranges – white cells

White cell type	× 10^9/litre (UK)	per mm³ (USA)	%
neutrophils (polymorphs)	2.5–7.5	2500–7500	50–70
basophils	< 0.2	< 200	≤ 3
eosinophils	0.04–0.44	40–400	≤ 5
lymphocytes	1.5–4.0	1500–4000	≤ 12–50
monocytes	0.2–0.8	200–800	3–15

are activated by platelet activating factor (released by endothelium of damaged blood vessels) to form a thrombus.

Platelet counts are often low in critical illness, from:

- loss from bleeding;
- impaired production;
- anti-platelet drugs (e.g. heparin, aspirin, clopidogrel).

Impaired blood flow and immobility expose ICU patients to high risk of deep-vein thrombosis (DVT) and pulmonary embolism (PE). All ICU patients should therefore be risk-assessed for DVT and thromboprophylaxis given unless there are specific contraindications to either (I.C.S., 2015). Thromboprophylaxis is discussed further in Chapter 26.

Critical illness frequently causes coagulopathies, usually with low platelet counts. Adequate coagulation can occur with surprisingly low numbers of platelets. If platelets are low, nurses should check whether anticoagulants are still required; most teams usually continue anticoagulants if platelet count exceeds 50.

Treatment. Platelets can be transfused if indicated. Routine transfusions are rarely indicated with platelet counts above 10–20, but platelet cover may be given, aiming for counts of 40–50, for procedures with high risk of bleeding (Estcourt *et al.*, 2017) – tracheostomy insertion, CVC insertion, epidural insertion or removal, surgery.

Albumin and total protein

Normal: albumin 35–50 grams/litre.
Total protein (TP): 60–80 grams/litre

Plasma proteins create most of the *colloid osmotic pressure* that retains normal plasma volume within the bloodstream. Low plasma protein levels therefore cause hypovolaemia and oedema. Proteins also:

- bind drugs and chemicals (see calcium, below);
- transport substances (e.g. bilirubin);
- are antioxidants.

Although there are many plasma proteins, more than half total protein concentration is albumin, and albumin exerts three quarters of plasma protein colloid osmotic pressure.

Hypoalbuminaemia and low levels of other plasma proteins is multifactorial, caused by:

- catabolism provoking protein metabolism;
- malnutrition (see Chapter 9);
- liver hypofunction (see Chapter 41).

Endogenous albumin half-life is normally 14–20 days (Bharadwaj *et al.*, 2016), so, although protein levels can be viewed as a marker of illness/recovery (Klek *et al.*, 2016), changes take days to occur. Low albumin correlates with muscle weakness (Malietzis *et al.*, 2016).

Treatment. Infusing albumin has relatively transient effects (see Chapter 33). Early nutrition (see Chapter 9) provides proteins needed in critical illness for tissue repair (McClave *et al.*, 2016), although serum albumin levels take many days before recovering.

Clotting

Normal APTT: 25–35 seconds.
PT: 10–12 seconds.
INR: normal 0.9–1.1.

In addition to platelet count, clotting is usually measured by some of:

- activated partial thromboplastin time (APTT or PTT), which measures the intrinsic clotting pathway (Reding and Cooper, 2012) – clotting factors already in blood;
- activated prothromin time (APT or PT), which measures the extrinsic clotting pathway (Reding and Cooper, 2012) – clotting factors released from vascular endothelium;
- international normalised ratio (INR), which indicates overall clotting time (intrinsic + extrinsic pathways).

Clotting is discussed further in Chapter 26.

Treatment. With anticoagulant therapy, target INR should normally be 2.5 (Keeling *et al.*, 2011). Clotting factors and blood products are sometimes needed. Thromboprophylaxis is discussed in Chapter 26.

D-dimers

Normal < 250 nanograms/ml (micrograms/litre), sometimes reported as "negative"

D-dimers are fibrin degradation products, released by fibrinolysis (clot breakdown). Raised levels therefore indicate either significant clot to break down (DVT or PE) or reduced (renal) clearance. Negative D-dimers can exclude DVT or PE (Task Force on the Diagnosis and Management of Acute Pulmonary Embolism of the European Society of Cardiology, 2008), but positive levels cannot confirm diagnosis (Rathbun *et al.*, 2004).

Treatment. Treat the disease – e.g. with therapeutic heparin.

Biochemistry

The main urea and electrolyte (U+E) results used in ICU, and the ones discussed here, are:

■ CRP (C-reactive protein)
■ sodium
■ chloride
■ potassium
■ glucose
■ phosphate
■ magnesium
■ calcium
■ creatinine
■ urea.

Most normal ranges below are Pathology Harmony – the UK national reference range for biochemistry.

C-reactive protein

Normal CRP = 0–10 mg/ml.

C-reactive protein (CRP) is an acute phase protein, serum levels rising within four to six hours after any inflammatory trigger (McWilliam and Riordan, 2010). Causes of inflammation are inferred from individual patient contexts; raised CRP usually indicates sepsis (Gucyetmez and Atalan, 2016). Failure to reduce within 48 hours of antibiotics probably indicates treatment failure (McWilliam and Riordan, 2010).

Treatment. Treat the disease – e.g. sepsis with antibiotics and system support.

Sodium (Na⁺)

Normal: 133–146 mmol/litre.

Sodium is the main intravascular cation. Acutely abnormal levels usually indicate hydration status:

■ hypernatraemia = (usually) dehydration (Alshayeb *et al.*, 2011);
■ hyponatraemia = (usually) water overload (Spasovski *et al.*, 2014) or fluid shifts from cell, where sodium concentration is normally about 14 mmol/ litre.

Extreme sodium levels are neurotoxic: below 120 causes encephalopathy (Sterns and Silver, 2016), while levels above 160 cause fitting. Hypernatraemia stimulates release of water-conserving hormones, such as vasopressin (antidiuretic hormone) and the renin–angiotensin–aldosterone cascade (Powell-Tuck *et al.*, 2008/2011). In moderate ill health, this may be useful compensation, but in patients with severe inflammatory responses (most ICU patients) this is likely to accelerate already-problematic oedema formation.

Treatment. If hyponatraemia is caused by water overload, restricting and/or removing fluid should resolve the problem. Otherwise, hyponatraemia can be corrected by giving sodium – usually as saline infusions, relying on kidneys to remove excess water while conserving salt. Hypernatraemia usually indicates dehydration, rehydration being achieved with water, usually as intravenous fluid.

Chloride (Cl⁻)

Normal: 95–108 mmol/litre.

A concentration of 0.9% sodium chloride is hyperchloraemic (154 mmol/litre chloride), so excessive saline infusions can cause hyperchloraemic acidaemia. Hyperchloraemia can also impair mental function and cause abdominal discomfort, headaches, nausea and vomiting.

Treatment. Hyperchloraemia is usually from excessive saline infusions, which should be discontinued. Hypochloraemia is rare and rarely problematic.

Potassium (K⁺)

Normal 3.5–5.3 mmol/litre.

Most (98%) body potassium is inside cells (Greenlee *et al.*, 2009). Serum potassium is used for cardiac conduction; hypokalaemia impairs conduction, so can provoke bradycardia and escape dysrhythmias, while hyperkalaemia can cause tachydysrhythmias. Traditionally, target levels for critically ill patients with cardiac history have usually been 4.0–5.0 or 4.5–5.5, but a recent meta-analysis suggests optimal level is 3.5–4.5 (Goyal *et al.*, 2012).

Most (90%) potassium loss is renal, so serum potassium levels usually reflect urine output: polyuria causes hypokalaemia, while oliguria causes hyperkalaemia. Haemofiltration causes rapid potassium loss, unless physio-logical levels are added to dialysate/replacement. Intracellular fluid contains about 150 mmol/litre, so extensive cell damage (such as major trauma) or large fluid shifts can cause hyperkalaemia. Haemolysis causes potassium leak from damaged blood cells, so haemolysed samples give falsely high levels. Haemolysis may make laboratory measurements higher than blood gas analysers (Parry *et al.*, 2010).

Treatment. Life-threatening hyperkalaemia (> 6 mmol/litre) should be urgently treated with intravenous glucose and insulin infusion, which transfers potassium into cells (Nyirenda *et al.*, 2009). Concurrent intravenous calcium (gluconate or chloride) stabilises cardiac conduction (Batterink *et al.*, 2015). Less severe hyperkalaemia (< 6 mmol/litre) may be treated with calcium resonium, given orally or rectally, which moves serum potassium into the gut for elimination in stools (Batterink *et al.*, 2015). If hyperkalaemia is caused by fluid shifts from severe dehydration, patients should be aggressively rehydrated. Salbutamol also transports potassium into cells, and together with glucose and insulin, this is the treatment Batterink *et al.* (2015) recommend, although they acknowledge the paucity of evidence for all interventions. As much supporting evidence for salbutamol is paediatric or from dialysis patients, and as salbutamol can cause gross tachycardia, using salbutamol to treat hyperkalaemia in adults is probably unwise. Resuscitation Council guidelines include an algorithm for treating hyperkalaemia.

Hypokalaemia is treated with potassium supplements. If the gut is functioning, oral/nasogastric supplements are often used. Strong potassium concentrations (such as 40 mmol in 100 ml) are often infused in ICU, but must be given through a central line, as peripheral infusion is both very painful and likely to cause severe thrombophlebitis. Strong potassium concentrations should only be used in critical care areas (N.P.S.A., 2002), where continuous ECG monitoring, potassium analysers and high staffing levels are available.

Glucose ($C_6H_{12}O_6$)

Normal: 3.5–8 mmol/litre (adult, non-diabetic (Diabetes UK, 2017)).

Glucose is the main source of intracellular energy (see Chapter 24), needing insulin to transport it into cells. Insulin deficiency or resistance therefore causes hyperglycaemia. In critically ill patients, stress responses and some drugs (e.g. corticosteroids) can cause mild hyperglycaemia.

Previously, mild hyperglycaemia was considered detrimental (Van den Berghe et al., 2001), but more recent studies consistently demonstrate that tight glycaemic control to achieve targets of 4.6–6.1 increases, rather than reduces, mortality (Wiener et al., 2008; Bilotta et al., 2009; NICE-SUGAR Study investigators; 2009; Preise et al., 2009; McCoy et al., 2016). Most ICUs now use Preiser et al.'s target of 7.8–10.0, although 7.8 is arguably too high for a lower limit. USA studies usually give levels in mg/decilitre; 10 mmol/litre = 180 mg/dL.

Arterial blood glucose is slightly higher than capillary/venous (Barrett et al., 2016). Whether this is clinically significant is debatable, especially if glycaemic control is managed solely by arterial blood gases. Poor peripheral blood flow can cause significant under- or over-readings (Kessler, 2009; Li et al., 2016), so is best avoided in most ICU patients.

Treatment. Hypoglycaemia is treated by giving glucose. Hyperglycaemia in the ICU is usually managed with sliding-scale actrapid insulin infusions, although usual insulin medication may be recommenced in diabetics before discharge. Most ICUs commence insulin infusions when blood sugar persists above 10 mmol/litre.

Phosphate (PO_4^{3-})

Normal: 0.80–1.50 mmol/litre.

Most phosphate is intracellular, especially bone cells (Gaasbeek and Meinders, 2005). Intracellular phosphate:

- is the main intracellular acid–base buffer;
- regulates enzymes (Ormerod et al., 2010);
- is needed for glycolysis to produce ATP (cell energy) (Ormerod et al., 2010);

■ is used for phagocytosis (Ormerod et al., 2010);
■ produces 2,3 DPG (assists oxygen dissociation from haemoglobin – see Chapter 18);
■ reduces free fatty acids.

Hyperphophosphaemia can cause calcium imbalance and dysrhythmias, but is rare in the ICU and rarely causes significant problems, so is not usually worth treating.

Low levels are very common, and contribute to a range of problems, including:

■ respiratory muscle weakness
■ cardiac failure
■ myopathy
■ delirium
■ seizures

(Ormerod et al., 2010)

Intake of phosphate may have been deficient prior to admission, but phosphate is lost in urine, so polyuria, diuretics and dialysis can cause low levels. It is not common practice to measure serum phosphate in many clinical areas, so undetected deficiencies often exist prior to admission.

Treatment. Hypophophataemia is usually treated by phosphate infusion (often 50 mmol over 24 hours), ideally infused through a central line. Intravenous phosphate has no known compatibility with any other drugs. Oral supplements are also available.

Magnesium (Mg⁺⁺ or Mg²⁺)

Normal: 0.7–1.0 mmol/litre.

Serum magnesium ("nature's tranquilliser") is a calcium antagonist, so it:

■ stabilises cell membranes;
■ reduces conduction – vasodilates and slows heart rate (hypotension, bradycardia).

It also bronchodilates, so may be nebulised or infused to treat bronchoconstriction (Sarhan et al., 2016).

Hypomagnesiumaemia, usually from malnutrition or excessive diuresis, occurs in 7–11% of hospitalised patients (Parikh and Webb, 2012). Hypermagnesiumaemia (> 3mmol/litre) is very rare and rarely a problem in ICU but may cause cardiac and/or respiratory arrest.

Treatment. In critical care, magnesium is usually infused intravenously; this can cause bradycardia and hypotension. Oral magnesium supplements are also available.

Calcium (Ca⁺⁺ or Ca²⁺)

Normal: total calcium 2.2–2.6 mmol/litre (laboratory results).
Ionised levels 1.1–1.3 mmol/litre (ABG results).

Like magnesium, only 1% of body calcium is in blood, but serum calcium facilitates:

- cardiac conduction
- muscle cell contraction
- cell function
- clotting.

About half of serum calcium is normally protein-bound, and half is free (*ionised*, or unbound). Only free (unbound) calcium is active. ICU patients almost invariably have low plasma protein (albumin) levels, which reduces protein-binding sites. Laboratories may "correct" calcium levels to reflect physiological activity of (ionised) calcium.

Treatment. Hypocalcaemia is treated with calcium supplements. Hyper-calcaemia is rare but can be countered with pamidronate.

Creatinine

Normal: female 49–90 micromol/litre, male 54–104 micromol/litre.

Creatinine, a waste product of muscle metabolism (hence gender differences), is normally cleared in urine. Unlike urea, creatinine is not produced by any other source, nor is it reabsorbed from glomerular filtrate. Creatinine therefore provides the best guide to renal function (Brochard *et al.*, 2010) and is used to estimate glomerular filtration rate (GFR).

Treatment. Low levels of creatinine are not significant. Raised creatinine (and urea, or low GFR) indicate kidney injury, so renal replacement therapy may be needed.

Glomerular filration rate (GFR)

Normal GFR > 90 ml/min/1.73m².

This is estimated from serum creatinine. Neither serum creatinine nor urine volume is an ideal marker of renal function – serum creatinine may remain normal when GRF is halved (Lee *et al.*, 2016), while tubular reabsorption can affect urine volume. Ideally, filtration across the glomerular bed would be measured, but, as this is impractical, estimated glomerular filtration rate (eGFR) is currently the best indicator.

Urea

Normal: 2.5–7.8 mmol/litre.

Urea is a waste product of (any) protein metabolism, normally cleared in urine. High urea and creatinine usually indicate kidney injury, but if uraemia

Table 21.3 Main biochemistry results

	Normal	(Normal) source	Loss	Main significance	Likely treatments if low	Likely treatments if high
CRP	< 10 mg/litre	liver (acute phase protein)		inflammatory marker		treat cause, not symptom
sodium	135–145 mmol/litre	diet	gut; urine loss regulated by aldosterone	sodium is the main extracellular cation	give sodium (e.g. 0.9% sodium chloride IVI)	sign of dehydration – give water
chloride	95–105 mmol/litre	diet	with salt	combines with sodium to form salt	not significant*	stop saline infusions
potassium	3.5–4.5 mmol/litre	diet (also cells – trauma, fluid shifts)	90% urine, 10% stools; lost with haemofiltration if not added to dialysate	cardiac conduction	potassium supplements	50 iu actrapid + 50 ml 50% glucose IVI
glucose	4.6–6.1 mmol/litre (non-diabetic, adult)	diet	glycolysis	cell energy: $C_6H_{12}O_6 + 6\ O_2 \rightarrow$ 36 molecules of ATP	glucose supplements	insulin
phosphate	0.80–1.45 mmol/litre	diet	urine/haemofiltration	cell energy (adenosine triphosphate has 3 phosphate molecules) and 2,3 DPG	phosphate supplements	not significant, very rare*
magnesium	0.75–1.0 mmol/litre	diet (especially greens)	urine/haemofiltration; gut loss (e.g. vomiting, loose stools/stoma)	energy; calcium antagonist – vasodilates bronchodilates, cardiac conduction	magnesium supplements	not significant; very rare*
calcium (total)	2.2–2.6 mmol/litre	diet	urine	cardiac conduction, clotting, cell repair	calcium supplements	rare*, can be treated calcium antagonists (e.g. pamidrinate; possibly magnesium) or calcium channel blockers
calcium (ionised)	1.1–1.3 mmol/litre	see calcium (total)	see calcium (total)	see calcium (total), but note ionised is the active calcium in blood	see calcium (total)	see calcium (total)
urea	2.5–7.8 mmol/litre	protein metabolism	urine	marker of renal function	not significant*	treat disease (AKI), not symptom
creatinine	female 49–90 male 64–104 micromol/litre	muscle metabolism – 50–100 micromol/day	urine	marker of renal function	not significant*	treat disease (AKI), not symptom

Note: * in critical illness

disproportionately exceeds creatinine (ratio is usually approximately 1:20), excessive protein metabolism is more likely, especially from digestion of blood following gastrointestinal bleeds. Uraemic patients are often disorientated/delirious; whether this is caused by urea or other neurotoxins is debated.

Treatment. As for creatinine.

Implications for practice

- low results are caused by: dilution, loss or failure of supply/to produce;
- high levels are caused by: dehydration (haemoconcentration), excessive intake/production, or failure to clear;
- optimum Hb for most critically ill patients is 70–90 grams/litre;
- key electrolytes in critical illness are usually potassium (aim 4–5.3 mmol/litre if cardiac history/problems), phosphate (aim > 0.8 mmol/litre) and magnesium (aim > 0.7 mmol/litre);
- mild hyperglycaemia commonly occurs with critical illness; in the absence of diabetes, upper target is usually < 10.0 mmol/litre.

Summary

Blood is the transport system of the body, so abnormal results indicate problems but may also cause further complications. Nurses usually download results before medical staff, so understanding main results and how abnormalities should be managed enables earlier treatment.

Further reading

Higgins (2013) provides an accessible book about laboratory investigations. While most medical/nursing articles explore specific aspects, occasionally overview articles appear in medical and sometimes nursing journals. Batterink *et al.* (2015) provide a Cochrane review of hyperkalaemia treatments, acknowledging the paucity of evidence for all interventions. Retter *et al.* (2012) review transfusion of blood and blood products. The British Society for Haematology provide guidelines, available from their website.

Clinical scenarios

Henry Duff is a 68-year-old known diabetic. He was admitted two days ago with bleeding gastric ulcers and has frequent episodes of melaena. He is self-ventilating on 28% oxygen via nasal cannulae, with a respiratory rate between 18 and 28 breaths/min. He has an intravenous infusion of omeprazole (80 mg over 10 hours) in progress. Henry appears to be hallucinating, reports visual disturbances, and is confused and at times agitated, with the following blood results.

217

Haematology		Biochemistry		Arterial blood gas	
Hb	9.2 g/litre	CRP	102 mg/litre	pH	7.48
WBC	18.7 x 10^{-9}/litre	Na$^+$	162 mmol/litre	PaCO$_2$	4.3 kPa
Neutrophils	15.2 x 10^{-9}/litre	K$^+$	4.7 mmol/litre	PaO$_2$	9.5 kPa
Lymphocytes	2.5 x 10^{-9}/litre	Cl$^-$	130 mmol/litre	HCO$_3^-$	25.7 mmol/litre
Platelets	234 x 10^{-9}/litre	Glucose	10.5 mmol/litre	Base Excess	1.1 mmol/litre
INR	1.2	PO$_4^{-3}$	0.74 mmol/litre	Lactate	1.5 mmol/litre
		Mg^{2+}	0.72 mmol/litre		
		Ca^{2+}	2.38 mmol/litre		
		Urea	18.6 mmol/litre		
		Creatinine	136 micromol/litre		
		Albumin	16 g/litre		

Q1. What are likely causes for abnormalities with Henry's blood results? Which ones are problems, which ones are symptoms and which ones are both problems and symptoms?

Q2. Which abnormalities should be treated? Choose the best treatments for Henry.

Q3. Identify rationales for your concerns and choice of treatments.

Chapter 22

ECGs and dysrhythmias

Contents

Fundamental knowledge

Myocardial physiology – automaticity, conductivity,
   rhythmicity
Normal limb electrode placement
Normal cardiac conduction (SA node, AV node,
   Bundle of His, Purkinje fibres)
Physiology of normal sinus rhythm
Current Resuscitation Council guidelines
Experience of using continuous ECG monitoring
   and taking 12-lead ECGs

Introduction

Some dysrhythmias are immediately life-threatening; others may compromise cardiac function by reducing stroke volume and increasing tachycardia and myocardial hypoxia. Dysrhythmias are usually symptoms of underlying problems and may be acute or chronic. Chronic dysrhythmias (atrial fibrillation being especially common) should be controlled but can rarely be reversed. Most acute dysrhythmias should actively be reversed if possible, necessitating close haemodynamic monitoring and support. This chapter focuses on acute rather than chronic problems.

Although ICU nurses seldom see the range of dysrhythmias encountered in coronary care units, ECG monitoring is standard, so nurses should be able to:

- identify dysrhythmias;
- identify likely causes from patients' histories;
- know usual management and treatment for commonly occurring dys-rhythmias.

As with almost all problems, early intervention reduces complication and improves survival and outcome, so ICU nurses should develop expertise in this fundamental aspect of critical care monitoring. Analysis by machines, while a potentially useful aid, is not fully reliable and should not be a substitute for interpretation by staff (Schläpfer and Wellens, 2017).

A parallel chapter in Woodrow (2016) includes some other dysrhythmias and focuses more on ward, rather than ICU, practice. Some commonly used drugs are mentioned, but practices vary, so users should consult summaries of product characteristics (SPCs) or pharmacopaedias for detailed information on drugs.

Normal conduction begins in the sinoatrial node, passing through atrial muscle to the atrioventricular node, then passing from the atrioventricular node through the ventricular conduction pathway and into ventricular myocytes. There are therefore three key stages in normal cardiac conduction and the ECG:

- atrial (P wave);
- atrioventricular node (PR interval);
- ventricular (QRS complex, ST segment, T wave).

The etymologically more accurate "dysrhythmia", rather than the more commonly used "arrhythmia", is used here as, except for asystole, rhythms are problematic rather than absent.

Basic principles of electrocardiography

An ECG is a time/voltage graph of myocardial electrical activity, representing three dimensional events in two. This section summarises basic principles for revision. Any parts unfamiliar to readers should be revised further before proceeding (e.g. from Hampton, 2013a or Woodrow 2016).

- on ECG graph paper, each small square is 1 mm × 1 mm and each large square is 5 mm × 5mm
- horizontal axes represent time;
- ECGs are normally recorded at 25 mm/second, making each large square = 0.2 seconds, each small square = 0.04 seconds. This text discusses timing in large and small squares, which would differ should recording time be changed;
- vertical axes represent voltage; a calibration square (normally 10 mm = 1 mV = 2 large squares) usually appears at the beginning or end of ECG printouts, and often on bedside monitors;
- a normal sinus rhythm complex (Figure 22.1) is labelled PQRST;
- SA and AV nodes have both sympathetic and parasympathetic nerve fibres, so are affected by brainstem control and vagal stimulation; hence suction can cause bradycardia/ectopics/blocks;
- limb electrodes are normally colour-coded:

  - red = right arm;
  - yellow = left arm;
  - green = left leg/hip;
  - black = right leg/hip.

Most ICUs use five-electrode monitors:

  - white = fourth intercostal space to right of sternum (modified chest lead 1: MCL-1);

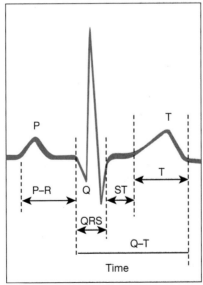

Normal wave form

■ *Figure 22.1 Normal sinus rhythm*

■ electrical "views" remain unchanged anywhere along limbs, or on a line between the limb joint and heart, so electrodes may be placed anywhere along the view line:

- lead I = right arm to left arm (bipolar);
- lead II = right arm to left leg (bipolar);
- lead III = left arm to left leg (bipolar);
- aVR = right arm (unipolar);
- aVL = left arm (unipolar);
- aVF = foot (left leg; unipolar);

■ limb lead II follows the normal "vector" (or "axis") of cardiac conduction, so is usually the default lead for single-lead monitors and rhythm strips on 12-lead ECGs;

■ chest (precordial) leads examine electrical activity from right atrium, through right ventricle, septum, left ventricle, to left atrium (Figure 22.2):

- C (or V) 1 (red): fourth intercostal space, to right of (patient's) sternum;
- C2 (yellow): fourth intercostal space, left of sternum;
- C3 (green): between C2 and C4;
- C4 (brown): fifth intercostal space, midclavicular line;
- C5 (black): between C4 and C6;
- C6 (purple): fifth intercostal space, mid axilla.

Colouring of chest leads almost follows colours in snooker.

■ normal times:

- P wave = 0.08 seconds (two small squares);
- PR interval = 0.12–0.2 seconds (three to five small squares) (measure PR intervals from beginning of the P wave to start of QRS);
- QRS = maximum 0.12 seconds (three small squares);
- T wave = 0.16 seconds (four small squares);

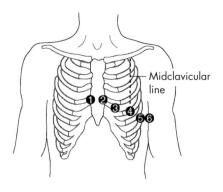

■ *Figure 22.2 Chest lead placement*

- QTc interval = (calculated by monitors) 0.48 seconds (Priori *et al.*, 2015);

■ sinus rhythm = technically, any rhythm origination from the sinoatrial node, although in practice the term is often used to describe regular rhythms of 60–100 beats per minute (bpm) originating from the SA node.

Table 22.1 provides a framework for ECG interpretation.

Action potential

At rest, the electrical charge (polarity) of myocyte membranes is about −90 millivolts (mV). Active movement of cations (positively charged ions) across the cell membrane changes this charge, making the cell electrically excitable

Table 22.1 **Framework for ECG interpretation**

Interpreting the ECG

Regularity
Is the rate regular?
If not, is rate:
■ regularly irregular (is there a pattern?)
■ irregularly irregular (no pattern)

1: P wave
Does the P wave appear before the QRS?
Is there one P wave for every QRS?
Is the shape normal?
Are P waves missing? (check for pacing spikes)

2: PR interval
Is the PR interval three to five small squares?

3: QRS complex
Is the QRS width within three small squares?
Is the axis normal ("positive QRS")?
Is the S wave deep ("negative QRS")?
Does it look normal?

4: ST segment
Does the isoelectric line return between the S and the T?
If not, is it:
elevated (> 1mm above isoelectric line)
depressed (< 0.5 mm below isoelectric line)

5: T wave
Does the T wave look normal?

6. QT interval
Is QTc within 0.48 seconds?
Tachycardia (> 100 bpm)
narrow complex (usually with P waves) = atrial (supraventricular)
broad complex (without P wave) = ventricular

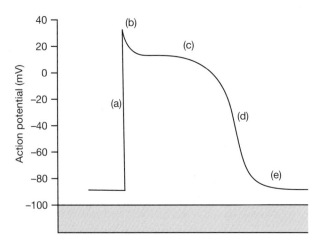

(a) Rapid depolarisation: influx via fast sodium channel (phase 0).
(b) Fast calcium channel open (phase 1).
(c) Plateau: slow calcium channel open (phase 2).
(d) Rapid depolarisation: potassium channel open (phase 3).
(e) Resting phase (phase 4).

Figure 22.3 Action potential

(*depolararisation*). When normal cation concentrations are restored, the charge is stabilised and electrical activity ends (*repolarisation*). Action potential is created by overlapping but sequential prominence of "channels" in myocyte membranes – sodium, calcium, potassium; the calcium channel creates both the peak and main duration of depolarisation, while activity ends with potassium influx. Hence, deranged serum calcium or potassium often causes ectopics and dysrhythmias. Figure 22.3 shows an action potential graph.

Lead changes

Each lead views cardiac conduction differently, so the aspect of the heart affected may be identified through leads viewing that aspect of the heart (see Figure 22.4).

Usual lead placement does not view posterior myocardium clearly, but posterior infarction is best seen in C1 and C2.

Six-step analysis

Using Figure 22.2, a six-step analysis is recommended.

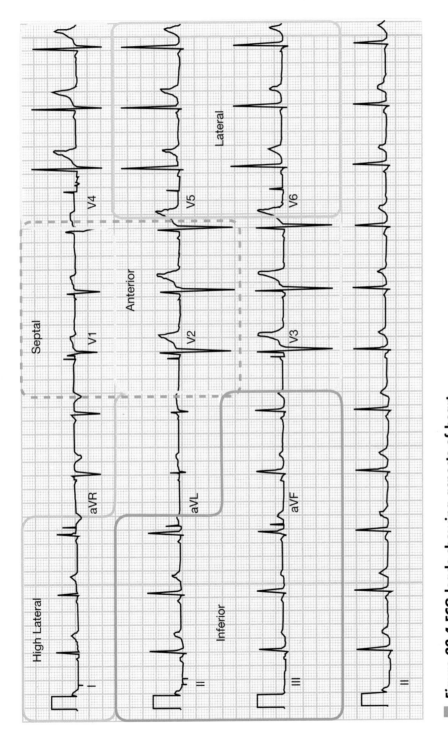

Figure 22.4 ECG leads showing aspects of heart

Step 1. P wave

The P wave represents atrial *depolarisation* (activity). P waves are normally small, resembling a "hump-back bridge". P wave abnormalities include:

- tall (peaked), usually right atrial hypertrophy;
- wide (often bifid, "notched", "P mitrale"), usually left ventricular hypertrophy;
- inverted – ectopic pacemaker.

Step 2. PR interval

Normal PR, measured from the start of the P wave, is three to five small squares, or no more than one large square. This represents the impulse crossing through the AV node. Abnormal PR intervals can only be:

- too short or
- too wide.

Short PR intervals are very rare. Long PR intervals are relatively common – see first-degree block below.

Step 3. QRS

This represents ventricular depolarisation. Being conducted through the Bundle of His, bundle branches and Purkinje fibres, it is quick, not more than three small squares wide.

Step 4. ST segment

From the S wave, ECG complexes should return almost vertically to the isoelectric line. Any ST elevation or depression should be noted and, if new, reported. Monitors used in ICU can usually detect ST abnormalities.

ST elevation (2 mm in chest leads, 1 mm in limb leads) in two or more consecutive leads usually indicates acute myocardial infarction. Classification of *acute coronary syndromes* into:

- ST elevation myocardial infarction (STEMI)
- non-ST elevation myocardial infarction (NSTEMI), and
- unstable angina (UA)

is discussed in Chapter 29.

- ST depression usually indicates ischaemia.
- T = ventricular *repolarisation* (end of activity).

Step 6. QT interval

The QT interval represents ventricular depolarisation. Monitors usually calculate "corrected" QT intervals (QTc) – what the QT interval would be if heart rate were 60 bpm. Normal QTc is 0.48 seconds (Priori *et al.*, 2015).

Long (QTc > 0.48 second) or short (< 0.34 second) QT results in excessive or insufficient proportions of the cardiac cycle with the ventricles being electrically active, which may trigger ventricular tachycardia (VT) (Priori *et al.*, 2015). Genetic abnormalities can cause "prolonged QT syndrome" but long QT intervals can also be triggered by:

- drugs (e.g. amiodarone, vancomycin, tricyclic antidepressants, soltalol);
- electrolyte imbalances (e.g. potassium, calcium, magnesium);
- hypothermia.

(Chevalier and Scridon, 2011)

U waves

These are seldom present, if present seldom seen, and if seen seldom significant. They appear like a second, smaller T wave. They may indicate electrolyte abnormality, such as hyperkalaemia or hypercalcaemia.

General treatments

Underlying causes (e.g. electrolytes – especially potassium and calcium) of dysrhythmias should be resolved, but otherwise asymptomatic dysrhythmias seldom require treatment. Haemodynamic compromise (hypotension) necessitates action.

Myocardial hypoxia is often present, so oxygen is usually a first-line treatment. But, since hyperoxia is tissue toxic (Eastwood *et al.*, 2016), oxygen should be given to achieve normal levels, which are usually SpO_2 94–98%, or 88–92% with COPD (B.T.S., 2017).

Most *drugs* ("chemical cardioversion") used either suppress myocardial automaticity or change AV node conduction (some increasing, others decreasing). New dysrhythmias may be caused by drugs, so drug charts should be reviewed – pharmacists are a useful source for advice about side effects. If possible, problem drugs should be discontinued – e.g. salbutamol may cause tachycardia; metochlopramide may cause bradycardia. Bradycardic dysrhythmias may need positive *chronotropes* (e.g. atropine). Tachycardic dysrhythmias are often caused by overexcitability. Amiodarone is often the first-line drug, as it reduces ventricular and supraventricular tachycardias. Ventricular conduction may be blocked with:

- beta-blockers (esmolol, sotalol, propanolol), which inhibit beta receptors (see Chapter 34);
- calcium channel blockers (e.g. diltiazem).

Poor cardiac output may necessitate positive inotropes, such as dobutamine (see Chapter 34).

If drugs fail, electrical cardioversion may restore stable rhythms. "Overpacing", using faster pacing rates, may also restore stable rhythms but is not generally used in most ICUs. Pacing can be used for bradycardias but significant problems are rare in ICU.

Problems likely to persist should be referred to cardiologists, as later ablation (destruction of abnormal pacemakers or conduction pathways) or other treatments may be needed.

Carotid massage is sometimes used to slow supraventricular tachycardias by stimulating the vagus nerve. It may be successful, but efficacy is unpredictable, and can cause thrombotic strokes in patients with vascular disease (many ICU patients). Carotid massage is therefore contraindicated with recent stroke or transient ischaemic attack – TIA (Ungar *et al.*, 2016) and is generally best avoided. If used, it should only be applied unilaterally, as bilateral massage can obstruct cerebral blood flow altogether.

Ectopics

Two key questions should be answered about ectopics:

- where do they originate?
- what is their timing?

There are three possible answers to the first question:

- atrial
- junctional/nodal
- ventricular,

And, provided underlying rhythms are regular, two possible answers to the second:

- *premature* (before expected impulses) or
- *escape* (expected complexes are absent, so ectopic impulses "escape" into gaps).

With irregularly irregular rhythms (e.g. atrial fibrillation), timing of ectopics cannot be identified.

Premature complexes indicate overexcitability. Escape ectopics indicate failed conduction. Likely causes of overexcitability or failed conduction include:

- damaged conduction pathways (infarction, oedema, hypoxia);
- drugs/stimulants;

■ electrolyte imbalance (especially potassium; also calcium, magnesium);
■ acidosis.

Escape ectopics provide pulses that would otherwise be absent, so provide "a friend in need" and should never be treated, although causes of the failed normal conduction should be resolved.

Treatment. Occasional ectopics seldom need treating, but underlying causes should (if possible) be resolved. Potassium imbalance is the most likely single cause, so serum potassium is usually maintained at 4–5.3 mmol/litre. Calcium and magnesium imbalances can also cause ectopics.

Frequent premature ectopics should be treated before they progress to dysrhythmias. Generally, amiodarone is the drug of choice for rhythm control in ICU, although rate control drugs such as calcium channel blockers, beta-blockers and other drugs (e.g. digoxin) may be used. Drugs used vary with focus and cause (see below).

Atrial ectopics (see Figure 22.5) have:

■ abnormal P waves;
■ possibly different PR intervals;
■ normal QRS, ST and T.

Junctional/nodel ectopics have:

■ no P wave (or occasionally inverted P waves, which may be before or after the QRS);
■ normal QRS, ST and T.

Ventricular ectopics (see Figure 22.6) have:

■ no P wave;
■ (usually) broad QRS (three small squares).

Complexes from a single focus ("unifocal") look alike; ectopics with different shapes originate from different foci ("multifocal"). A sequence of three or more ectopics is sometimes called a *salvo*.

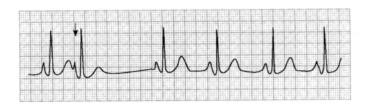

■ *Figure 22.5 Premature atrial ectopic*

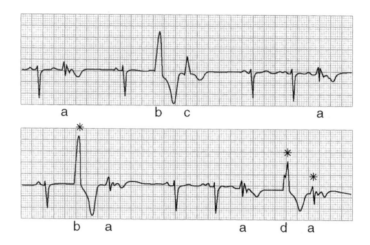

Figure 22.6 Multifocal ventricular ectopics

Atrial dysrhythmias

Sinus arrhythmia (see Figure 22.7) occurs in a few young, usually athletic, people. Inspiration significantly increases venous return, and so heart rate. Sinus arrhythmia is rarely seen in ICU, is rarely problematic and should not be treated.

Sinus bradycardia. Although any sinus rate below 60 bpm is technically sinus bradycardia, significant problems usually only develop with rates below 50.

Treatment. Sinus bradycardia is only treated if symptomatic or problematic – rare in ICU. Obvious causes should be removed, so oxygen should be optimised. Rate may be increased with atropine or other drugs, but if problems persist pacing may be needed.

Sinus tachycardia. Tachycardia is any sinus rate > 100 bpm. Although normal in young children, tachycardia is abnormal with adults, but many critically ill patients have compensatory mild tachycardias. Rates up to 130 bpm usually provide effective compensation; faster rates result in significantly reduced

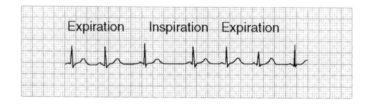

Figure 22.7 Sinus arrhythmia

stroke volumes and are often called *supraventricular tachycardia*. Most positive inotropes are also positive chronotropes (= increase heart rate).

Supraventricular tachycardia (see Figure 22.8) is any tachycardia originating above the ventricles, although usually implies rates exceeding 130 bpm, where decompensation causes hypotension. Narrow-complex tachycardia must be SVT, but not all SVTs have narrow complexes: ventricular depolarisation abnormalities can cause broadening of the QRS. More specific terms, such as "atrial tachycardia" (i.e. originating in the atrium but not sinus), are sometimes used.

Treatment. In the ICU, SVT is usually treated with amiodarone. Other drugs, such as beta-blockers, may sometimes be tried.

Atrial fibrillation (AF) (see Figure 22.9) occurs in approximately half of hospitalised patients. The key question is whether it is new or "old". Atrial fibrillation should be classified as:

- first diagnosed (regardless of duration or symptoms);
- paroxysmal: spontaneous termination, usually within 48 hours, can persist seven days;
- persistent: not self-terminating;
- long-standing: > 1 year;
- permanent ("accepted"): no cardioversion attempted,

(Task Force, 2016b),

the first four being "new", where the aim is to stop fibrillation. With "old" (permanent, accepted, chronic), the AF cannot be reversed, so the aim is to control it.

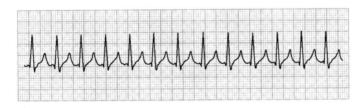

Figure 22.8 Supraventricular tachycardia

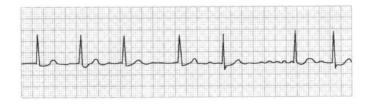

Figure 22.9 Atrial fibrillation

231

New-onset AF may be provoked by disease or surgery. If not self-resolving, AF should be reversed if possible. Permanent/established ("chronic") AF should be controlled.

AF causes chaotic atrial activity, seen by either a chaotically wavy or almost flat line between ventricular electrical activity. QRS complexes, ST segments and T waves are normal (unless there are other cardiac problems), but timing (space) between ventricular contractions (QRS complexes) is erratic – irregularly irregular. Loss of atrioventricular synchrony ("atrial kick") reduces stroke volume by 5–15% (Task Force, 2010a), which usually provokes compensatory tachycardia.

Treatment. New-onset AF should be cardioverted either electrically or chemically, the preferred chemical usually being amiodarone (Camm *et al.*, 2012). Other drugs, or electrical cardioversion, are occasionally used. Controlling permanent AF necessitates both:

- rate control: aim < 110 bpm (Task Force, 2016b) and
- anticoagulation: aim INR 2.5 (Keeling *et al.*, 2011).

Traditionally, rate control was most often achieved with digoxin, but digoxin may increase AF mortality (Vamos *et al.*, 2015); Task Force (2016b) recommends beta-blockers or calcium channel blockers for rate control.

Passive blood flow through atrium can cause a thrombus, and therefore possible thromboembolism. Stroke risk is increased fivefold by AF (Camm *et al.*, 2012), hence the importance of anticoagulation.

Atrial flutter (see Figure 22.10). An ectopic pacemaker in the atrium causes rapid atrial waves with distinctive sawtooth shapes ("F" or flutter waves), typically 300 bpm. This rate exceeds possible AV nodes conduction, so a regular block occurs, usually of an even ratio (e.g. 2:1, 4:1, 6:1 or 8:1). A 4:1 AV block with atrial rates of 300 creates ventricular responses of 75 bpm. But blocks can change suddenly, creating gross tachycardia (2:1 block = ventricular rate 150/minute) or bradycardia.

Treatment. Generally, electrical cardioversion is usually preferred, but chemical cardioversion (e.g. amiodarone) may restore sinus rhythm. Where pacing wires are already inserted, such as following cardiac surgery, "over-pacing" may be preferred.

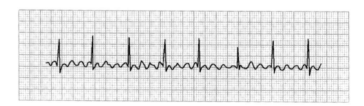

Figure 22.10 Atrial flutter

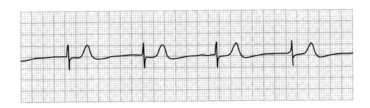

■ *Figure 22.11* **Nodal/junctional rhythm**

Junctional (or "nodal") rhythm (see Figure 22.11) describes impulses originating in the AV node or atrioventricular junction. Rate is often (but not always) slower than sinus/atrial rhythms. P waves are not usually seen, but if present are inverted, and may appear after QRSs. Irritation (oedema, mechanical – e.g. central lines in the right atrium) may cause junctional ectopics. Oedema from cardiac surgery often causes transient junctional rhythms, hence epicardial pacing wires.

Treatment. Junctional rates are often sufficient to support life but should be closely monitored. If bradycardia becomes symptomatic, treat as sinus bradycardia above – atropine, pacing.

Atrioventricular blocks

Any conduction pathway may be blocked by:

- infarction
- oedema
- ischaemia.

If oedema or ischaemia resolve, blocks usually disappear. Infarction usually causes permanent block. Blocks may occur at the atrioventricular node (first-, second- or third-degree) or in one of the bundle branches.

First-degree (AV node) block (see Figure 22.12), delayed atrioventricular node conduction, prolongs PR intervals beyond 0.2 seconds (five small squares). Despite delay, every impulse is conducted, so a QRS complex follows each P wave. Acute blocks may be caused by disease or drugs. Chronic first-degree

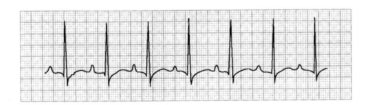

■ *Figure 22.12* **First-degree block**

block is usually from age-related sclerosis of the atrioventricular node, and is rarely problematic.

Treatment. Acute blocks should be monitored, but only treated if bradycardia causes problems. Chronotropes (e.g. atropine) or pacing can resolve symptomatic bradycardia.

Second-degree block, or incomplete heart block, occurs when at regular intervals there is an unconducted P wave. There are two types of second-degree block:

■ Mobitz type 1, also called "Wenkebach": progressive lengthening of PR intervals until an atrial impulse is unconducted (see Figure 22.13);
■ Mobitz type 2: constant PR intervals, with regular unconducted P waves (e.g. 2:1; see Figure 22.14).

Mobitz type 2 is less common, but more serious, than type 1, as it is more likely to progress into third-degree block or asystole (Vogler *et al.*, 2012; Houghton and Gray, 2014).

Treatment. If new and/or symptomatic, optimise oxygen and remove causes (e.g. any drugs blocking conduction). Chemical cardioversion may help, but pacing is often needed.

Third-degree block (see Figure 22.15), also called complete heart block, causes complete atrioventricular dissociation. Any atrial activity (e.g. P waves) is unrelated to QRS complexes; some P waves may be "lost" in QRS or T waves. Patients with third-degree block more often have atrial fibrillation, in which case dyssynchrony may be less obvious. Ventricular pacemakers usually cause broad, regular but slow QRS complexes – often 30 bpm). Cardiac output and blood pressure are usually compromised.

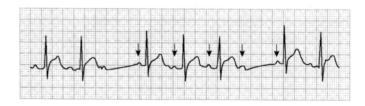

■ *Figure 22.13 Second-degree block (type 1)*

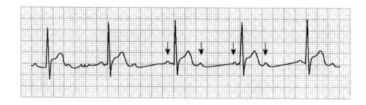

■ *Figure 22.14 Second-degree block (type 2)*

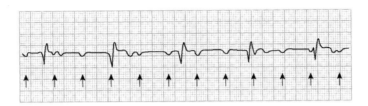

■ *Figure 22.15* **Third-degree block**

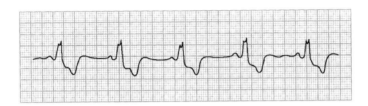

■ *Figure 22.16* **Bundle branch block**

Treatment. Unless transient, pacing is almost invariably needed. Until pacing is commenced, optimise oxygen.

Bundle branch blocks

This occurs (see Figure 22.16) when conduction through one of branches from the Bundle of His, or one or more of the left hemibranches, is blocked. This creates two QRS complexes – a normal one from the intact branch, and a broadened ventricular-shaped complex from impulses spreading across the septum. This RSR, or biphasic QRS, wave creates the characteristic M or W shapes on ECGs.

Left bundle branch block causes a W in early, and an M in late chest leads; right bundle branch block reverses this picture. The mnemonics WiLLiaM and MaRRoW may be useful:

■ WiLLiaM: W in C1 and W in C6 = LBBB;
■ MaRRoW: M in C1 and (often) W in C6 = RBBB.

New left bundle block (i.e. not on previous ECGs) indicates myocardial infarction, is classified as STEMI (ST wave elevated myocardial infarction – see Chapter 29), necessitating urgent pPCI. New right bundle branch block often necessitates management of heart failure but may be treated with PCI.

Ventricular dysrhythmias

Ventricular impulses originate in ventricular muscle, so usually travel from muscle fibre to muscle fibre rather than through conduction pathways, making

235

progress relatively slow, giving them typically broad QRS complexes. Impulses originating in or near conduction pathways may have narrow complexes. Rates typically commence slowly (about 30 bpm), but myocardial hypoxia rapidly accelerates rate, often to gross tachycardia.

Bigeminy (Figure 22.17) and *trigeminy* are sinister extensions of ventricular ectopics, occurring regularly. Bigeminy is one ventricular ectopic every other complex; trigeminy is one ventricular ectopic every third complex. Ectopics are usually unifocal, usually from hypoxia or digoxin toxicity.

Treatment. Trigeminy is not usually treated. Provided underlying causes are resolved, bigeminy can be treated with rhythm stabilisers.

Ventricular tachycardia (see Figure 22.18) is a regular rhythm, with rapid unifocal impulses (typically 200–250 bpm). Asymptomatic VT rarely persists, either reverting or progressing after a few minutes.

Treatment. Ventricular tachycardia with a pulse may respond to drugs (e.g. amiodarone), but pulseless VT is a shockable rhythm, necessitating immediate resuscitation.

Torsades de pointes (see Figure 22.19), a rare type of multifocal ventricular tachycardia, causes ECG traces to "twist" around isoelectric baselines, creating an irregular broad-complex tachycardia. If prolonged or untreated it leads to ventricular fibrillation. It may be caused by drugs (e.g. amiodarone,

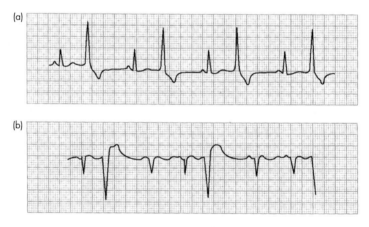

Figure 22.17 Bigeminy and trigeminy

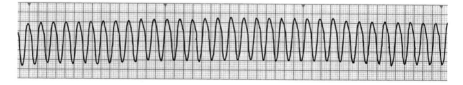

Figure 22.18 Ventricular tachycardia

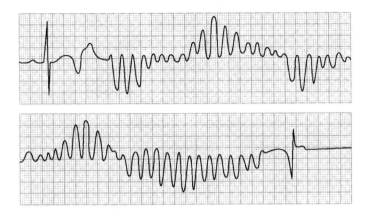

■ *Figure 22.19* **Torsades de pointes**

vancomycin, soltolol), severe electrolyte imbalance (especially hypokalaemia, hypomagnesaemia), subarachnoid haemorrhage, myocardial infarction, angina, bradycardia, sinoatrial block or congenital abnormality.

Treatment. Electrolyte imbalances or underlying causes should be treated, and drugs that prolong QT intervals should be stopped. It often results from hypomagnesiumaemia, so magnesium is usually the first-line drug for torsades (Houghton and Gray, 2014; Priori *et al.*, 2015). If drugs fail, temporary atrial or ventricular pacing or cardiopulmonary resuscitation may be necessary.

Ventricular fibrillation (VF) (see Figure 22.20) is almost invariably fatal in two to three minutes. VF may be coarse or fine; fine ventricular fibrillation may appear like asystole, so increasing gain on ECGs shows whether "f" waves are present.

Treatment. Ventricular fibrillation is a shockable rhythm, necessitating immediate resuscitation.

Asystole (= ventricular standstill), literally absence of systole, appears as an uninterrupted isoelectric line, although progression from dysrhythmias to asystole may persist for considerable time ("dying" heart), with occasional atrial or ventricular complexes. Chest wall movement from breathing (including mechanical ventilation) typically causes slow undulations to the isoelectric line.

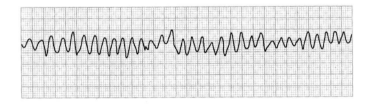

■ *Figure 22.20* **Ventricular fibrillation**

Absence of any cardiac function is an arrest situation. Absence of complexes on ECGs may be caused by:

- disconnection/failed electrodes (e.g. dry gel): typically causes a perfectly horizontal isoelectric line;
- fine VF – increasing height ("gain") of ECG may reveal fibrillation.

Arterial line and/or pulse oximetry monitoring may indicate pulses, but if only ECG is being monitored; both the above should be checked.

Treatment. Asystole is not a shockable rhythm. Cardiac compressions and drugs (following the Resuscitation Council algorithm) are essential to maintain effective circulation. If P waves are present, external or transvenous pacing may be used, but, whatever treatments are tried, resuscitation is seldom successful.

Pulseless electrical activity (PEA) results in whatever electrical activity is seen not being translated into pulses and arterial blood pressure traces. ECG traces are usually abnormal, often showing tachycardia and with low amplitude complexes. PEA is typically caused by one of the "4Hs and 4Ts" reversible causes:

- Hypoxia
- Hypovolaemia
- Hyper/hypokalaemia
- Hypothermia
- Tension pneumothorax
- Tamponade
- Toxic/therapeutic disturbances (drug overdose)
- Thrombi (PE, MI).

Causes are usually obvious from patients' histories.

Treatment. Pulseless electrical activity is not a shockable rhythm. Cardiac compressions and drugs should be given. Underlying causes should be reversed.

Implications for practice

- most dysrhythmias are only treated if problematic, but underlying causes (e.g. hypoxia, electrolytes) should be resolved;
- chest pain, together with either ST elevation (1 mm in chest leads, 2 mm in limb leads) in two or more consecutive leads or a new left bundle branch block indicates acute myocardial infarction – STEMI;
- ectopics may originate from any part of the heart. Atrial ectopics have abnormal P waves, but normal QRS. Junctional ectopics have no P wave, but normal QRS. Ventricular ectopics have no P wave, and broad and bizarre QRS;
- isolated ectopics are insignificant, but frequent premature ectopics indicate overexcitability. Escape ectopics are "a friend in need" so should not be treated. Causes of failed conduction should be resolved;

■ ST depression usually indicates ischaemia;
■ nurses should know current Resuscitation Council guidelines.

Summary

Critical illness exposes ICU patients to various symptomatic dysrhythmias, so ICU patients are usually continuously monitored; ICU nurses should therefore be able to recognise common dysrhythmias and initiate appropriate action. Many drugs are used in cardiology, but most acute problematic dysrhythmias respond to amiodarone. ICU staff should already be familiar with basic electrocardiography, so this chapter has discussed dysrhythmias most likely to be seen in ICU, together with standard treatments.

Further reading

Current Resuscitation Council guidelines can be downloaded from the UK Resuscitation Council website. The European Society of Cardiology produce guidelines for many common dysrhythmias, which can be downloaded from their website. There are many books, articles and internet resources for ECG interpretation. Hampton (2013a) provides a useful overview, with supplementary detail in Hampton (2013b) and examples for practice in Hampton (2013c). Houghton and Gray (2014) is also useful. Campbell *et al.* (2017) provide national guidelines for recording ECGs.

Clinical scenarios

Q1. Describe how you would perform a 12-lead ECG on an ICU patient who is awake. Include how you would explain the procedure, position the patient and apply electrodes to ensure an accurate and optimal ECG tracing.

Q2. For continuous bedside ECG monitoring in ICU, which lead is usually chosen for waveform analysis? Have you seen other leads used, and if so why?

Q3. Have you witnessed external carotid massage for tachycardia? Identify why this was used, risks and limitations, and issues of professional accountability. List alternative strategies that can be used to reduce life-threatening tachycardia, together with their benefits and limitations.

Chapter 23

Neurological monitoring

Contents

Fundamental knowledge

Brainstem function
Cerebral blood supply – carotid arteries, Circle of Willis
Cerebral autoregulation
Sedation (see Chapter 6)

Introduction

Many ICU patients have acutely altered neurological function, whether from chemical sedation, disease of other organs/systems, or specific neurological disease/damage. Patients unconscious on admission may have suffered hypoxic brain damage, which can only be fully assessed on waking. Some ICUs specialise in neurosurgery or neuromedicine, but most units receive patients with head injuries and cranial pathologies. Many conditions, such as meningitis, hepatic failure, can increase intracranial pressure, causing both acute confusion and physiological complications. Nurses should therefore assess and monitor neurological function.

The nervous system can be differentiated between central and peripheral. The central nervous system is the brain and spinal cord. Peripheral nerves link the spinal cord to all other organs and tissues. Either, or both, parts of the nervous system may be dysfunctional, and therefore assessment should measure whichever part of the nervous system is a cause for concern.

The simplest way to assess neurological function is whether someone is responding appropriately and in their normal manner. Unfortunately, diseases and treatments prevent normal responses in many ICU patients, but with conscious patients their actions and communication (non-verbal as well as verbal) should be assessed. Acute neurological changes may be caused by abnormal biochemistry, especially glucose (Hare *et al.*, 2008), so biochemistry should be assessed. Other non-invasive assessments can indicate:

- consciousness (Glasgow Coma Scale);
- cranial nerve function (pupil responses, gag, cough, facial movements);
- spinal nerve function (limb movement).

Invasive neurological monitoring is largely limited to neurological centres, although is sometimes used elsewhere. Technological developments have increased availability of less invasive and non-invasive alternatives. However neurological function is assessed, it should be understood by staff and beneficial to patients. Assessments recorded and reported should remain factual, and any limiting factors noted with the report. For example, intubated patients cannot make a verbal response, and pupil size or muscle strength may be evaluated differently by different observers. Where assessors are uncertain about their evaluation, they should seek a second opinion.

Intracranial pressure

Most of the total adult intracranial volume (average 1.7 litres) is brain tissue, the remaining 300 ml being divided between blood and cerebrospinal fluid – CSF (March and Hickey, 2014). Because the skull is rigid and filled to capacity with essentially noncompressible contents (the *Monro-Kellie hypothesis*), increasing one component necessarily compresses others. Small and transient increases of intracranial contents may be compensated for (*compliance*) by

241

displacing blood and CSF into the spinal column, so coughing, straining or sneezing do not usually cause problems. But sustained pressure, once compliance is exhausted, inevitably causes intracranial hypertension (see Figures 23.1 and 23.2). Any pressure on vital centres may affect vital signs, so neurological assessment should be evaluated in the context of vital signs, especially pulse and blood pressure.

Normal adult intracranial pressure is 0–10 mmHg (Carney *et al.*, 2016). Increased intracranial contents, such as cerebral oedema or bleeding, increase intracranial pressure, causing neurological dysfunction. Sustained intracranial pressures of 20–30 mmHg may cause injury. Sustained intracranial pressure above 60 mmHg causes irreversible ischaemic brain damage and is usually fatal (Bahouth, 2018). Progressive cell damage (see Chapter 24) causes a vicious cycle of intracranial hypertension and tissue injury (see Figure 23.3).

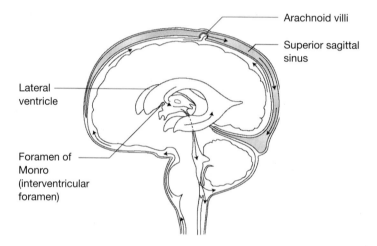

Figure 23.1 Cross-section of the cranium

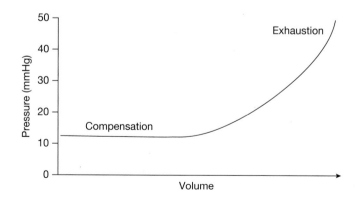

Figure 23.2 Pressure/volume curve

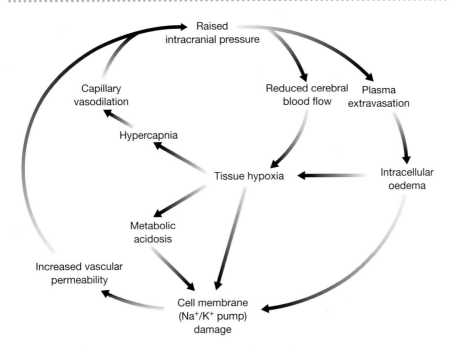

Figure 23.3 Intracranial hypertension and tissue injury: a vicious circle

Cerebral blood flow

The brain normally receives about 15% of cardiac output. The single main factor affecting cerebral perfusion is mean arterial pressure. Brain cells have high metabolic rates, yet unlike most cells have no ATP (energy) stores. Therefore, without constant supplies of oxygen and glucose, ischaemic damage rapidly occurs. In health, autoregulation maintains relatively constant cerebral blood flow, if necessary depriving other tissues to supply the brain. But cerebral damage can cause autoregulation to fail (Ho, 2016), resulting in excessively high or low CPP. Cerebral perfusion pressure (CPP) is also limited by the inability of the skull to expand, and so CPP is the difference between mean arterial pressure (MAP) and intracranial pressure:

$$CPP = MAP - ICP$$

Monitors can calculate CPP from ICP. The arterial transducer should be at aortic root level, not head level. It can also be estimated by non-invasive transcranial Doppler, although Cardim *et al.* (2016) found differences of ±12 mmHg compared with invasive methods, which given normal ranges of ICP make this currently impractical.

CPP should be high enough to fully perfuse the brain without increasing intracranial pressure – Carney *et al.* (2016) tentatively suggest that normal CPP is 60–70 mmHg, and higher CPP should be avoided because of risks of respiratory depression. Initial symptoms of insufficient or excessive CPP may include acute confusion and fitting, but sustained high or low CPP is likely to cause cell death.

Cerebral oxygenation is also influenced by oxygen carriage (e.g. hypoxia, anaemia). So management of intracranial hypertension should consider total trends and factors affecting cerebral demand and supply, rather than focusing on single measurements or parameters.

Hypocapnia may cause cerebral vasoconstriction, and so ischaemia, while hypercapnia increases intracranial pressure. Ventilation should therefore aim for normocapnia – $PaCO_2$ 4.6–6.0 kPa (Carney *et al.*, 2016; Hunningher and Smith, 2006).

Cerebral oedema

Intracranial hypertension is usually caused by cerebral oedema (May, 2009), which can be:

▪ interstitial or
▪ intracellular

but is usually:

▪ vasogenic.

Interstitial and intracellular oedema formation is discussed in Chapter 33.

Vasogenic hypertension is caused when blood/brain barrier failure causes excessive blood flow into capillaries, forcing proteins across capillary walls. Proteins in tissue spaces draw further fluid into already oedematous tissue.

Glasgow Coma Scale

Normal: 14–15.

The Glasgow Coma Scale (GCS) (Teasdale and Jennett, 1974) is an established means of assessing level of consciousness by evaluating eye, verbal and motor responses. Eye opening is regulated by the brainstem, mediated through nerves passing between the two hemispheres; Voice is controlled by two speech centres in the left hemisphere, and motor responses are controlled by the cerebral cortex, so GCS achieves simple and quick assessment of much of the brain.

As each item scores one point more than the box below, the minimum score is 3 and the maximum 15. Scores below 14 indicate impaired consciousness:

▪ 13 = mild impairment;
▪ 9–12 = moderate impairment;
▪ 3–8 = severe impairment (coma).

Scores of 8 or below indicate a high risk of airway obstruction from impaired consciousness, placing airway at risk, so usually necessitating intubation (Riley and de Beer, 2014). Assessment should include distinguishing purposeful from reflex responses – e.g. eyes opening spontaneously may be a reflex. In 2014 Teasdale modified some wording of the scale to reduce ambiguity; the updated scale is shown in Figure 23.4.

Response to painful stimuli may already have been observed, such as localising irritation from oxygen masks or endotracheal tubes/suction. Inflicting pain conflicts with fundamental values of nursing, so should only be used when therapeutic benefits outweigh humanitarian considerations. Pain may also cause physiological harm, such as increasing intracranial pressure and stress responses. As peripheral stimuli may elicit spinal reflex responses of guarding or withdrawal, central stimuli should be used to assess consciousness (Cree, 2003). Central stimuli include:

- suborbital pressure (running a finger along the bony ridge at the top of the eye);
- trapezium squeeze (pinching trapezius muscle, between head and shoulders);
- sternal rub (grinding the sternum with knuckles);
- mandibular pressure – pushing upwards and inwards on the angle of the patient's jaw for maximum 30 seconds (Waterhouse, 2005).

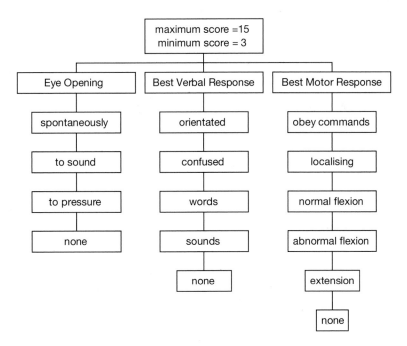

Figure 23.4 Glasgow Coma Scale

Source: Adapted from Teasdale, 2014.

Peripheral stimuli, such as nail bed pressure, may elicit central responses (Lower, 2003), such as grimacing, or peripheral reflexes (see below).

Different stimuli may be appropriate for different patients and situations. Painful stimuli should not be inflicted if patients respond to clear commands (Dougherty and Lister, 2015). The trapezium squeeze should not be used if patients have neck injury, although the opposite shoulder to one-sided injury should be considered. Suborbital pressure should be avoided with skull fractures. The two remaining listed stimuli should only be used in extreme circumstances. Once widely used, the sternal rub is now discouraged as it can cause severe bruising and skin damage; if there is cervical spine injury, that may cause responses to be absent. Mandibular pressure is more difficult, and may dislocate the jaw, so is again not recommended. If response from one stimulus is unclear, other stimuli should be attempted.

Neurological crises may occur rapidly; secondary damage occurring before intermittent measurement (e.g. Glasgow Coma Scale) detects deterioration. Frequency of GCS monitoring varies greatly. In the ICU, GCS is generally assessed each shift, or more frequently if there are neurological concerns.

GCS does not measure peripheral nerve function or effectiveness of chemical sedatives, and in the ICU eye responses may be impaired by disease or drugs. Although it does not measure pupil reaction or cardiovascular function, these are both affected by brainstem function, so are important adjuncts to GCS assessment. Other limitations of GCS include the following:

■ The overall score combines three separate assessments, so as well as the cumulative score, the score for each component should be recorded.
■ Being intermittent, deterioration can occur between assessments. Frequency of assessments should therefore be determined by risk of deterioration.
■ One of the three areas assessed is verbal response, but intubation prevents a verbal response. Dysphasia and aphasia may remain after acute crises have passed.
■ Scores may be inconsistent between different users (Green, 2011).

Like any observation, GCS assessment may be useful but is only part of the overall situation.

Pupil size and response

Normal: PERTL; normal size varies with light level.

Normally, pupils constrict in light and dilate in darkness. Pupil response is best assessed in a darkened area (if possible) to dilate the pupils. Both eyes should be assessed for:

■ pupil size (in millimetres);
■ whether both pupils are equal (PE).

Eyelids may need to be gently raised. A bright light (e.g. pentorch) should then be moved from the corner to the centre of the eye, assessing:

■ how briskly pupils react to light (RTL).

Light is sensed by the optic nerve (cranial nerve II), to which pupil reaction is regulated through the occulomotor nerve (cranial nerve III). Although we can consciously close individual eyelids, light sensed by one eye causes bilateral constriction. Constriction to light is normally brisk, so sluggish responses indicate either brainstem damage or cranial nerve III dysfunction. 10% of people have unequal pupils (Amide, 2017); otherwise, dilated, fixed or (significantly) unequal pupils are usually late signs of intracranial hypertension (Waterhouse, 2005). Drugs affecting pupils include atropine (dilate) and opioids (pinpoint constriction).

Owing to discrepancies between different assessors, Olson *et al.* (2016) recommend pupilometry, technology which measures the Neurological Pupil Index (NPi; normal = 3–5), quantifying pupil reaction. Chen *et al.* (2011) recommends pupilometry as a non-invasive alternative to assess intracranial hypertension. Whether precise quantification adds to patient prognostication and outcome, or merely fulfils clinicians' pursuit of objectivity, remains to be seen.

Limb assessment

Normal: equal + strong.

Limb movement requires both peripheral nerve and muscle function. Peripheral motor nerves may respond to either:

■ painful peripheral stimuli, transmitted through sensory nerves and causing spinal reflexes, or
■ central nervous stimuli (response to commands).

Both legs and both arms should be tested together, by:

■ asking patients to lift their limbs;
■ holding feet/hands and asking patients to push you away;
■ asking patients to grip your hands;
■ if unable to move limbs, test ability to localise sensation – initially light sensations such as touch, but if these elicit no response, painful peripheral stimuli may be needed (e.g. fingernail pressure).

Assessment should evaluate:

■ strength (strong, medium, weak);
■ co-ordination;
■ any unilateral weakness.

Many people are slightly stronger on their dominant side, and for GCS assessment the stronger motor response should be scored, but significant weakness on one side may indicate a stroke or other problem, so should be noted and reported. Ability to raise legs when lying supine in bed also indicates significant muscle strength, and probable ability to breathe without ventilator support.

If not over-ridden by central nervous control, peripheral stimuli should cause guarding/defensive spinal reflexes, such as *flexion* (withdrawal). Central nervous system damage may cause abnormal peripheral responses, such as *extension* (pushing towards the stimulus) or *decorticate* posture (limbs flexed rigidly outwards).

Near infrared spectroscopy (nirs)

Normal cerebral StO_2: 60–80% (Samraj and Nicolas, 2015).

Spectroscopy measures tissue (venous) oxygenation (StO_2) using infrared light, and has potential to measure organ oxygenation, including cerebral (Biedrzycka and Lango, 2016). For cerebral measurement, probes are placed on the temples. Experimentally, spectroscopy has been used to assess both systemic and tissue oxygenation – effectively oxygen demand and supply, which has potential benefits for surgery, interventions and disease management in diverse parts of the body. StO2 only indicates oxygenation in the area beneath the probe, and much of the skull is unsuitable for probe placement, so localised injury elsewhere may remain undetected (Samraj and Nicolas, 2015).

Jugular venous bulb saturation (SjO₂)

Spectroscopy via jugular vein catheterisation can measure cerebral oxygen uptake – jugular bulb saturation (*SjO2*). As this is blood returning from cerebral oxygenation, it indicates global cerebral uptake. Low levels are often artefactual but may indicate cerebral hypoperfusion. High, and rising, SjO_2 often indicates increased cerebral blood flow, and very high levels (> 85%) usually indicate imminent death. Owing to high cerebral oxygen uptake, SjO_2 is lower than StO_2 elsewhere – Samraj and Nicolas (2015) suggest normal systemic StO_2 is 65–90%. Being non-invasive, it is an attractive option, but has not significantly been adopted into clinical practice, partly owing to lack of randomised controlled trial (RCT) evidence of efficacy (Samraj and Nicolas, 2015).

Intracranial pressure measurement

Normal: 0–15 mmHg.

Intraventricular catheters, usually fibre-optic, can be connected to most ICU monitors to display a waveform (see Figure 23.5).

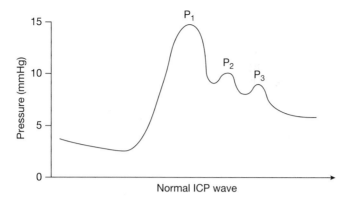

Figure 23.5 Normal ICP waveform

Mean intracranial pressure is usually recorded. Arterial pulses affect intracranial pressure, creating waves that should have three peaks (March and Hickey, 2014) (see Figure 23.5):

- P1: *percussion wave*: sharply peaked, with fairly constant amplitude, produced by arterial pressure transmitted from choroids plexus to ventricles;
- P2: *tidal wave*: shape and amplitude is more variable, but like an arterial waveform ends on the dicrotic notch. P2 indicates cerebral compliance (Ross and Eynon, 2005);
- P3: *dicrotic wave*: from aortic valve closure.

Like other pressure monitoring waves, dampened shape indicates unreliable measurement. Probes are normally reliable, but once inserted cannot be recalibrated inserted. Suspected inaccuracy (doubtful waveforms) can be tested by lowering the patient's head, which should increase pressure and thus waveform amplitude.

ICP monitoring is highly invasive, and, although used in neurological centres, is not usually used in other ICUs (Cardim *et al.*, 2016). There is no evidence that routine ICP monitoring improves outcomes compared with clinical assessment (Forsyth *et al.*, 2010; Chesnut *et al.*, 2012).

Other technologies

Intracranial monitoring is necessarily invasive, and penetrating the skull for monitoring largely limits use to specialist neurological centres. Almost inevitably, technological developments will bring some less- or non-invasive device that is sufficiently accurate for wider use. Geeraerts *et al.* (2008) found non-invasive ocular sonography correlated with invasive ICP.

Implications for practice

- abnormal blood glucose levels are a common cause of acute behavioural changes;
- nearly all units receive patients with head injuries, so need some means to assess and monitor neurological status;
- because the skull is rigid, any increase in contents (bleed, oedema) increases intracranial pressure, impairing cerebral perfusion;
- aspects of central nervous system function can be inferred from:

  - Glasgow Coma Scale (with pupil responses);
  - spinal reflexes;
  - blood tests (glucose, electrolytes, gases);
  - mean arterial pressure;

- ICP should be 0–15 mmHg, but transient rises are insignificant;
- CPP should be sufficient to perfuse the brain, without increased intracranial pressure – 60 mmHg is usually aimed for;
- continuous display is valuable for evaluating effects of all aspects of care.

Summary

Intracranial hypertension can occur in many ICU patients; monitoring neurological status (outside neurological ICUs) often relies on the Glasgow Coma Scale, which assesses level of consciousness rather than cerebral perfusion. More invasive methods of assessment inevitably incur greater risks but may provide more useful information to guide treatment. As with monitoring any aspect of patient care, benefits and burdens of each approach should be individualised to patients and justified by the extent to which they can safely be used and usefully guide treatments and care given. Management of patients with intracranial hypertension is discussed in Chapter 36.

Further reading

Hickey (2014) remains the key text for neurological nursing. Specialist journals include the *Journal of Neuroscience Nursing*, the *Annals of Neurology* and the *Journal of Neurology, Neurosurgery and Psychology*.

Clinical scenarios

Mr Michael Roberts is a 54-year-old who was admitted to the ICU unconscious. He sustained a head injury from a fall down stairs at home and was found by his partner. Mr Roberts is a known insulin-dependent diabetic who drinks approximately eight units of alcohol a day and has epilepsy. On examination Mr Roberts had a large scalp haematoma over the right parietal region, another over his right eye and bruising to his right elbow.

Mr Roberts' initial results:

Both pupils' response to light is sluggish, equal, size 4 mm:

Glasgow Coma Scale (GCS) 6 (E1, V1, M4)
All limbs flexing spontaneously without any stimuli
Both pupils' response to light is sluggish, equal, size 4 mm
Respiration rate 26 breaths / minute, audible gurgling breath sounds
SpO_2 100% on 15 litres of oxygen
BP 232/120 mmHg
HR 100 beats/minute
Capillary refill < 2 seconds with warm peripheries

Mr Roberts was intubated and sent for a head CT scan, which revealed a large right subdural haematoma with midline shift (9 mm) to the left side of his brain, widespread subarrachnoid haemorrhage, fracture to right parietal skull and several focal intracerebral contusions. He underwent emergency craniotomy for evacuation of subdural haematoma and insertion of ICP bolt. He was invasively ventilated, sedated with propofol and fentanyl infusions.

Mr Roberts's post-operative results:

Glasgow Coma Scale (GCS) 4 (E1, V1, M2)
Right pupil not assessed as eye closed from local swelling, left pupil size 2 mm, sluggish response to light
ICP 35 mmHg
BP 132/65 mmHg
HR 68 beats/minute
Capillary refill < 2 seconds
Central temperature 34.4°C
Blood sugar 14.0 mmol/litre

Q1. Explain why the GCS is used in Mr Roberts's initial and post-operative neurological assessment and what his score represents. Consider how accuracy can be ensured, frequency of assessment and most appropriate type of stimuli for Mr Roberts.

Q2. Calculate Mr Roberts's cerebral perfusion pressure (CPP = MAP − ICP). What is the significance of this for his care? What are likely causes and significance of his temperature and hyperglycaemia?

Q3. List complications and risks associated with ICP monitoring. How could these be managed with Mr Roberts? What surrogate markers could guide care if these are not available?

Part IV

Micropathologies

Chapter 24

Cellular pathology

Contents

Fundamental knowledge

Oxygen delivery to cells
Glycolysis

Introduction

Focus on visible macrophysiology (systems and organs) has increasingly been replaced by recognition that disease processes originate primarily at micro-physiological levels; organ/system failure follows widespread cell failure. Cell function relies on chemical reactions, which require both oxygen and energy. Absence of oxygen and energy sources (mainly blood glucose) therefore quickly leads to cell damage and failure. Restoring oxygen and energy supplies to failing cells may enable cell survival, reversing critical illness.

In health, hundreds of chemicals produced by the body maintain homeostasis. In ill health, these same chemicals can contribute to or cause critical illness. A few of the most significant chemicals are identified in this chapter, which therefore outlines pathological mechanisms underlying most critical illnesses. Readers may find sections in this chapter more useful as reference points for later use. This chapter begins with brief revision of cell physiology. If unfamiliar, this should be supplemented from anatomy texts.

Cell membrane

Cell membranes are a single layer of phospholipid, interspersed with proteins and cholesterol. This phospholipid creates an oil-like film which is both flexible and self-sealing and which separates internal structures of cells from their external environment. Although some passive movement of fluid and solutes does occur across cell membranes, most movement is actively regulated by various "pumps", "channels" or "gates" in cell membranes. Probably the best-known is the sodium–potassium pump, but many others exist, including calcium channels mentioned in Chapter 22. Influx of excessive calcium into cells is one of the main mechanisms of necrosis (Karch and Molkentin, 2015). Calcium channel blockers manipulate this channel in cardiac and vascular cells. Active

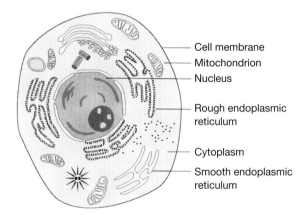

Cell membrane
Mitochondrion
Nucleus

Rough endoplasmic reticulum

Cytoplasm
Smooth endoplasmic reticulum

■ *Figure 24.1 Cell structure*

movement through these pumps and channels maintains normal, healthy intracellular environments. Cell failure, discussed below, affects all parts of cells, including membranes.

Mitochondria

Mitochondria produce adenosine triphosphate (ATP), the type of energy which cells use. ATP is normally mainly produced from metabolism of glucose and oxygen (Krebs' cycle):

$$C_6H_{12}O_6 + 6O_2 \rightarrow 36 \text{ ATP molecules} + \text{waste}$$

Anaerobic metabolism significantly reduces ATP production, so cells attempt to compensate by shunting pyruvate to lactate to produce more ATP (Greaves *et al.*, 2012). Lactate is discussed in Chapter 19.

The hypoperfusion that typically causes anaerobic metabolism also fails to remove metabolic waste (acids and carbon dioxide), creating a toxic environment for failing cells. Oxygen radicals (see below) accelerate cell and organ failure. Cells with high metabolic rates (including cardiac and brain cells) are especially vulnerable to hypoxic damage (Clay *et al.*, 2001).

Cell death

There are essentially two mechanisms for cell death:

- apoptosis
- necrosis.

Apoptosis, "cell shrinkage" is the normal way cells die, encapsulating powerful intracellular chemicals in the shrinking membrane. Necrosis, pathological cell death, is an inflammatory process (Karch and Molkentin, 2015), damaging mitochondria and releasing potentially toxic chemicals such as tumour necrosis factor alpha (TNFα) and interleukins into surrounding tissues. Cell necrosis causes many pathologies seen in ICU, so underlies discussion in many subsequent chapters.

Autophagy, the "quality control" mechanism by which cell components are destroyed, has been found to malfunction in various diseases such as cardiomyopathy and cancer, causing pathological remodelling (Sridhar *et al.*, 2012).

Inflammatory response

This homeostatic mechanism forms part of non-specific immunity. Damaged tissue releases pro-inflammatory cytokines (especially TNFα and interleukin 1), which trigger a "cytokine cascade" of vasoactive chemicals (inflammatory mediators), which:

- vasodilate (e.g. from histamine, and many interleukins);
- increase capillary leak (e.g. from leukotrienes);
- activate other defences, such as mast cells.

Increased blood flow and leakier capillaries enable leukocytes and other defences to migrate into infected tissue, and destroy invading bacteria. The area becomes swollen (oedema), red (increased blood flow from vasodilatation) and painful (pressure on nerves). Pus is often formed (from dead neutrophils and bacteria). When confined to an area of local damage, this homeostatic response helps recovery and healing; but when extensive inflammatory responses occur, extensive vasodilatation and massive capillary leak cause hypovolaemia, shock and organ failure (see Chapter 32).

There are many chemical mediators. Appropriate responses to threats, such as infection, help restore health. Imbalanced responses can either be:

- insufficient, so diseases can cause harm or death, or
- excessive, responses becoming pathological.

Critical illness usually provokes excessive inflammatory responses; key mediators are discussed below.

Cytokines ("cell killers") are mainly mediators of the immune system, released by macrophages and other cells. Tumour necrosis factor alpha (TNFα) is usually the first cytokine to be released, initiating the cytokine cascade. Systemic release of large quantities of TNFα, which occurs in septic shock, is:

- negatively inotropic
- pyrogenic
- coagulopathic.

(Abbas *et al.*, 2015)

Interleukins are powerful mediators released by white cells, especially monocytes and macrophages. There are many interleukins but they may be divided between pro-inflammatory and anti-inflammatory. Pro-inflammatory interleukins, major mediators of critical illness, include interleukins (IL) 1, 6, 8 and 10.

Nitric oxide is the main endogenous vasodilator release by vascular endothelium in response to tissue hypoxia, so once sufficient blood flow delivers oxygen, the mechanism triggering its release is removed. Insufficient nitric causes ischaemia and hypertension, while excessive release (which typically occurs in sepsis) causes systemic vasodilatation and so hypotension. With tissue ischaemia, such as angina, nitric oxide release can be increased by nitrates (Singh *et al.*, 2017), such as glyceryl trinitrate and isosorbide mono-/dinitrate.

Leukotrines are mediators also released by leukocytes. They increase capillary leak. Excessive leukotrine release in sepsis causes extravasation of blood water resulting in tissue oedema and hypovolaemia.

Acute phase proteins

Infection initiates early release of proteins, including *fibrinogen, alpha-1 protinase inhibitor, C-reactive protein* (CRP – see Chapter 21) and *serum amyloid associated protein* to assist phagocytosis.

Radicals

Cells need oxygen. Lack of oxygen and the generation of oxygen radicals are key mechanisms in cell necrosis (Karch and Molkentin, 2015). Free radicals are molecules with one or more unpaired electrons in their outer orbit; this makes them inherently unstable and highly reactive. Any biochemical reaction can release free radicals (e.g. micro-organism lysis by neutrophils, Krebs' cycle). Although radicals only exist for microseconds, they trigger chain reactions which are typically thousands of events long, causing tissue damage – the autocatalysis underlying most critical illnesses.

Reactive oxygen species (ROS) and oxygen radicals can cause oxidative stress (damage) to tissues. In health balanced release between oxygen radical release and antioxidant defences can contribute to muscle-building and angiogenesis, but, if ROS production exceeds defences, oxidative stress can contribute to cardiovascular disease, acute lung injury and many other diseases (Gomes *et al.*, 2012), including most critical illnesses.

Oxygen metabolism occurs intracellularly, inevitably releasing some radicals. The few radicals normally produced are destroyed by antioxidants, such as vitamin E, vitamin C, and albumin. But hyperpoxia, from oxygen therapy, produces more radicals (Knight *et al.*, 2011; Ward *et al.*, 2011), while critically ill patients usually have depleted antioxidant defences (Ghashut *et al.*, 2016). Massive production of oxygen radicals overwhelms endogenous antioxidant defences. Antioxidant therapy, seemingly logical, has few benefits.

Reperfusion injury is caused when oxygen radicals and other toxic chemicals are released owing to ischaemia (Frank *et al.*, 2012). These chemical mediators can cause myocardial stunning, resulting in transient ventricular tachycardia, other dysrhythmias and ectopics. Although reperfusion injury can occur following any ischaemia, and is relevant to many pathologies discussed in the remainder of this book, it becomes especially significant following myocardial, infarction accounting for up to half of final infarct size (Frank *et al.*, 2012).

Implications for practice

■ most critical pathologies originate at microcellular rather than macrosystem level; understanding these processes enables nurses to understand pathologies and treatments covered in most other chapters (e.g. pressure sores, oxygen toxicity, fluid and electrolyte balance);

■ cells need energy and oxygen. Microcirculatory resuscitation requires:

● oxygen delivery to cells (tissue perfusion);
● nutrition;
● ventilation;

- high FiO$_2$ (above 0.5) is potentially toxic (see Chapter 18), so prolonged use should balance needs for oxygen delivery against risks of potential toxicity;
- reperfusion injury can cause secondary damage, so recovery requires close observation of effects (e.g. dysrhythmias) and prompt intervention.

Summary

The microscopic nature of cell function and dysfunction make these less easy to understand than function and dysfunction of major organs, but understanding cell dysfunction is a valuable basis for understanding pathophysiologies described in the remainder of this book. Most critical illnesses originate and progress at cellular level; macroscopic symptoms are accumulations of microscopic problems. Cell function is complex, and knowledge of cell function and potential medical interventions is rapidly increasing. Abnormal figures (e.g. disordered arterial blood gases) may be tolerated to assist cell recovery (e.g. permissive hypercapnia – see Chapter 27). Currently, our ability to manipulate cell function in clinical practice is limited, but the future is likely to bring new microphysiological treatments; while some of these will disappoint, others will probably become embedded in practice. As microphysiological knowledge will therefore become increasingly necessary for critical care nursing, this chapter has given an overview of cellular pathology and some of the more significant mediators.

Further reading

Current attempts to target problems from cell dysfunction prompt frequent articles in medical and scientific journals, although complexities of this aspect of science limits value of most articles for most nurses. Fewer articles have appeared in nursing journals. Normal cell physiology can be revised from recent and appropriate anatomy texts, such as Marieb and Hoehn (2016). Abbas *et al.* (2015) is a classic textbook about cellular pathology. Frank *et al.* (2012) review reperfusion injury.

Clinical scenarios

David Roberts, 33 years old with a history of poorly controlled asthma, is admitted to the ICU following a respiratory arrest. On endotracheal suction his sputum is thick and mucopurulent and arterial blood gases indicate severe respiratory acidosis.

His blood results include abnormalities in white blood cells and other blood results:

WBC	27.3 x 10^{-9}/litre
Platelets	277 x 10^{-9}/litre
Neutrophils	23.4 x 10^{-9}/litre
Eosinophils	1.6 x 10^{-9}/litre
Basinophils	0.8 x 10^{-9}/litre
Monocytes	0.7 x 10^{-9}/litre
Lymphocytes	0.7 x 10^{-9}/litre
Hb	76 grams/litre
CRP	372 mg/litre

Arterial blood gases are:

pH	7.26
$PaCO_2$	8.08 kPa
PaO_2	8.78 kPa
HCO_3^-	24.2 mmol/litre
Base excess	0.1 mmol/litre
Lactate	2.3 mmol/litre

Q1. Identify which results are:

- symptoms
- problems
- both symptoms and problems.

What treatments are likely to be changed/initiated for results which are problems?

Q2. What do the counts of subtypes of white cells indicate?

Q3. David develops systemic hypotension and acute lung injury. What cellular processes contribute to his respiratory condition (e.g. effect of hypoxia and hypercapnoea on cellular function, mitochondrial ATP production, cell membrane potential, mediators triggered, function and systemic effects of these mediators, causes of capillary permeability, role of basophils, implications of associated histamine release)?

Chapter 25

Immunity and immunodeficiency

Contents

Fundamental knowledge

Physiology of normal immunity

Introduction

The immune system enables us to resist many potential pathogens, but most critically ill patients are immunocompromised. This chapter describes normal immunity, illustrating dysfunction through human immunosuppressive virus (HIV) and AIDS-related complex (ARC).

Immunity

Immunity may be:

- non-specific (innate)
- specific (adaptive).

Non-specific immunity is any defence mechanism not targeting specific micro-organisms. Much human non-specific immunity is present at birth. Specific immunity is necessarily acquired through exposure to various organisms or antibody vaccination.

Non-specific immunity includes:

- stickiness of mucous membrane and cilia (trapping airway particles smaller than two micrometres);
- body "flushes" (tears, saliva), many including antibacterial substances such as lysozyme;
- sebrum (from sebaceous glands) preventing bacterial colonisation of skin;
- acidity/alkalinity of gastrointestinal tract;
- pyrexia (see Chapter 8);
- inflammatory response – increases and activates phagocyte and *complements*;
- interferon – inhibits viral replication and enhances action of killer cells;
- lactoferrin – binds iron (needed by microbes for growth);
- the steroid hormone cortisol (hydrocortisone) released from the adrenal glands and the glucocorticoid hormone cortisone released from the liver.

Non-specific chemical defences inhibit bacteria and viruses, but can cause or complicate disease; for example:

- inflammatory responses complicate most critical illnesses;
- stress ulceration is more likely with critical illness;
- graft versus host disease (GvHD – see Chapter 43) threatens viability of transplanted tissue (foreign protein), necessitating immunosuppression.

Logically, immunosupression would help recovery, but in sepsis, and probably most critical illnesses, steroids do not help recovery (Annane *et al.*, 2009).

Specific immunity involves recognition of specific antigens by antibodies (lymphocytes, part of the agranulocyte group of white cells – see Chapter 21). T-lymphocytes to respond to (non-specific) protein by producing various cytokines; B-lymphocytes are antigen-specific. Excessive or inappropriate responses can cause:

- allergy
- anaphylaxis

Or, if the body's own tissue is identified as the antigen,

- autoimmunity.

Immunodeficiency

Failure of the immune system is usually secondary to either autoimmune pathologies (e.g. HIV, leukaemia, hepatic failure) or drug-induced (e.g. steroids, ciclosporin/tacrilimus, chemotherapy). The immune system can also be overwhelmed by infection or complex surgery/invasive treatment, exposing patients to opportunistic infections (e.g. *MRSa*) that may colonise, but not infect, healthier people (e.g. staff). Older people (most ICU patients) have decreased immunity (Li *et al.*, 2011; Valiathan *et al.*, 2016).

HIV

Since initial reports of human immunosuppressive virus (HIV) in 1981, some people were colonised by the virus while remaining disease-free. HIV+ therefore means that the virus is present, regardless of whether infection exists. Once the virus causes pathological responses, the person has Autoimmune Disease Syndrome (AIDS), immunity exposing people to various complications, often called AIDS-Related Complex (ARC – see below).

In the 1980s, survival of ventilated HIV+ patients was poor, so ICU admission was often denied. Largely owing to highly active antiretroviral therapy (HAART), mortality has fallen, resulting in more people living longer with HIV – one third of people accessing HIV care in the UK are now aged over 50 (Public Health England, 2016b). Survival to hospital discharge continues to improve (Powell *et al.*, 2009), outcome being comparable to other medical admissions to ICU (Dickson *et al.*, 2007). HIV is usually classified as type 1 (HIV-1) or type 2 (HIV-2), HIV-1 being prevalent in the West.

HIV primarily attacks CD4 (T helper) lymphocytes, causing progressive problems with immunodeficiency. Once inside host cells, HIV transmits genetic information as a single *RNA* strand. Using the enzyme reverse transcriptase, it then replicates RNA into a DNA copy (hence "retrovirus"). This clumsy arrangement is complicated by inaccuracies of enzyme replication, causing on average one mutation each replication cycle (Wainberg, 1999).

ARC

Autoimmune dysfunction exposes patients to opportunistic infections:

- respiratory
- gastrointestinal
- central nervous system.

Respiratory failure remains the main cause of ICU admission (Wittenberg *et al.*, 2010), usually caused by bacterial pneumonia (Barbier *et al.*, 2009). The virus *Pneumocystis jirovici*, previously called *Pneumocystis carinii*, causes pneumonia (PJP; sometimes still abbreviated as PCP – *Pneumocystis carinii* pneumonia). PJP is the single main micro-organism causing respiratory failure (Miller *et al.*, 2006), although incidence is declining (Wittenberg *et al.*, 2010). *P. jirovici* forms cysts in alveoli and interstitial lung tissue, which often progress to *ARDS*. Tuberculosis (TB) infection is the main cause of mortality in ARC (W.H.O., 2014a), a problem aggravated by development of resistant strains (Gandhi *et al.*, 2010; W.H.O., 2016a).

Cardiovascular failure is often from sepsis, but prolonged antiretroviral therapy can cause dyslipidaemias, insulin resistance and diabetes (Huang *et al.*, 2006).

Gastrointestinal dysfunction includes malnourishment and increased motility – diarrhoea, vomiting and nausea. Early nutrition, often with vitamin supplements, significantly improves outcome. Anti-emetics and antidiarrhoeal drugs can restore comfort and dignity. Mouthcare provides comfort and helps prevent opportunist infection. Viral hepatitis disproportionately affects people with ARC (W.H.O., 2014a), making hepatic dysfunction more likely.

Central nervous system damage and encephalitis are usually seen at post-mortem. Neurocognitive disorders commonly occur with HIV (Focà *et al.*, 2016). Many patients suffer both cognitive and behavioural changes, such as memory loss, apathy, poor concentration and (very) early dementia. Depression and anxiety are common (W.H.O., 2014a). HAART has not reduced incidence of neurological disease (Wittenberg *et al.*, 2010). Cognitive changes can be especially distressful for families and friends.

Psychological stressors include:

- stigma surrounding HIV/AIDS
- anxieties about dying.

Psychological distress needs human care and interaction, spending time with people and allowing them to express their needs. Anxieties and stigma surround HIV and ARC often increasing psychological needs of patients and families and friends.

Ethical and health issues

HIV and ARC have raised more ethical dilemmas and issues than any other disease in recent years. Often, HIV status is undiagnosed on admission to ICU (Blackwell and Guido-Sanz, 2016). Non-consensual touch is (legally) assault, so undertaking tests on patients unable to give informed consent, or receive the counselling that would usually be given before HIV testing, risks charges of assault. Although this applies to any tests, most tests in the ICU are justifiable as being in patients' best interests. Treatment for HIV is relatively long-term, and knowing HIV status would often not alter their care on the ICU, so tests should usually wait until they are fully conscious and can make an informed decision.

Relatives may discover diagnosis of HIV/ARC from death certificates, having been unaware, and perhaps disapproving, of the deceased's lifestyle. Duty of confidentiality to patients is absolute (apart from specific legal requirements), extending beyond death of patients. Dilemmas raised through clinical practice can usefully be discussed among unit teams, contributing to the professional growth of all involved.

Implications for practice

- many ICU pathologies and treatments impair immunity, so high standards of infection control are needed to protect patients from opportunistic infections;
- respiratory failure is the main reason for patients with ARC being admitted to ICU; outcome is comparable to most other patient groups, so HIV/ARC should not prejudice admission;
- informed consent should be gained before testing for HIV;
- people with HIV/ARC may experience prejudice and stigma. Nurses have a duty of care to all their patients, and should promote positive attitudes among other staff;
- ARC often causes various gastrointestinal symptoms. Nurses should assess nutritional needs and bowel function, feeding early, and providing appropriate care and support;
- HIV+ patients and their families may need additional psychological support; many trusts employ specialist HIV nurses.

Summary

Most patients in ICU are immunocompromised. Treatments and interventions increase infection risks, but proactive infection control can reduce risks from nosocomial infection.

HIV and ARC have created medical and ethical challenges for healthcare. The unique role of nurses in the ICU team enables them to challenge and resolve stigmas and negative attitudes to meet the psychological and physiological needs of their patients.

Support groups

- National AIDS helpline, 0800 567123.
- Terrence Higgins Trust, 0808 802 1221.

Further reading

HIV has focused and rekindled many ethical dilemmas surrounding treatment and attitudes to certain diseases. Goffman's (1963) classic work on stigma (written before HIV was identified) and Sontag's (1989) outstanding investigative journalism into HIV offer useful sociological/historical insights. Reports and guidelines for HIV frequently appear, such as W.H.O. (2014a) and UKHIVA (2016), although these have little direct application to the ICU. Occasionally ICU-specific articles are published, such as that by Blackwell and Guido-Sanz (2016).

Clinical scenario

Vanessa Warring, a 27-year-old single mother of two small children, was admitted to intensive care for ventilatory support following rapidly deteriorating respiratory function from right lung pneumonia. Vanessa refused consent for a HIV test pre-intubation. Microbiology results confirmed presence of *Pneumocystis jirovici* pneumonia (PJP). Her CD4 count on admission was < 20 cells/mm³. Over the next 10 days, Vanessa continued to deteriorate despite therapy, she became colonised with several opportunistic organisms and it was obvious that she was dying. Her children were being cared for by a social worker.

Q1. If working with a student nurse, how would you explain differences in immune response between HIV-positive and HIV-negative people on exposure to opportunistic organisms, such as *Pneumocystis jiroveci*? Why is an HIV-positive person more susceptible to develop pneumonia?

Q2. Analyse interventions available to support Vanessa, including benefits and limitations of these interventions (e.g. protective isolation, drug therapies of antibiotics, antiviral, antifungal, nutrition, psychological support, therapeutic relationships). Reflect on your experiences of using these with HIV+ patients on your unit.

Q3. Consider the ethical and legal issues associated with this situation. Should Vanessa's children be tested for HIV? Who should make this decision and how would this be justified? What local policies, structures and support (e.g. clinical nurse specialists) does your hospital have for patients with HIV/AIDS?

Haemostasis

Contents

Fundamental knowledge

Normal clotting – intrinsic, extrinsic and common
  coagulation pathways

Introduction

In health, clotting involves a complex pathway combining intrinsic and extrinsic clotting factors. Intrinsic factors are those already in blood, produced by the liver; extrinsic are those released by vascular endothelium, so are sometimes called "tissue-dependent factors".

Critical illness usually involves excessive inflammatory responses, causing pro-inflammatory cytokines to disrupt normal clotting. "Virchnow's triad" predisposing to thromboembolism is:

- venous stasis
- vessel wall damage
- hypercoagulability.

(Wolberg *et al.*, 2012)

The first two commonly occur in critically ill patients. Clotting is usually disrupted, and can be hypercoagulable, but is more often prolonged. Coagulopathies are relatively common in critical illness; this chapter illustrates problems through some rare, but extreme, coagulopathies:

- disseminated intravascular coagulation (DIC);
- haemolytic uraemic syndrome (HUS);
- thrombotic thrombocytopenia purpura (TTP);
- heparin-induced thrombocytopenia and thrombosis syndrome (HITTS).

Other haemoglobinopathies – sickle cell disease, leukaemia, thalassaemia – are discussed in Woodrow (2016).

Most hospitalised patients are at risk of VTE, but venous stasis from immobility places ICU patients at especially high risk of deep-vein thrombosis (DVT) (I.C.S., 2015). Venous thromboembolism (VTE) prophylaxis, which is usually "routine" for all ICU patients, is also discussed. Major haemorrhage is discussed in Chapter 40.

DIC – pathophysiology

This group of disorders is triggered when a primary problem, most commonly sepsis, acute leukaemia and solid cancers (Asakura, 2014), causes excessive fibrin-mediated intravascular microthrombi (Boral *et al.*, 2016; Onishi *et al.*, 2016), leaving insufficient clotting factors to maintain haemostasis (Liaw *et al.*, 2016). DIC progresses rapidly, often occurring within a few hours of the trigger. Relatively rare in most hospitalised patients, Singh *et al.* (2013) suggest it causes 9–19% of ICU admissions, with mortality rates of 45–78%.

There is no single diagnostic test for DIC (Squizzato *et al.*, 2016), but stabilising clotting takes priority over confirming suspected diagnosis.

Signs

Early symptoms of DIC are typically non-specific, such as:

- *breathing* – mild hypoxia, dyspnoea;
- *circulation* – petechial bleeding (especially trunk), mucocutaneous bleeding (especially gut), purpura, minor renal dysfunction;
- *disability* – mild cerebral dysfunction (e.g. confusion);
- *exposure* – skin rashes, mottled, cool;

As DIC progresses, symptoms become more severe. DIC prolongs *clotting times*, with high levels of fibrin degradation products, such as D-dimers, and reduced levels of antithrombin and many clotting factors, especially fibrinogen, platelets and antithrombin. Patients bleed from multiple sites, including arterial and venous cannulae.

Treatment

DIC is always secondary to an underlying problem, so underlying causes should (if possible) be resolved (Squizzato *et al.*, 2016).

Clotting factors should be replaced. With active bleeding, platelets should be transfused to maintain platelet counts above 50×10^9/litre, or above 30 in the absence of bleeding (Squizzato *et al.*, 2016). Other clotting factors, especially fresh frozen plasma (FFP), may also be needed.

Various anticoagulants have been used to release clotting factors. Heparin may be useful (Levi *et al.*, 2009; Onishi *et al.*, 2016). Exogenous antithrombin, previously called antithrombin III, is not beneficial but increases risk of bleeding (Allingstrup *et al.*, 2016).

System failure often necessitates support (e.g. ventilation, inotropes, haemofiltration). Various other symptoms may also require treatment (e.g. antibiotics and cytoprotective drugs to prevent gastric bleeding). The pro-inflammatory state often also causes vasodilatation and so hypotension. Aggressive fluid resuscitation is often necessary but will further dilute already scarce clotting factors.

Related pathologies

HUS

Haemolytic uraemic syndrome (HUS), relatively common in children, is a rare disorder in adults. In children, it is often caused by *E. coli* infection, but in adults is usually caused by genetic disorders (Cataland and Wu, 2014). Both forms cause thrombocytopenia, which can be treated with platelet transfusions. The adult form often results in acute kidney injury and potentially end-stage renal failure, so is best treated with eculizumab (anti-C5) (Boral *et al.*, 2016).

Thrombotic thrombocytopenia purpura (TTP), also rare, is a medical emergency caused by deranged (over-large) von Willebrand factor, resulting in systemic platelet aggregation (Boral *et al.*, 2016), and therefore similar effects to DIC.

Symptoms typically include purpura, neurological deficits, multifocal neuropsychiatric disturbances and kidney injury. TTP is usually treated by plasma exchange (Norfolk, 2013) and supportive therapies.

Heparin-induced thrombocytopenia and thrombosis syndrome (HITTS; HIT) is caused by antibody reaction to heparin, especially unfractionated rather than low-molecular-weight heparin (Onishi *et al.*, 2016). Like DIC, HITTS can cause major organ infarction (e.g. myocardial, cerebral). Unfractionated heparin is now rarely used, making HITTS a relatively rare phenomenon in ICUs.

Nursing care

Bleeding can occur anywhere, internally or externally. Nurses should therefore:

- observe skin for bruising, petechial or purpuric haemorrhages;
- observe any invasive sites for oozing/bleeding (e.g. intravenous cannulae, drains, wounds);
- observe and test any body fluids for blood (nasogastric aspirate, vomit, stools, urine).

Daily urinalysis may also reveal protein. Any abnormal findings should be reported.

Although DIC is a medical problem, and treatments will be medically prescribed, nursing care can significantly reduce complications from trauma, sepsis and bleeding. Many nursing interventions may provoke haemorrhage:

- endotracheal suction;
- turning;
- cuff blood pressure measurement;
- enemas;
- rectal/vaginal examinations;
- plasters/tape;
- shaving;
- mouthcare.

Some interventions may be necessary, although alternative approaches should be considered. For example, if the patient possesses an electric razor, this should be used in preference to giving a wet shave. Similarly, foam sticks are less traumatic than toothbrushes. Lubrication of skin and lips (e.g. with yellow soft paraffin) helps prevent cracking. Invasive cannulae and procedures should be minimised to reduce risks of haemorrhage.

Small bleeds which may be physiologically insignificant can cause great distress, and possible fainting. Visitors should be warned about the possible sight of blood, escorted to the bedside and observed until staff are satisfied about their safety. If patients sense their relatives are distressed, they may themselves become distressed, aggravating their disease.

Deep-vein thromboses (DVTs)

Risk of thromboembolism is significantly increased with immobility and infection. DVTs can be fatal – pulmonary emboli are almost invariably from DVTs (Berthomier *et al.*, 2016). Failure to initiate thromboprophylaxis is a major cause of preventable deaths in hospitals (Donaldson *et al.*, 2014). Thromboprophylaxis may be:

- pharmacological (e.g. low-molecular-weight heparin – LMW heparin);
- mechanical (e.g. compression).

Many ICUs combine both forms of thromboprophylaxis, although I.C.S. (2015) states that pharmacological thromboprophylaxis should be prescribed unless contraindicated. Kakkar *et al.* (2011) found that adding LMW heparin did not reduce mortality when compression stockings were used. As with other conditions, treatment is not without risks. All ICU patients should be risk-assessed for DVTs, and appropriate treatments prescribed.

Development of DVT is significantly reduced with subcutaneous low-molecular-weight heparin and thromboembolism deterrent stockings ("TEDS") (N.I.C.E., 2010d). Unless there are specific contraindications, such as excessively prolonged clotting, all patients in ICU should have:

- daily subcutaneous low-molecular-weight heparin;
- daily clotting screens;
- knee-length thromboembolism deterrent stockings;
- twice-daily removal and remeasuring of stockings.

With DIC, VTE prophylaxis with low-molecular-weight heparin should be discontinued if the patient is bleeding or platelet count is below 30×10^9/litre (Squizzato *et al.*, 2016).

Mechanical compression devices are equally effective at preventing DVTs (Weinberger and Cipolle, 2016) and can be useful if TEDS are contraindicated.

Implications for practice

- DIC is a rare, but often fatal, complication of critical illness;
- if patients have prolonged/deranged clotting, nurses should be especially vigilant to minimise any interventions that may cause trauma/bleeding;
- unless specifically contraindicated, all ICU patients should receive DVT prophylaxis (anticoagulants, TEDS);
- TEDS should be removed twice daily, and remeasured before replacing.

Summary

Deranged haemostasis often occurs with critical illness. Extreme pathologies, such as DIC, are rare but too often fatal. Management is largely conservative: replacing clotting factors and treating symptoms to buy time while underlying pathologies are treated. Nursing care should focus on avoiding complications of trauma, while minimising anxiety to both patients and relatives.

Patients in ICU are at especially high risk of developing deep-vein thrombosis owing to often prolonged immobility and pro-coagulant diseases and syndromes. DVT prophylaxis is, and should be, routine for all ICU patients, unless there are specific contraindications. Prophylaxis generally includes daily subcutaneous injection of low-molecular-weight heparin, knee-length anti-thrombotic stockings, and daily clotting screens.

Further reading

Squizzato *et al.* (2016) provide guidelines for managing DIC. N.I.C.E. (2010d) guidelines for DVT prophylaxis should be followed. BCSH (2012) provides guidelines for thrombocytopenic purpura.

Clinical scenarios

Gary Williams is a 56-year-old Afro-Caribbean man admitted with a coagulopathy of unknown cause. Initial investigations revealed deranged clotting, 15–20 ml/hr of cloudy urine with casts, pyrexia (37.7°C), tachypnoea (44 breaths/minute), and tachycardia (124 beats per minute) with hypotension (84/58 mmHg) and severe metabolic acidosis. He has bloodshot eyes and rectal bleeding.

Gary's blood investigations values include:		Laboratory reference range:
INR	1.5	0.9 to 1.1
Thrombin Time (seconds)	21	10 to 12
Fibrinogen (grams/litre)	1.5	2 to 4
D-dimer (mg/litre)	8.48	0.0 to 0.3
Platelets (10⁹/litre)	26	150 to 400
Hb (grams/litre)	78	130 to 180
WCC (10⁹/litre)	23.1	4.0 to 11.0
Neutrophils (10⁹/litre)	22.4	1.7 to 8.0
Lymphocytes (10⁹/litre)	0.7	1.0 to 4.0
Monocytes (10⁹/litre)	0.1	0.24 to 1.1
HCT	0.24	0.41 to 0.52
Urea (mmol/litre)	12.9	2.5–7.8
Creatinine (micromol/litre)	517	64 to 104 (male)
Creatine kinase (units/litre)	15571	40–320 (male)
CRP (mg/litre)	244	0–10
Troponin T (ng/litre)	20	< 35 (male)

Q1. Interpret Gary's blood result, noting clinical significance of abnormal values. Which results indicate (a) intrinsic and (b) extrinsic clotting pathways?

Q2. Which coagulopathy do you think Gary's has? What is the most likely primary cause? How might diagnosis be confirmed?

Q3. Three units of blood, cryoprecipitate, fresh frozen plasma and platelets are prescribed. Outline the rationale for this treatment and nursing approaches which can maximise their therapeutic benefits – e.g. sequence of administration, storage, temperature, minimising bleeding points and/or further fibrinolysis.

Part V

Respiratory

Chapter 27

Acute Respiratory Distress Syndrome (ARDS)

Contents

Fundamental knowledge

Respiratory anatomy and physiology – alveoli, pulmonary blood flow
V/Q mismatch; pulmonary shunting

Introduction

Acute Respiratory Distress Syndrome (ARDS) is a syndrome causing life-threatening respiratory failure, occurring within one week. Chest X-rays show bilateral opacities in at least three quadrants that cannot be fully explained by pleural effusions, atelectasis and nodules. Echocardiography may be needed to exclude cardiogenic causes for oedema (ARDS Definition Task Force, 2012). Severity is classified by PaO_2/FiO_2 ratio:

■ mild: < 40, or < 60, with PEEP or CPAP ≥ 5 cmH_2O;
■ moderate: < 20, or < 40 with PEEP ≥ 5 cmH_2O;
■ severe: > 20 with PEEP ≥ 5 cmH_2O.

(if PaO_2 measured in kilopascals)

Inflammation, neutrophil infiltration, and diffuse oedema cause gross oedema, extensive atelectasis, and cell necrosis.

Like most critical illnesses, the cost (mortality and financial) of ARDS is high, and evidence for benefits of specific management strategies is often limited and controversial. Prolonged stay and poor prognosis may increase psychological needs of ICU patients and families.

Mortality remains high – 35–65% (Petrucci and De Feo, 2013). Many patients are young, and survivors often suffer long-term limitations to function (McCormack and Tolhurst-Cleaver, 2017).

Ventilation

Severe lung injury is usually fatal without artificial ventilation, yet positive pressure ventilation can cause ventilator-induced lung injury (VILI), once called "ventilator lung". Large tidal volumes can cause "volutrauma" (or "volotrauma"). Lung protection strategies include:

■ small tidal volumes: 3–5 ml/kg ideal body weight (Fanelli et al., 2013);
■ limiting peak (plateau) pressure to 25–30 cmH_2O (Fanelli et al., 2013);
■ permissive hypercapnia.

Peak, but not mean, airway pressure causes over-distension of alveoli. Ventilation mode and settings may therefore be adjusted to maximise mean airway pressure and volume while limiting peak pressure. Maintaining adequate oxygenation for survival may necessitate compromise of these ideals.

Permissive hypercapnia may create life-threatening respiratory acidosis, so should be used cautiously or avoided with:

■ raised intracranial pressure;
■ anoxic brain injury (e.g. following MI);
■ severe ischaemic heart disease;
■ hypotension;
■ dysrhythmias.

Hypercapnia being a respiratory stimulant, neuromuscular blockage may be needed.

Mode of ventilation may affect outcome. As with other aspects of managing ARDS, options remain controversial, but spontaneous modes, such as airway pressure release ventilation, are more likely to reverse atelectasis (Yoshida *et al.*, 2009).

Previously, high PEEP (> 5 cmH$_2$O) was advocated to increase alveolar recruitment, but there is no evidence that high PEEP improves outcome (Briel *et al.*, 2010), although Gattinoni and Quintel (2016) recommend using higher PEEP in preference to high tidal volumes. Increasingly, "open lung" approaches have been adopted to prevent the sequential alveolar closing that can cause atelectasis. In part, this is achieved through PEEP, but modes of ventilation such as APRV (see Chapter 4), and more controversially some of the modes discussed in the next chapter, can achieve this.

Rescue therapies

High mortality from ARDS has encouraged various attempts to improve outcome, often with more enthusiasm than evidence. Rescue therapies for ARDS include:

- prone positioning;
- inverse ratio ventilation.

Other rescue therapies are discussed in the next chapter.

Prone positioning is probably the most established of interventions in this list. It may enable limitation of tidal volumes (Gattinoni and Quintel, 2016). Whether it reduces mortality (Sud, Friedrich *et al.*, 2010; Guérin *et al.*, 2013; Park *et al.*, 2015) or not (Taccone *et al.*, 2009) is less clear.

Prone positioning is not without problems. It is relatively labour-intensive, although Bein *et al.* (2016) suggest that centres familiar with using proning use three to four staff, and have few complications, whereas centres less familiar with it use more staff and have more complications. Major risks are listed in Table 27.1. Harcombe (2004) recommends:

- pre-oxygenation before turning;
- placing ECG electrodes on the back;
- supporting genitalia on a pillow.

Limbs should be placed in a "swimmer's" position. Proning may reduce absorption but angling the whole bed with the head up reduces reflux. To reduce risks of aspiration, Drahnak and Custer (2015) recommend stopping enteral feeds at least an hour before proning, but Blaser *et al.* (2017) recommend not delaying enteral nutrition for proning. Wright and Flynn (2011) recommend a reverse Trendelenburg position (bed tilted so the mattress remains flat but angled head-upward), which would reduce aspiration risk. They do not

Table 27.1 Complications of prone positioning

extubation and line disconnection
pressure sores, especially on the thorax, head, iliac crest, breast and knee
oesophageal reflux and vomiting
need for more sedation
airway obstruction requiring suction
facial and orbital oedema
ocular damage ("ventilator eye")
increased need for sedation and muscle relaxants
transient desaturation
hypotension
dysrhythmias
need for sufficient staff
difficult to resuscitate

recommend a specific angle, but the 30° minimum adopted for most other patients seems logical.

Prone positioning tends to be an intervention either favoured or avoided by different ICUs. Duration of proning has been widely discrepant between studies, but most studies have adopted the majority of the day; Guérin *et al.*'s (2013) study used at least 16 consecutive hours. Various devices have been marketed to assist either positioning or supporting prone, but many units do not use these.

Inverse ratio ventilation increases mean (but not peak) airway pressure: prolonging inspiratory time increases alveolar recruitment, while shorter expiratory phases prevent atelectasis. But inverse ratio ventilation can cause air trapping (auto-PEEP), and is usually distressing, requiring additional sedation and causing further hypotension. While physiologically attractive, inverse ratio ventilation is distressing, so usually impractical without deep sedation, and its safety/effects currently remain unproven (Kotani *et al.*, 2016).

Reducing pulmonary hypertension

Intra-alveolar damage increases pulmonary vascular resistance, causing pulmonary hypertension. Systemic vasodilators, such as glyceryl trinitrate (GTN) may cause problematic hypotension.

The rapid progression of ARDS, together with shortage of both donor organs and centres performing lung transplants, usually prevents lung transplantation being a viable option.

Fluid management

Fluid management in ARDS necessitates balancing problems from pulmonary oedema against perfusion needs. Measuring extravascular lung water (EVLW – see Chapter 20) has refined fluid assessment, but unfortunately optimum targets remain unclear – conservative fluid management reduces ventilator time but makes no difference to outcome (National Heart, Lung, and Blood Institute Acute Respiratory Distress Syndrome (ARDS) Clinical Trials Network, 2006).

Paralysing agents

Neuromuscular blockade may improve oxygenation and outcome from severe ARDS (Morange *et al.*, 2010) but, while this may be necessary for oxygenation, adverse effects of paralysing agents should be considered (see Chapter 6).

Psychological support

Patients with ARDS may remain on the ICU for weeks, exposing them and their family to prolonged anxiety and stress, which may exhaust their coping mechanisms. Prolonged stays can enable close rapport between families and staff but can become stressful for both; both bedside nurses and nurse managers need to recognise distress. Families may seek hope where little exists, placing excessive trust/reliance/expectations on individual members of staff. As well as being a symptom of denial, this can be particularly stressful for staff.

ARDS also has poor cognitive, psychological and social outcomes. Briegel *et al.* (2013) found that one quarter of survivors of ARDS had cognitive impairment six years later; Herridge *et al.* (2016) suggest this occurs in nearly all survivors. Kamdar *et al.* (2017) found that nearly half of previously employed people remained unemployed one year later.

Implications for practice

- ARDS is caused by inappropriate (excessive) inflammation in lungs;
- ARDS may be suspected with increasing need for ventilatory support; other signs may include increasing airway pressure, new left ventricular failure and bilateral infiltrates on chest X-ray;
- early recognition enables optimal treatment, so nurses should be able to recognise likely signs of developing ARDS, and report concerns;
- while increased ventilator support may benefit oxygenation, it may cause ventilator-associated lung injury (VALI), so strategies such as permissive hypercapnia may be adopted;
- prevention is better than treatment, and may be achieved by lung protection strategies – low tidal volume, lung rest/open lung strategies;
- evidence supporting active treatments, such as steroids, surfactant and prone positioning remains weak and controversial;
- if prone positioning is used, angle the whole mattress head up at 30° (reverse Trendelenburg);
- after initial fluid resuscitation, fluid restriction is probably beneficial;
- cardiac output (flow) monitoring may be needed to guide fluid management, extravascular lung water being especially useful.

Summary

ARDS is a relatively common complication of critical illness. Mortality remains high and panaceas remain elusive. The mainstay of treatment is system support and attempting to prevent further lung injury. Prolonged ICU stay can place families, friends and nursing staff under considerable stress.

Further reading

The Berlin definition of ARDS (Ranieri *et al.*, 2012) is currently accepted internationally. Publication of this spawned a flurry of articles, of which Fanelli *et al.*'s (2013) review is one of the most authoritative. Being a major pathology in ICUs, ARDS is included in almost all ICU texts, and many conferences.

Clinical scenarios

Ann O'Reilly, a 45-year-old mother of six children who weighs 104 kg, was admitted to hospital for elective ligation of fallopian tubes using fibre-optic surgery. Initially Mrs O'Reilly was making a good recovery on the ward, but on the fourth post-operative day she presented with severe shortness of breath, fever and abdominal pains. Investigations revealed perforated bowel. Mrs O'Reilly became septic, developed ARDS and was transferred to the ICU for invasive ventilation and organ support.

In the ICU pressure-controlled inverse ratio ventilation was commenced:

PEEP 10 cmH$_2$O
Pressure Control 30 cmH$_2$O
FiO$_2$ 0.8
Rate 16 per minute
Tidal volumes 600 ml
I:E ratio of 2:1

Arterial blood gases on these settings were:

pH	7.25
PaO$_2$	6.53 kPa
PaCO$_2$	8.47 kPa
HCO$_3^-$	16 mmol/litre
Base excess	−5.8 mmol/litre

Q1. What signs and symptoms led to Ann's diagnosis of ARDS?
Q2. Ann is nursed prone to improve alveolar gas exchange. Analyse rationales for this, and resources in your own clinical area. Devise a plan for staff needed for the procedure and how risks will be minimised.

Q3. Ann's gas exchange improves, allowing reduction in FiO_2 to 0.6. What are potential adverse effects from proning for Ann? What nursing strategies might minimise or prevent occurrence (e.g. abdominal wound healing, pressure areas, breast, eye, mouthcare, and psychological effect on Ann and her family).

Chapter 28

Alternative ventilation

Contents

Fundamental knowledge

Alveolar physiology, gas exchange and pulmonary
  function
Surfactant production and physiology
V/Q mismatch

Introduction

Mortality from severe respiratory failure, especially ARDS, remains frustratingly high, prompting searches for alternative ways to oxygenate and remove carbon dioxide from patients. Although some of these options bypass the lungs, this chapter uses "alternative ventilation" as a convenient, if technically inaccurate, means of encompassing these "rescue therapies". Owing to limited use, there is often limited, and dated, evidence for most options discussed. Modes discussed in this chapter are:

- extracorporeal membrane oxygenators (ECMOs);
- interventional lung assist (iLA);
- Heliox;
- inhaled vasodilators;
- hyperbaric oxygenation;
- high-frequency ventilation (HFV), especially oscillatory (HFOV) and jet (HFJV);
- liquid ventilation (perfluorocarbon – *PFC*),

although availability of most is often confined to specialist units.

Alveolar recovery is optimised if:

- inflated sufficiently to prevent further atelectasis;
- movement is minimised (low tidal volumes, to minimise volutrauma);
- over-distension (high peak inflation pressures – barotrauma) is avoided.

Optimal ventilation would provide adequate gas exchange without causing actual or potential harm. No ideal ventilator exists, and most modes described in this chapter have been found problematic, so are not generally used. But the history of ECMO, described here, illustrates how a mode once largely considered obsolete has again been found useful. Future developments are not always predictable, and some of the other modes not currently recommended may witness resurgence.

1. Extracorporeal lung support (ECLS)

ECMO

Extracorporeal membrane oxygenation (ECMO), initially developed as "bypass" for open-heart surgery (see Chapter 30), can replace or augment conventional ventilation ("respiratory ECMO"). It can also be used for cardiac support, including cardiac arrest (Fagnoul *et al.*, 2014), although Hung *et al.* (2012) suggest that "cardiac ECMO" survival is lower than "respiratory ECMO", presumably because underlying conditions often have less reversibility. Like haemofiltration, ECMO pumps blood extracorporeally through semipermeable membranes. Concurrent lung ventilation is usually maintained during ECMO to prevent atelectasis, but, as ECMO efficiently removes carbon dioxide, lung protection strategies are used – E.L.S.O. (2017) suggests FiO_2 below 0.4 and peak airway pressures below 25 cmH$_2$O. Schmidt et al. (2013) recommend tidal volumes of 3–4 ml/kg, although they comment that optimal strategies remain unknown.

Martinez and Vuylsteke (2012) recommend using ECMO for ARDS when other therapies fail. Use for treating severe influenza resulted in reasonable survival in patients for whom mortality would otherwise have been almost certain (The Australia and New Zealand Extracorporeal Membrane Oxygenation (ANZ EMO) Influenza investigators, 2009; Peek et al., 2009 – the "CESAR" trial), so together with improvements in technology it is likely that ECMO may increasingly be accepted as an intervention available in general, as well as specialist, ICUs. Stewart et al. (2012) question whether the CESAR trial has proved safety and efficacy of ECMO. Studies identify varying mortality rates – Brogan et al. (2009) measured 50% mortality when used to treat severe acute respiratory failure, a figure similar to mortality in older studies, but Schmidt et al. (2014) found mortality while in ICU was only 29%. ECMO is likely to remain a rescue therapy rather than standard treatment. Tramm et al. (2015) conclude that, although ECMO use with newborns and infants is established, efficacy for adults remains uncertain. The American Extracorporeal Life Support Organization guidelines (E.L.S.O., 2017) recommend considering ECMO when mortality risk from respiratory failure reaches 50%, and recommend always using it when risk reaches 80%. Paradoxically, adult ECMO is more effective when used early (Brogan et al., 2009).

Complications of ECMO include:

■ *bleeding*. Pumped circuits cause physical trauma to platelets (as with haemofiltration), compounding problems from anticoagulants and underlying pathologies (Gaffney et al., 2010; Martinez and Vuylsteke, 2012). Manipulation of major vessels may cause vascular trauma, perforation and haemorrhage (Hung et al., 2012; Tramm et al., 2015), while cannulation can cause limb ischaemia (Bein et al., 2013), so access to specialised cardiothoracic and vascular surgery is essential (Martinez and Vuylsteke, 2012).
■ *thrombosis*. Interaction between blood and artificial surfaces can cause thrombi, the other main complication of ECMO (Gaffney et al., 2010).
■ *cost*. From equipment, staff and extending the life (or death) of very sick patients.

While most recent studies suggest ECMO reduces severe ARDS mortality, unsurprisingly fibrosis and other tissue damage often persist, limiting long-term quality of life (Lindén et al., 2009).

ECMO variants

ECMO requires high blood flow, requiring cannulation of major vessels, which, with anticoagulation, significantly contributes to risks of haemorrhage and infection. Various devices, sometimes called extracorporeal lung assists (ECLAs), mimic a smaller, less aggressive ECMO. Many of these function in similar ways to haemofiltration circuits, but compared with ECMO use smaller cannulae in smaller vessels, with less anticoagulation, removing carbon dioxide efficiently but with less effective oxygenation (Baker *et al.*, 2012; Tiruvoipati *et al.*, 2013). As technology has become smaller and more portable, circuits options often include:

- arterial-venous (often without an artificial pump);
- venous-arterial;
- venous-venous.

Venous-venous avoids cannulating an artery, so is safer, but increases risks of thrombi from cannulae or exchange membranes (Baker *et al.*, 2012).

Limiting tidal volumes to avoid barotrauma has often necessitated accepting permissive hypercapnia. Respiratory acidosis reduces myocardial contractility and mean arterial pressure, while causing pulmonary hypertension (Tiruvoipati *et al.*, 2013), so if carbon dioxide can be removed without increasing ventilation cardiovascular stability might be improved. One of the earliest ECMO variants, extracorporeal carbon dioxide removal (ECCO$_2$-R), improves carbon dioxide clearance, enabling lower tidal volumes (3 ml/kg in Bein *et al.*'s (2013) study), so potentially reducing ventilator-induced lung injury.

Many devices used pumped circuits, but interventional lung assist (iLA) uses the patient's own cardiac output (Tiruvoipati *et al.*, 2013), thus avoiding some of the complications of pumped circuits. iLA is probably the most widely used ECMO variant at present, although Tramm *et al.* (2015) were unable to recommend whether or not to use ECMO.

Attempts to oxygenate via intravenous oxygenators (IVOXs) were disappointing; this technology is largely obsolete.

2. Gases

Heliox

Like air, Heliox contains 21% oxygen but replaces air's nitrogen with helium. Helium has a low density (three times less than air and eight times less than oxygen) so, being less affected by airway resistance, reduces the work of breathing (Harris and Barnes, 2008). With airway obstruction, where the work of breathing is excessive, Heliox may enable adequate oxygenation. It should be given through a non-rebreathe mask so that it is not diluted with room air (Kass, 2003). Benefits should occur within minutes, buying time to resolve the underlying problem (Calzia and Stahl, 2004). Its value beyond one hour is limited (Ho *et al.*, 2003). It has been advocated for use with COPD (Tassaux *et al.*, 2005; Eves and Ford, 2007). Heliox is supplied in gas cylinders (brown, with white tops), so although relatively expensive it is also readily available. But few ventilators (invasive or non-invasive) are designed to work with Heliox (Calzia and Stahl, 2004), and it may affect ventilator monitoring.

Heliox is inert, colourless, odourless and tasteless. It disperses quickly, so should not significantly affect anyone nearby. Helium affects vocal cords, so they should be warned about a temporary high-pitched, squeaky voice.

Inhaled vasodilators

With severe acute lung injury (ALI), pulmonary vasodilatation may enable effective oxygenation with lower levels of inspired oxygen and therefore less risk of oxygen toxicity, and possible alveolar damage. Delivering vasodilators either as a gas or nebuliser has attracted intermittent interest, partly because delivery is to ventilated parts of the lungs, optimising V/Q match (Teman et al., 2015). Chemicals used include nitric oxide (NO; as iNO = inhaled nitric oxide), prostaglandin (epoprostenol, also called prostaglandin I_2 – PGI_2; alprostadil, also called prostaglandin E – PGE) and sildenafil (Viagra) (Gall et al., 2016). Using drugs outside manufacturers' licences raises questions of account-ability. Coagulopathies, frequently complicating ARDS, may be aggravated by prostacyclin.

Like many rescue therapies for ARDS, practice has largely been imported from paediatrics, with limited supporting evidence, and assumptions that effective therapies for infant respiratory distress syndrome (IRDS) will work with ARDS.

As an endogenous vasodilator, nitric oxide appears attractive but it can produce toxic metabolites such as nitrogen dioxide, and change haemoglobin structure to methaemoglobin, which impairs oxygen delivery (Bhatraju et al., 2015; Wright, 2015). While Adhikari et al. (2014) found nitric oxide harmful, Bhatraju et al. (2015) consider that it does not have significant side effects. Fuller et al. (2015) consider there is insufficient evidence to support use of prostaglandins. Fanelli et al. (2013) found it improved oxygenation but not outcome. Currently, the use of inhaled vasodilators is likely to be limited largely to clinical trials.

Hyperbaric oxygenation

Ratios between gases in air remain constant; if temperature remains constant, water content (volume) of humidified air also remains constant. This means that changes in atmospheric pressure alter the volume of each gas that can be dissolved in plasma. At sea-level atmospheric pressure (approximately one bar), only small volumes of oxygen are dissolved in plasma (3 ml oxygen per 100 ml blood). If haemoglobin carriage is prevented (e.g. carbon monoxide poisoning), tissues rely on plasma carriage.

21% oxygen at 2.8 bar (= 18 metres depth of water) increases oxygen pressure from 21 kPa to 284 kPa, providing sufficient plasma carriage to meet normal metabolism (Pitkin et al., 1997). Hyperbaric oxygen of 3 bar reduces the half-life of carbon monoxide from 320 minutes in room air to 23 minutes (Blumenthal, 2001), although the benefits are controversial and, unless hyperbaric oxygen is readily available, its use for carbon monoxide poisoning cannot be supported (Juurlink *et al.*, 2005). Hyperbaric chambers can be *single patient*, or *rooms* which staff and equipment can enter. Hyperbaric pressure can be discontinued once haemoglobin oxygen carriage is available (at most, usually a few hours). Oxygen toxicity was first identified in contexts of hyperbaric oxygen therapy (Gerschman *et al.*, 1954), but Sinan *et al.*'s (2016) laboratory study suggests that hyperbaric oxygen does not cause oxidative stress to erythrocytes.

Complications of hyperbaric oxygen include:

- *high atmospheric pressures*: these cause barotrauma to ears and sinuses, oxygen toxicity, tonic-clonic seizures and visual problems such as myopia and cataracts (Wagstaff, 2014);
- *monitoring*: as oxygen is not being carried by haemoglobin, pulse oximetry has no value;
- *infusions*: pressure may affect infusion pumps (Hopson and Greenstein, 2007), and tubing should be pressure-resistant (Bailey *et al.*, 2004);
- *access*: single-person chambers may prevent equipment (including ventilators) being used, while transfer of equipment (e.g. emergency equipment) between normal and hyperbaric pressures may be restricted or delayed. This may affect ventilation, inotropes and other infusions/mechanical support;
- *scarcity*: few units have hyperbaric chambers, necessitating the long-distance transfer of hypoxic patients.

Hyperbaric oxygen may provide support, enabling short-term survival; Gibson and Davis (2010) found that hyperbaric oxygen improved neurological outcome if stroke occurred following cardiac surgery, but Scheinkestel *et al.* (1999) did not find any reduction of neurological complications with use following carbon monoxide poisoning. Sample sizes for studies into this and other rarely available options are almost inevitably small, and so findings have limited reliability.

3. High-frequency ventilation (HFV)

This includes various infrequently used modes, which have largely failed to establish a place in practice. Frequent but small tidal volumes prevent alveoli closure, so may prevent ventilator-associated lung injury (Carney *et al.*, 2005).

Complications of most high-frequency modes include:

- *safety*: chest wall movement and air entry are barely perceptible, spirometry is impractical, and some ventilators have few alarms. Blood gas analysis and pulse oximetry are among the few remaining means of monitoring;
- gas trapping/shunting;
- peak intra-alveolar pressures are higher than measurable peak airway pressure. Excessive pressure may impair perfusion, so increasing mean airway pressure may exacerbate V/Q mismatch;

■ noise: high-frequency modes are usually noisy, provoking stress responses, disrupting sleep and contributing to sensory overload.

High-frequency oscillatory ventilation (HFOV)

Adding oscillation (3–15 hertz (Hz)) to modified CPAP circuits or near-conventional ventilators achieves a form of high-frequency ventilation that potentially keeps alveoli open for oxygenation, while creating a sufficient number of small tidal volumes (180–900 breaths each minute) to clear carbon dioxide. Henderson-Smart et al. (2007) found insufficient evidence to support its use in paediatrics; while Sud, Sud et al.'s (2010) meta-analysis suggested it could significantly reduce ARDS mortality, and Young et al. (2013) found that HFOV improved oxygenation, more recent studies suggest no overall benefit from HFOV, and even increased mortality (Ferguson et al., 2013; Malhotra et al., 2013; Young et al., 2013; Marini et al., 2015). While not recommending routine use for ARDS, Facchin and Fan (2015) suggest it may be a useful rescue therapy.

Lungs should be auscultated, but low tidal volumes prevent clear air entry sounds. Abdominal chest wall movement ("wiggle") should be monitored – change indicating altered lung compliance or airway resistance. Suction causes alveolar deflation and possible atelectasis, so should only be performed if specifically indicated, and if possible avoided completely for the first 12 hours. On chest X-rays, at most eight pairs of ribs should be visible; if more appear, lungs are overdistended.

High-frequency jet ventilation

HFJV (or "jet") uses tidal volumes of 1–5 ml/kg – with most adults, approximately the same volume as physiological dead space. Rates of 100–300 are usually used (Keogh and Cordingley, 2002). HFJV can be delivered through mini-tracheostomy (Allison, 1994), preventing many complications of intubation.

Carbon dioxide clearance is efficient. Pulmonary secretions are mobilised, presumably due to constant chest wall "quivering" resembling physiotherapy, so increasing alveolar surface area and gas exchange. Lack of recent evidence for jet ventilation reflects lack of use.

4. Liquid ventilation

Perflurocarbons are very efficient oxygen carriers, dissolving nearly 20 times more gases than water (Tremper, 2002). Perfluorocarbon is also anti-inflammatory, creating fewer oxygen-free radicals (Lange et al., 2000; Haitsma and Lachmann, 2002). Although total liquid ventilation is possible, partial liquid ventilation – instilling perfluorocarbon into lungs then using conventional ventilation in the remaining lungfields – appeared attractive. While liquid ventilation improves oxygenation (Dernaika et al., 2009), it also increases ventilator days and mortality (Kacmarek *et al.*, 2006), so cannot currently be recommended.

Implications for practice

- highly invasive modes (e.g. ECMO) may cause haemorrhage; cannulae should (where possible) be easily visible;
- other modes discussed in this chapter are rarely seen outside specialist units; where used, staff should take every opportunity to become familiar with their use;
- modes discussed are usually "rescue therapies", so individual complications of each mode are compounded by complications of severe pathophysi-ologies; nursing care should be actively planned to optimise safety for each patient;
- visitors and patients may be anxious about use of rarer modes, or frightened by particular aspects (e.g. liquid ventilation = "drowning"), so should be reassured;
- monitoring facilities are often limited with unconventional modes, so nurses should optimise remaining facilities (e.g. pulse oximetry, blood gases), which may need to be measured more frequently;
- with limited evidence to support use of these modes, units should consider practitioners' accountability before adopting them;
- Heliox may provide adequate oxygenation despite airway obstruction, so can usefully buy time for other interventions.

Summary

Options discussed in this chapter have the potential to oxygenate and remove carbon dioxide while enabling lung rest. Tempting as it is to seek alternatives when conventional ventilations fails, the safety and complications of extra-corporeal lung support remain largely speculative (Del Sorbo *et al.*, 2014). Some modes discussed are currently rarely used, but like ECMO may be revived if technical improvements and/or evidence of efficacy become available. The only thing certain about the future is that it is uncertain. Some options discussed are available in specialist centres to which patients may be transferred, for subsequent repatriation. This chapter provides an introduction to these modes for staff unfamiliar with them or new to units where they are used. More experienced users will wish to pursue supplementary material.

Whenever rarer modes/treatments are used, unidentified complications may occur, so decisions to use (or suggest) alternatives should be tempered by considerations of patient safety:

- how will the patient benefit?
- what are the known complications?
- what is the likely risk from unidentified complications (research base)?
- are staff competent to use the mode safely?

Further reading

Brogan *et al.* (2009) and Peek *et al.* (2009) both report major ECMO trials, while Schmidt *et al.* (2013) provide a useful summary through meta-analysis. Young *et al.*'s (2013) study describes how HFOV works and its theoretical benefits and measured effects. Tramm *et al.* (2015) provide a Cochrane review of ECMO, although, unsurprisingly in view of the paucity of evidence, their main recommendation is for more studies.

Clinical scenarios

Mrs Margaret Sheppard is a 60-year-old known asthmatic who was admitted to a respiratory ward with community-acquired pneumonia. Her respiratory function continued to deteriorate over nine days. She was then admitted to ICU with a diagnosis of ARDS, intubated and commenced on conventional ventilation. Despite maximal conventional ventilation, she continues to deteriorate.

Q1. Which, if any, of the options discussed in this chapter are available in your region? Which would you advocate for Mrs Sheppard, and why?

Q2. Locate any local criteria/guidelines to assist choices. If none are available locally, find out what is available from your tertiary centre, their criteria for acceptance, and requirements for transfer.

Q3. Following improvement, what strategies are likely to be used on your unit following Mrs Sheppard's repatriation from your tertiary centre? If your unit has guidelines for this, reflect on your experience of seeing them implemented.

Part VI

Cardiovascular

Chapter 29

Acute coronary syndromes

Contents

Fundamental knowledge

Coronary arteries – structure and location
Coagulation cascade
Renin-angiotensin mechanism
Reperfusion injury (Chapter 24)

Introduction

Coronary heart disease causes more UK deaths than any other disease (Townsend *et al.*, 2012). In cardiothoracic ICUs, interventions for coronary artery disease are usually the reason for admission (discussed further in Chapter 30). Elsewhere, coronary artery disease more often complicates other pathologies, necessitating ICU admission.

Coronary artery disease is an atherosclerotic process, with stable and unstable periods. During unstable periods, local inflammatory responses release vasoactive mediators that can cause *acute coronary syndromes*:

- ST elevation myocardial infarction (STEMI);
- non-ST elevation myocardial infarction (NSTEMI);
- unstable angina (UA).

If myocardial infarction is suspected, or the person has chest pain which may be cardiac, a 12-lead ECG should be taken. Sedated patients may not show signs of chest pain, although most ICU monitors detect ST segment abnormalities. If the ECG shows persistent ST elevation in two or more consecutive leads (2 mm in chest leads, 1 mm in limb leads) or a new left bundle branch block (i.e. not on the previous ECG), the patient has had a *STEMI*. If neither of these ECG abnormalities is present, troponin (or alternative cardiac markers) should be measured. Troponin positive indicates a *NSTMI*. Negative troponin indicates unstable angina, although if chest pain (or suspicion of MI) persists, troponin should be rechecked within three hours (Thygesen *et al.*, 2012). Persistent is defined as more than 20 minutes, to exclude possible transient causes; it would obviously be inappropriate to wait this length of time before initiating action. This diagnosis is summarised in Figure 29.1.

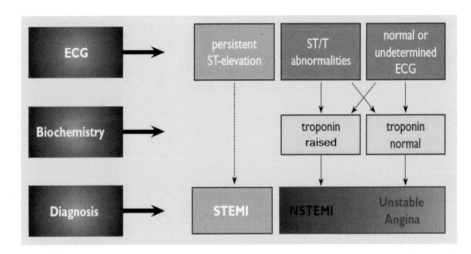

Figure 29.1 Acute coronary syndromes

Source: Adapted from EC, 2011

Myocardial oxygen supply

Myocytes have high metabolic rates, necessitating large quantities of oxygen. The right and left coronary arteries are the first arteries to leave the aorta, delivering one twentieth of cardiac output to the myocardium. The left artery divides into the *left anterior descending* and *circumflex* (see Figure 29.2). At rest, the myocardium normally extracts nearly all available oxygen, leaving little reserve for oxygen debt. In health, increased oxygen demand is met either through vasodilatation or tachycardia (or both). Diseased coronary arteries produce little nitric oxide (Kalucka *et al.*, 2017), preventing significant vaso-dilatation. Critically ill patients typically already have compensatory tachycardias. Gross tachycardia (> 130 bpm) reduces stroke volume, making myocardium work harder (increased oxygen demand) while further reducing oxygen supply.

While supplementary oxygen is usually needed, hyperoxia can cause cardiac and brain damage, including coronary artery vasoconstriction (Conti, 2011), so oxygen should be given to achieve target saturations of 94–98% (Nolan *et al.*, 2015; B.T.S., 2017).

Treatment

STEMI is usually caused by complete artery occlusion (Task Force, 2011), so ideally should be treated by primary percutaneous coronary intervention (pPCI – see Chapter 30). If patients are too unstable to transfer for pPCI, thrombolysis (see below) is an acceptable alternative (N.I.C.E., 2013a).

Hospitals usually have local ACS protocols to guide medication, but key drugs for NSTEMI and unstable angina are:

- nitrates, such as glyceryl trinitrate;
- beta-blockers;
- anti-platelet drugs, such as clopidogrel and aspirin.

(Task Force, 2016c)

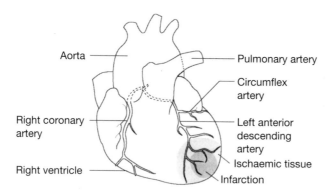

Figure 29.2 Coronary arteries, with anterior myocardial infarction

Cardiac markers

Injured cells release chemicals. Identifying and measuring these chemicals enables diagnosis of cell damage. The most useful chemical marker to identify cardiac damage remains troponin (T or I) (Task Force2016c), although for heart failure B-type natriuretic peptide, or its precursor N-terminal pro-B-type natriuretic peptide, are recommended (N.I.C.E., 2014a; Priori *et al.*, 2015). Myoglobin is not sensitive or specific enough as a cardiac marker (Task Force, 2016c). Creatine kinase (CK) and its isoenzymes, the main cardiac biomarker before troponin, can usefully assess skeletal muscle damage (e.g. with rhabdomyolysis), but are not normally now used to assess myocardial infarction.

High-sensitivity *troponin* has enabled earlier detection of myocardial infarction (Lee *et al.*, 2016), resulting in current ranges being lower than previously. Significant levels may differ between trusts, and will probably continue to be lowered, so readers should check what is currently used in their own trust. There are many reasons for "false positives", mostly respiratory and cardiac diseases that are not infarction, but probably most importantly renal failure (Task Force, 2016c), as troponin is cleared via the kidneys. Provided reasons for false positives can be excluded, higher levels indicate greater damage.

Cardiac myosin-binding protein C (cMyC)

Unique to the heart, more abundant than troponins and released earlier, this protein may enable earlier diagnosis (Kaier *et al.*, 2017). Kaier *et al.*'s study used levels below 10 nanograms/litre to exclude infarction, and levels above 120 to confirm diagnosis.

B-type Natriuretic peptide

Natriuretic peptides are hormones which increase renal sodium excretion ("natrium" = sodium), so raised levels indicate cardiac remodelling (Natriuretic Peptides Studies Collaboration, 2016). Levels above 100 nanograms/litre indicate heart failure (N.I.C.E. 2014a) but should not be used to diagnose acute coronary syndromes (N.I.C.E., 2010e).

Myoglobin (see also Chapter 38)

This is released following muscle damage, including myocardial infarction. Normal serum myoglobin is < 72 (male) and < 58 (female) nanograms/millilitre (Walsh-Irvin, 2013).

Creatine kinase (CK)

This is also released from brain and skeletal muscle. There are three isoenzymes: CK: MM (skeletal muscle), MB (heart) and BB (brain). With availability of troponin tests, most laboratories no longer test isoenzymes.

Thrombolysis

STEMI, and arguably NSTEMI, should be treated by pPCI where possible. If pPCI is unavailable or impractical, urgent thrombolytics should be given. Streptokinase (the oldest and cheapest) and t-PA/rt-PA (recombinant tissue plasminogen activator), both of which necessitate continuous infusions, have largely been replaced by third-generation thrombolytics which can be given by bolus, such as tenecteplase (Metalyse). Urokinase, a weak thrombolytic, is useful for dissolving thrombi in vascular devices and shunts but not for treating myocardial infarction.

Other drugs

Many drugs are used in cardiology; ones frequently seen in ICU include:

- *nitrates* (e.g. glyceryl trinitrate – GTN, isosorbide mono-/dinitrate) stimulate endogenous nitric oxide release, relaxing smooth muscle, which vasodilates (Agewall *et al.*, 2016; Singh *et al.*, 2017), which:
  - reduces preload;
  - reduces afterload;
  - dilates coronary arteries,

  thus reducing cardiac work and increasing myocardial oxygen supply (Thacker and Patel, 2017). In crises, GTN infusions are usually commenced. Isosorbide dinitrate can be given sublingually, enabling ready access and quick absorption.
- *aspirin.* A single dose of 300mg aspirin can reduce or prevent infarction, but this is unlikely to be useful in ICU. Optimal daily cardiac dose is 75–81 mg, with no clear benefit to doses above 100 mg (Steinhubl *et al.*, 2009). Like colleagues elsewhere, ICU nurses should ensure that patients and their families understand the prescribed dose – some patients self-medicate one 300 mg aspirin tablet each day, and should understand the risk this poses of gastric bleeding.
- *Clopidogrel,* or alternative anti-platelet drugs such as prasugrel or ticagrelor (Wenger, 2012), should be given to all ACS patients, unless platelet counts are very low. Most teams will probably only omit antiplatelet drugs when platelet count is below 50, although it is worth checking with counts below 100.
- beta-blockers (drugs ending in -olol) inhibit beta stimulation of the heart, so reducing blood pressure (Chen *et al.*, 2010) and myocardial work. Beta-blockers are also often used to control atrial fibrillation.
- *ACE inhibitors* (drugs ending in –pril) inhibit *a*ngiotensin *c*onverting *e*nzyme. Angiotensin is a more powerful vasoconstrictor than noradrenaline, so inhibiting the enzyme necessary for its activation prevents hypertension. This allows coronary artery "remodelling".

- *calcium channel blockers* (e.g. nifedipine, amlopidine, diltiazem, verapamil) regulate the calcium channel of action potential (see Chapter 22). This reduces myocardial excitability and vasodilates arteries.
- *statins* lower circulating lipid levels, thus reducing morbidity and mortality from coronary artery disease (Heart Protection Study Collaborative Group, 2012; Jellinger *et al.*, 2017). Used for long-term treatment, they are unlikely to be commenced in the ICU, but patients already taking statin therapy should resume their treatment as soon as practical. Most statins, including simvastatin, should be given at night (6 pm or 10 pm), as most cholesterol is synthesised overnight, although some, including atorvastatin, may be given at any time. Statins interact with many drugs, so doses may need reducing. If in doubt about timing or dose of statins, check with the unit pharmacist.

Post cardiac arrest syndrome

The three major complications following resuscitation are:

- brain injury;
- myocardial dysfunction;
- systemic ischaemia/reperfusion responses.

Myocardial dysfunction causes cardiogenic shock (see Chapter 31), responsible for most deaths within the first two to three days, after which brain injury causes most later deaths (Nolan *et al.*, 2015). Seizures occur in one third of patients who remain comatose following cardiac arrest (Nolan *et al.*, 2015). Ischaemia and reperfusion responses cause oxidative stress, and so inflammation, which results in vasodilatory (distributive) shock. Post cardiac arrest syndrome combines cardiogenic and vasodilatory shocks, a syndrome often progressing to multi-organ dysfunction syndrome (de Chambrun *et al.*, 2016).

Reducing morbidity from post cardiac arrest syndrome therefore targets these three areas. Brain injury may be reduced by targeted temperature management, although optimum temperature has proved controversial (see Chapter 8); currently preferred targets often range from 33–36°C, with drugs being used to stop shivering, which would increase metabolic oxygen demand (Nakashima *et al.*, 2017). Myocardial dysfunction is treated by ways familiar from general ICU care, primarily maintaining MAP with fluids and vasopressors (Nakashima *et al.*, 2017), while perfusion responses are minimised by avoiding both hypoxia and hyperoxia (Nakashima *et al.*, 2017).

Psychology

Physical or psychological stress stimulates catecholamine release (see Chapter 1), which causes vasoconstriction, hypertension and other detrimental effects. While stress responses can be life-preserving for healthy people faced by physical danger in the community, stress has long been associated with cardiovascular disease. Coronary heart disease is often associated with depression (Dhar and Barton, 2016; Osler *et al.*, 2016); although Potijk *et al.* (2016) found that while childhood stressors influenced physical health, the only link in adulthood was through behaviours, such as smoking, that increase risks of cardiovascular disease. Patients with cardiac disease, and needing major cardiac interventions, are prone to depression, which as well as being psychologically undesirable also increases mortality (Lichtman *et al.*, 2014; Osler *et al.*, 2016).

Health promotion

Most trusts produce information leaflets, and the British Heart Foundation produce a range of useful booklets that are available in most hospitals. Most trusts also employ heart failure nurses and offer rehabilitation programmes for patients following myocardial infarction. If patients are not transferred to a coronary care unit, local resources should be identified and offered to patients and their families.

Patients and families are often receptive to health information following infarction and should be offered advice to reduce risks of further attacks. Advice should be patient-specific, but is likely to include lifestyle changes such as:

- stopping smoking;
- exercising;
- reducing alcohol – there is widespread belief, but little evidence, that mild drinking may be cardioprotective (Foster, 2016), but heavy drinking contributes to atherosclerosis;
- reducing weight;
- maintaining a healthy diet – reducing animal fats; fish oils and other sources of polyunsaturated fatty acids (PUFAs) are cardioprotective; dietician referral may be useful;
- keeping good control of chronic co-morbidities (e.g. diabetes).

Patients and partners should also be warned of the risks of sexual intercourse provoking further infarction.

Implications for practice

- hypoxic myocardium needs oxygen, but hyperoxia increases risks of cardiac and brain damage, so oxygen should be given to achieve 94–98% saturation;
- troponins are the best marker for myocardial infarction;
- STEMI should be treated by primary percutaneous coronary intervention (pPCI) if reasonably possible. If patients are too unstable to transfer, thrombolysis is the next best option;
- NSTEMI should be managed initially by treating heart failure. Angiography, possibly proceeding to percutaneous coronary interventions or open-heart surgery, may be needed later;

■ infarction risk is greatest between 06.00–10.00, so avoid early-morning strenuous stimulation (e.g. bedbaths) with all patients (unless requested by the patient);

■ pain relief is important both for humanitarian reasons and to prevent further stress responses; opioid analgesics are usually needed, and their efficacy should be assessed.

Summary

Coronary heart disease is endemic in Western societies. Cardiovascular disease kills more people in the UK than any other single disease. Acute coronary syndromes may necessitate admission to ICU (usually if there are other system complications) or occur in patients already on the unit. In addition to technical aspects, an important part of nursing care is health promotion.

Further reading

The European Society of Cardiology publishes various guidelines, both on its website and in the *European Heart Journal* (e.g. Task Force 2016c). Readers should be familiar with the current UK Resuscitation Guidelines (currently, 2015). Nolan *et al.* (2015) provide updated guidelines for patients admitted to ICU following cardiac arrest. Outhoff (2016) reviews statins.

Clinical scenario

Mr Howard Gray is a 52-year-old insurance broker scheduled for a laparoscopic cholecystectomy when he developed inverted T waves. Troponin was 230 nanograms/litre. Surgery was therefore postponed, and he is admitted to ICU for observation, further assessment and optimisation.

Mr Gray has a six-month history of indigestion and abdominal pain, exacerbated by eating, and he has recently lost weight; one year ago he weighed 82 kg. He normally has hypertension, for which he takes bisoprolol and atorvastatin. He is a smoker (20 pack years) and occasional drinker. His wife states that lived an active life until problems with pain.

On arrival in ICU his ECG shows sinus tachycardia with ST elevation in leads I, aVL and V_2-V_6, with ST depression in II, III and aVF.

Vital signs include:

HR 128 beats/minute
BP 93/65 mmHg (MAP 74 mmHg)
temperature 35.8°C

Q1. Using Chapter 22 and the description of the ECG, identify which part of Mr Gray's myocardium are damaged. Which coronary arteries supply this area?

Q2. Mr Gray is transferred for pPCI. Using guidelines and practice from your trust, what you would prepare to facilitate this transfer?

Q3. Following successful stenting, Mr Gray returns to ICU. Immediate post-pPCI care is discussed in the next chapter, but what advice, information and follow-up services can you offer to patients like Mr Gray? What other resources are available within your trust/locality for health promotion, advice and cardiac rehabilitation for both Mr Gray and his family?

Chapter 30

Cardiac surgery and interventions

Contents

Fundamental knowledge

Cardiac anatomy – arteries and valves
Coronary artery disease

Introduction

Coronary artery and valve disease (see Chapter 29) remain major causes of UK mortality, especially among older people. ST elevation myocardial infarction (STEMI) should be treated by urgent transfer for primary percutaneous coronary intervention (Antman *et al.*, 2008; Di Mario *et al.*, 2008). With other cardiac disease, when drug therapies cannot support cardiac failure, percutaneous intervention or open-heart surgery may be needed either to repair or replace damaged tissue. Outcomes (survival and quality of life) for both are good. Percutaneous and open surgery may be used to repair or bypass occluded coronary arteries or repair valves. This chapter also describes heart transplants. Intra-aortic balloon pumps and ventricular assist devices (means to support failing hearts) are described in Chapter 31. Immediate post-procedure nursing care largely follows from actual and potential problems created by procedures.

Percutaneous coronary interventions (PCIs)

PCI is a generic term for procedures using catheters inserted into the vascular system which enter the coronary circulation. PCI has increasingly replaced open-heart surgery. Procedures include:

- percutaneous transluminal coronary angioplasty (PTCA),
- coronary angiogram (diagnostic, although may proceed to PTCA),

and increasingly:

- valve repair

and some other interventions. Previously usually inserted into the groin, whenever feasible radial approaches are now usually used. PCI tends to be preferred for single- and two-vessel disease, but with multivessel disease morbidity and mortality are lower with open-heart surgery (Sipahi *et al.*, 2014). Angioplasty forces plaque back against the vessel wall and, unless vessels are especially tortuous, stents are inserted to maintain patency. Drug-eluting stents (DESs) are usually inserted, as they provide better outcomes (Dind *et al.*, 2017), although Greenhalgh *et al.*'s (2010) Cochrane review suggested they did not reduce mortality and there was no evidence they were cost-effective.

Most studies, such as Pyxaras *et al.* (2016) found outcomes between open and percutaneous repair were similar.

Primary percutaneous coronary angioplasty is the first-line treatment for ST elevation myocardial infarction (STEMI), provided "call to balloon" time does not exceed 120–150 minutes (D.O.H., 2008a), although European guidelines suggest that maximum time should be two hours (Task Force, 2010b). With the potential for therapeutic hypothermia to reduce cerebral damage for out-of-hospital arrests, patients may be transferred significant distances to centres offering pPCI, with almost inevitable post-procedure admission to ICU.

Non-ST elevation myocardial infarction (NSTEMI) has traditionally been treated conservatively, supporting systems, with possible later, but not primary, PCI. Wallentin *et al.* (2016) reported improved mortality from early PCI with NSTEMI.

Catheters for PCI occluding already severely diseased coronary arteries, procedures can induce myocardial infarction (MI) – Prasad and Hermann (2011) found 5–30% suffered periprocedural, classified as types 4 and 5 myocardial infarction by Thygesen *et al.* (2012).

Open-heart surgery

Open-heart surgery necessitates opening the thorax by sternotomy. Historically, this involved cross-clamping the aorta and vena cavae, using a blood pump oxygenator (see extracorporeal membrane oxygenator – ECMO, Chapter 28), arresting the heart with cardioplegia to enable surgery, and using moderate hypothermia to reduce metabolic oxygen demand. After completing surgery, the great vessels would then be reconnected, heartbeat restarted with DC shock, and hypothermia reversed. Some of these techniques are still used but have been increasingly abandoned or replaced.

Traditional concerns surrounding pump oxygenators included:

- neurological complications, including strokes and delirium;
- respiratory failure, including atelectasis;
- inflammatory responses;
- kidney injury;
- blood cell damage.

Although pump oxygenators' pump designs have improved, most open-heart surgery is now *"off-pump"* coronary artery bypass – OPCAB, which has similar outcomes (Lamy *et al.*, 2012; van Harten *et al.*, 2012), although Møller *et al.*'s 2012 Cochrane review suggests that OPCAB entails greater risks. For OPCAB, the heart is usually slowed to about 40 bpm with beta-blockers.

Cardioplegia, a potassium-rich crystalloid (Alexander and Smith, 2016) used to arrest myocardium and so reduce metabolic oxygen demand, can cause post-operative dysrhythmias. Traditionally, cold cardioplegia (4–10°C) was used to reduce metabolism, but "warm" (normothermic) cardioplegia is generally considered more cardioprotective, so is now usually used.

Hypothermia reduces metabolic oxygen demand and causes peripheral vaso-constriction (reducing venous capacity). To prevent hypervolaemia with vasoconstriction, two units of blood are usually removed for post-operative *autologous* transfusion. Post-operative rewarming causes vasodilatation, necessitating fluid monitoring and replacement. Many centres have abandoned inducing perioperative hypothermia. Targeted temperature management is discussed in Chapter 8.

Sternotomies are closed with permanent wire loops (usually five, visible on X-rays).

Coronary artery bypass grafts

Occluded coronary arteries can be bypassed by grafts to restore myocardial blood supply. The saphenous vein, which is easy to remove, is often used, although arteries provide more effective grafts. The most commonly grafted arteries are the internal mammary artery (*IMA*, especially left – LIMA) (Alexander and Smith, 2016), and increasingly radial artery (Valgimigli *et al.*, 2015). Arterial grafts can cause more pain, both from arterial spasm and from the graft site.

Valve surgery

Mitral valve disease, historically a late complication of rheumatic fever, has decreased in Western countries, although incidence of age-related aortic stenosis is increasing (Blackburn and Bookless, 2002).

Diseased valves can be repaired or replaced. Replacement valves are either:

■ biological (human cadaver, xenografts – porcine, bovine, baboon);
■ prosthetic.

Biological valves are less thrombogenic, not requiring lifelong anticoagulation therapy but are likely to need earlier replacement (Stasseno *et al.*, 2009).

Valves can be replaced percutaneously (Coeytaux *et al.*, 2010), enabling post-operative recovery of uncomplicated cases in high-dependency units (Dewhurst and Rawlins, 2009). Mitral stenosis can be resolved by percutaneous balloon valvuloplasty (Chandrashekhar *et al.*, 2009).

Post-operative nursing

In addition to needs of any post-operative patient, cardiac surgery creates specialised needs. Complications vary, partly with procedures – normothermic and off-pump surgery avoid some problems. Common post-operative complications include:

A – airway management is the same as for all patients
B – ventilation
C –
    ■ blood pressure management
    ■ bleeding
    ■ temperature
    ■ dysrhythmias
    ■ metabolic
    ■ kidney function
D –
    ■ pain control
    ■ neurological complications
    ■ psychological considerations

E –
- skincare
- normalisation.

Most patients undergoing cardiac surgery have only single organ failure, so recovery is usually rapid, most patients being transferred to stepdown units the following day. Seeing and helping patients progress rapidly can be very rewarding for nurses. Emphasis should therefore focus on normalisation, promoting homeostasis and encouraging patients to resume normal activities of living.

Ventilation

If therapeutic hypothermia is used, weaning from ventilation and extubation are usually delayed until normothermia is achieved. Otherwise, extubation usually occurs at the end of surgery/procedure, or very soon after. *Hypoventilation* and *impaired cough* may be caused by:

- pain;
- fear;
- impaired respiratory centre function;
- pleural effusion.

With adequate analgesia cover, patients should be encouraged to breathe deeply and cough. Good pain management and patient education can prevent many complications. Sternal instability, suffered by one sixth of patients undergoing coronary artery bypass grafts (CABGs) via median sternotomy (El-Ansary *et al.*, 2000), can cause "clicking" sounds. Although not painful, external stabilisation with hands or a single-patient-use support, such as a "cough lock", helps deep breathing and coughing. Incentive spirometry is often useful.

Exudative pleural effusions occur in half of patients (Light *et al.*, 2002). Brims *et al.* (2004) drained on average one litre of fluid from each patient, which significantly improved oxygenation.

Blood pressure management

Initial hypertension from hypothermic vasoconstriction may damage anastomoses, causing bleeding. Medical staff usually indicate upper limits for systolic pressure, frequently 100–120 mmHg, prescribing vasodilators (e.g. glyceryl trinitrate – GTN) or inodilators (see Chapter 34). Persistent hypertension unresponsive to nitrates indicates neurological damage.

Early hypotension is usually due to:

- hypovolaemia on rewarming
- myocardial dysfunction.

Once adequately fluid-resuscitated, inotropic support may be needed to maintain tissue perfusion. Hypotension can also result from cardiogenic shock (see Chapter 31), which is likely to be exacerbated rather than resolved by giving fluids.

Bleeding

Significant bleeding usually occurs from:

- anastomoses;
- fibrinolysis and other coagulopathies (Pleym *et al.*, 2006).

Re-exploration for haemorrhage increases morbidity and mortality (Pleym *et al.*, 2006), so is avoided if possible.

Any sutures can fail, but aortic (from CPB) and myocardial sutures are exposed to high pressure and heartbeat/pulse movement. Arterial spasm with IMA grafts usually cause more bleeding. Pericardial bleeding may cause rapid *tamponade*. Two/three drains are inserted:

- pericardial
- mediastinal
- pleural (if pleura injured).

Tamponade causes obstructive shock (see Chapter 31); emergency treatment is drainage – needle thoracocentesis. On arrival, volumes in each drain should be marked. Drainage, usually recorded hourly, should gradually reduce, becoming more serous. Sudden cessation may indicate thrombus obstruction, with likely tamponade; if patency of drains cannot be re-established, report this urgently, as emergency thoracotomy may be needed.

Coagulopathies are multifactorial (e.g. heparinsation using CPB), being monitored through full blood count and clotting studies. Haemostasis may require platelets/FFP and/or other clotting factors.

Temperature

If hypothermic, gradual rewarming should bring central within 2°C of peripheral (pedal) temperature – avoid measuring pedal temperature on limbs from which saphenous veins are harvested. Warming hastens homeostasis and may prevent shivering (which increases metabolic rate, and so increasing oxygen consumption).

Dysrhythmias

Various dysrhythmias (often multifocal) often occur following cardiac (especially valve) surgery. Resolution is usually spontaneous and relatively quick. Causes include:

- chronic cardiomyopathy;
- oedema (from surgery, disrupting conduction pathways);
- acidosis;
- electrolyte imbalance;
- hypoxia/ischaemia;
- mechanical irritation (e.g. drain/pacing wire removal);
- hypothermia.

Only symptomatic and problematic dysrhythmias normally need treatment (drugs, pacing or resuscitation).

Atrial fibrillation occurs post-operatively in 20–40% of patients (Cavolli *et al.*, 2008).

Other post-operative dysrhythmias include *bradycardias*, *blocks*, *junctional* and *tachydysrhythmias*. Persistent blocks often require pacing, hence perioperative placement of epicardial wires. Epicardial wires are unipolar, a negative pole being created by inserting a subcutaneous needle. Pacing wires usually remain in place until dysrhythmias become unlikely – usually five to 10 days.

Myocardial infarction may necessitate emergency thoracotomy/sternotomy and internal massage/defibrillation. Staff should therefore know where thoracotomy packs are situated. Internal defibrillation avoids transthoracic bioimpedance, so uses less energy (e.g. 20–50 joules).

Metabolic

Anaerobic metabolism from hypoperfusion causes metabolic acidosis. Although acidosis is closely monitored through blood gas analysis, it is not usually necessary to treat acidosis following cardiac surgery.

Target potassium levels should be identified and maintained. Infusions are often needed.

Kidney function

Acute kidney injury occurs in nearly one third of patients undergoing cardiac surgery (O'Neal *et al.*, 2016), owing to both hypoperfusion and other insults such as oxidative stress, reperfusion injury and nephrotoxic drugs (Thiele *et al.*, 2015). Perfusion should be optimised post-operatively but some patients later require haemofiltration (see Chapter 39). Urinary catheters can normally be removed the day after surgery.

Pain control

Pain control is central to intensive care nursing, but with cardiac problems sympathetic nervous stimulation from pain is likely to cause additional complications, prolonging recovery. Opioid infusions are therefore usually necessary.

Thoracic nociceptor innervation being relatively sparse, patients often experience relatively less pain from thoracic than saphenous incisions (Fisher *et al.*, 2002), although arterial graft spasm (e.g. IMA) can cause angina, and IMA harvest disrupts richly innervated tissue. Pain is individual so should be individually assessed rather than stereotyped by operations performed. Nitrates (e.g. GTN) dilate arteries, reducing spasm pain and tension on newly grafted vessels.

Neurological complications

Stroke remains the single greatest risk following cardiac surgery, occurring in 1–2% of patients (Alexander and Smith, 2016). Other neurological deficits may include:

- impaired peripheral nerve function;
- cerebral/cognitive deficits;
- uncontrollable hypertension (injury to vital centres).

Cognitive function should therefore be assessed as soon as possible and any deficits reported.

Psychological considerations

The heart, more than any other body organ, carries emotional connotations for most people – people "love with their heart". Both coronary artery disease and cardiac surgery increase incidence of depression (Wellnius *et al.*, 2008; Perrotti *et al.*, 2016). Post-operatively, mood is often labile, euphoria (induced by opioids and survival) being followed (days two to four) by reactive depression. Anxiety and depression often persist long after ICU discharge (Gallagher and McKinley, 2009) and may provoke further, potentially fatal, infarction.

Stress provokes tachycardia, hypertension and hyperglycaemia (see Chapter 3), all impairing recovery in patients least able to tolerate such insults. Providing information, optimising pain control, relieving anxieties and minimising sensory imbalance are therefore important aspects of holistic nursing care. Psychological distress, and sleep problems, may be reduced with off-pump surgery (Hedges and Redeker, 2008).

Skincare

Wound breakdown or skin ulceration may occur from poor perfusion, peri- or post-operative immobility and other factors. Pain and anxiety often make patients reluctant to move.

Wound dressings are usually removed within 24 hours; if clean and dry, they are then usually left exposed. Sternal wound dehiscence is rare, occurring in 0.4% of patients (Alexander and Smith, 2016) but potentially fatal (Chan *et al.*, 2016), especially following IMA grafts (which can reduce sternal blood supply by up to 90%); deep sternal dehiscence necessitates surgical debridement (Chan et al., 2016).

Perfusion of graft sites (especially radial artery grafts; also arteriovenous shunts) should be protected, so pressure (e.g. blood pressure cuff, tourniquet) should be avoided.

Normalisation

Nurses can experience considerable satisfaction from assisting rapid post-operative recovery following cardiac surgery. Normalisation should be encouraged. Families and friends should be encouraged to visit, as they would on a surgical ward. The day following surgery, patients may enjoy breakfast before transfer. Early mobilisation should be encouraged.

Transplantation issues

Severing of sympathetic and parasympathetic pathways causes loss of vagal tone, resulting in resting heart rates of about 100 beats/minute. Denervation also (usually) prevents angina, increasing risk of silent infarction, but partial albeit unpredictable renervation does occur (Thajudeen et al., 2012).

Loss of sympathetic tone impairs cardiac response to increased metabolic demands, making atropine ineffective.

Surgery preserves recipients' right atrium, which can cause two P waves (one intrinsic, one graft).

Implications for practice

- care of patients following cardiac interventions shares much in common with care of other post-operative patients, but requires continuing full individual assessment;
- long-standing cardiovascular disease and acute responses to cardiac surgery necessitate close monitoring and system support – especially ECG and blood pressure;
- persistent problematic dysrhythmias may necessitate temporary pacing – epicardial wires are usually inserted perioperatively;
- cardiac drains should be measured on arrival, and excessive or sudden cessation of drainage reported;
- nurses should know where thoracotomy packs are kept, what they contain and what will be expected of them in the event of emergency thoracotomy;
- patients should be encouraged to take deep breaths and cough periodically, especially following extubation;
- neurological events may prove fatal, so neurological state should be assessed as soon as possible after surgery, and any concerns reported;
- physical and psychological pain cause various complications; patients should receive adequate analgesia, its effect being monitored by frequent assessment;

- nursing care should focus on normalisation;
- disease and interventions with the heart often cause greater anxiety than with other organs, so patients should be reassured and supported psychologically.

Summary

Patients with single organ failure usually recovery rapidly from either open-heart surgery or percutaneous interventions, often not needing admission to ICU. Rapid recovery, often overnight, can be both rewarding and time-consuming for nurses. But heart failure may have caused multi-organ failure, necessitating ICU support. Even if complications have not occurred, potential for post-repair complications remain, necessitating close observation. Outcomes from both open surgery and percutaneous repair are good, with little evidence of either being superior.

Further reading

Most articles examine specific aspects of surgery interventions and care. Dind *et al.* (2017) review pPCI. Alexander and Smith (2016) describe coronary artery bypass grafting.

Clinical scenarios

Johnny Doyle is a 57-year-old man with a history of angina, hypertension, insulin-dependent diabetes and weighing 110 kg. He was admitted to ICU following off-pump coronary artery bypass grafts × 2 using saphenous vein and left IMA to right ascending vein. Mr Doyle's blood sugar is 7.5 mmol/litre and managed by an intravenous infusion of 50% glucose at 20 ml/hour and insulin infusion running at 8 units/hour.

Q1. Describe Mr Doyle's pre-operative preparation and explain relevance to ICU care (e.g. type of investigations, patient information, pre-admission visits, diabetes control).

Q2. Examine the nursing priorities and identify potential complications in the first 24 hours post CABG surgery for Mr Doyle.

Q3. Mr Doyle develops dehiscence of his sternal wound and can feel his sternum moving on deep breaths and coughing. Review causative factors for this complication and propose a plan of care to stabilise sternum, promote healing and recovery (evaluate various treatments approaches, pharmacological/surgical interventions, approaches used to stabilise sternum, blood sugar control).

Chapter 31

Shock

Contents

Fundamental knowledge

Cellular pathology (see Chapter 24)

Cardiac anatomy, including the mitral valve and
   pericardium

Autonomic nervous system – sympathetic and
   parasympathetic regulation, especially the vagus nerve

Baroreceptors + chemoreceptors

Renin–angiotensin–aldosterone mechanism

Normal inflammatory responses (increased capillary
   permeability, leucocyte migration, vasoactive
   mediators release)

Introduction

In health, normotension is maintained by matching blood volume to blood vessel capacity. This is achieved through autonomic reflexes and endocrine responses.

1. Hypotension is sensed by *baroreceptors* in major arteries. Baroreceptor stimulation activates the *hypothalamic–pituitary–adrenal axis* (the stress response – fight or flight), causing more adrenocorticotrophic hormone (ACTH) release from the pituitary gland, which stimulates adrenal production of adrenaline and noradrenaline, causing vasoconstriction and increased heart rate, which therefore increases blood pressure. HPA axis activation also increases glucocorticoid secretion (O'Connor *et al.*, 2000).
2. Intrarenal hypotension initiates the *renin–angiotensin–aldosterone* mechanism:

renin (released by kidney)
activates angiotensinogen (in liver)

↓

angiotensin 1
mild vasoconstriction; changed by *angiotensin-converting enzyme* in (lungs) to:

↓

angiotensin 2
powerful vasoconstrictor – eight times more powerful than noradrenaline; also increases adrenal production of:

↓

aldosterone (adrenal gland)
increases renal sodium reabsorption

3. The pituitary gland releases more *antidiuretic hormone*, increasing renal water reabsorption.

So (1) reduces blood vessel capacity and (2) mainly reduces blood vessel capacity, while (3) together with increased aldosterone production (2) increases blood volume.

Adjusting these opposite responses enables the body to compensate for problems. Shock, inadequate blood flow to tissues, or perfusion failure occurs when compensatory mechanisms are exhausted or fail.

There are four types of shock:

- cardiogenic
- obstructive
- hypovolaemic
- distributive.

Some of these types can be caused by different pathologies. This chapter provides an overview of effects of shock, symptoms and main treatments. The first three types of shock (cardiogenic, obstructive and hypovolaemic) are then discussed. Some causes of distributive shock are discussed, but the main type seen in ICU is sepsis, discussed in the next chapter.

Stages of shock

Shock is often classified into four stages, reflecting its progression and homeostatic responses:

- *Initial* (hypodynamic): poor cardiac output causes systemic hypoperfusion. Cells resort to anaerobic metabolism. Lactic acid begins to rise. Pulse oximetry may fail to detect a pulse.
- *Compensation* (hyperdynamic): neuroendocrine responses increase circulating catecholamine levels, causing:
    - tachycardia;
    - increased stroke volume (palpitations);
    - tachypnoea;
    - oliguria.

  Neurological signs at this stage usually include:
    - dilated pupils, still responsive to light;
    - confusion, lethargy or agitation;
    - clammy/moist skin.

- *Progression* (hypotensive): compensation fails (although tachycardia usually increases), causing hypotension. Arteriolar and precapillary sphincters constrict, trapping blood in capillaries. This activates inflammatory responses, including histamine release from mast cells, creating oedema. Signs include
    - hypotension;
    - increasing tachycardia;
    - hyperkalaemia (from cell damage – see Chapter 24);
    - worsening metabolic acidosis;
    - myocardial ischaemia (ECG changes);
    - severely impaired consciousness;
    - cold/cyanotic skin;
    - progressive multi-organ failure.

Death often occurs at this stage, but shock may progress to a final stage:

- *Refractory* (irreversible): symptomatic multi-organ failure, with no response to any treatments, death becoming inevitable within a few hours.
- Early detection and appropriate treatment of shock may prevent progression, reduce complications, and improve outcome.

Perfusion failure

Perfusion may fail due to:

- insufficient circulating volume;
- inadequate cardiac output;
- excessive peripheral vasodilatation.

However caused, perfusion failure deprives cells of glucose and oxygen. Tissue cells need energy – adenosine triphosphate (ATP), which is produced in their mitochondria. Without glucose and oxygen, mitochondria metabolise alternative energy sources (body stores – fat and muscle protein), and metabolism becomes anaerobic. Both anaerobic metabolism and metabolism of alternative energy sources are inefficient, producing relatively little energy and large amounts of waste, including lactate. Without perfusion, waste products of metabolism (carbon dioxide, water and metabolic acids) are not removed, creating an increasingly hostile, acidic internal and external environment which, together with reduced energy production, progressively destroys cells. Shock therefore starves tissue cells of the oxygen and glucose they need for normal, healthy (aerobic) metabolism.

Anaerobic metabolism of alternative energy sources produces little energy but much waste, including metabolic acids (especially lactate, which forms lactic acid). Shock therefore causes metabolic acidosis:

- pH < 7.35, bicarbonate < 22 mmol/litre, base excess < 2.0;
- raised lactate.

Progressive cell failure causes leakage of intracellular contents into blood. Normal intracellular and intravascular concentrations of many substances being very different (see Chapter 24), this causes many abnormalities, especially:

- hyperkalaemia.

Progressive cell failure in organs causes progressive organ failure. Early symptoms of shock should therefore be aggressively treated with urgent micro-circulatory resuscitation (oxygen and fluids) to prevent organ failure.

System failure

Cardiovascular. In health, hypoperfusion triggers neuroendocrine compensatory responses (described above):

- hypothalamic–pituitary–adrenal axis;
- renin–angiotensin–aldosterone mechanism;
- antidiuretic hormone release.

Complex pathologies (most ICU patients) cause imbalance and failure of compensatory and autoregulation mechanisms. Reduced cardiac output induces myocardial hypoxia, which usually triggers tachycardia. Tachycardia increases myocardial oxygen consumption but reduces ventricular filling time and myocardial oxygenation time, so may make myocardium more ischaemic, provoking dysrhythmias and infarction.

Respiratory. Metabolic acidosis, from systemic hypoperfusion, stimulates a compensatory respiratory alkalosis (tachypnoea). Pulmonary hypoperfusion increases pathological dead space and V/Q mismatch. Severe shock therefore increases work of breathing without improving tissue oxygenation. Ischaemic surfactant-producing cells in alveoli fail to produce surfactant, while increased capillary permeability causes pulmonary oedema, progressing to *ARDS* (once called "shock lung").

Renal. Prolonged renal ischaemia (volume-responsive acute kidney injury) causes intrarenal oedema and necrosis (see Chapter 38), increasing toxic levels of active metabolites (e.g. urea contributes to confusion/coma).

Hepatic. The liver has a very high metabolic rate, so is particularly susceptible to ischaemic damage, although symptoms often appear later than with other major organs. The liver has many functions (metabolic, digestive, immune, homeostatic), so hepatic dysfunction causes many problems, including:

- delayed clotting;
- immunocompromise causing opportunistic infections, including sepsis;
- hypoalbuminaemia, contributing to oedema.

Pancreas. Serum amylase and lipase become elevated. Pancreatic cell death releases myocardial depressant factor, further exacerbating shock. Production of insulin and the pancreatic hormones may be impaired.

Types of shock

Sturgess (2014) suggests there are four types of shock:

- hypovolaemic
- cardiogenic
- obstructive
- distributive.

Hypovolaemic (haemorrhagic) shock is caused by a rapid and large loss of blood volume, resulting in perfusion failure. Haemorrhagic shock causes more than half of deaths from trauma, and is the most common cause of shock in hospitalised patients. Hypovolaemia may be caused by:

- acute haemorrhage (trauma, surgery, gastrointestinal bleeding);
- other excessive fluid loss (e.g. diabetic ketoacidosis);
- insufficient fluid replacement if patients have difficulty drinking or are nil-by-mouth.

With compensation, people may survive loss of two fifths of blood volume, but, without compensation, losing one fifth of blood volume over 30 minutes may be fatal (Hall, 2016). When compensation fails, venous return falls, inevitably reducing stroke volume. Compensatory tachycardia may restore blood pressure, but increased myocardial oxygen consumption can cause ischaemia, dysrhythmias and infarction.

Hypovolaemic shock should be treated or (even better) prevented by giving adequate fluid. Ambulance transfer can provoke hypovolaemic shock, as acceleration and deceleration during transport exaggerate blood pressure in hypovolaemia, so blood volume should be optimised before transfer.

Major haemorrhage may necessitate massive transfusion together with tranexamic acid (Hunt *et al.*, 2015); readers should familiarise themselves with local major haemorrhage guidelines.

Cardiogenic shock is caused by failure of the heart to pump sufficient blood. The most common cause of cardiogenic shock is myocardial infarction ("coronary cardiogenic shock"), occurring after 5–10% of myocardial infarctions (Unverzagt *et al.*, 2014). Other causes of cardiogenic shock include:

- valve disease, especially mitral regurgitation;
- congenital defects (e.g. ventricular septal defects);
- and various other cardiac problems, collectively called "non-coronary cardiogenic shock".

Cardiogenic shock follows extensive left ventricular damage; Rosenberger *et al.* (2018) suggest more than 40%. Left ventricular dysfunction causes systemic hypotension, myocardial hypoperfusion and hypoxia, and pulmonary congestion (pulmonary oedema). Compensatory tachycardia may increase myocardial oxygen supply but also increases consumption. Extensive left ventricular damage is rapidly fatal. Between 20 and 40% of people with cardiogenic shock will die (Power, 2014), usually fairly quickly. Survivors often develop congestive cardiac failure, necessitating cardiac surgery.

Treatment attempts to increase systemic perfusion pressure while limiting myocardial hypoxia. Inotropes may be necessary to increase cardiac output but they also increase myocardial workload. As with sepsis (see Chapter 32), increased nitric oxide production causes vasodilatation, so contributing to hypotension (Nicholls *et al.*, 2007).

Obstructive shock is caused by any obstruction to blood flow through the heart:

- raised intrathoracic pressure (positive pressure ventilation, PEEP);
- obstructed intrapulmonary flow (ARDS, pulmonary emboli, pneumo/haemothorax);
- cardiac tamponade.

Tamponade is direct continuous compression of the heart, usually caused by pericardial effusions, Accumulation forces myocardium inward, reducing intraventricular space and so stroke volume.

Tamponade can develop slowly or quickly. Slow tamponade may accumulate up to two litres of blood, whereas a fast bleed can cause tamponade with as little as 150 ml (Schairer and Keteyian, 2016). Rapid tamponade typically occurs following cardiac surgery or trauma, and is an emergency, usually causing imminent cardiac arrest once compensatory tachycardia and vaso-constriction fail.

Rapid tamponade necessitates urgent needle aspiration of pericardial fluid, under echocardiographic or fluoroscopic guidance (Task Force, 2015). Following pericardial aspiration, patients should be closely monitored for further accumulation (ECG, drainage).

Distributive shock occurs when normal vasoregulation fails. Normally only one quarter of capillaries are open at any time (Deroy, 2000). Blood flow into capillaries is controlled by capillary sphincters. Excessive peripheral vasodilatation increases blood vessel capacity, so existing blood volume is maldistributed, excessive volume pooling in peripheral circulation at the expense of central blood volume and pressure.

The most frequent cause of distributive shock seen in ICU is sepsis, discussed in the next chapter. Other types of distributive shock include:

- neurogenic
- spinal
- anaphylaxis
- toxic shock syndrome.

Massive inflammatory responses, such as can occur with severe pancreatitis and severe burns, can also cause a sepsis-like distributive shock in the absence of infection.

Neurogenic shock occurs with severe central nervous system injury – brain damage or high thoracic spinal cord injury. Sympathetic tone, which increases heart rate and vasoconstriction, is generally absent, while vagal (parasympa-thetic) regulation, which reduces both heart rate and vasoconstriction, usually remains intact. Respiratory failure often occurs due to nerve damage, necessitat-ing artificial ventilation.

Failure of autonomic response usually makes inotropes ineffective. Volume replacement can compensate for increased blood vessel capacity. Unresponsive sudden hypotension usually indicates a stroke, which, with critical illness, may prove fatal. Patients with spinal cord injury are usually transferred urgently to spinal injury units. Ruiz *et al.* (2017) found that most patients with neurogenic shock were also hypovolaemic.

Spinal shock is also caused by spinal cord injury, but usually implies damage at slightly lower levels (below T5). Pathology is similar, but usually less immediately life-threatening.

Autonomic dysreflexia, a potentially fatal complication of spinal cord injury, is discussed in Chapter 36. Patients with spinal cord injury are usually transferred urgently to spinal injury units, which are more familiar with managing these problems.

Anaphylactic shock occurs when T-lymphocytes (antibodies) recognise antigens, initiating an antigen–antibody reaction. This stimulates a massive release of histamine and other pro-inflammatory chemicals (Zilberstein *et al.*, 2014), which:

- vasodilate (e.g. interleukins, prostaglandins);
- increase capillary pore permeability (e.g. histamine);
- trigger clotting (e.g. platelet activating factor).

Increasing capillary capacity together with increasing capillary leak (reduced blood volume) rapidly causes hypovolaemia, triggering tachycardia. Histamine also induces bronchoconstriction, which causes respiratory distress.

Anaphylaxis typically occurs with second doses of drugs, but "first doses" may not be danger-free – previous exposure to antigens (e.g. drugs) may be unrecorded. Incidence of anaphylaxis in the UK is increasing (Gibbison *et al.*, 2012).

Anaphylactic shock is an emergency, necessitating adrenaline to restore circulating blood pressure (Simons and Simons, 2010; Simons *et al.*, 2011). Traditionally, antihistamines (chlorphenamine) and steroids (hydrocortisone) have also been used, although their efficacy for treating anaphylaxis remains unproved (Simons *et al.*, 2011). Massive extravasation from inflammation often necessitates fluid resuscitation. Oxygen and other system supports may be needed.

Toxic shock syndrome is a rare form of sepsis. Arguably, the term should be obsolete, as current sepsis guidelines (Rhodes *et al.*, 2017) discourage use of any terms outside "sepsis" and "septic shock", and ICU management would not change from standard sepsis care (see Chapter 32), although the term is occasionally still used. Toxic shock syndrome is typically from poor tampon hygiene, but can be from any skin-surface staphylococci invading the body, such as through wounds or dressings. Necrotising fasciitis (see Chapter 12) causes toxic shock syndrome. The rarity of toxic shock syndrome may delay recognition when it occurs, especially if unconscious women admitted to ICU have tampons in place.

Rescue therapies

If other therapies fail, intra-aortic balloon pumps (IABPs), ventricular assist devices (VADs) and extracorporeal membrane oxygenators (ECMOs – see Chapter 28) can support perfusion with life-threatening heart failure (de Chambrun *et al.*, 2016; den Uil *et al.*, 2017; van Nunen *et al.*, 2016), "buying time" for interventions such as transplantation (Shuhaiber *et al.*, 2010) PCI/surgery or spontaneous recovery.

Ventricular assist devices (VADs – "artificial hearts") may be biventricular (BiVAD – see Figure 31.1) or left ventricular assist devices (LVADs) (Task Force, 2010b). Percutaneously implantable devices have so far proved disappointing (Task Force, 2010b), and most ICUs do not have access to external VADs.

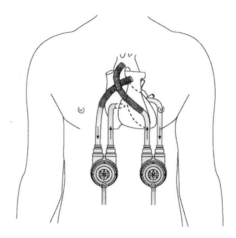

Figure 31.1 Ventricular assist devices (left and right)

Intra-aortic balloon pumps use a catheter inserted into a femoral artery, passing up into the descending aorta (see Figure 31.2). On R waves of ECGs (end of diastole), the balloon inflates, displacing blood down into the renal arteries and forcing blood ejected from the left ventricle to perfuse the coronary and carotid arteries, the only arteries remaining between the ventricle and occlusion.

Increased systemic pressure is visible as augmented pressure waveforms on arterial blood pressure traces (see Figure 31.3).

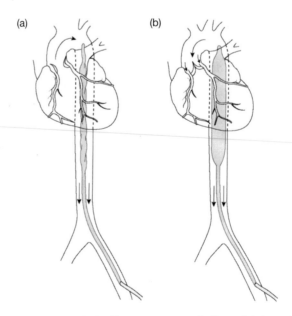

Figure 31.2 Intra-aortic balloon pump – deflated (a) and inflated (b)

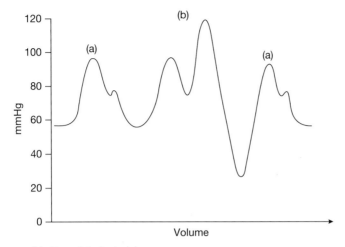

(a) Unassisted arterial pressure
(b) Augmented pressure with inflation increasing
pressure after closure of the aortic valve creating
a second pressure wave after the dicrotic notch

Figure 31.3 Arterial pressure trace, showing augmented pressure from use of an intra-aortic balloon pump

IABP has been used to treat cardiogenic shock refractory to inotropic support, although Thiele *et al.*'s (2013) post-revascularisation study found no significant mortality benefit with IABP, and routine use for cardiogenic shock is no longer recommended (Ponikowski *et al.*, 2016). As a rescue therapy it is less invasive, and more likely to be available outside tertiary centres, than ventricular assist devices or ECMO (den Uil *et al.*, 2017).

Among its more serious complications is limb ischaemia, sometimes necessitating amputation, so peripheral pulses should be assessed. Other complications include:

- bleeding at insertion site;
- infection.

Balloon rupture (rare) or gas diffusion through the balloon mixes gas used with aortic blood, so soluble gases (e.g. helium) are used. Helium causes rapid coagulation, so tubing should be frequently inspected for black flecks (clots). Gas cylinders maintain constant pressures to compensate for leaks. Alarms should sound before reserve gas in cylinders is exhausted, but nurses should still check cylinder volume and know how to replace them. While enabling survival, highly invasive devices expose severely immunocompromised patients to risks from infection and thromboembolism. If standby mode is used for prolonged periods (30 minutes), thrombi may have formed so the IABP catheter should be changed. IABPs have high electrical consumption, which limits battery life during transfer.

In the event of cardiac arrest, cardiac pressure trigger on IABPs augments compressions during cardiopulmonary resuscitation, and is vital for pulseless VT or PEA.

As the catheter is inserted into the femoral artery, clotting time should be checked before removal; this will usually be measured by activated clotting time (ACT), a simple bedside test. Prolonged and high pressure is needed to stop femoral artery bleeds, usually using mechanical devices.

Implications for practice

- shock causes inadequate tissue perfusion at capillary (microcirculatory) level, so treatments should target microcirculatory resuscitation – primarily oxygen (aim SaO_2 94–98%) and fluid resuscitation;
- oxygen delivery can be assessed by comparing SaO_2 with SvO_2 (see Chapter 18);
- once blood volume is optimised, cardiac output can be increased with inotropes;
- unreversed shock will cause acute kidney injury. Volume-responsive acute kidney injury needs volume, and should not be treated with diuretics (Davenport and Stevens, 2008);
- sudden shock may be caused by tamponade, especially following cardiac surgery. If cardiac chest drains are present, patency should be restored. Otherwise, needle aspiration by medical staff may be necessary.

Summary

Many pathologies can cause shock. But, however caused, shock results in inadequate perfusion to tissues which, if not reversed, will cause progressive cell damage. Cells with high metabolic rates, such as cardiac and brain cells, are especially susceptible to perfusion failure. Once sufficient cells in an organ fail, the organ will fail to function adequately. Priorities of care therefore focus on microcirculatory (capillary) resuscitation:

- oxygen
- fluids
- system support.

Underlying causes of shock should, where possible, be treated. Close monitoring and observation by ICU nurses, with an understanding of probable mechanisms of shock, enables prompt treatment.

Further reading

Shock is discussed in most nursing and medical texts. Guidelines, such as Task Force (2015) and Simons *et al.* (2011), although these are not ICU-specific. Readers should be familiar with their local massive transfusion protocol. Shekar *et al.* (2016) review various mechanical supports for failing hearts.

Clinical scenarios

Mr Reece Owen is a 71-year-old gentleman admitted to hospital with acute exacerbation of COPD. Despite respiratory support and antibiotic therapy his physical condition deteriorated. He became confused with a low GCS, unstable ECG and was transferred to ICU for monitoring, intubation and mechanical ventilation (PSIMV, PEEP of 8 cmH$_2$O, FiO$_2$ 0.4).

Observations on admission include:

Temperature	34.5°C
Heart rate	135 beats/minute
Rhythm	Sinus tachycardia with multifocal ventricular ectopics
BP	106/55 mmHg
CO	4.72 litres/minute
CI	2.55 litres/minute/m^2
SV	35 ml
SVI	19 ml/beat/m^2
SVR	1000 dynes/second/cm^5
SVRI	1850 dynes/second/cm^5/m^2
SvO$_2$	68%
SVV	21%

Blood results are:

Haematology		Biochemistry		Arterial blood gases	
Hb	9.2 g/dl	CRP	129 mg/litre	pH	7.13
WCC	25.5 x 10^{-9}/litre	Na$^+$	142 mmol/litre	PaCO$_2$	7.13 kPa
Neutrophils	23.5 x 10^{-9}/litre	K$^+$	4.9 mmol/litre	PaO$_2$	14.67 kPa
Lymphocytes	0.2 x 10^{-9}/litre	Albumin	11 grams/litre	HCO$_3^-$	16.3 mmol/litre
Platelets	334 x 10^{-9}/litre	Creatinine	251 micromol/litre	Base excess	−10.1 mmol/litre
INR	1.5	Urea	14.2 mmol/litre	Lactate	1.5 mmol/litre
APTT ratio	> 5.0			Glucose	10.5 mmol/litre
Troponin T	130 nanograms/litre			Cl$^-$	110 mmol/litre
APTT	> 100 secs				

Q1. Which type of shock is present? What other investigations might help confirm diagnosis and treat Mr Owen's problems?

Q2. Explain the physiology underlying Mr Owen's abnormal results. Comment on his organ and tissue perfusion.

Q3. Which interventions can optimise his cardiovascular function? Identify any additional tests or monitoring which may be useful.

Chapter 32

Sepsis

Contents

Fundamental knowledge

Vascular anatomy – function of tunica intima
Cellular pathology (see Chapter 24), especially inflammatory
  response
Shock (see Chapter 31)
Immunity (see Chapter 25)

Introduction

Sepsis remains the most common reason for ICU admission (I.C.S., 2015), and the leading cause of death in critically ill patients (Hunter and Doddi, 2010). Other than development of antibiotics, there were relatively few advances in sepsis management during the twentieth century, the first international guidelines being published as recently as 2004. Since then, a plethora of national and international reports and guidelines have been published; in 2017 the World Health Organization passed a resolution to make sepsis a global priority, requiring a report to be written in 2018. While critical care has focused much on sepsis, patients and caregivers often lack awareness and understanding of sepsis (Gallop *et al.*, 2015).

The prevalence and problems of sepsis have prompted many searches for panaceas, which have remained largely elusive. Organ failure needs system supports – many aspects of which have been discussed in previous chapters. This chapter summarises progressive pathology, prognosis, and issues specific to sepsis.

What is sepsis?

Sepsis occurs when bloodstream infection provokes a host response. Ibeh *et al.* (2012) suggest that blood is normally sterile; the presence of foreign organisms in blood provoke defensive inflammatory responses. If balanced, this response is defensive; if excessive, it becomes pathological, causing systemic activation of pro-inflammatory mediators which:

- vasodilate (hypotension) (Hunter and Doddi, 2010);
- increase capillary leak (hypovolaemia and oedema);
- (over-)activate endothelium (e.g. deranged clotting).

Extent of inflammatory responses determine the severity of sepsis. Hypoperfusion of organs often results in progressive organ failure; each main organ/system failure carries approximately a 25% mortality risk.

In the past, the term "severe sepsis" was used to distinguish the stage between sepsis developing and septic shock occurring. Consensus revision to international guidelines (Singer *et al.*, 2016) recommend limiting terminology to "sepsis" and "septic shock".

Early identification of sepsis improves outcome (Rhodes *et al.*, 2017). Unfortunately, symptoms are non-specific, often delaying diagnosis. Singer *et al.* (2016) recommend using qSOFA (quick sequential organ failure assessment), which is any two of:

- respiratory rate 22/minute or greater;
- altered mentation;
- systolic blood pressure 100 mmHg or less;
- qSOFA is quick; whether it is specific enough is questionable. Seymour *et al.* (2016) found it useful for use outside ICU, but less useful in ICU.

Inflammation

Tunica intima forms an active part of the cardiovascular system, releasing many vasoactive mediators, such as tumour necrosis factor (TNF), interleukins, cytokines, nitric oxide, leukotrienes and platelet activating factor.

Excessive (systemic) response becomes pathological, reducing perfusion to all tissues (pathological cell death – necrosis) and triggering neutrophils and macrophages to release reactive oxygen species (ROS) to destroy antigens. If ROS release exceeds antioxidant defences, which it usually does in critical illness, tissue damage occurs (Gomes *et al.*, 2012). Periodic "cytokine bursts", also called "septic showers" make blood pressure labile, and often challenging to control.

MODS

Sepsis may progress to **Multi-Organ Dysfunction Syndrome** (MODS, sometimes called "multi-organ failure" – MOF). The sequence of organ failure varies, but often starts with respiratory failure, a major cause of ICU admission. Sepsis impairs respiratory muscle function (Lanone *et al.*, 2005). Cardiac dysfunction frequently follows. This is largely from vasodilatation and capillary leak (see above) but is compounded by sepsis, reducing ejection fraction (Hunter and Doddi, 2010). If cardiac output is poor, dobutamine is the recommended inotrope (Rhodes *et al.*, 2017). Cardiovascular failure typically causes acute kidney injury (AKI) and low-grade liver failure; sepsis is the most common cause of AKI (Lai *et al.*, 2013; Alobaidi *et al.*, 2015). The liver is often one of the last main organs to show signs of failure. Up to 70% of septic patients develop encephalopathy (Smith and Meyfroidt, 2017), which can cause long-term neurological and psychological problems (Heming *et al.*, 2017).

There is no single treatment for MODS, but system support is attempted around each problem. A problem facing all systems is microcirculatory hypo-perfusion, so tissue perfusion should be optimised, assessing needs through cardiac output study monitoring and resuscitating with fluids to deliver oxygen to tissues.

Treatments

Human and financial cost of from sepsis remain high, so much research has been invested to find solutions. This creates the temptation to promote and use expensive therapies which may have limited benefits. Survival has improved but remains poor, and solutions remain largely evasive. Treatment focuses primarily on treating symptoms and preventing complications. The 2013 guidelines (Dellinger *et al.*, 2013) identify two care bundles (see Table 32.1).

Sepsis is caused by infection, usually but not always bacterial (N.C.E.P.O.D., 2015a). So, urgent antimicrobial agents, usually antibiotics, are fundamental to treatment. Survival is reduced by 7.6% for each hour's delay in starting antibiotics (Kumar *et al.*, 2006), yet inappropriate initial antimicrobial therapy

Table 32.1 Surviving sepsis campaign bundles

Three-hour bundle:
measure lactate
obtain blood cultures (within 45 minutes) before giving antibiotics
broad-spectrum antibiotics (within one hour)
30 ml/kg crystalloid for hypotension or if lactate ≥ 4 mmol/litre

Six-hour bundle:
apply vasopressors (for hypotension not responding to initial fluid resuscitation) to maintain MAP ≥ 65 mmHg
if persistent hypotension after initial fluid resuscitation or initial lactate ≥ 4 mmol/litre, reassess volume status & tissue perfusion (see website for details)
remeasure lactate if initial measure was elevated

Note: Current guidelines (Rhodes et al., 2017) have devolved care bundles to an educational group. Current bundles, appearing on the Surviving Sepsis Campaign website remain the 2015 update from the 2013 guidelines, summarised here. Items are compatible with the 2017 guidelines.

Source: Dellinger et al., 2013.

occurs in up to one fifth of patients (Kumar et al., 2009). Blood cultures should be taken before giving antibiotics.

Effectiveness of antibiotics can be assessed by procalcitonin levels (Rhodes et al., 2017), enabling earlier changes from antibiotics that prove ineffective. Calcitonin is a hormone, or "hormokine", which regulates calcium and phosphate in bone metabolism. Normal levels of its precursor, procalitonin (PCT), are < 0.5 nanograms/millilitre. Levels rise within hours of bacterial or fungal (but not viral) infection, peaking at six hours, allowing rapid evaluation of effectiveness of antimicrobial agents. Its half-life being less than 34 hours, levels should be monitored daily. Procalcitonin levels do not predict outcome (Hillas et al., 2010). Levels are not affected by steroid therapy.

However caused, shock results in tissue hypoperfusion. Shock creates a syndrome of microcirculatory hypoperfusion, creating an "oxygen debt". Reversing oxygen debt improves survival. Despite improvements in monitoring technology, oxygen debt (the difference between oxygen demand and oxygen delivery) cannot directly be measured. Where possible, causes are identified and treated and systems supported. Treatment should focus on early and aggressive resuscitation to normalise vital signs, achieve mean arterial pressure ≥ 65 mmHg, and normalise lactate (Rhodes et al., 2017).

Vasodilatory mediators and capillary leak cause profound hypotension. Aggressive fluid and vasopressors are often needed, although gross inflammatory responses too often result in infused fluid quickly shifting into interstitial spaces – oedema, including pulmonary oedema; fewer than 40% of patients with septic shock are fluid-responsive (Marik and Bellomo, 2016). Once adequately filled, vasopressors such as noradrenaline can reverse inappropriate vasodilation.

Septic shock usually necessitates ICU admission for mechanical ventilation. Risk of ARDS is high. Artificial ventilation may necessitate neuromuscular blockade – Steingrub *et al.* (2014) found this improved outcome, a finding which conflicts with general trends in ICU practice for the last quarter century.

Steroids should theoretically reduce inflammatory responses, but evidence is weak to support its use in sepsis, so intravenous hydrocortisone should only be given if septic shock fails to respond to fluid resuscitation and vasopressors (Rhodes *et al.*, 2017).

Haemofiltration (see Chapter 39) may remove mediators of sepsis, although there is currently insufficient evidence to support using plasma exchange solely to remove mediators (Rimmer *et al.*, 2014). The Surviving Sepsis Campaign recommends continuous filtration to facilitate management of fluid balance (Rhodes *et al.*, 2017). CytoSorb cartridges may be added to standard circuits to increase removal of cytokines, but very limited usage (evidence) and high costs (N.I.C.E., 2016b) make this currently difficult to justify.

Prognosis

Despite its frequency among ICU patients, and some recent progress, sepsis remains a major challenge, causing significant morbidity and mortality. Yealy *et al.* (2014) suggest that one-month mortality from sepsis is about 20%.

Critical care follow-up, together with research, has increasingly identified multiple residual problems in survivors of sepsis, all of which impair quality of life, and aggravate depression. Problems persisting include:

- acute kidney injury, which can progress to chronic kidney disease, needing dialysis (N.C.E.P.O.D., 2015a);
- muscle weakness (Gallop *et al.*, 2015);
- chronic pain and fatigue (NHS England. 2014);
- the long-term cognitive impairment suffered by more than half of survivors (Iwashyna *et al.*, 2010; Annane and Sharshar, 2015; Gallop *et al.*, 2015);
- post-traumatic stress disorder, which is relatively common (Iwashyna *et al.*, 2010; N.C.E.P.O.D., 2015a);
- sepsis-related brain dysfunction, causing delirium (Burkhart *et al.*, 2010);
- feeling a burden on family and friends (O'Brien *et al.*, 2009);
- ongoing financial costs from morbidities (O'Brien *et al.*, 2009).

Over one fifth of survivors from sepsis have complications when discharged from hospital (N.C.E.P.O.D., 2015a).

Implications for practice

- sepsis, the most common pathology in most ICUs, causes inappropriate, systemic activation of inflammatory responses. This results in excessive vasodilatation, massive capillary leak, and coagulopathy;
- vasodilatation usually necessitates vasoconstriction with vasopressors such as noradrenaline;
- capillary leak may necessitate initial aggressive fluid resuscitation, to maintain perfusion and prevent further organ dysfunction; once initially fluid-resuscitated, ongoing capillary leak predisposes to counterproductive oedema formation;
- multi-organ dysfunction syndrome results from pathological processes initiated at cellular level;
- monitor cumulative fluid balance;
- mortality rates from MODS remain very high, increasing with each organ that fails, but early intervention to support failing systems (especially microcirculatory resuscitation) can improve survival;
- maintaining high standards of fundamental aspects of care, especially infection control, can reduce complications;
- mortality reflects the number of major organs failing; multidisciplinary teams should consider whether prognosis justifies continued treatment (is death being prolonged?); nurses should be actively involved in team decisions.

Summary

Sepsis often begins before ICU admission. The Sepsis Care Bundle has been widely promoted, although Yealy *et al.* (2014) found no benefit from protocol-based approaches. Multi-organ dysfunction complicates many ICU admissions, incurring high human and financial costs. Mainstays of sepsis treatment remain vasopressors (e.g. noradrenaline) for excessive vasodilatation and beta stimulants (e.g. dobutamine) for poor cardiac output. High incidence and paucity of curative, rather than supportive, treatment encourages searches for novel solutions which may have few benefits and high costs. Progression from single to multi-organ failure remains the greatest challenge facing intensive care.

Further reading

The Surviving Sepsis Campaign provides evidence-based international guidelines (Rhodes *et al.*, 2017). This decade has seen many national reports and responses, including N.C.E.P.O.D., 2015a) and N.I.C.E. (2016a). N.I.C.E./National Collaborating Centre for Cancer (2012) has published guidelines for neutropenic sepsis. It is likely that during the shelf-life of this book international guidelines will be further updated, and further national reports will be issued. The W.H.O. 2018 report will probably also provide useful information, although at the time of writing this has yet to be published.

Clinical scenarios

Tricia Downes, 38 years old, is admitted after being rescued from a house fire. She suffered smoke inhalation and extensive burns down the right side of her head and body. She was intubated by paramedics, then transferred to A&E before undergoing extensive and prolonged surgery. Post-operatively she is admitted to ITU where a CVC is inserted.

She is ventilated on spontaneous mode, with PEEP 8, FiO_2 0.45, PS 12.

Following these procedures, vital signs include;

Heart rate	SVT 130 beats/minute, regular
BP	100/78 mmHg (MAP 86)
PPV	14%
Temperature	39.3°C

Q1. Which signs indicate Ms Downes's fluid status? What further information would you like to confirm thoughts about fluid balance? How should her fluid balance be managed? – include details such as drugs/fluids/rates.

Arterial blood gas		Blood results		Cardiac output studies	
pH	7.37	Hb	135 grams/litre	CO	7.3 litres/min
$PaCO_2$	3.08 kPa	WCC	$13.9 \times 10-9$/litre	CI	4.6 litres/min/ m^2
PaO_2	14.2 kPa	Platelets	$83 \times 10-9$/litre	SV	95 ml
HCO_3	15.3 mmol/litre	INR	2.6	SVI	52 ml/beat/m^2
BE	-8.6 mmol/litre	Na+	124 mmol/litre	SVR	900 dynes/sec/ cm^5
COHb	48%	K+	7.2 mmol/litre	SVRI	1950 dynes/ sec/cm^5/m^2
Na	127 mmol/litre	Creat	193 micromol/litre	SvO_2	79%
K	6.8 mmol/litre	Albumin	17 grams/litre	DO_2I	360 ml/min/m^2
Glucose	11 mmol/litre	PO4	1.2 mmol/litre		
Lactate	2.7 mmol/litre	Mg	1.1 mmol/litre		
CRP	147 mg/litre				

Q2. Explain the physiology underlying Ms Downes's abnormal results. Comment on her organ and tissue perfusion.

Q3. Which interventions can optimise her cardiovascular function? Identify any additional tests or monitoring which may be useful. How useful is, and what dangers may be caused by, cardiac output monitoring?

Fluid management

Contents

Introduction

Fluid therapy has long been a topic of passionate, often conflicting, views. Evidence to support assertions is often limited, and mixed. One extreme is that any fluid bolus given for hypovolaemia may be harmful (Maitland *et al.*, 2011). While this does not reflect current practice, practice is variable, debatable, and liable to change.

Most (60–80%) of the body is water. Water is distributed unevenly between:

■ extracellular and
■ intracellular

fluid, with potential "third spaces" that normally contain no or insignificant volumes of fluid (e.g. 10–20 ml pericardial fluid), but which with disease can contain significantly more. Extracellular fluid is divided between:

■ intravascular
■ interstitial

compartments. In health, water distribution is approximately as shown in *Figure 33.1*:

Perfusion

Tissue perfusion is needed to supply nutrients to cells and remove waste products of metabolism. Tissue perfusion relies on pressure gradients across capillary walls. These gradients are the sum of:

■ resistance in tissues;
■ (mean) arterial blood pressure (MAP);
■ colloid osmotic pressure.

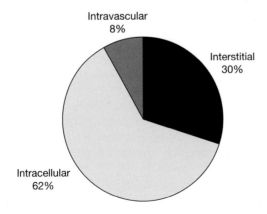

Figure 33.1 Normal distribution of body water

In health, each day nearly five times total blood volume moves in and out of the cardiovascular system (Barrett *et al.*, 2016). Movement is largely regulated by pressures. Osmotic pressure exerted within the bloodstream is called *colloid osmotic pressure (COP)*. Colloid osmotic pressure is normally mainly created by plasma proteins, especially albumin. Capillaries are semipermeable: thin, sqauemous (= scale-like) epithelium, with gaps between cells. At the arteriolar end, intracapillary pressure (average: 30 mmHg (Hall, 2016)) exceeds combined interstitial and COP, forcing fluid into tissues. In health, homeostasis maintains normal fluid balance. With ill health, gross and problematic fluid imbalance can occur.

Starling's (1896) research established the effects of osmotic and hydrostatic pressures on fluid movement, forming the basis for twentieth-century approaches to fluid management. These beliefs included that colloid osmotic pressure drew extravascular back near venule ends of capillaries. It is now known that most fluid returns to the cardiovascular system via lymphatics (Delaney, 2016). Otherwise, Starling's findings remain largely true for the healthy body, but failure of resuscitation fluids to behave as predicted raised suspicions that other factors also influenced fluid distribution. One factor is clearly the inflammatory response, contributing to capillary leak. But more recently glycocalyx has been increasingly studied. Glycocalyx is a polysaccharide ("sugary slime") that coats many cells to protect them and enable them to function. Many bacterial cell membranes contain glycocalyx. Vascular glycocalyx contributes to homeostatic and defensive cardiovascular functions, including capillary blood flow (Reitsma *et al.*, 2007) and permeability to water and electrolytes (Becker *et al.*, 2010). Dysfunction of vascular glycocalyx has been identified in many inflammatory diseases (Woodcock and Woodcock, 2012), and contributes to:

- cytokine release (Becker *et al.*, 2010);
- hypoxia, ischaemia and oxidative stress (Annecke *et al.*, 2011);
- increased leucocyte adhesion, capillary leak and oedema (Annecke *et al.*, 2011; Marik and Lemson, 2014);
- possible increased nitric oxide production (Reitsma *et al.*, 2007), which vasodilatates.

Capillary permeability varies greatly, ranging from the blood–brain barrier (least permeable) to renal glomerulus (most permeable). Glomeruli may filter positively charged substances up to 70 kilodaltons (kDa), although clearance rate reduces as molecular size increases.

All treatments, all drugs and all fluids have risks, so selection should depend on balancing risks and benefits in the context of each patient. Fluids used clinically have generally changed little in decades, but knowledge about their effects, benefits and problems has grown. Choice depends partly on whether the prime target is:

- maintenance;
- intravascular rehydration (resuscitation);
- whole-body rehydration (especially intracellular).

Many patients are hypovolaemic on arrival in ICU, so initial fluid resuscitation is often needed, but with the almost invariable capillary leak of ICU patients, continued infusion of large volumes too often results in gross interstitial oedema, including excessive extravascular lung water, while only transiently increasing intravascular volumes (Marik and Bellomo, 2016). After initial resuscitation, fluid administration should therefore be cautious, and closely monitored, including recording cumulative fluid balance.

Fluids for intravenous infusion were traditionally divided into two main groups: crystalloids and colloids. Crystalloids have small-molecule solutes, which extravase rapidly, hydrating mainly the extravascular spaces. Colloids have larger molecules, so were traditionally viewed as remaining longer in the bloodstream, but evidence does not support this traditional division, and there are significant differences between different fluids in each group. Increasingly, debate has shifted to difference between chloride-rich and "balanced" or "buffered" fluids. Duration of fluids' effect, like drugs, is measured by *half-life*, although effect in critically ill people is often noticeably shorter.

While maintenance rates should be individualised to each patient, according to needs and loss, N.I.C.E. (2013c) recommends that resuscitation volume should be 500 ml within 15 minutes.

Fluid responsiveness

Incidence of heart failure in hospitalised patients is high (N.I.C.E., 2014a), so infused fluids will only improve perfusion if the heart is able to pump it into arteries. While continuous blood pressure monitoring usually facilitates this in the ICU, raising one leg quickly returns approximately one litre of blood to the heart enabling rapid assessment of whether the heart will respond to volume (Marik and Lemson, 2014).

What's in the water?

All intravenous fluids are mainly water. They also include solutes and sometimes other chemicals suspended in them. While many people have passionate views favouring or disliking particular fluids, too often these views are founded on very limited knowledge of the fluid.

Three key questions to ask about any fluid are its:

- pH
- contents – solutes and chemicals
- osmolatily,

remembering the normal levels of blood pH, solutes and osmolality. Pathology Harmony identify normal plasma osmolality as 275–295. Where any of these are abnormally low or high for normal serum levels, these effects should be considered, especially in patients whose diseases cause abnormal levels – for example, sicker patients often have acidoses.

Many of these aspects are identified in sections about individual fluids in this chapter; while reading through this chapter, it will be useful to complete the table in Time Out 1 (below), using resources such as this text, information printed on IVIs in your clinical area, and other resources such as the internet. Depending on fluids available and used on your unit, you may wish to adapt columns. There can be minor differences between products from different manufacturers.

Time Out 1

Table 33.1 Table for different fluids

	pH mOsm	Contents (including amounts in mmol/litre)	Normal blood levels? (mmol/litre)	When seen used, and why? Potential benefits?	When seen avoided, and why? Potential problems?
0.9% sodium chloride					
1.8/2.7% sodium chloride					
Glucose/saline (percentages vary, so identify which used)					
5% glucose					
kJ? Balanced solutions (e.g. Ringer's, Hartmann's, Plasma-Lyte 148)					
(exclude acetate + gluconate) Gelatins (e.g. Gelofusine, Volplex)					
which crystalloid?					

Crystalloids

Crystalloids rapidly extravase, quickly passing into extravascular (interstitial and intracellular) spaces, where most body water is. Half-life is usually about 20–40 minutes (Htun, 2015; Hahn and Lyons, 2016). Crystalloids are therefore effective for maintaining whole-body hydration. Traditionally, their rapid extravasation was considered to cause more rapid oedema than colloids (Brochard *et al.*, 2010). Most crystalloids are also acidic, likely to exacerbate the acidosis that usually accompanies critical illness.

0.9% sodium chloride mostly extravases into interstitial spaces, where it largely remains; sodium is primarily an extracellular cation, being repelled by sodium–potassium pumps in cell membranes. Its 154 mmol/litre of chloride is much higher than normal plasma levels (95–108 mmol/litre); hyperchloraemia draws hydrogen ions from water, producing acid, so excessive saline infusion can cause hyperchloraemic metabolic acidosis (Cortés *et al.*, 2014; Krajewski *et al.*, 2015). Chloride-rich solutions, such as 0.9% saline, vasoconstrict glomerular arterioles, predisposing to acute kidney injury (Choudhury *et al.*, 2012; Bellomo *et al.*, 2012; Shaw *et al.*, 2014; Krajewski *et al.*, 2015), although Young *et al.* (2015), comparing saline with buffered solutions, found no difference in incidence of acute kidney injury, while Cortés *et al.* (2014) suggest that there is mixed evidence whether saline impairs renal function. Chloride-rich fluids are also associated with greater need for blood transfusion and longer need for mechanical ventilation (Krajewski *et al.*, 2015).

Hypotonic and hypertonic saline solutions (different percentages) are available, providing different osmotic "pull", but currently are seldom used in most UK ICUs. Hypotonic saline can cause potentially fatal hyponatraemia (Wang *et al.*, 2014).

Compared with normal plasma, saline does not have a normal:

- pH;
- sodium concentration;
- chloride concentration;
- osmolality.

The term "normal saline" was coined from studies of the 1880s which showed that 0.9% did not cause erythrocyte lysis; it is now known that plasma saline is 0.6% (Myburgh, 2014). The B.N.F. (2017) explicitly states that the term "normal saline" should not be used; referring to it as "normal" perpetuates misconceptions.

5% glucose is a little glucose (5 grams per 100 ml; about one sachet of sugar) and water. Not being salt water, this water therefore moves freely across cell membranes into intracellular fluid, where most body water should normally be. Glucose solutions are therefore excellent intracellular rehydration solutions, but should be avoided with raised intracranial pressure where they may increase cerebral oedema (Haddad and Arabi, 2012).

"Balanced solutions". The unphysiological nature of saline was recognised by Sidney Ringer in the nineteenth century (Hahn, 2014). His compound sodium lactate solution ("Ringer's") was modified by Hartmann in the 1930s, which has since been further modified into Plasma-Lyte (Hahn, 2014). Although electrolyte contents are closer to normal plasma, the main "balance" is pH: balanced solutions contain a buffer precursor, so that, even if solutions are acidic in the bag, once infused they metabolise to buffers, hence the alternative group name "buffered solutions". Variable metabolism makes pH variable. Most balanced solutions contain a normal serum concentration of potassium, which may be a concern with hyperkalaemia.

Ringer's and Hartmann's use lactate, relying on the body to metabolise lactate into bicarbonate. Compared with saline, balanced solutions reduce inflammation, endothelial activation, and kidney injury (Wu *et al.*, 2011; Zhou *et al.*, 2014; Mårtensson and Bellomo, 2015), may achieve more effective volume resuscitation (Feldheiser *et al.*, 2013), and have a lower associated mortality when used for resuscitation (Shaw *et al.*, 2014), although Young *et al.*'s (2015) findings suggest choice of crystalloid does not affect mortality. The older balanced solutions are referred to by name as if only one formulation exists, but both Ringer and Hartmann originally used various formulations, and Ringer's is manufactured in both lactate and acetate buffers.

Plasma-Lyte 148 is slightly more "normal" physiologically than Hartmann's or Ringer's, but most importantly replaces lactate buffering with acetate and gluconate, which are metabolised into bicarbonate (Baxter, 2015), although currently little is known about whether either have adverse effects (Cortés *et al.*, 2014). Lactate is often a concern with critically ill patients, so infusing lactate-based fluids seems illogical. More significantly, infused lactate relies largely on metabolism by the liver for conversion into bicarbonate, but many critically ill patients have impaired liver function. Labelling suggests that Plasma-Lyte 148 has a pH of 7.4, but smaller print identifies a variable range of 6.5–8.0.

Colloids

Colloids have large molecules. They may be natural (e.g. blood and blood products, of which albumin is sometimes used for treating hypovolaemia) or artificial (e.g. gelatins). In the past, colloids were preferred to crystalloids for fluid resuscitation, as it was believed a smaller infusion volume was needed to maintain blood volume. This traditional hypothesis is incorrect (Bayer *et al.*, 2011), and resuscitation with crystalloids is as effective (Perel *et al.*, 2013), probably less harmful (Reinhart *et al.*, 2012) and cheaper. Most units have therefore largely abandoned use of artificial colloids. They are included in this chapter for the benefit of readers who may encounter them. This chapter also describes oxygen-carrying artificial fluids, which have little effect on COP, are not colloids, and are not yet currently licensed for UK use.

Blood

Blood for transfusion can be obtained from:

- donors;
- recycling (usually perioperative "cell savers");
- autotransfusion.

Problems/risks of transfusing blood and blood products include:

- limited supply;
- infection risk (low in UK);
- transfusion-related acute lung injury (TRALI);
- reactions (usually mild, but can include anaphylaxis).

People can survive an 80% loss of erythrocytes, but only a 30% loss of blood volume, so hypovolaemia can usually be effectively treated with crystalloids. Increasing haemoglobin increases oxygen-carrying capacity, but increased viscosity reduces perfusion; survival from critical illness is highest if Hb between 70–90 grams/litre (Hébert *et al.*, 1999), although there is some evidence that older people benefit from slightly higher levels (N.C.E.P.O.D., 2010b) – often assumed to be 80–100 grams/litre. Norfolk (2013) recommends a transfusion threshold of 80 grams/litre to asymptomatic patients. For a 70–80 kg patient, one unit of blood raises haemoglobin by approximately 10 grams/litre (Norfolk, 2013).

Recombinant erythropoetin may slightly reduce need for blood transfusion but it does not improve survival from critical illness (Rhodes *et al.*, 2017).

Albumin

Exogenous albumin is available as 4.5% or 5% (isotonic, various volumes up to 500 ml) and 20% (hypertonic/salt-poor, 100 ml). Hypertonic albumin has a high osmotic pressure, drawing extravascular water into the bloodstream. Although claimed benefits for albumin include:

- oxygen radical scavenging
- binding toxic substances
- anti-inflammatory (Woodcock and Woodcock, 2012),

evidence is mostly weak. In contrast to artificial colloids, Hartog *et al.* (2011) consider albumin to be safe. Albumin solutions are suspended in saline, so being chloride-rich may cause acute kidney injury (Yumos *et al.*, 2012). Infusing albumin has relatively transient benefits – endogenous albumin half-life is usually 14–20 days (Bharadwaj *et al.*, 2016), infused albumin half-life is 12–16 hours (Hahn and Lyons, 2016).

Other blood products

Most blood components are available individually for transfusion but should not be transfused unless specifically indicated. More commonly used blood products include fresh frozen plasma (FFP) and platelets.

Gelatins

Gelatins (e.g. Gelofusine, Volplex) have mean molecular weights of 30,000–40,000, about half the molecular weight of albumin, and lower than renal threshold. Like most fluids, gelatins are iso-osmotic, only expanding blood by the volume infused. Most, gelatins are suspended in 0.9% sodium chloride, such as those mentioned above, but gelatins suspended in "balanced" solutions have been marketed.

Among cautions for gelatins listed by the B.N.F. (2017) are:

- cardiac disease
- liver disease
- renal impairment,

although whether gelatins improve (Saw *et al.*, 2012) or impair (Bayer *et al.*, 2011) renal function is unclear, probably because reversing hypotension should reverse volume-responsive acute kidney injury. There is some evidence that gelatins may impair clotting (Niemi *et al.*, 2006).

Dextran

Dextran 70 (number refers to molecular weight) is rarely used. Hypertonic saline dextran (HSD -7.5% sodium chloride + 6% dextran 70) draws fluid from the extravascular spaces, increasing blood volume by four times the amount infused, and sustains intravascular volume for three to six hours. HSD also contains oxygen-free radical scavengers which reduce inflammation (Bradley, 2001). Dextrans are rarely used now.

Starches

Hydroxyethyl starch (HES) exerts a high colloid osmotic pressure, and owing to larger molecule size should have a far longer half-life than other artificial colloids. Concerns that starches may cause acute kidney injury led to restricting their indications to very few conditions, few of which are relevant to ICU. Choudhury *et al.* (2014) suggests that starches suspended in saline cause acute kidney injury, but starches suspended in balanced solutions do not, so their use may be further reappraised. The B.N.F. (2017) continues to list some starches, but states that:

> they should only be used to treat hypovolaemia due to acute blood loss when crystalloids fail to resuscitate.

Oxygen-carrying fluids

Fluids discussed above initially increase blood volume without increasing oxygen-carrying capacity but can cause dilutional anaemia. Blood transfusion creates hazards, and supply and shelf-life are limited. Oxygen-carrying fluids might resolve both problems.

Oxygen-carrying fluids may be grouped as:

- haemoglobin derivatives;
- chemical (e.g. perfluorocarbon – see Chapter 28).

There are three types of haemoglobin derivatives:

- free haemoglobin (from expired human bank blood or bovine sources);
- recombinant haemoglobin (genetically engineered *E. coli*);
- modified haemoglobins (e.g. cross-linked haemoglobins).

While haemoglobin derivatives carry oxygen, clinical trials revealed multiple serious complications, including acute kidney injury (Lumb, 2017), so, outside the context of research, oxygen-carrying fluids are unlikely to be encountered in the near future.

Implications for practice

- prescription of fluid remains a medical decision, but nurses are professionally responsible and accountable for all fluids they administer, so should be aware of efficacy and adverse effects;
- 0.9% sodium chloride mainly hydrates interstitial spaces; 5% glucose mainly hydrates cells, but both are acidic;
- contents of "balanced" solutions are closer to normal plasma than other crystalloids and, importantly, buffer acidosis;
- weight of recent evidence suggests crystalloids are as effective, and less harmful, than artificial colloids.

Summary

Critical illness usually predisposes to fluid imbalances, necessitating intravenous fluids, but also causes complications for many fluids. The traditional division between crystalloids and colloids is of limited value and has been largely replaced by debate between "balanced" and chloride-rich solutions. Although usually prescribed by doctors, fluids are usually administered by nurses, who therefore should be aware of likely benefits and problems of commonly used fluids. While this chapter has outlined main effects, and often suggests half-lives, performance of fluids will differ between individual patients and conditions.

Further reading

Most textbooks include chapters on fluid management. Among recent medical reviews, Cortés *et al.* (2014) provides a useful meta-analysis, highlighting the paucity and poor quality of evidence for all fluids. N.I.C.E. (2013c) has published guidelines for fluid therapy. Blood and blood products are authoritatively reviewed in national guidelines (Norfolk, 2013).

Clinical scenarios

Mr Kenneth McDowall is a 48-year-old smoker who had spent an afternoon drinking alcohol and watching sports with friends. While preparing an outdoor barbeque later that day, he collapsed onto the grill, which overturned, dropping hot charcoal onto him. He sustained extensive burns down the right side of his head and body.

Mr McDowall was admitted unconscious, vasoconstricted and diaphoretic with full thickness burns. His ECG on admission revealed a large left ventricular infarcted area. Other results included tachycardia (130 beats/minute), BP 100/78 mmHg, PPV 14%, tachypnoeic (26 breaths/min). Arterial blood gas showed good oxygenation with uncompensated respiratory acidosis, Na+ 148 mmol/litre, K+ 4.5 mmol/litre, blood glucose 12 mmol/litre. He is cannulated with one peripheral cannulae and quadruple lumen CVC in his left jugular vein.

Q1. What signs indicate Mr McDowall needs fluid management.
Q2. Which fluid would you recommend? Why? What would be an appropriate rate?
Q3. How are fluid challenges administered in your unit? – type, volume, rate, route? Does your unit/trust have guidelines for fluid management?

Chapter 34

Inotropes and vasopressors

Contents

Fundamental knowledge

Sympathetic nervous system
Negative feedback and parasympathetic effect
Renin–angiotensin–aldosterone mechanism

Introduction

By far the most common pathology in general ICUs is sepsis, necessitating chemical support of blood pressure. Blood pressure is the sum of volume (cardiac output) multiplied by resistance (systemic vascular resistance, or "afterload"). Cardiac output is the amount of blood ejected by the left ventricle each minute, so is heart rate multiplied by stroke volume. So:

$$BP = HR \times SV \times SVR$$

Provided other factors remain constant, increasing one factor necessarily increases blood pressure.

Inotropes (*inos* = "fibre" in Greek) alter stretch of cardiac muscle fibres but, more commonly in the ICU, vasopressors (also called "vasoconstrictors") are needed to reverse excessive vasodilatation. These effects are mediated through stimulation of the sympathetic nervous system.

Inotropes can be classed as *positive* if they increase stretch and cardiac output, and *negative* if they reduce stretch and output. Negative inotropes include beta-blockers, and many chemical mediators such as tumour necrosis factor, but without a prefix "inotrope" usually implies positive inotropes. This chapter discusses only vasopressors and positive inotropes.

Vasoactive drugs may be divided into two main groups:

■ adrenergic agonists (inoconstrictors);
■ phosphodiesterase inhibitors (inodilators).

In the ICU, adrenergic agonists are usually used.

Although the UK has now adopted international names for most drugs, it retains the traditional UK names for adrenaline (elsewhere, "epinephrine") and noradrenaline (elsewhere, "norepinephrine")

Indications

Inotropes and vasopressors are used to increase blood pressure. Blood volume should be optimised before using drugs. Increasing cardiac work when there is insufficient circulating volume can cause myocardial ischaemia. Many patients are hypovolaemic on admission to ICU.

Receptors

The heart and blood vessels contain various types of receptors, many of which have subtypes.

Alpha (α) receptors are located primarily in arterioles, especially in peripheries. Alpha stimulation (e.g. with noradrenaline) causes arteriolar vasoconstriction, so increasing systemic vascular resistance. Alpha stimulation has little effect on cerebral, coronary and pulmonary blood flow, so maintaining perfusion to vital organs.

Alpha stimulation may adversely affect many major organs:

- heart (dysrhythmias, ischaemia, infarction);
- pancreas (reduced insulin secretion, contributing to hyperglycaemia);
- liver (accentuating immunocompromise and coagulopathies);
- kidneys (vasoconstriction, causing acute kidney injury);
- gut (ischaemia, causing translocation of gut bacteria);
- skin (peripheral blanching or cyanosis; extreme ischaemia may cause gangrene, necessitating amputation of digits).

Alpha stimulants are usually given to counter excessive vasodilatation.

Beta (β) receptors are primarily in the heart and lungs. Beta$_1$ receptors in pacemaker cells cause *chronotropic* effects, while in other myocardial cells they increase spontaneous muscle depolarisation (stretch), so β_1 stimulation:

- increases contractility;
- improves atrioventricular conduction;
- hastens myocardial relaxation;
- increases stroke volume;
- increases heart rate (with potential dysrhythmias),

so increasing cardiac output. Hypertension being a common problem in society, negative inotropes, such as beta-blockers, are widely used in healthcare; critical illness presents the less usual challenge of needing positive inotropes.

β_2 receptors are found mainly in bronchial smooth muscle, but a significant minority are also found in myocardium. β_2 stimulation is especially chronotropic, increasing myocardial workload and predisposing to dysrhythmias (hence the tachycardic/dysrhythmic effects of bronchodilators such as salbutamol). β_2 receptors are also found in other smooth muscle, such as blood vessels and skeletal muscle. When stimulated, these β_2 receptors vasodilate arterioles and reduce systemic vascular resistance (afterload).

Main receptor sites targeted are summarised in Table 34.1, although no inotropes purely target only one receptor.

Safety

The half-lives of most inotropes and vasopressors used in the ICU is very short – often two to five minutes; noradrenaline's half-life is one to two minutes (Argettant, 2013). Rapid changes in blood pressure necessitate use being limited to areas where:

- blood pressure and ECG can be monitored continuously (or at least every five minutes);
- sufficient staff are available to observe monitors;
- staff have sufficient knowledge to understand significance of observations and know how to resolve excessive or insufficient effects.

Appropriate alarm limits should be set on monitors. Effectively, this usually limits positive inotrope and vasopressor use to ICUs and a few other designated specialist areas, such as CCUs and theatres.

When patients are dependent on large doses, interruptions when changing infusions, or syringe drivers taking up "slack" in the mechanism when new syringes are inserted, can cause life-threatening hypotension. This risk can be reduced by:

- double pumping – commencing new infusions before switching off old ones, some units only switching off the old once blood pressure begins to increase;
- switching technique – running new infusions before connecting to patients, then turning off old ones as the new is connected (Llewellyn, 2007).

While both methods seem equally effective, the quick change technique is faster, easier and more cost-effective, so double pumping is not recommended (De Barbieri *et al.*, 2009). If changing strength of infusions, deadspace in lines contains a small volume of the previous concentration. Using volumetric pumps rather than syringe drivers overcomes problems of delays/overlap, provided a new bag is available in time. Drugs being generally heavier than the solutions they are mixed with, may settle at the base of bags, resulting in stronger concentrations near time of commencing infusions. Whether this is a practical, or just theoretical, problem is questionable.

Some inotropes and vasopressors should only be mixed with 5% glucose. Most units dissolve all inotropes in glucose solutions, both reducing risks of error and enabling often limited venous access to be shared by more than one drug.

Although some inotropes can be infused peripherally, in practice they are usually given centrally as poor peripheral circulation and possible alpha vasoconstriction may cause pooling of drugs in peripheries and extravasation into tissues. Lines should be clearly labelled, and no bolus or short-term drugs given through lines containing inotropes.

mcg/kg/min

Inotropes are usually measured in micrograms (*mcg* or *μcg**) per kilogram per minute (see below):

$$\text{mcg/kg/minute} = \frac{\text{mg}}{\text{ml}} \times \frac{1000}{\text{patient's weight}} \times \frac{\text{infusion rate (ml/hour)}}{60}$$

*use of μ is generally discouraged; "micro" or "mcg" is generally preferred.

This formula can be expressed in various other ways, e.g.

$$\frac{\text{mcg/kg/minute}}{1000} \times \frac{\text{ml}}{\text{mg}} \times \text{patient's weight} \times 60 = \text{infusion rate}$$

Most syringe drivers and volumetric pumps used in ICU can calculate doses once patient and drug details are entered.

Such calculations are complex, and with drugs that have such short half-lives and are titrated to a continuously monitored target, it is questionable whether a simpler way would be preferable, enabling quicker dosage changes. For safety, the Intensive Care Society (I.C.S., 2017a) recommends standard concentrations for drugs; this document also identifies whether or not drugs can be given peripherally.

Adrenaline (epinephrine)

Adrenaline, the main adrenal medullary hormone, stimulates alpha, β_1 and β_2 receptors, triggering the "fight or flight" stress response via the sympathetic nervous system:

- vasoconstriction (alpha receptors);
- increased cardiac output (β_1, β_2),

together increasing blood pressure. Traditionally, adrenaline was believed to dilate coronary and cerebral arteries (Jowett and Thompson, 2007), although this is now questioned. Adrenaline remains the recommended first-line drug for resuscitation from cardiac arrest (Resuscitation Council (UK), 2015), where immediate short-term restoration of systemic blood pressure and circulation is essential. Its bronchodilatory qualities (β_2) make nebulised adrenaline useful during asthma crises, especially with children (Sireesha *et al.*, 2018). This combination of effects makes it less useful in ICU.

Adrenaline can cause gross tachycardia, ventricular dysrhythmias, hyper-glycaemia, oliguria, increased lactate, hypokalaemia, hypophosphataemia and other metabolic complications, so is not widely used in most ICUs. Rhodes *et al.* (2017) recommend adding adrenaline if noradrenaline fails to reverse hypotension from sepsis.

Noradrenaline (norepinephrine)

Noradrenaline is the first-choice vasopressor for sepsis (Rhodes *et al.*, 2017). Theoretically, doses would ideally be titrated to systemic vascular resistance measurements from cardiac output studies; there is scant evidence that cardiac output studies improve outcome, and low diastolic blood pressure indicates vascular resistance, while mean arterial pressure indicates organ perfusion. Nurses should therefore observe peripheries for perfusion, and delayed capillary refill, pale/mottled skin or cold digits should be reported.

Noradrenaline appears to have fewer metabolic complications (e.g. lactate, glycaemia) than adrenaline. Noradrenaline is highly acidic – pH 3.0–4.0 (Argettant, 2013), so extravasation of noradrenaline can cause necrosis and peripheral gangrene, necessitating central venous administration. Vasoconstriction can cause reflex bradycardia (Charlton and Thompson, 2016).

Growing evidence suggests noradrenaline is useful for treating refractory cardiogenic shock, perhaps because it improves right ventricular perfusion (Gupta *et al.*, 2015).

Dobutamine

Dobutamine, a synthetic analogue of dopamine, is primarily a β_1 stimulant. It does have some β_2 and α effects, but is less chronotropic and dysrhythmic than most β_1 inotropes. It reduces systemic vascular resistance, so together with increased cardiac output, increases oxygen delivery to cells. Provided euvolaemic, it is the first-line choice for poor cardiac output (Rhodes *et al.*, 2017).

Metraminol

An α_1 agonist, with some β effect, metraminol causes peripheral vasoconstriction, so is often used during a hypotensive crisis, and as an emergency drug during transfer. It is metabolised hepatically, so renal failure does not limit its usage. Its duration is 20 minutes to one hour, considerably longer than adrenaline, so it is usually given as a bolus. It can also be given subcutaneously and intramuscularly, although slower absorption limits usefulness of these routes in crises.

Dopexamine (hydrochloride)

Dopexamine, a synthetic dopamine derivative, primarily causes arterial vasodilatation (β_2 agonist) with weak β_1 and dopaminergic effects. Claimed renal and splanchnic benefits appear doubtful (Renton and Snowden, 2005), and mortality is not reduced by its use (Gopal *et al.*, 2009), so it has largely fallen into disuse. It can be given peripherally but, being an irritant, should be given through a large vein. Its half-life is five to 10 minutes.

Dopamine

Dopamine is an endogenous catecholamine and noradrenaline precursor. There are specific dopamine receptors (DA_1), but dopamine also stimulates alpha and beta receptors. Exogenous dopamine impairs immunity (Van den Berghe and de Zegher, 1996; Grebenik and Sinclair, 2003) and gut motility (Dive *et al.*, 2000). As a vasopressor, it has similar mortality to noradrenaline, but is highly dysrhythmic (Gupta *et al.*, 2015), is associated with more adverse events (De Backer *et al.*, 2010), and provides no protection against gut ischaemia (Azar *et al.*, 1996) or kidney injury (Australian and New Zealand Intensive Care Society Clinical Trials Group, 2000; Marik, 2002). It is therefore rarely used in ICU.

Insufficient brainstem production causes neurotransmission failure in Parkinson's disease, but dopamine cannot permeate mature blood–brain barriers (Van den Berghe and de Zegher, 1996), so intravenous dopamine does not affect cerebral receptors.

Table 34.1 Main target receptors for drugs

	α	β₁ (heart)	β₂ (mainly lungs)
Effect of stimulation	Vasoconstriction	Increased cardiac output	Bronchodilation
adrenaline	✓	✓	✓
noradrenaline	✓		
metraminol	✓	some	some
argipressin	✓		
dobutamine	✓		
dopexamine	some	some	✓
dopamine	✓	✓	

Inodilators

Traditionally, treatment has focused on maintaining perfusion by optimising arterial blood pressure as a surrogate indication of capillary flow and delivery of oxygen to tissues. Arteriole vasoconstriction may achieve arterial blood pressure targets at the expense of tissue oxygen delivery. Adrenoreceptor stimulation, such as with dobutamine, increases myocardial oxygen demand (Belletti *et al.*, 2017). An alternative strategy could be to increase cardiac output and vasodilate, using inodilators such as levosimenden and milrinone.

Primarily calcium sensitisers, these drugs enhance calcium binding to troponin, so improving contractility (Jonkman *et al.*, 2017). They can also be classified as phosphodiesterase inhibitors (PDIs). Phosphodiesterase is an intracellular enzyme which prolongs cardiac and coronary artery contraction. Inhibiting phosphodiesterase therefore:

- increases ventricular filling;
- improves myocardial oxygenation;
- vasodilates (reduces afterload).

PDIs are protein-bound, giving them half-lives of about 45 minutes, but also usually necessitating loading doses. Half-life is increased with renal impairment. Comparing levosimendan with dobutamine for septic shock cardiomyopathy, Meng *et al.* (2016) found levosimendan resulted in lower biomarker levels but no difference in clinical outcome, while Gordon *et al.* (2016) suggest that it may delay weaning and result in more supraventricular tachycardias. Belletti *et al.* (2017) consider levosimendan the most promising treatment for septic shock, although they acknowledge there is currently insufficient evidence to recommend its use. Mebazaa *et al.* (2007) found that levosimendan had no mortality benefit compared with dobutamine. It is more expensive than dobutamine (Rhodes *et al.*, 2017) and is currently not licensed in the UK.

Haemodynamic management is inevitably limited by availability of haemodynamic monitoring. Development of minimally invasive tissue oxygenation monitoring (De Santis and Singer, 2015) may facilitate therapies that optimise tissue oxygenation rather than arterial blood pressure.

Argipressin

Various drugs have been used to "test" response to, or augment, noradrenaline, but most have fallen into disuse. Vasopressin (antidiuretic hormone) may be used if noradrenaline fails to reverse septic shock (Rhodes *et al.*, 2017), usually given in its synthetic form of argipressin.

Unlike most drugs discussed in this chapter, argipressin can be given peripherally (I.C.S., 2017a). In some ICUs, argipressin infusions are added if noradrenaline fails to achieve targets.

Implications for practice

- before commencing drugs to increase blood pressure, blood volume should be optimised (avoid "dry drive");
- most inotropes and vasopressors should be diluted in 5% glucose (to prevent oxidation) before preparation;
- some inotropes may be given peripherally, but for safety most units give all inotropes and vasopressors through central lines, especially as they are usually being used in patients whose peripheral blood flow is often problematic;
- within prescribed limits, doses should be titrated to achieve desired effects, while minimising adverse effects;
- dobutamine increases cardiac output;
- adrenaline increases both systemic vascular resistance and cardiac output
- vasopressors increase systemic vascular resistance; the main vasopressor used in ICU is noradrenaline, but hypotension refractory to noradrenaline may be treated additionally with other vasopressors such as argipressin;
- most inotropes and vasopressors (but not phosphodiesterase inhibitors) have half-lives of only a very few minutes, so should only be used where continuous blood pressure and ECG monitoring is available, where there are sufficient staff to observe monitors, and where staff are familiar with using the drugs;
- with alpha stimulants (e.g. noradrenaline), monitor peripheral perfusion (e.g. capillary refill time);
- many patients become highly dependent on inotropes, rapidly becoming hypotensive when infusions are changed; changes should therefore minimise risks (e.g. have a "spare" ready, and use a quick change technique).

Summary

Central blood pressure can be increased by increasing heart rate (chronotropes), increasing stroke volume (β_1 stimulation or phosphodiesterase inhibition) or increasing systemic vascular resistance (alpha stimulation).

For β_1 stimulation, most units use dobutamine. Alpha stimulation (from adrenaline or noradrenaline) can usefully raise central blood pressure by increasing systemic vascular resistance. Most ICUs use noradrenaline to counter inappropriate vasodilatation (sepsis) and dobutamine to increase cardiac output (cardiogenic shock).

Further reading

Other than studies of specific drugs, there have been very few articles about inotropes in recent years, but Charlton and Thompson (2016) provides a useful overview. Pharmacology texts, including from the B.N.F., can provide useful information. Manufacturers' summaries of product characteristics should be followed. Many units provide local guidance about vasopressors and inotropes. I.C.S. (2017a) offers guidance on drug concentrations and whether or not drugs can be infused peripherally.

Clinical scenarios

Mrs Caroline Williams, 53 years old, is admitted following an emergency laparotomy for faecal peritonitis. During induction she had a cardiac arrest and three cycles of CPR performed. Mrs Williams has no previous cardiac history, is 1.6 m tall and weighs 70 kg. Four days after her operation she remains sedated and invasively ventilated with signs of septic shock. Arterial blood gas indicates severe metabolic acidosis with pH of 6.9.

Her haemodynamic results include:

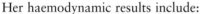

Temperature	38.5°C
BP	135/72 mmHg (MAP 93 mmHg)
HR	108 beats/minute, sinus rhythm
PPV	16%
Stroke volume	52 ml
Cardiac index	2.92 litres/minute/m²
SVRi	1600 dynes/sec/m⁻⁵/m²
DO_2I	455 ml/minute/m²

Mrs Williams has continuous infusions of noradrenaline (at 0.19 mcg/kg/minute) and dobutamine (1.0 mcg/kg/minute) in progress.

Q1. Describe the therapeutic actions of Mrs Williams's vasoactive drug infusions. Explain their action on specific receptor sites and intended effects.

Q2. What other parameters should be assessed and recorded when evaluating effectiveness (and monitoring for adverse effects) of Mrs Williams's treatment?

Q3. Over the day, noradrenaline and dobutamine infusion rates are increased. Are there any alternative actions or considerations that could reverse the increasing need for inotropic support?

Chapter 35

Vascular surgery

Contents

Fundamental knowledge

Pathology of atherosclerosis
Thrombolysis (see Chapter 29)
Sternotomy (see Chapter 30)
Anatomy and physiology of large arteries (including aorta, femoral, carotid, renal artery)
Pathology of connective tissue disease
How and where to assess pedal pulses

Introduction

Vascular disease is common, frequently needing medical or surgical interventions, only a few of which usually necessitate ICU admission:

- aneurysm repair;
- carotid artery repair.

In addition to needs created by often prolonged and major operations, surgery on major arteries creates risks from:

- major bleeds;
- organ and tissue damage from perioperative ischaemia distal to the repair
- thrombus/embolus formation (especially strokes);
- patients often having extensive vascular and other co-morbidities that complicate recovery.

Aneurysms

"Aneurysm" means "widening" (Greek). Once believed to be simple stretching, aneurysms are now known to be caused by remodelling (Baxter, 2004), usually from atherosclerosis. Progressive deposits eventually separate the wall's layers, causing haemorrhage and rupture. Potentially any part of the aorta can widen, but ascending aortic aneurysms and aneurysms of the aortic arch are relatively rare, and surgery is especially complex, so is performed in relatively few specialist centres. Descending aneurysms, widening exceeding 50% (E.S.V.S., 2017), are more common, less difficult to repair, with surgery available in most trusts. A significant minority have both descending and ascending aneurysms (Larsson et al., 2011).

Aneurysms are usually asymptomatic (Nilsson et al., 2017), usually being found by chance. Pain is usually a symptom of rupture (E.S.V.S., 2017), necessitating urgent surgery. Without repair, rupture is usually fatal (Braithwaite et al., 2015), and even with surgery mortality exceeds 40% (Tambyraja and Chalmers, 2009). Vascular disease elsewhere typically creates significant co-morbidities, especially diabetes (Bath et al., 2017), cardiovascular disease (Bath et al., 2017) and renal failure (Lilja et al., 2017). Co-morbidities may necessitate ICU admission.

Atherosclerosis is an inflammatory process; vascular leak from inflammation frequently causes pleural effusions. Immediate treatment of aneurysms usually includes antihypertensives, such as beta-blockers, but earlier drug interventions may prevent or limit atherosclerosis. A minority of aneurysms are caused by trauma, bacterial or fungal infections, and other problems.

Renal compromise, both from the disease and surgery/repair, stimulates the renin–angiotensin–aldosterone cascade (Adembri et al., 2004), exacerbating problems from hypertension. Open surgery necessitates cross-clamping the aorta. Most abdominal aneurysms occur below the renal artery, so clamps can normally be placed below the renal artery, preserving renal perfusion. But higher aneurysms necessitate clamping above the renal artery, which may cause acute kidney injury. With endovascular repair, intrarenal damage may be caused by obstruction from the endograft or nephrotoxic dyes, and so damage may accelerate after admission to ICU.

Mortality and morbidity from ascending aortic repair is very high, partly because it precedes the carotid arteries but also because it usually involves aortic valve disease, resulting in simultaneous aortic valve replacement. Repair is therefore usually undertaken in specialist centres by cardiothoracic, rather than vascular, surgeons. The ascending aorta stretches from the aortic valve to the carotid arteries and is especially susceptible to aneurysm in people with Marfan's syndrome (Price *et al.*, 2016) and other connective tissue disease. Surgery compromises cerebral perfusion, unless cardiopulmonary bypass is used. Endovascular approaches may offer a viable alternative provided valve replacement is not needed.

Traditionally, surgery involved grafting a synthetic prosthesis (aortic tube graft) into the vessel, but major vessels are now often repaired through endovascular insertion of fabric or metal stents, inserted through catheters similar to those used for angioplasty. N.I.C.E. (2008) cautiously recommended laparoscopic vascular surgery, including aortic repair. Most studies suggest EVAR has lower early mortality and morbidity (The United Kingdom EVAR Trial Investigators, 2010; E.S.V.S., 2017), although Patel *et al.* (2016) found that, while EVAR may offer better early outcomes, open aneurysm repair had lower long-term mortality than EVAR.

While open aneurysm repairs are usually admitted to Level 3 facilities, EVAR repairs are usually admitted to Level 2.

Carotid artery disease

Atheromatous plaques frequently form in carotid arteries, especially in older people. About one tenth of people aged over 80 have carotid artery stenosis (Carrell and Wolfe, 2005). Stenosis reduces cerebral blood flow, predisposing to ischaemic strokes (Naylor, 2009), while thrombi may cause thrombotic strokes, so with severe disease repair is usually needed. Stenting carries greater risk of peri-procedure stroke but endarterectomy carries greater risk of periprocedure myocardial infarction (Brott *et al.*, 2010), making carotid endarterectomy the treatment of choice (International Carotid Stenting Study Investigators, 2010).

False aneurysms

Also called pseudoaneurysms, these occur when damage to an artery wall, often from medical/surgical procedures, enables a haematoma to develop. It usually requires vascular intervention.

Nursing care

In addition to system support, specific individual needs and standard post-operative care, such as observing wound site/dressings, patients with vascular disease are especially susceptible to complications from perfusion failure. Vascular surgery creates the problem of maintaining sufficient perfusion pressure in patients who usually have extensive vascular disease, while preventing graft damage from excessive pressure – patients needing vascular surgery usually have a history of hypertension. The most common cause of post-operative death is myocardial infarction, often from unidentified coronary artery disease (Carrell and Wolfe, 2005). Clonidine is useful for both its anxiolytic and antihypertensive properties (Schneemilch *et al.*, 2006). Extensive vascular disease often causes ischaemia and chronic pain. Immediate post-operative pain is usually managed with epidural analgesia.

E.S.V.S. (2017) cite suggestions of maintaining post-operative mean arterial pressures of MAP 80–100 mmHg, although support this from a 2001 reference. Following aneurysm repair, pPerfusion is also monitored through urine output (aim > 0.5 ml/kg/hour) and observing peripheral pulses both by touch and Doppler. Interruption to perfusion from vascular intervention in patients who usually have a long history of vascular disease predisposes most organs and tissues to risks of complications. Main medical complications from open repair are listed in Table 35.1.

Vascular surgery may cause bleeding from surrounding tissue, so drains should be clearly labelled or numbered, volume marked or measured on arrival, and drainage initially monitored hourly. If vacuum drains are used, vacuum should be checked hourly.

"Endoleak" – blood flowing within the aneurysm sac but outside the graft – is more common following EVAR than open surgical repair (Stather *et al.*, 2013).

Patients with vascular disease are at high risk of developing pressure sores (Scott *et al.*, 2001). Common post-operative complications include acute kidney injury (Castagno *et al.*, 2016) and spinal cord injury (Puchakayala, 2006). Endovascular surgery has a high incidence of spinal cord ischaemia (Riambau *et al.*, 2017).

Although the carotid artery is relatively superficial, repair exposes patients to additional specific risks:

- neurological deficit from occlusion, thrombi or emboli;
- oedema, compressing the vagus nerve, causing bradycardia, hypotension and possible heart-blocks;
- displacement of the trachea.

Nurses should therefore observe:

- neurological function, reporting any inappropriate or deteriorating responses;

Table 35.1 Main complications: open surgery to the aorta

neurological – paraplegia, paraparesis, stroke
cardiac – myocardial ischaemia, myocardial infarction
respiratory failure
acute kidney injury
sepsis
limb ischaemia

Source: After E.S.V.S., 2017.

■ airway patency. Tracheal shift will probably be detected on X-ray, but any respiratory problems in extubated patients should be reported;

■ ECG, heart rate and blood pressure, setting appropriate alarms and reporting any signs of excessive vagal stimulation.

Drains used with carotid surgery are usually small, so more likely to occlude and fill quickly. Arterial flow to, and venous drainage from, the head should not be occluded.

Unlike most post-operative patients, thromboembolism deterrent stockings (TEDS) are not usually used, as patients are at high risk of bleeding rather than clotting following vascular surgery, and pressure on any femoral incisions may occlude perfusion.

Once stabilised (especially fluids optimised and clotting normalised) and extubated, recovery is usually quick. Provided no complications are present, patients are often discharged to vascular wards the day following surgery.

Implications for practice

■ pulses, colour and warmth should be monitored on limbs distal to surgery;

■ mean arterial pressure should be maintained > 70 mmHg, but hypertension avoided;

■ urine output should be maintained > 0.5 ml/kg/hour;

■ pain should be assessed, together with side effects of epidurals or whatever analgesia is used (see Chapter 7);

■ following carotid artery repair, pressure to the opposite side of the neck should be avoided;

■ anticoagulant therapy is usually omitted post-operatively, and thromboembolism deterrent stockings (TEDS) are usually not used.

Summary

Most vascular surgery does not necessitate ICU admission, unless patients develop complications or other problems or have open aneurysm repair. But, following surgery on the aorta or carotid artery, patients are usually admitted to Level 2 facilities for observation. The main post-operative dangers are:

- stroke;
- graft/vessel occlusion;
- kidney injury;
- haemorrhage or bleeding from graft leak.

Post-operative recovery focuses on stabilisation, observation, symptom control and system support.

Further reading

Vascular surgical journals include *Journal of Vascular Surgery* and *Journal of Vascular Nursing*. The European Society for Vascular Surgery (E.S.V.S., 2017) has published guidelines, although these are medically focused.

Clinical scenarios

Mr Owen Fowler is an 81-year-old gentleman with hypertension. He has been diagnosed with an abdominal aortic aneurysm (AAA) of 5.2 cm diameter. This was repaired under fluoroscopic guidance using digital subtraction angiography (DSA) to insert an endograft through his femoral arteries. During the endovascular repair, Mr Fowler lost two litres of blood and was transfused with six units of packed red cells. He was admitted to ICU for further fluid and cardiovascular management, with Hb of 62 grams/litre, a platelet count of 50×10^9/litre and a BP of 110/58 mmHg. He has two vacuum drains located in the right and left groin incision wounds.

Q1. Identify the potential complications for Mr Fowler following his endovascular repair. Why might these occur and consider the effects of contrast dye, position and type of endograft etc.?

Q2. Plan nursing interventions which monitor and enhance tissue perfusion for Mr Fowler (e.g. fluids, blood products, vasopressors, drain management, limb assessment, use of Doppler, thromboprophylaxis).

Q3. How would you describe relative benefits and risks between open and endovascular aortic aneurysm repair to a student nurse?

Part VII

Neurological

Chapter 36

Central nervous system injury

Contents

Introduction

Although neurology services are usually focused in regional centres, patients with acute neurological injuries and complications may be admitted to general ICUs, sometimes for stabilisation before transfer. Traumatic brain or spinal injury can cause life-threatening respiratory and cardiovascular failure, necessitating urgent ICU admission.

This chapter discusses:

- traumatic brain injury;
- diabetes insipidus;
- spinal cord injury;
- autonomic dysreflexia;
- epilepsy;
- intracranial haemorrhage.

Stroke is discussed in Woodrow (2016). There are some similarities, but also many differences, about complications from and treatments for this diverse group of pathologies. Patients with severe traumatic brain injury or spinal cord injury will usually be transferred to regional specialist centres, but initial stabilisation may occur on general ICUs, which are not able to provide specialist interventions such as craniotomy, specialist monitoring such as intracranial pressure monitoring, and whose staff have less experience of neurology. Some patients may remain in general ICUs owing to poor prognosis, injury being relatively minor, or lack of beds.

The "golden hour" of trauma care applies to central nervous system injury. Primary damage is largely irreversible, so focus of treatment should be preventing secondary damage (Sanfilippo *et al.*, 2014). Immediate priorities are preserving life:

- Airway
- Breathing
- Circulation
- Disability (neurological),

with special emphasis on neuroprotection: hypoxia and hypotension are the most likely causes of death.

Airway

Airway obstruction may be caused directly by trauma or impaired consciousness. Anyone with a Glasgow Coma Scale Score of 8 or below may be unable to maintain their own airway, so should be intubated (Riley and de Beer, 2014). Securing of endotracheal tubes should avoid impairing venous drainage, which could contribute to intracranial hypertension.

Breathing

Unlike cells elsewhere, brain cells do not store ATP, so need constant supplies of oxygen. Severe traumatic brain injury therefore usually necessitates artificial ventilation. Diaphragmatic nerves usually exit the spinal cord at C3–C5, so spinal injuries involving or above these may cause apnoea, necessitating ventilation. Even if able to self-ventilate, hypopnoea and weak cough reflexes expose patients to greater risk of chest infection. Other indications for artificial ventilation may include:

- lung injury from multiple trauma– contusion, pneumothorax, fractured ribs;
- hypercapnia – carbon dioxide vasodilates, so controlling levels (target 4.0– 4.5 kPa) limits intracranial hypertension.

Sedation is usually needed, for humanitarian reasons, to facilitate effective ventilation and to reduce brain activity (neuro-protection). Propofol, being short-acting, is usually the sedative of choice. Paralysing agents may be necessary to facilitate ventilation or reduce metabolism, especially to stop shivering, but there is insufficient evidence to support or confound their use with traumatic brain injury (Sanfilippo et al., 2014).

Increased intrathoracic pressure impairs cerebral venous drainage, so unnecessary coughing and straining at stool should be prevented if possible. Anti-tussive drugs and early tracheostomy may help prevent coughing. Constipation should be prevented through good bowel care, which usually necessitates laxatives (see Chapter 9).

Circulation

With traumatic brain injury, labile systolic blood pressure is associated with poor outcome, so Manning et al. (2014) recommend keeping systolic blood pressure consistently below 140 mmHg.

Hypovolaemia causes cerebral vasospasm, further reducing perfusion. Fluid resuscitation should aim to maintain mean arterial pressure $\geq$ 80 mmHg (N.I.C.E., 2014b), thus maintaining cerebral perfusion pressure.

Glucose solutions should be avoided, as their "free water" can transfer into cells, causing cerebral oedema and potentially fatal intracranial hypertension (Haddad and Arabi, 2012). Once adequately filled, blood pressure optimisation may necessitate inotropes.

Disability (neurological)

Traumatic brain injury, but not spinal cord injury, causes breakdown of tight junctions in the blood–brain barrier, allowing protein leak into brain tissue, which causes vasogenic oedema (Nag *et al.*, 2011) and intracranial hypertension, the most life-threatening secondary complication. Medical imaging, such as computerised tomography (CT), is therefore a priority to identify whether neurosurgical intervention is necessary. Otherwise, secondary brain damage may be minimised by:

- sedating, to reduce cerebral oxygen consumption – identified above;
- (sometimes) paralysing;
- minimising intracranial pressure,

while identifying additional risks, such as:

- base of skill fracture;
- fitting.

Blood glucose is often labile with neurological pathologies, potentially exacerbating brain damage (Smith and Meyfroidt, 2017), so should be closely monitored and controlled.

Because there is essentially no passive movement across the blood–brain barrier, draining cerebral *oedema* necessitates either drain insertion or hyperosmolar fluid infusion. Hypertonic saline (e.g. 2.7%) (Kamel *et al.*, 2011; Ropper, 2012) is generally the first choice, although mannitol is still sometimes used. Being hypertonic, these fluids are thrombophlebitic, so ideally should be given centrally, or at least through a large vein.

Cranial venous drainage can be optimised by *positioning* patients at angles of 15–30° (E.A.S.L., 2017; Winkeleman and Hilton, 2018), although Ledwith *et al.* (2010) and Kim *et al.* (2013) showed that the position needs to be individualised to each patient, which is currently impractical in units that lack intracranial pressure monitoring. Restriction of drainage by overly tight endotracheal tube holders and unnecessary rigid neck collars should be avoided.

Base of skull fractures are not visually obvious, and may not have been diagnosed, but may still exist. With any cranial trauma, base of skull fracture should be suspected until excluded, and no equipment should be inserted nasally until excluded. Base of skull fractures may cause leakage of cerebrospinal fluid (CSF) from the nose (rhinorrhoea) or ear (otorrhoea). CSF stains linen yellow. Signs of bleeding may be visible through bruising around eyes ("racoon eyes") (Venkatesh, 2014) or behind the ear ("battle sign") (March and Hickey, 2014).

Up to one quarter of patients develop *fitting*. Likely causes (e.g. hypoxia) should be treated and if fitting persists, antiepileptics are usually needed.

If the spine is uninjured but soft tissue injury is suspected, collars should be used for moving, and CT/MRI scans arranged when stable.

Traumatic brain injury (TBI)

Traumatic brain injury is the most common cause of death and injury in people under the age of 40 (N.I.C.E., 2014b). Classification follows Glasgow Coma Scale scoring:

- mild = GCS 13–15;
- moderate = GCS 9–13;
- severe = GCS 3–8.

Trauma may cause externally visible fracture and bruising, but may also cause internal injuries, such as:

- haematoma (extradural, subdural);
- contusion;
- contre-coup (the brain hits the opposite side of the skull to the original injury);
- rotation (the brain rotates within the skull, wrenching away nerves and other brain tissue);
- diffuse axonal injury.

Victims of TBI often suffer multiple injuries to other parts of the body, so need multisystem support. Some injuries may not be immediately obvious, so nurses should continually assess all body systems and functions.

Following initial stabilisation, severely injured patients (GCS < 8) should be urgently transferred to specialist centres (N.I.C.E., 2014b). Priorities of medical management are summarised in Table 36.1.

Preventing raised intracranial pressure

In addition to immediate care above, nurses have an important role in providing therapeutic care and environments for their patients, primarily by limiting

Table 36.1 Possible main aspects of medical management of moderate/severe head injury

- diagnostic investigations (computerised tomography – CT, magnetic resonance imaging – MRI, lumbar puncture)
- surgical (e.g. evacuation if haematoma, ventricular drainage to remove excess/blocked CSF)
- artificial ventilation, keeping $PaCO_2$ 4.5–5.0 kPa; muscle relaxation sedation + short-term sedation (N.I.C.E., 2014b)
- osmotic diuretics (mannitol) and/or barbiturates to reduce cerebral oedema and ICP
- fluid management
- stabilise electrolytes and blood glucose
- ICP monitoring, maintaining ICP 0–10 and CPP > 70 mmHg
- system support (e.g. vasoactive drugs to normalise blood pressure)

stimuli that may increase intracranial pressure. Ideally, normal intracranial pressure (ICP) and cerebral perfusion pressure (CPP) should be maintained – normal ICP 0–10 mmHg, normal CPP 60–70 mmHg (Carney *et al.*, 2016).

Preventing *pain* has humanitarian and physiological benefits, as stress responses increase intracranial pressure. Codeine phosphate is less likely to mask neurological (diagnostic) signs than other opioids, but once diagnosis is established pain is usually controlled with standard opioids, such as fentanyl. Limbs should be kept in comfortable alignment. Skincare and pressure area care can help prevent pressure sore development, which both cause discomfort and expose patients to potential complications.

Nutrition

Malnutrition increases risks of infection and delayed rehabilitation in all patients, but head injury significantly increases catabolism (Hunningher and Smith, 2006). Early nutrition should be given (Blaser *et al.*, 2017), which may necessitate prokinetics, such as metoclopramide.

Electrolyte imbalances may occur from fluid shifts and loss. Levels should be checked and monitored, with supplements given as necessary.

Blood sugar is often labile following head injury, so should be monitored frequently (e.g. two- to four-hourly). Hypoglycaemia starves neurones of the main fuel used to produce energy. Maintenance fluids should be saline solutions, not glucose (see above).

Positioning

Most ICU patients are at risk of developing pressure sores. Traumatic brain or spinal injury usually cause or necessitate immobility. Pressure area care interventions should be planned against risks from stimulation. Aggressive manual handling can significantly increase intracranial pressure.

Severe spasticity is common (Iggulden, 2006), so assessment and care planning should include active consideration of:

- active/passive exercises;
- positioning;
- physiotherapy;
- removing any stimuli that reduce muscle tone (e.g. constipation).

Although these aspects will be the focus of later rehabilitation, neglect during the acute phase may prolong or limit rehabilitation.

Pituitary damage

Although rare, direct trauma from head injury by central nervous system infection (meningitis) or raised intracranial pressure can cause pituitary damage. The pituitary gland regulates the endocrine system, so damage can cause diverse problems, including diabetes insipidus, while damage to the adjacent hypothalamus may cause pyrexia.

Diabetes insipidus is caused when the hypothalamic pituitary damage results in insufficient antidiuretic hormone ADH (Bajwa and Haldar, 2015). ADH affects renal reabsorption of water, and lack causes polyuria. Damage might be permanent, but is more often transient, from oedema. Once oedema subsides, diabetes insipidus usually resolves. Until resolution, fluid balance should be carefully monitored, and adequate volume replacement prescribed.

Pyrexia in contexts of neurological injury is usually caused by hypothalamic damage/disruption (Niven and Laupland, 2016). Autonomic nervous system dysfunction may cause inappropriate responses. Pyrexia increases cerebral oxygen consumption and hydrogen peroxide (a free radical) production (Kuffler, 2012), may provoke fitting. Temperature should therefore be closely monitored, and antipyretic drugs (e.g. paracetamol) prescribed prophylactically, or "as required" for neuroprotection.

Therapeutic hypothermia does not affect outcome (Andrews, 2015; Atia and Abdel-Rahma, 2016), so is generally not recommended for TBI (Urbano and Oddo, 2012; Carney *et al.*, 2016), although it may be beneficial with intracranial haematoma (Atia and Abdel-Rahma, 2016).

Epilepsy

Epilepsy is common (N.I.C.E., 2012a), occurring in many patients, especially if admitted with cerebral trauma, oedema or hypoxia. Seizures may be:

- partial – involving only one hemisphere of the brain;
- generalised – involving both hemispheres, and causing loss of consciousness,

with subclassifications of each group. Generalised seizures, usually more problematic, are described in terms of motor (muscle) symptoms:

- tonic – increased muscle tone;
- clonic – increased reflex activity;
- atonic – sudden loss of tone;
- absence – no motor symptoms.

Most generalised seizures are tonic-clonic seizures (previously called *grand mal*). Absence seizures (previously *petit mal*), typically causing a blank expression, are usually idiopathic, and occur mainly in children. Status epilepticus is prolonged fitting, often defined as lasting 30 minutes, although fitting that persists beyond five minutes is unlikely to self-resolve (Meierkord *et al.*, 2010; Glauser *et al.*, 2016).

Patient safety is a priority. If at risk of falling patients may need to be repositioned. Pillows or other padding should be placed between patients and anything on which they may hurt themselves (e.g. cotsides). Tonic-clonic seizures almost invariably cause apnoea, so intubated patients should be fully ventilated and sedated. Facemask ("Ambu-bag") ventilation may be necessary if patients are not intubated. If fitting persists, sedatives (e.g. propofol or benzodiazepines,) often control seizures (Meierkord *et al.*, 2010; Oddo *et al.*, 2016). If fitting persists, antiepileptic drugs may be needed. Fits should be observed, and duration, appearance and effects recorded. Priorities of care are listed in Table 36.2.

Spinal cord injury

Spinal cord injury may be traumatic (e.g. road traffic accidents) or non-traumatic (e.g. degeneration, tumours). Recovery from spinal injury is highest if patients are treated at trauma centres (Macias *et al.*, 2009), but initial management and stabilisation in ICU may be needed. Nearly all patients with complete SCI develop respiratory complications (March, 2005). Even if not admitted with identified spinal injury, multiple trauma may have caused unidentified/unconfirmed injury, so should always be presumed present until excluded. The spinal cord forms the lowest part of the central nervous system, and so damage affects function of all systems and organs regulated by nerves below the injury. Typically, injuries to:

- cervical vertebra 1 (C1) to thoracic vertebra 1 (T1) cause tetraplegia;
- T2 to lumbar vertebra 1 (L1) cause paraplegia,

and injuries above T12 usually cause spasticity and hyperreflexia. Injury above C3 causes complete paralysis, with loss of respiratory function (March, 2005).

Spinal injury necessitates supine positioning and may require special ("spinal") beds. Controls for adjusting angles of the head or foot of the bed should be locked, if possible. If not possible, control panels should be clearly labelled to identify which controls may and may not be used (with most controls, only the vertical elevation control is safe to use).

Moving can cause further spinal injury, so spinal column alignment should be maintained. Specific instructions about positioning should be clearly visible in the bed area – for example, multiple trauma may involve the thoracic spine, necessitating maintenance of leg alignment as well. Most ICUs have guidelines for nursing and positioning patients with spinal injury. Sufficient staff should

Table 36.2 Priorities of care during fitting

- summon help
- provide safety and privacy
- maintain clear airway (e.g. remove saliva/vomit, insert artificial airway)
- give 100% oxygen (intubation and artificial ventilation if apnoeic)
- antiepileptics
- reassure family
- observing fits: duration, which parts of the body are affected, and record observations

be gathered to safely log-roll patients. Before rolling, a team leader should be identified (normally the person holding the head), readiness of all staff involved should be identified, instructions clarified, and the destined angle specified. Additional staff may be required to manage specific injuries or equipment. Cervical and upper thoracic spine injury (C1 to T4) necessitates additional stabilisation of the head with a hard collar or head immobiliser, and one additional person holding just to maintain head alignment. Position changes, usually two-hourly, should be recorded on observation charts.

Venous stasis causes high risk of thrombus formation, so thromboprophylaxis should be prescribed unless contraindicated. Risk of intracranial bleed from thromboprophylaxis is small and is usually outweighed by risks of developing DVTs (Hunningher and Smith, 2006).

Thermoregulation is impaired and labile due to:

- inappropriate cutaneous vasodilatation (hypothermia);
- inability to shiver (hypothermia);
- impaired sweating predisposes (hyperthermia).

Spinal injury care is often prolonged, benefitting from inclusion of various specialists. Neurophysiotherapists should be actively involved in care of spinal injury patients, treating and advising about mobilisation, spasticity (Burchiel and Hsu, 2001), foot drop and other complications caused by loss of peripheral nervous system control. Many patients develop severe pain and spasticity, so pain control specialists should be consulted.

Acute spinal cord injury causes bowel flaccidity, necessitating manual evacuation (Thumbikat et al., 2009). Complete lesions below T12/L1 affect bowels (Ash, 2005), causing permanent problems with elimination. For many patients, faecal incontinence is the most distressing aspect of their injury (Ash, 2005).

Autonomic dysreflexia ("hyper-reflexia")

The autonomic nervous system regulates homeostasis, including vasodilation/constriction and heart rate. Most patients with higher spinal cord injury, generally above T6, experience autonomic dysreflexia (Ahuja et al., 2017; Sharif and Hou, 2017), where underlying excessive parasympathetic-induced bradycardia and hypotension are interrupted by excessive sympathetic reflex responses, causing hypertensive crises. Symptoms include pounding headaches, profuse sweating, blurred vision, flushing of skin above lesions, with pallor below, nausea and nasal congestion.

Although usually occurring after transfer to spinal injuries units, ICU nurses may encounter it, so should be able to recognise it should it occur in ICU and be able to provide appropriate information for patients and their families.

Almost any cutaneous or visceral stimulus may trigger crises, but distended bladder or bowels are the most common causes (National Patient Safety Agency – N.P.S.A., 2004b; Sharif and Hou, 2017). Unable either to sense stimuli or move, spinal reflexes occur without normal protective responses (e.g. changing position).

Treating crises requires urgent intervention – immediately elevating the bed-head to reduce intracranial hypertension and removing possible causes (e.g. straightening creased sheets). All acute hospitals treating patients with spinal cord injury should have bowel care protocols to prevent hyper-reflexic crises (N.P.S.A., 2004b). Constipation may require manual evacuation (N.P.S.A., 2004b). Antihypertensives (e.g. hydralazine) may be used, but once sympathetic stimuli for hypertension are resolved, circulating drugs and bradycardia may cause excessive rebound hypotension.

Gentle bladder irrigation with 30 ml sterile water may be attempted (van Welzen and Carey, 2002) but blocked urinary catheters usually need to be replaced urgently.

Autonomic dysreflexia occurring during rehabilitation from spinal injury, patient and carer education become progressively important. Tetraplegia creates continuing dependency on carers for fundamental aspects of living, including movement. Pressure area care regimes are carefully staged to build skin tolerance until patients can remain in one position for prolonged periods, possibly all night, without developing sores or dysreflexic crises.

Carers should be increasingly involved in aspects of care, which they will have to perform following discharge (e.g. changing urinary catheters, performing manual evacuations). While later stages of rehabilitation are unlikely to be reached before transfer to spinal injury units, ICU nurses may initiate reha-bilitation, and should therefore supply appropriate information to patients and carers, as well as being able to recognise and treat complications of autonomic dysreflexia.

Haemorrhage

Major intracranial haemorrhage is usually caused by severe traumatic brain injury or spontaneous rupture of cerebral blood vessels, usually from aneurysms (Wilson *et al.*, 2005). Haemorrhage may be:

- subdural;
- extradural;
- subarachnoid (SAH).

Haemorrhage is ideally treated by either surgical or endovascular coiling or neurosurgical clipping (Molyneux *et al.*, 2015), necessitating transfer to neurological centres. Cerebral perfusion should be maintained, while avoiding hypertension. Gupta *et al.* (2010) recommend:

- head elevation;
- sedation;
- mannitol/hypertonic saline;
- hyperventilation;
- barbiturate coma;

Prognosis

Prognosis of major CNS pathologies is often complex, with significant mortality and often unpredictable outcome. With traumatic brain injury, memory problems persist in about one tenth of patients (Terrio *et al.*, 2009). Nearly half of survivors from subarachnoid haemorrhage suffer long-term cognitive impairment (Suarez *et al.*, 2006), and a significant minority develop major depressive disorders (Bombardier *et al.*, 2010). Many patients experience amnesia, often having no memory of events immediately before the injury (Watkins, 2000). Even with minor head injury, post-discharge CT scans show brain damage (Ling *et al.*, 2013). This may be psychologically protective but can also be psychologically distressing.

Following traumatic brain injury, sleep/wake cycles are frequently disturbed, so Ouellet *et al.* (2015) recommend cognitive-behavioural therapy and medication, although these may be initiated after ICU discharge.

Rehabilitation can be a long and often frustrating process for both patients and their relatives, so planning for rehabilitation should begin early. Once their condition has stabilised, patients may be transferred to specialist rehabilitation centres.

Epilepsy carries restrictions on driving, insurance policies and other aspects affecting quality of life. Patients and their families may therefore be fearful of the label, or its potential effects on their lifestyle.

Personality changes

In addition to general psychological stressors from critical illness and ICU admission, central nervous injury, prolonged recovery and fears about their future can affect psychological function and cause depression (Bénony *et al.*, 2002). Traumatic brain injury can cause temporary or permanent changes in behaviour due to damage; on waking, patients may exhibit:

- lack of inhibition;
- inflexible thinking;
- memory deficits;
- irritability.

(O'Neill and Carter, 1998)

Frontal lobe damage is especially likely to cause aggressiveness and loss of inhibition. Damage to other areas of the brain may cause other problems, such as dysphasia. Personality and mood changes are especially distressing for families (Powell, 2004), so family should be warned in advance about possible behavioural change. Victims of road traffic accidents or assault may be anxious about litigation or police involvement. Nurses should therefore assess psychological needs of both patients and families.

Family care

Prolonged, unpredictable and incomplete recovery exposes families to continuing distress. Families need help to enable them to cope (O'Neill and Carter, 1998). ICU staff can offer useful advice and support in the early stages. Social workers, support groups, counsellors or other social supports may be beneficial.

Family and friends often bring comfort but might cause distress. Where visitors do cause undue distress, nurses may need to intervene to enable patients to rest, but visits that provide therapeutic benefits should be encouraged. Nursing documentation and handover should identify effects of visitors on patients.

While their prime duty is to their patients, care of relatives is an important, albeit secondary, nursing role. Relatives usually appreciate being given appropriate information. They also need adequate rest themselves; they may feel obliged to stay by the bedside, exhausting both themselves and the patient, so planning care with the next of kin can prove beneficial to all. Providing somewhere to stay and access to catering facilities can greatly reduce the stress experienced by relatives.

Legal aspects

Admissions caused by road traffic accidents or other potentially criminal actions may involve the police. There are certain requirements in law for nurses to disclose information, but they are few in number and often require a court order. In the absence of any specific legal requirement, nurses should remember their duty of confidentiality to patients (N.M.C., 2015). If in doubt about whether the police or other authorities have a right to information or specimens, nurses should seek the advice of their line manager, and may need to consult their employer's legal department. Details of legal obligations can be found in Dimond (2015).

Implications for practice

- complications and death from patients admitted with central nervous system injury is usually caused by hypoxia or cerebral ischaemia, so immediate priorities are:
  - airway and breathing – artificial ventilation;
  - cardiovascular – fluid resuscitation, aiming for CPP 60 mmHg;
  - disability – neuroprotection (sedation, preventing intracranial hypertension);
- following traumatic brain injury, patients should be nursed at 15–30°, with head and neck alignment maintained, and nothing (e.g. endotracheal tapes) restricting venous drainage from their head;
- therapeutic hypothermia is not recommended;
- spinal injury patients should be nursed supine, with their spine in alignment;

■ spinal injury patients should be turned at least two-hourly. Manual patient handling should always use log-rolls, with sufficient staff to safely turn the patient and manage equipment;

■ autonomic dysreflexia occurs with most spinal cord injuries above T6, so staff should observe for hypertensive crises, know how to manage them, and appropriate bowel care protocols should be available;

■ rehabilitation is often prolonged and may remain incomplete. Patients and families often experience psychological distress, so nurses should assess both patients' and relatives' psychological needs, and refer to appropriate support agencies;

■ there are a few instances where police or other authorities have rights to access confidential information; if in doubt, nurses should seek advice before disclosing anything.

Summary

Neurological admissions may be transferred to regional specialist centres, but early ICU care is more often managed on general units, significantly affecting outcome. When specialist centres consider they cannot offer additional care, patients remain on general units. Head injury can range from mild to severe, and skilled nursing care significantly contributes to survival and recovery following head injury. Prognosis is considerably worse with spinal cord injury and subarachnoid haemorrhage. With all central nervous system pathologies, priorities remain cerebral oxygenation and perfusion. Secondary deaths are often from complications, which should be prevented if possible. Additional aspects of nursing care include supporting fundamental activities of living, co-ordinating care, and providing psychological support to patients and families.

Further reading

Guidelines for traumatic brain injury have been published by N.I.C.E. (2014b, updated 2017) and Brain Trauma Foundation (Carney *et al.*, 2016). N.I.C.E. has also published guidelines for epilepsy, although Glauser *et al.*'s (2016) US guidelines are more recent. Hickey (2014) remains the key text on neurological nursing.

Clinical scenarios

Claire Healy is 56 years old and sustained a severe head injury after falling 10 feet from an attic. She experienced loss of consciousness for an unknown length of time. Claire was admitted to ICU via A&E wearing a cervical collar with spinal immobilisation. The results from a neurological examination revealed:

GCS	7 (E: 2, V: 1, M: 4) which changed to GCS 3 (E: 1, V: 1, M: 1)
Pupil response	sluggish, equal response, size 3 mm diameter
	Cough and gag reflex present
	Blood discharging from both ears; active bleed in left ear, old dried blood in right ear

Other observations included:

Respiratory rate	29 breaths/minute
BP	150/96 mmHg (mean BP 114 mmHg)
HR	74 beats/minute
Central temperature	36.0°C
Blood sugar	10.5 mmol/litre

A head CT scan confirmed fractures of basal skull, left occipital, left and right mastoid with a small left subdural haematoma.

Q1. Which results indicate head injury? Explain underlying physiology for these.

Q2. The aim of ICU management is to anticipate, prevent and treat secondary physiological insults. Prioritise a plan of care, including neuroprotection strategies and cerebral perfusion pressure optimisation.

Q3. How are head and spinal injured patients positioned and moved in your unit? List equipment, personnel and any other resources. Does your unit/trust have guidelines for managing these patients?

Chapter 37

Peripheral neurological pathologies

Contents

Fundamental knowledge

Nerve anatomy and conduction – myelin, nodes of Ranvier

Introduction

Peripheral nervous system problems can cause many diseases but are only likely to necessitate ICU admission if respiratory muscles are affected. This chapter describes Guillain-Barré Syndrome, the most common peripheral nervous system pathology to necessitate ICU admission. But patients already in ICU can also develop peripheral nervous system problems, the most common being "ICU-acquired weakness", which too often delays rehabilitation and can contribute to longer-term morbidity. Many of the problems, and some treatments, discussed in this chapter apply to other causes of peripheral neuropathy, such as myasthenia gravis. Myasthenia gravis is a relatively rare disease, so is not specifically discussed, but effects and management are similar to Gullain-Barré Syndrome.

Nursing patients with neurological complications can be labour-intensive and stressful. Patients need care and support with many activities of living, but neuromuscular weakness also exposes them to complications. Nursing care is therefore especially valuable for patients with these conditions. Physiotherapy is beneficial for almost all critically ill patients (Schweickert *et al.*, 2009), but has an especially important role in rehabilitating patients with severe muscular weakness (I.C.S, 2015).

Management of both conditions centres on:

- attempts to remove underlying causes;
- preventing complications;
- system support.

Intensive care unit-acquired weakness

More than half of ICU patients develop weakness that appears to be a complication of their disease and/or treatments (TEAM Study Investigators, 2015). Appleton and Kinsella (2012) identify three pathologies:

- critical illness polyneuropathy (CIP);
- critical illness myopathy (CIM) – subdivided by histology into cachectic myopathy, thick filament myopathy, necrotising myopathy;
- critical illness neuromyopathy (CINM).

Although incidence varies between studies and units, outcomes are poor, with increased length of ICU and hospitals stays, increased costs, and increased mortality (Hermans and Van den Berghe, 2015) – Appleton and Kinsella (2012) suggest 45% die before discharge home, with a further 20% dying within one year.

Various causes for weakness have been suggested, but most dismissed. Among drugs implicated are muscle-paralysing agents and steroids (Annane, 2016), although, as problems have persisted despite reduced use of these drugs, it seems unlikely that the problem is primarily drug-related. There is no simple way to prevent or reverse weakness, but intensive physiotherapy and early mobilisation are helpful (N.I.C.E., 2009; Appleton and Kinsella, 2012; Herridge *et al.*, 2016).

Guillain-Barré Syndrome (GBS)

More than a century after being first described, Guillain-Barré remains the most common and most severe acute paralytic neuropathy (Willison *et al.*, 2016). This syndrome describes a group of similar pathologies which disrupt nerve conduction:

- acute inflammatory demyelinating polyneuropathy (AIDP);
- acute motor axonal neuropathy (AMAN),

and some rarer variants, such as:

- Miller Fisher syndrome.

(Willison *et al.*, 2016)

In Europe and North America AIDP is the main cause of severe GBS (Willison *et al.*, 2016). Loss of motor function ascends from peripheries, a quarter of patients developing respiratory failure (Dua and Banerjee, 2010; Willison *et al.*, 2016), the reason for ICU admission. One fifth remain severely disabled, and 5% die (Yuki and Hartung, 2012).

Chronic inflammatory demyelinating polyneuropathy (CIDP) is a similar, but longer-lasting, disease, previously called "chronic GBS". Disease is usually preceded by mild upper respiratory tract viral infections, often *Campylobacter jejuni* (Yuki and Hartung, 2012; Kuwabara and Yuki, 2013). Although vaccinations have sometimes been blamed for causing the disease, infections being vaccinated against are more likely to cause Guillain-Barré Syndrome (Kwong *et al.*, 2013).

Treatments are mainly supportive, although intravenous gamma globulin (IVIg) and plasma exchange hasten recovery (Willison *et al.*, 2016).

Muscle weakness and autonomic dysfunction can cause:

- *pain*, usually severe which can persist for months (Willison *et al.*, 2016), and is often exacerbated by touch and anxiety. Opioids are usually needed, but adjuvants, such as analgesics for neuropathic pain, are often useful. Pain contributes to depression (Kogos *et al.*, 2005).
- *respiratory failure*. If possible, non-invasive ventilation is usually attempted first, to reduce risks of ventilator-associated pneumonia, but many patients deteriorate to need intubation and invasive ventilation. Intensive chest physiotherapy may limit respiratory failure.
- *hypotension* caused by extensive peripheral vasodilatation from autonomic nervous system dysfunction (Willison *et al.*, 2016).

- *hypertensive* episodes caused by failure of normal negative feedback opposition to sympathetic stimuli.
- *dysrhythmias* (sinus tachycardia, bradycardia, asystole) frequently occur due to similar failure of neuroregulation.
- *thrombosis*. Risk of thromboembolism is high due to hypoperfusion and venous stasis from immobility, so thromboprophylaxis is a priority (Willison *et al.*, 2016).
- *limb weakness*, ascending from distal to proximal muscles, affects hands, feet or both. Passive exercises may prevent contractures and promote venous return.
- *hypersalivation* and loss of swallow from autonomic dysfunction necessitate oral care, and often suction, for comfort and to prevent aspiration.
- *bilateral facial muscle weakness* may cause causing dribbling of saliva and ophthalmoplegia, distressing both patients and relatives.
- *sweating*, from autonomic dysfunction, is often profuse, so frequent washes and changes of clothing help provide comfort.
- *incontinence* if not catheterised, from bladder muscle weakness.
- *psychological* problems from progressive and prolonged weakness. Mentally fit (often young) adults forced to rely on others to perform fundamental and intimate activities of living causes distress, compounding environmental stressors of the ICU (see Chapter 3), while fears about prognosis often cause psychoses and acute depression (Kogos *et al.*, 2005). Most develop severe fatigue (Dua and Banerjee, 2010)
- *immunocompromise* is multifactoral, aggravated by factors such as hepatic dysfunction, reduced functional residual capacity, sleep disturbance, stress responses, and depression, as well as treatments such as intubation. Infection control and preventing opportunistic infection are therefore especially important.
- *catabolism*, necessitating aggressive (and early) nutrition to limit muscle wasting.

Depression reduces motivation, needed with protracted debility. Antidepressants are often useful but should not become a substitute for active human and humane nursing (e.g. making environments as "normal" as possible). Psychological support should be extended to family and friends.

Implications for practice

- peripheral nervous failure causes many problems, including dysregulation of cardiovascular homeostasis, but respiratory failure is usually the cause of ICU admission;
- prolonged admission makes nursing care an especially important factor in recovery for these patients;
- holistic assessment enables many complications to be avoided;
- depression and sensory imbalance can easily occur; psychological care should be optimised;

■ neurological deficits impair normal homeostatic mechanisms, so nurses should avoid interventions or lack of interventions that may provoke crises;

■ providing information to patients and families can help them cope and develop any skills they may need following discharge.

Summary

This chapter has described the two most common peripheral system pathologies encountered in ICU. Recovery from both is relatively slow, in ICU terms; discharge typically takes weeks, and sometimes months. Subsequent rehabilitation is also usually slow, and too often incomplete (Willison *et al.*, 2016). For all staff, these conditions can create very real challenges, but more so than many other pathologies are largely resolved by nursing and physiotherapy rather than medical interventions.

Support group

ICUsteps 0300 3020121.

Further reading

Hickey (2014) remains the classic neurology nursing text. Useful medical articles on Guillain-Barré Syndrome include Yuki and Hartung (2012) and Willison *et al.* (2016). European guidelines for autoimmune neuromuscular disorders (Skeie *et al.*, 2010) also contain useful information.

Clinical scenarios

Donald McLean, 58 years old, presented with a 10-day history of dysphagia, progressive tachypnoea with increasing oxygen requirements, difficulty swallowing, weak cough, slurred speech, general fatigue, deep tendon reflexes absent in all limbs with numbness in both legs and tips of fingers in both hands. When examined the following results were noted:

Respiratory rate	42 breaths/minute
SpO_2	91% on 15 litres of oxygen
Vital capacity	380 ml
BP	150/100 mmHg
HR	80 beats/minute
Temperature	36.0°C

Chest X-ray reveals right middle and lower lobe pneumonia. Arterial blood gas analysis shows uncompensated respiratory acidosis with hypoxia.

In the previous month Mr McLean had flu-like symptoms and was recovering from an upper respiratory tract infection. Acute post-infective polyneuropathy or Guillain-Barré Syndrome is suspected and Mr McLean was admitted to the ICU for respiratory support.

Q1. What are the most suitable types of respiratory support for Mr McLean? Provide rationales for your suggestions.

Q2. Identify additional complications associated with polyneuropathy that Mr McLean may experience during his ICU stay. What specific nursing interventions may minimise these? What other treatments may be useful while Mr McLean is in ICU?

Q3. What resources are available locally to support Mr McLean and his family, both for short-term needs and potential longer-term problems?

Part VIII

Abdominal

Chapter 38

Acute kidney injury

Contents

Fundamental knowledge

Renal anatomy and physiology (including
   glomeruli and nephrons)
Urea + creatinine (see Chapter 21)

Introduction

Acute kidney injury (AKI) occurs in 13–18% of hospitalised patients (N.I.C.E., 2013b), usually as a result of systemic hypotension (Pallet, 2017). Incidence generally increases with acuity of illness, so it may occur in up to two thirds of ICU patients (Perazella, 2012), usually due to sepsis and hypotension (Hoste et al., 2015). Insufficient perfusion of the kidney causes both ischaemia of kidney tissue and oliguria. Ischaemia causes inflammation, which may progress to necrosis.

Oliguria causes:

- fluid retention;
- electrolytes imbalances (especially potassium);
- retention of toxins, and metabolites of drugs and hormones;
- metabolic acidosis.

This chapter describes acute kidney injury and rhabdomyolysis. Haemofiltration is discussed in Chapter 39.

Oliguria (< 0.5 ml/kg/hour) is often a sign of kidney disease, but functional failure can occur despite "normal" or "polyuric" urine volumes. Oliguria may be:

- volume-responsive AKI;
- intrinsic (intrarenal);
- postrenal

in origin.

Volume-responsive AKI

Volume-responsive AKI is caused by failure to perfuse kidneys; glomeruli and renal tubules remain undamaged. This is the most common cause of AKI (N.C.E.P.O.D., 2009). Failure to treat volume-responsive acute kidney injury with early and adequate volume almost inevitably causes intrinsic acute kidney injury.

Intrinsic AKI

Intrinsic AKI is caused by damage to glomeruli and nephrons. Damage may be caused by:

- ischaemia
- inflammation
- nephrotoxicity.

Many drugs are nephrotoxic, including ACE inhibitors, gentamicin and metformin (Nee et al., 2016). Radiocontrast dyes used for CT scans can cause nephropathy; while the risk is low (Moos *et al.*, 2014), radiographers should be made aware of any renal impairment, and short-term (e.g. overnight) elective haemofiltration may be initiated to prevent contrast nephropathy. Hyperchloraemia from chloride-rich fluids such as 0.9% saline can vasoconstrict afferent arterioles – see Chapter 33. Whereas volume-responsive AKI is immediately reversible, intrinsic AKI persists until oedema subsides and cells recover.

Pathology typically begins with hypoperfusion, which causes oxidative stress (Joannidis *et al.*, 2010; Perazella, 2012). This causes inflammation and oedema, which with expansion limited by the tough fibrous outer capsule of the kidney quickly increases intrarenal pressure, obstructing renal tubules. Prolonged perfusion failure causes oedema and potentially cell necrosis – intrarenal acute kidney injury. Release of vasoactive cytokines from failing cells provokes further intrarenal vasoconstriction.

Oliguria usually occurs within two days of precipitating events. If still at the oedematous stage, recovery may typically take a week, but if significant cell necrosis has occurred, recovery usually takes longer.

As tubular cells readily regenerate, they are initially immature, so tubular reabsorption and solute exchange remain poor, causing large volumes of poor-quality urine; serum urea and creatinine remain elevated – "polyuric renal failure". When tubule cells mature, normal function is recovered, urea and creatinine levels fall, urine volumes return to normal, and electrolyte balance is restored.

Vasculitis, a systemic autoimmune disease of unknown aetiology, can reduce glomerular filtration. It can be detected by testing for ANCA (antineutrophil cytoplasmic antibodies) (Berden *et al.*, 2012). If detected, patients would almost inevitably be referred to renal teams.

Postrenal kidney injury

Postrenal kidney injury is usually caused by mechanical obstruction to flow of urine – such as tumours, stones (calculi), strictures or enlarged prostate. Postrenal obstruction is the main cause of acute kidney injury in the community, but unlikely to occur in ICU unless already present on admission. Postrenal problems are reversed by removing the obstruction, usually needing surgery, but seldom needing ICU admission.

Monitoring renal function

There are many, but no ideal, ways to monitor function, including:

- urine volume;
- bloods – creatinine, urea, glomerular filtration rate (GFR);
- urinalysis (below).

Urea and creatinine are described in Chapter 21. Like most body systems, healthy kidneys have large physiological reserves; once serum creatinine rises,

GFR is less than half of normal (Nee *et al.*, 2016). Kidney injury typically becomes apparent once three quarters of nephrons are non-functional. End-stage chronic kidney disease occurs when GFR is < 15 and irreversible (Marieb and Hoehn, 2016), so there is a narrow margin between initial signs of AKI and potentially terminal failure. Glomerular filtration rate is estimated (eGFR) by laboratories from serum creatinine. Normal adult GFR is > 90 ml/minute/1.73 m^2 (Murphy and Robinson, 2006).

Urinalysis

While reagent-strip urinalysis has limitations, it is a simple, non-invasive test that should be undertaken at an early stage for all acute hospital admissions (N.C.E.P.O.D., 2009).

Unless identified otherwise, normal levels for all aspects listed is negative/zero.

Blood/leukocytes

Like plasma proteins, blood cells are not normally filtered by the glomerulus. Inflammatory disease may allow cells to pass into urine, or trauma to the urinary tract (e.g. stones, cancers, catheterisation) may cause bleeding. If haematuria (blood in urine) is present, protein will inevitable also be detected. Leukocytes (white blood cells) are part of the immune system and are usually only found in urine if infection is present (urinary tract infection – UTI).

Nitrite

Bacteria convert nitrate, which is normally in urine, to nitrite (Memişoğulları *et al.*, 2010; Monte-Verde and Nosanchuk, 2016), so nitrite will only be found if urine is infected. A few bacteria, such as *Enterococci* and *Streptococci*, do not convert nitrate, giving false negative readings, although these bacteria are responsible for less than one tenth of urinary tract infections (Monte-Verde and Nosanchuk, 2016).

Urobilinogen/Bilirubin

Bilirubinuria is only likely to occur if blood bilirubin levels are significantly raised. Bilirubin is a waste product of erythrocyte metabolism. Normally converted by the liver into bile which flows to the gall bladder, gall bladder disease causes bilirubin loss in urine (Wilson, 2005). Bilirubinuria usually causes urine to look dark.

Protein

Being negative charged, plasma proteins are repelled by negatively charged sialoproteins in glomerular beds, so protein is not normally filtered. Proteinuria usually indicates glomerular inflammation (Birn and Christensen, 2006; Steggall, 2007).

pH (normal: 5–6)

Renal function significantly affects metabolic acid–base balance by transferring hydrogen ions from into filtrate. Urinary pH varies according to physiological needs, but is almost always acidic, whereas blood, from which urine is made, is slightly alkaline. Provided renal function is reasonable, high pH may reflect alkalaemia, while low pH may reflect acidaemia.

Specific Gravity (normal: 1.002–1.035)

Urine is mainly water. The specific gravity of pure water is 1.0 (= low SG), so urine normally is just slightly more concentrated. High specific gravity suggests more water is being reabsorbed by the kidney, usually in response to dehydration – i.e. volume-responsive AKI. Intrinsic and postrenal failure often causes low specific gravity, as damaged renal tubules lose their ability to concentrate urine (Barratt, 2007).

Ketones

Ketones are waste products of fat metabolism (see Chapter 45). The two main reasons for this are:

- lack of insulin (diabetic ketoacidosis – see Chapter 45);
- starvation.

As well as indicating problems, ketones may form ketoacids, a cause of metabolic acidosis.

Glucose

The kidney filters blood sugar, but normally reabsorbs it all provided blood sugar is below 11 mmol/litre (Gerich, 2010). Glycosuria therefore usually indicates hyperglycaemia. Glucose has a high osmotic pressure, reducing water reabsorption, causing polyuria and dilute urine (low specific gravity). Diabetes is often initially detected from routine urinalysis. Acute illness and many drugs (especially cardiac) can cause transient hyperglycaemia.

Effects

Kidney disease disrupts homeostasis, main complications being:

Cardiovascular

- hyperkalaemia
- acidosis
- dysrhythmias.

Nervous system

- confusion ("uraemia")
- twitching
- coma.

Respiratory

- tachypnoea – compensatory respiratory alkalosis
- pulmonary oedema
- hiccough.

Gut

- nausea
- vomiting
- diarrhoea.

Metabolic

- electrolyte imbalances
- acidosis
- toxicity from active drug metabolites.

Potassium

Most potassium loss is normally from urine, so oliguria usually causes hyperkalaemia, while polyuria causes hypokalaemia (see Chapter 21).

Management

Poorly managed volume-responsive AKI usually progresses to intrinsic AKI. Kidney function can be protected by optimising perfusion with *fluids*. Once blood volume and pressure are optimised, a *fluid challenge* helps identify whether oliguria is volume-responsive (urine volume increases) or caused by intrinsic injury (no significant increase in urine). Large volumes should be infused rapidly – 500 ml over 15 minutes (N.I.C.E., 2013c).

If kidneys fail to respond to fluid challenges, then medical options are mainly *drugs* (below) and/or *continuous renal replacement therapy* (see Chapter 39). Renal replacement therapy buys time until recovery.

Diuretics

Furosemide, a loop diuretic, blocks sodium reabsorption in the ascending loop of Henle; and as water follows sodium urine output is increased. Furosemide is an effective way of treating fluid overload, but should not be given with hypovolaemia or to prevent acute kidney injury (Joannidis *et al.*, 2017). Furosemide is ototoxic (Ho and Power, 2010), so intravenous administration should be slow – 4 mg/minute. Large doses are therefore best given through a syringe driver or volumetric pump. Furosemide can cause hypokalaemia, so with large doses ECG should be monitored and serum potassium levels checked.

Rhabdomyolysis

Extensive muscle damage, such as from crush injuries, major burns, severe infection/sepsis or prolonged immobilisation, can cause rhabdomyolysis, leading to acute kidney injury. Various speculated mechanisms of kidney disease from rhabdomyolysis include:

- blockage of tubules with myoglobin precipitate;
- myoglobin-induced vasoconstriction of renal arterioles;
- oxygen-free radicals, mainly from iron-containing haem molecules, damaging renal tubules (Cooper *et al.*, 2006).

Hydrogen ion excretion into renal tubules changes ultrafiltrate from alkali to acid, creating the acid environment in which myoglobin can precipitate. As myoglobin contains iron, urine looks distinctively rusty. Rhabdomyolysis is diagnosed by clinical suspicion but confirmed by elevated serum creatine kinase (CK – see Chapter 29) (Sharp *et al.*, 2004). Some trusts can test for myoglobin.

Rhabdomyolysis is treated by fluid resuscitation to flush out myoglobin. In the past, to reduce precipitation and free radical damage the osmotic diuretic mannitol and/or alkalinisation with sodium bicarbonate infusion was advocated (Sever *et al.*, 2006), but neither is now recommended (Zimmerman and Shen, 2013). Diuretics such as furosemide may accompany aggressive fluid therapy to "flush out" precipitate. Extensive muscle cell damage may cause life-threatening hyperkalaemia (Hunter, 2002).

Implications for practice

- renal function should be determined by the ability of the kidneys to achieve and maintain homeostasis, not simply by the amount of urine produced;
- creatinine, and its derivative eGFR (estimated glomerular filtration rate), is the most useful biochemical marker of kidney function;
- factors outside the kidneys (e.g. metabolism) may affect glomerular filtration of urea, so blood urea alone is not a reliable marker;
- the most common cause of acute kidney injury in ICU patients is hypovolaemia;
- volume-responsive AKI can often be prevented by fluid resuscitation to maintain perfusion;
- most potassium is excreted in urine, so oliguria may cause hyperkalaemia, while polyuria may cause hypokalaemia;
- kidney disease limits excretion of hydrogen ions from the body, so causing metabolic acidosis;
- diuretics may restore urine volumes, and are useful for offloading excess fluid, but should be avoided with hypovolaemia.

Summary

Acute kidney injury frequently complicates other pathologies in ICU patients. While mortality from primary kidney disease is encouragingly low, mortality from multi-organ dysfunction remains depressingly high. Mortality from AKI remains unchanged at about 50% (Ympa *et al.*, 2005). So, if the incidence of progression to acute kidney injury can be reduced, mortality and morbidity among ICU patients will significantly decrease.

Kidney disease causes failure of renal function, resulting in fluid overload, electrolyte imbalances, acid–base imbalances and other metabolic disturbances; these causing further complications. Nurses therefore need knowledge of physiology and effects to optimise prevention and provide holistic care.

Further reading

Most applied physiology texts include overviews of kidney function and disease, although recent changes in practice limit the value of older texts. Thomas (2014) remains the key renal nursing text. Joannidis *et al.* (2017) provide ICU-specific guidance, while general guidance can be found in K.D.I.G.O. (2012), N.C.E.P.O.D. (2009) and N.I.C.E. (2013b). Vanmassenhove *et al.* (2017) provide a recent medical review.

Website

www.kdigo.org.

Clinical scenarios

Mr James Roger is 67 years old, has type 2 diabetes and underwent aortic valve replacement three months previously. He was found collapsed at home and was subsequently admitted to the ICU with abnormal clotting and diagnosed with sepsis secondary to endocarditis. Mr Roger had received high dose intravenous antibiotics including gentamicin, vancomycin, rifampicin, cefotaxime and had been taking oral warfarin. His last recorded weight is 74 kg.

James's U+Es include:

Urea	28.4 mmol/litre
Creatinine	255 micromol/litre
Creatine kinase	294 units/litre
Sodium	142 mmol/litre
Potassium	4.0 mmol/litre
Chloride	119 mmol/litre

Arterial blood gas results while invasively ventilated on FiO$_2$ of 0.5

pH	7.2
PaCO$_2$	7.05 kPa
PaO$_2$	9.3 kPa
SaO$_2$	96.1%
Bicarbonate	17 mmol/litre
Base excess	5.8 mmol/litre
Lactate	4.7 mmol/litre

Vital observations with a noradrenaline infusion at 0.5 mcg/kg/minute were:

Temperature	36.2°C
Heart rate	107 beats per minute
Rhythm	Atrial fibrillation
BP	76/46 mmHg
Cardiac index	2.1 litres/minute/m^2
Urine	10–20 ml/hour for the last four hours

Q1. Is Mr Roger's developing volume-responsive, intrinsic, or postrenal acute kidney injury? List results and risk factors which suggest the cause.

Q2. Compare Mr Roger's results to normal values. Which results are caused by, rather than indicate, renal impairment? Identify physiological rationales for your choice.

Q3. What effects, if any, can hypoxaemia, hypercapnia, acid–base disturbances and mechanical ventilation have on Mr Roger's sympathetic nervous system and ADH release. What actions could be taken to improve renal blood flow and renal function?

The same patient is used in scenario for Chapter 39: Haemofiltration.

Haemofiltration

Contents

Fundamental knowledge

Normal renal anatomy and physiology
Acute kidney injury (see Chapter 38)

Introduction

Acute kidney injury (AKI) is a common complication of critical illness, and about one fifth of ICU patients developing AKI need renal replacement therapy (Truche *et al.*, 2016). While renal units mainly use intermittent haemodialysis for renal replacement therapy, this is usually unsuitable for critically ill, hypotensive patients; conversely, the continued bedrest usually necessitated by haemofiltration is not problematic in the ICU but would be problematic for renal unit patients. Continuous renal replacement therapies (CRRTs) avoid aggressive reductions in blood pressure, so continuous veno-venous haemo-filtration/haemodiafiltration (CVVH/CVVHDF) is the main CRRT used in ICUs.

Filtration

In the human kidney, glomerular capillaries filter large volumes of blood (minus blood cells and plasma proteins) to form *ultrafiltrate*. This ultrafiltrate is then concentrated into urine in the renal tubule, with active movement of solutes to conserve electrolytes and micronutrients and remove waste. Haemofilters act like a large glomerulus, the filter removing large volumes of ultrafiltrate. Provided they are smaller than pore size, solutes move across semipermeable membranes to form an equal concentration on either side (*convection*). Blood flowing through nephrons, or haemofilters, has a higher pressure than ultrafiltrate, so filtered solutes (and fluid) flows on through the system, making filtration a one-way process. Solutes exert an osmotic pressure, drawing water with them ("solvent drag"). In practice, ultrafiltration (see Figure 39.1) and convection (see Figure 39.2) are inseparable. But, whereas human renal tubules actively reabsorb water, electrolytes and micronutrients, haemofilters cannot do this. So replacement fluid aims to replace water and important electrolytes.

Continuous veno-venous haemofiltration (CVVH) uses only ultrafiltration and convection. While this effectively removes volume, as solute concentration

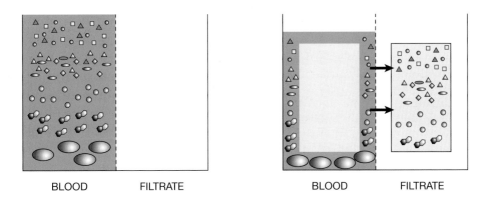

BLOOD   FILTRATE   BLOOD   FILTRATE

■ *Figure 39.1* Ultrafiltration and convection

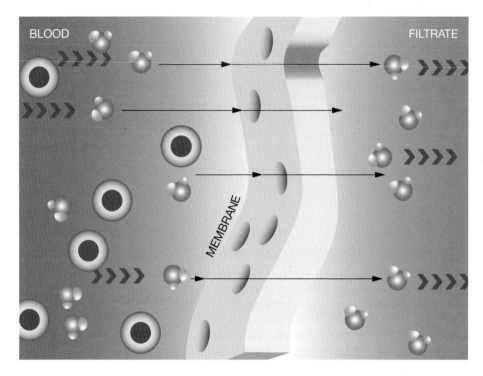

Figure 39.2 Convection

within the haemofilter increases, solute clearance is limited by the volume being removed. So CVVH is relatively inefficient in removing toxins and is rarely used now on ICUs.

Continuous veno-venous haemodiafiltration (CVVHDF) uses:

- ultrafiltration
- convection
- dialysis.

Dialysis is movement of solutes across a concentration gradient, so CVVHDF adds *dialysate*, running in an opposite direction (counter-current) to the blood. This "washes out" solutes, so increasing removal. To prevent electrolyte imbalances, dialysate fluid contains normal serum concentrations of many electrolytes (although little/no potassium).

Preparation

Haemofilters use high blood flow, so a large double-lumen cannula (e.g. Vaccath) is inserted into a large vein – usually internal jugular or femoral. Blood is drawn from one side, normally coloured red and called *afferent*, into the circuit. Blood is returned to the patient through the other lumen, normally coloured blue and called *efferent*. Early haemofilters lacked pumps, so using arterial and venous cannulae drove circuits with patients' blood pressure. Colouring, and sometimes naming ("arterial", "venous"), of lines reflects this obsolete practice.

Haemofilter pore sizes vary, but many have a similar pore size to human glomeruli – 65–70 kiloDaltons (kDa). Hollow-fibre haemofilters typically contain more than 20,000 fine capillary tubes, creating a large surface area for filtration while using small blood volumes.

Priming volumes are usually two litres to remove air emboli and potentially toxic chemicals used to protect filters during storage and transportation. Users should check local protocols and manufacturers' recommendations for priming.

Predilution, infusing volume before the filter, reduces viscosity within filters, so reducing need for anticoagulants and prolonging filter life (I.C.S., 2009b; at the time of writing, these guidelines are identified as due for review).

Anticoagulation helps reduce thrombus formation within filters, so prolonging their life. Thrombus formation is increased by slow blood flow. Signs of thrombus formation include:

- high transmembrane pressure;
- dark blood in circuits;
- kicking of lines.

Anticoagulation may be unnecessary with s prolonged clotting. Anticoagulants are below filter threshold, but some inevitably reaches patients, aggravating coagulopathies. I.C.S. (2009b) suggest avoiding anticoagulation with any of:

- INR > 2–2.5;
- APTT > 60 seconds;
- thrombocytopenia (e.g. platelet count $< 60 \times 10^9$/litre);
- high risk of bleeding;
- activated protein C.

Clotting times should be checked at least daily.

Citrate is now the preferred anticoagulant (K.D.I.G.O., 2012), although alternative anticoagulants include heparin and prostacyclin (epoprostenol; prostaglandin I_2 – PGI_2). Prostacyclin inhibits platelets, and causes vasodilation. Although much prostacyclin is removed by the filter, systemic vasodilatation does occur (Kanagasundaram, 2007).

Citrate chelates calcium, a chemical used for clotting. Infusing citrate before the filter, together with calcium after the filter to maintain systemic levels of calcium, results in lower risk of bleeding and prolonged filter life (Hetzel *et al.*, 2011, Bai *et al.*, 2015; Chowdhury *et al.*, 2017). Systemic and post-filter ionised calcium need to be frequently checked – usually one hour after commencing the filter, and every six hours thereafter. The ratio between total calcium and ionised calcium should also be checked periodically, usually daily.

Extracorporeal circulation causes convection of heat, so may cause *hypothermia*, especially if circuits hold relatively large volumes of blood. Most manufacturers produce blood warmers for circuits.

Afferent pump speed should be commenced slowly (e.g. 100 ml/minute) as some patients develop acute hypotensive crises. If stable, speeds should usually be increased within 10 minutes, usually to the full target/prescribed speed, although readers should check local protocols.

Monitoring

Filtration relies on *blood flow* through filters and *pressure gradients* across the semipermeable membrane. While blood flow (blood pump) is adjustable, pressure gradients are created by settings for blood pump speed, fluid removal, and resistance across the filter (transmembrane pressure – see below).

Blood flow is created by the blood pump speed. Because this draws blood into the circuit, it creates a negative pressure. If inadequate blood can be obtained from the cannulae, an alarm will sound. Likely reasons for blood pump alarms are:

- occluded flow from patient position, especially with femoral cannulae;
- afferent lumen against vessel wall;
- thrombus in the catheter or at the tip.

So troubleshooting solutions include:

- position – change;
- lumen against vessel wall – swap afferent and efferent connections to catheter;
- thrombus – try aspirating, but this is unlikely to succeed; flushing is not recommended, as this may create an embolus; although the catheter may be saved with urokinase, by the time this works the haemofilter will probably clot.

Ultrafiltrate rate is regulated by the ultrafiltrate pump speed setting (fluid removal). Brochard *et al.* (2010) recommend rates of 20 ml/kg/hour, as faster speeds provide no benefit, although the Intensive Care Society (I.C.S., 2009b) recommend using minimum exchanges of 35 ml/kg/hour. High-flow exchanges:

- increase costs (each treatment cycle necessitates a new circuit);
- increase workload;
- expose hypotensive patients to potentially greater haemodynamic instability.
                (Renal Replacement Therapy Investigators, 2009)

While overall mortality rates are similar, continuous modes provide better renal recovery than intermittent treatment (Bell *et al.*, 2007; VA/NIH acute kidney injury trial network, 2008; Palevsky, 2009), so intermittent treatments are not recommended, and not used by most units.

Fluid aim should be ascertained daily from medical staff. Fluid removal can be programmed hourly on most haemofilters. If aiming for a negative balance, later hypotension may limit removal, so it is wise to aim for higher initial removal. Drug volumes and other inputs should be included when calculating volume to be removed.

Transmembrane pressure (TMP – the pressure across the membrane inside the filter) gradients are created by:

- driving pressure;
- resistance;
- oncotic/osmotic pressure.

Maximum transmembrane pressure should not exceed 100 mmHg. Rising pressure usually suggests significantly decreased filtration surface area from thrombus formation and is usually an indication to discontinue filtration. High transmembrane pressure can rupture ("blow", "burst kidney") the filter, necessitating immediate cessation of filtration. Haemofilter rupture typically causes a sudden massive drop in TMP, blood may be seen in the filtrate, and usually machines will alarm and stop. If a filter ruptures, no attempt should be made to return blood ("washback"), as fragments of membrane may be washed back with blood. Machines usually measure pressure drop – the loss in pressure from the top to the bottom of the filter, so rises with clotting of fibres.

Biochemistry. Efficacy of haemofiltration is usually measured through daily bloods, such as serum creatinine levels. If circuits fail to achieve aims (removal of volume and/or solutes), they are consuming nursing time and exposing patients to needless risks.

Manufacturers' warranty usually limits circuit life to 72 hours. Although circuits have been used for longer, they are major sources for infection, most filters containing biofilm (Moore *et al.*, 2009). Exceeding manufacturers' warranty exposes users to litigation risks.

Troubleshooting

While circuit volume is usually relatively small (often < 100 ml), patients may develop transient hypotension when commencing haemofiltration, and dysrhythmias can occur, so haemodynamics should be closely observed when commencing filtration. Filters are biocompatible, to minimise cytokine release, but biocompatibility is relative rather than absolute.

Drug clearance by haemofiltration is complex, requiring advice from unit pharmacists. Increased clearance may result in under-dosing, so whenever possible drugs should be titrated to desired effects. Any substance below filter pore size may be filtered; this includes most electrolytes and micronutrients (e.g. potassium, magnesium, phosphate).

Haemofiltration limits mobility, so pressure areas should be checked carefully.

Many, but not all, patients being haemofiltered are oliguric/anuric. In addition to the underlying kidney injury that is often the cause of filtration being needed, removal of fluid is likely to stimulate antidiuretic hormone in an attempt to conserve body water. If urine is minimal or absent, it is usually wise to remove urinary catheters to reduce infection risks.

Haemofiltration machines are designed to be safe. They monitor many aspects of filtration, and have many alarms, many of which stop circuits. Problems should be resolved urgently, and if the circuit has been stopped, it should be restarted as soon as it is safe to do so, before the circuit clots.

Outcome

Haemofiltration in ICU is largely used as a means for normalising blood chemistry and/or removing fluid while underlying diseases, such as sepsis, are resolved. Duration of haemofiltration is therefore usually limited to a few days.

While acute kidney injury usually resolves, problems may persist, potentially becoming chronic, so if intrarenal pathologies are suspected, ultrasound will usually be requested, and renal physicians involved. Zarbock *et al.* (2016) argue that early initiation of filtration improves outcome from acute kidney injury, although Gaudry *et al.* (2016) found no mortality benefit between early and delayed haemofiltration.

Implications for practice

■ haemofilters resemble human nephrons, so although machines can appear daunting, follow through circuits comparing them with nephron function;

■ when checking circuits, start from the beginning of the afferent line and work through the circuit until the end of the efferent line;

■ check the circuit and equipment at the start of each shift and whenever necessary;

■ large fluid balance errors can quickly accumulate; fluid balance should be kept as simple as possible; recheck calculations and running totals;

■ the minimal optimal rate is probably 20 ml/kg/hr; a minority of guidelines recommend 35 ml/kg/hr;

■ hypotension can occur quickly, especially when commencing filtration, so haemodynamic status should be closely monitored, and blood pumps commenced at 100 ml/hr;

■ most alarms halt circuits; identify and resolve problems urgently, restarting the system before coagulation blocks the filter;

■ small substances, including electrolytes and trace elements, are removed through haemofilters, so blood levels should be checked at least daily – especially potassium, magnesium and phosphate;

■ involve unit pharmacists to identify how therapeutic drugs are affected by filtration;

■ nurses who have not used haemofiltration equipment should take every opportunity to learn how to manage it before caring for patients being haemofiltered;

■ if patients are anuric, urinary catheters should be removed.

Summary

Renal replacement in most ICUs is provided by haemofiltration/haemodiafiltration, although hospitals with renal units may use haemodialysis. Haemofiltration has proved a valuable medical adjunct to intensive care. While technology has made circuits and machines safer, haemofiltration is highly invasive, exposing patients to various complications and dangers. Kidney injury in ICU patients is usually secondary, so caring for patients receiving haemofiltration can create high nursing workloads. Care should be prioritised to ensure a safe environment. Nurses unfamiliar with using haemofiltration are encouraged to find out how to use it in practice before having to care on their own for patients receiving haemofiltration.

Further reading

Much relevant literature appears in renal journals, but I.C.S. (2009b; currently scheduled for update) provides comprehensive guidelines. Staff should familiarise themselves with handbooks for equipment used on their units. Most ICUs have local guidelines/protocols.

Clinical scenarios

Mr James Roger is 67 years old and developed acute kidney injury from sepsis secondary to endocarditis. Mr Roger had received high dose intravenous antibiotics including gentamicin, vancomycin, rifampicin, cefotaxime and had been taking oral warfarin prior to admission.

He is commenced on continuous veno-venous haemodiafiltration (CVVHDF) with 3 litre fluid exchanges. The pump speed is 250 ml/minute; venous pressure 97 mmHg and transmembrane pressure 60–70 mmHg. Mr Roger has delayed clotting (INR 3.4). Standard citrate anticoagulation is being used.

Q1. What alternatives does your unit have for CRRT? Would you recommend changing anticoagulation? If so, why, and to what?

Q2. Venous pressures increase over the first 24 hours to 250 mmHg, with transmembrane pressures of 150 mmHg. What do these changes indicate, and what (if any) actions might you take?

Q3. What nursing interventions can help maintain effectiveness and patency of CRRT? Using filters from your unit, list controls (settings), displayed monitoring and alarms. Find out the significance of each. Familiarise yourself with haemofiltration fluids used on your unit, and why and when each one is used.

Chapter 40

Gastrointestinal bleeds

Contents

Fundamental knowledge

Gastrointestinal anatomy
Hepatic portal pressure

Introduction

Gut failure is increasingly recognised as a problem in critically ill patients. It is often part of multi-organ dysfunction syndrome (see Chapter 32) but is one of the last vital organs to show symptoms. Supporting the system, such as through early enteral nutrition (see Chapter 9), may prevent complications. But the gut can also cause primary pathologies, such as GI bleeds.

Gastrointestinal bleeding is one of the commonest medical emergencies, usually causing haemorrhagic shock (N.C.E.P.O.D., 2015b). Being highly vascular, the gastrointestinal (GI) tract is prone to bleeding. Risk factors include:

- stress responses increasing gastric acid secretion;
- impaired gut perfusion;
- inflammatory responses impair vascular endothelium function, which releases most extrinsic clotting factors;
- lack of enteral feeding;
- anticoagulation therapy, especially with thrombolytic therapy for acute coronary syndrome or pulmonary embolism;
- impaired liver function – intrinsic clotting factors are produced by the liver; alcoholic liver disease poses an especially high risk,

and many other factors – for example, patients with arthritis are often prescribed non-steroidal anti-inflammatory drugs (NSAIDs), which impair clotting. Major haemorrhage may cause or complicate admission, necessitating massive transfusion together with tranexamic acid (Hunt *et al.*, 2015); readers should familiarise themselves with local major haemorrhage guidelines. While clotting is usually measured daily in most patients, and patients' history may suggest risk factors, visible signs of ulceration are only likely to be seen once bleeding occurs. While the focus of critical care is usually on other major systems, gut function and integrity should be assessed, any signs of bruising noted.

Peptic ulcers

Although most upper GI bleeds are from peptic ulcers (N.C.E.P.O.D., 2015b), these seldom necessitate ICU admission. Gastric mucosa maintains wide pH differences between gastric acid (or alkaline bile) and epithelium. While most ulcers stop bleeding spontaneously (Sung, 2010), a few necessitate endoscopic treatment, which may take place on the ICU.

Helicobacter pylori

Most gastric ulcers in people not taking NSAIDs are caused by the bacterium *Helicobacter pylori*, one of the most common chronic bacterial infections in humans (Chey *et al.*, 2017). To produce the alkaline environment they need to survive, *H. pylori* produce carbon dioxide, so breath tests are usually used to detect *H. pylori*. Like eradication, this is unlikely to be undertaken before ICU discharge.

403

Stress ulceration

Once a major complication of critical illness, incidence of stress ulceration has declined, possibly owing to increased use of enteral nutrition. Previously, ventilator care bundles included stress ulcer prophylaxis (Hellyer *et al.*, 2016). The only licensed drugs for ulcer prophylaxis in acutely ill patients are H$_2$-blockers (e.g. ranitidine, cimetidine) (N.I.C.E. 2012b updated 2016). H$_2$-blocker doses differ with oral and intravenous routes, and are usually reduced with renal impairment. Although not licensed for prophylaxis, many ICUs use PPIs. For active gastric ulcers, N.C.E.P.O.D. (2015b) recommends proton pump inhibitors (PPIs, e.g. omeprazole, lansoprazole, esomeprazole); if given for treatment rather than prophylaxis, they are usually infused continuously. Compared with H2 blockers, such as ranitidine, PPIs increase risks of GI bleeding, pneumonia, and *Clostridium difficile* infection (Buendgens *et al.*, 2014; MacLaren *et al.*, 2014), while increasing mortality (Xie *et al.*, 2017). The Intensive Care Society now recommends risk assessment for gastric bleeding, with judicious use of stress ulcer prophylaxis (Hellyer *et al.*, 2016).

Variceal bleeding

11% of upper GI bleeds are from varices (N.C.E.P.O.D., 2015b). Varices are collateral vessels, which develop to relive the portal hypertension caused by hepatic obstruction. Varices typically surround the lower oesophagus and sometimes upper parts of the stomach (Tripathi *et al.*, 2015). Rupture causes massive haemorrhage, which without urgent endoscopy is often fatal (Kapoor *et al.*, 2016).

Urgent treatment should:

- stop haemorrhage;
- restore blood volume (fluid resuscitation);
- replace clotting factors.

Haemorrhage is usually stopped by endoscopy (banding and/or injection), but emergency stabilisation may also be achieved with balloon tamponade. With critically ill patients, endoscopy is usually performed in ICU. Once haemorrhage is stopped, antihypertensives will usually be needed.

Medical treatments

Endoscopy is the first-line treatment for upper GI bleeds (N.C.E.P.O.D., 2015b). Endoscopy therapies include:

- banding
- injection (sclerotherapy).

Injection alone is not recommended (N.I.C.E., 2012b), but it is a useful optional adjunct to banding.

Vasopressin (antidiuretic hormone) and derivatives (desmopressin, terlipressin) cause splanchnic arterial vasoconstriction, so reducing portal hypertension.

Balloon tamponade (see Figure 40.1) is rarely used but offers an effective "first aid" intervention to stop bleeding when endoscopy fails. Tamponade places direct pressure on varices. Tubes are often incorrectly called "Sengstarken" tubes; Sengstarken tubes have only three lumens and have virtually been replaced by the four-lumen "Minnesota":

- oesophageal balloon (to stop bleeding);
- oesophageal aspiration port (omitted on three-port Sengstarken tubes);
- gastric balloon (to anchor tubes);
- gastric aspiration port.

While balloon tamponade usually stops bleeding, half of patients rebleed on balloon deflation (Tripathi *et al.*, 2015). Deflation should not therefore be performed by nurses.

Pressure should be sufficient to control haemorrhage; recommended pressures vary, up to 50–60 mmHg (Sung, 2014). Desired pressure should be identified and documented. External traction, which can further compress varices with the gastric balloon (Sabol and York, 2018b), should only be used on documented medical instructions. Balloon tamponade should be limited to a maximum of 24 hours (Garcia-Tsao and Bosch, 2015).

Beta-blockers (e.g. propanolol) reduce cardiac output, and constrict mesenteric arteries, so reducing portal pressure and therefore risk of bleeding (Tripathi *et al.*, 2015). They should be inserted when OGD fails to stop variceal

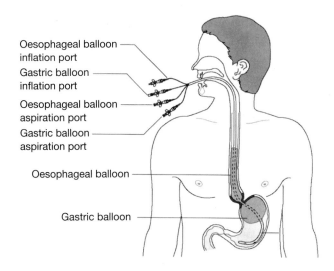

Oesophageal balloon
inflation port

Gastric balloon
inflation port

Oesophageal balloon
aspiration port

Gastric balloon
aspiration port

Oesophageal balloon

Gastric balloon

Figure 40.1 Tamponade ("Minnesota") tube

bleeding. Creating a shunt between the hepatic portal vein and the inferior vena cava bypasses the hepatic obstruction, reducing portal vein hypertension (N.C.E.P.O.D., 2015b). Shunted blood bypasses to relieve portal hypertension, but because the blood is not detoxified, encephalopathy often persists (Bercu *et al.*, 2015; Pereira *et al.*, 2015), which may compound other neurophysiological and psychological problems.

Surgical oesophageal transection or implantation of portocaval shunts, such as a transjugular intrahepatic portosystemic shunt (TIPS), reduce risk of further bleeding, but are unlikely to occur before ICU discharge and are usually undertaken in tertiary centres.

Nursing care

While nursing care largely follows from medical interventions, and many specific aspects to these interventions are included above, as with any emergency, ABCDE assessment facilitates prompt and appropriate care:

- A – is the airway patent? If not protected by an endotracheal tube or tracheostomy, patients may need to be placed in the recovery position until intubated; if a Ryles or balloon tamponade tube is in place, gastric aspiration can be performed. Is cuff pressure sufficient to prevent aspiration?
- B – has the patient aspirated? if so, ventilatory support may need increasing.
- C – monitor vital signs – especially heart rate and blood pressure. Is Hb satisfactory?
- D – if neurological state is acutely altered, reasons for this should be assessed. With vascular disease, possibilities of strokes should be considered.
- E – seeing blood or blood-stains can distress patients and/or relatives, so if reasonably possible soiled bedding should be quickly replaced, and relatives warned of the possibility of seeing blood.

Lower GI bleeds

One fifth of gastrointestinal bleeds are from the lower tract (Fearnhead, 2011), but these are rarely acutely life-threatening. Most stop spontaneously, seldom necessitating ICU admission. Many ICU patients have coagulopathies, so may bleed from the highly vascular lower GI tract.

Stools should be observed for frank blood; occult bleeding can be confirmed by testing. Observations should be recorded and reported; samples may be required for testing. Bleeding may be fresh (red; usually lower GI bleeds) or old (black, tarry; usually upper GI bleeds).

Most bleeds are small, but if large bleeds do not resolve spontaneously, early surgery (e.g. hemicolectomy) may be needed.

Implications for practice

- the gut is highly vascular, so prone to bleeding;
- all critically ill patients are at risk of gut dysfunction, and many have lesions visible on endoscopy;
- upper gastrointestinal haemorrhage can be massive and life-threatening, requiring urgent fluid resuscitation and close haemodynamic monitoring;
- with major bleeds, follow ABCDE assessment; fluid resuscitation forms a major aspect of management;
- endoscopy is the preferred treatment for major upper GI bleeds;
- balloon tamponade quickly stops bleeding from oesophageal varices, but is only a temporary measure, and removal often restarts bleeding;
- lower gut bleeds are more often insidious, and can increase morbidity, but are seldom life-threatening; the first sign of lower gut bleeds may be frank blood in stools, or melaena;
- seeing blood can make patients and families especially anxious; psychological support/care can help them cope and warn them about possibly seeing/smelling blood; if possible, remove soiled linen;
- signs of significant bleeding should be recorded and reported.

Summary

Many factors can contribute to coagulopathies and bleeds in critical illness, but major haemorrhage may also cause ICU admission. Immediately life-threatening situations necessitate urgent resuscitation, but predisposing factors may be prevented by nursing assessment and observation of risks. While lower gut bleeds are not usually life-threatening, they may be detected by melaena.

Further reading

Although not ICU-specific, N.I.C.E. (2012b updated 2016) and N.C.E.P.O.D. (2015b) provide authoritative perspectives, while Tripathi *et al.* (2015) provide national guides for variceal bleeds. Szura and Pasternak (2015) provide a medical overview of upper GI bleeds. Hunt *et al.* (2015) provide national guidelines for major haemorrhage, although readers should familiarise themselves with local policies.

Clinical scenarios

Victor Newton is a 51-year-old known alcoholic who was admitted to ICU via A&E with a three-week history of melaena, recent large-volume haematemesis that morning and severe epigastric pain. He had previous episodes of melaena and haematemesis over the Christmas holiday season and was awaiting an out-patient endoscopy appointment.

Q1. List nursing priorities when preparing for and admitting a patient with an emergency GI bleed. Include resources needed such as equipment, drugs, investigations, specialists.

An emergency endoscopy is performed which confirms three bleeding oesophageal varices that were banded. Mr Newton had a further bleed, so balloon tamponade was inserted. Current medications include intravenous omeprazole infusion at 8 mg/hour.

Q2. Identify nursing interventions following balloon tamponade tube insertion which monitor effectiveness and minimise potential complications (e.g. checking tube placement, type of traction methods, free drainage or not, sputum clearance, saliva removal, aspiration pneumonia, tissue pressure necrosis, melaena, metabolic effects of blood in lower GI tract).

Q3. The balloon tamponade tube is to be removed after 12 hours. How should this be managed to minimise risk of rebleeding?

Mr Newton's experience of haematemesis and emergency intervention have made him very anxious. Review possible causes of his ruptured varices and the risk of reoccurrence. What liver function investigations may he undergo?

Develop a plan of care for Mr Newton, focusing on reducing anxiety and risks of rebleeding in ICU, following transfer to ward and after discharge from hospital care.

Advice should include the reason for and practical strategies regarding:

- avoiding vigorous coughing and sneezing;
- recognition of early signs and symptoms of rebleeding;
- relaxation techniques;
- drug action affected by his condition and hepatic impairment, e.g. benzodiazepines, aspirin, paracetamol, some antibiotics, alcohol, cigarettes/nicotine;
- lifestyle changes;
- use of specialist nurses, referral groups.

Chapter 41

Liver failure

Contents

Fundamental knowledge

Hepatic anatomy and physiology
Liver macrophages

Introduction

The liver has more, and more diverse, functions than any other major organ, including:

■ nutrition (synthesis of plasma proteins, glucogenesis);
■ immunity;
■ heat production;
■ synthesis of homeostatic regulators (most intrinsic clotting factors, angiotensin 1);
■ detoxification (ammonia, drugs, hormones),

so hepatic failure affects most other major systems. Symptoms of liver dysfunction often appear later than respiratory, cardiac or renal dysfunction, and usually occur with co-morbidities from other systems.

Except for specialist liver centres, liver failure or poor function more often complicates than causes ICU admission. Poor liver function is relatively common in ICU, and some patients are admitted with pre-existing chronic failure. As with most systems, compensation for liver failure can maintain apparent health for a considerable time. But because it has so many functions, once decompensation occurs, many other systems are likely to be compromised. This chapter describes pathophysiologies, major complications and treatments. Main liver function tests are identified, but because liver function is so diverse, no single test exists to identify liver failure. Severe hepatic failure may necessitate transfer to specialist centres.

Acute failure

Acute liver failure is usually defined as the presence of hepatic encephalopathy in patients with no pre-existing liver failure (Donnelly *et al.*, 2016). The European Association for the Study of the Liver (E.A.S.L., 2017) adopts the 1999 classification for acute liver failure:

■ *hyperacute*: lasting less than 10 days;
■ *fulminant*: lasting 10–30 days;
■ *subacute*: lasting five to 24 weeks,

with jaundice usually being the first sign of failure. Life-threatening failure usually indicates the need for urgent liver transplantation (Bachir and Larson, 2012).

Until transfer, priorities are stabilisation:

■ Airway – intubation;
■ Breathing – invasive ventilation;

■ Cardiovascular – fluid resuscitation, optimising blood pressure and perfusion, stabilise coagulopathy with clotting factors, treat infections/sepsis, support kidneys and other vital organs;
■ Disability – treat cerebral oedema.

(summarised from Nilles and Subramanian, 2012).

Paracetamol (acetaminophen) remains the most common cause of acute liver failure in the UK and USA (Lancaster *et al.*, 2015), although because the liver detoxifies blood it is also susceptible to acute damage from many other drugs, chemicals, viruses and other factors. Although acute liver failure from other drugs is rare, most drugs that do cause acute failure are over-the-counter medicines and dietary/herbal remedies (Goldberg *et al.*, 2016), but the potency and range of drugs used in the ICU makes it likely that rises in serum transaminases after admission to the ICU are drug-related, so prescriptions should be reviewed. Recent paracetamol overdose should be treated with acetylcysteine (Parvolex) (Commission on Human Medicines, 2012; Lancaster *et al.*, 2015). Paracetamol overdose is discussed further in Chapter 46.

Chronic failure

In the UK, chronic liver disease is usually caused by:

■ alcohol;
■ non-alcoholic fatty liver disease (NAFLD)/non-alcoholic steatohepatitis (NASH);
■ hepatitis B or C (HBV, HCV);
■ primary hepatocellular carcinoma,

but can develop from acute failure, and sometimes causes are unknown. Chlordiazepoxide is useful for alcohol withdrawal.

Alcohol remains the main chemical cause of chronic liver failure (APPHG, 2014), and alcohol-related admission to ICU continues to increase (McPeake *et al.*, 2016). But not all liver failure is alcohol-related. In contrast to the UK, non-alcoholic fatty liver disease (NAFLD) is emerging as the main cause of liver failure in Western Europe, with incidence increasing (LaBrecque *et al.*, 2014; Yki-Järvinen, 2014, Than and Newsome, 2015). NAFLD is the hepatic manifestation of metabolic syndrome (see Chapter 45), with fat being deposited in liver cells (E.A.S.L., 2017). Up to one quarter of cases progress to NASH, which causes hepatitis and makes development of cirrhosis more likely (Than and Newsome, 2015). 20% to 30% of the UK population have NAFLD, and 2–3% of the population have NASH (N.I.C.E., 2016c). Hepatitis can be caused by many viruses, although in the UK the main viral causes are HBV and increasingly HCV. In the developing world, liver failure is usually viral (Bernal *et al.*, 2010).

Complications from chronic failure include:

- portal hypertension;
- oesophageal varices and bleeding (see Chapter 40);
- cirrhosis – scarring and so obstruction of channels between liver cells – "obstructive liver disease".

Cirrhosis impairs detoxification of drugs, hormones and other chemicals in blood, and so patients admitted to ICU with pre-existing cirrhosis have very poor prognoses (Weil *et al.*, 2017).

Liver function tests

Diversity of liver functions is reflected by various tests, including:

- clotting (especially INR);
- bilirubin;
- albumin; total protein;
- transaminases.

See Table 41.1.

With severe acute failure, *INR* rises rapidly, potentially exceeding 10. Clotting is discussed in Chapter 21.

Bilirubin, a waste product of erythrocyte metabolism, is normally metabolised by the liver into bile. Obstructive liver disease causing bilirubinaemia and jaundice.

Jaundice is both a symptom and a problem, often causing pruritis. Skincare and dressings should be selected to minimise irritation. If pruritis occurs, drugs such as antihistamines may be useful.

The liver metabolises dietary *proteins* into plasma proteins, so liver hypofunction contributes to low plasma protein levels. Low serum albumin contributes to hypovolaemia and oedema. Albumin levels are unlikely to significantly rise until many days after ICU discharge.

Table 41.1 Main liver function tests

Liver function tests	Normal range
Bilirubin (Bil)	< 21 mol/litre
Alkaline phosphatase (Alk Phos)	30–130 units/litre
Aspartate aminotransferase (AST)	< 40 units/litre
Alanine aminotransferase (ALT)	< 40 units/litre
Gamma glutamyl transpeptidase (GGT)	10–48 units/litre
Albumin	35–50 grams/litre
Total protein (TP)	60–80 grams/litre

Transaminases are intracellular enzymes released by damaged hepatocytes (Giannini *et al.*, 2005), just as damaged myocytes release troponin. Transaminases are also found elsewhere in the body (Agarwai and Cottam, 2009; Chen *et al.*, 2016; Sookoian *et al.*, 2016)), so two transaminases are usually measured, usually two of:

- alkaline phosphatase (Alk Phos/ALP);
- aspartate aminotransferase (AST);
- alanine aminotransferase (ALT);
- gamma glutamyl transpeptidase (GGT).

Levels do not correlate with extent of liver damage, so cannot be used to predict outcome.

Decompensation

Progressive liver failure causes failure of homeostasis, especially:

- encephalopathy;
- gross ascites;
- hypotension;
- haemorrhage (especially gastrointestinal – see Chapter 40).

The liver detoxifies many substances, including ammonia. Raised serum ammonia and other toxins cross the blood–brain barrier, exerting an osmotic pull which causes cerebral oedema and hepatic *encephalopathy*, as well as generating oxygen radicals (Suraweera *et al.*, 2016). Cerebral oedema can cause neurological symptoms such as irritability, reversed sleeping patterns, and fitting. Severe hepatic encephalopathy can be rapidly fatal, necessitating urgent hepatic transplant (E.A.S.L., 2017). Even mild neurological symptoms are often distressing for relatives. Serum ammonia can be measured, but check requirements with your laboratory before taking samples.

Cerebral oedema may be prevented or reduced by keeping the head aligned (to facilitate venous drainage), nursing patients at a 30° angle (E.A.S.L., 2017), treating underling infections, and reducing gut bacterial production of ammonia with lactulose (Nilles and Subramanian, 2012) or non-absorbable antibiotics (Patton *et al.*, 2012). Gluud *et al.*'s (2016) Cochrane review found no evidence of either treatment being preferable. Cerebral oedema is discussed in Chapter 36. Psychological care should include:

- frequent, simple explanations;
- calm, low voice;
- avoiding/minimising conflict;
- supporting relatives.

Ascites compresses the liver, lungs and other major organs, as well as contributing to hypovolaemia. Large ascetic collections are drained (paracentesis), with 20% albumin being infused to reverse the osmotic pull of any remaining protein-rich ascites. Intra-abdominal pressure measurement (see below) is useful to prevent liver damage from mechanical compression. Heart rate and cardiac output may increase, but hypovolaemia causes *hypotension*, mainly due to:

■ vasodilatation and increased capillary permeability (inflammatory responses);
■ hypoalbuminaemia;
■ bleeding – most intrinsic clotting factors are produced in the liver.

Angiotensinogen, the precursor of angiotensin (see Chapter 31), is produced in the liver, so hepatic failure causes failure of the renin–angiotensin–aldosterone mechanism, contributing to vasodilatation.

Prolonged hypotension results in tissue hypoxia, anaerobic metabolism, widespread cell dysfunction and death, and eventually multi-organ dysfunction. Hypotension should therefore be treated with aggressive fluid resuscitation.

The liver synthesises most clotting factors, so bleeding may be an early symptom of acute hepatic failure. ICU nurses should therefore minimise trauma and observe for bleeding during invasive interventions such as endotracheal suction. Oozing around cannulae, or healing of sites after removal, may also cause problems. Cannulae, especially arterial, should remain visible whenever possible.

The liver contributes significantly to immunity through:

■ producing complements;
■ liver macrophages.

Liver dysfunction therefore causes *immunocompromise*. Most patients with liver failure develop infection (Bachir and Larson, 2012), often progressing to sepsis (O'Brien *et al.*, 2007; Forrest, 2009).

Acute *kidney injury* usually occurs with acute liver failure (Tujios *et al.*, 2015), often from hypotension, so should be prevented by optimising perfusion with fluid management.

The liver has over 500 metabolic functions, so failure causes complex disorders, including:

■ *electrolytes*, including low potassium, magnesium, phiosphate and calcium;
■ metabolic *acidosis* – the liver is the main site for bicarbonate synthesis;
■ *hypoglycaemia* (Rylah and Vercueil, 2010) due to depleted glycogen stores and elevated circulating insulin.

The liver is a major digestive organ, so liver failure often causes various deficits and complications. Enteral *nutrition* is recommended, although may be to be commenced to low rates (Blaser *et al.*, 2017).

Intra-abdominal pressure

Pressure in the abdomen affects perfusion and function of abdominal and other organs, including lungs, liver, kidneys and gut. Normal intra-abdominal pressure (IAP) is 5–7 mmHg. although it will be increased by positive pressure ventilation (Ashraf *et al.*, 2008), PEEP and obesity (De Keulenaer *et al.*, 2009). While pressure below 15 mmHg rarely causes problems, pressures of 16 or above cause gut ischaemia and necrosis (Kaussen *et al.*, 2012). Intra-abdominal hypertension, defined as ≥ 12 mmHg (Maddison *et al.*, 2016), significantly increases risk of organ failure, and abdominal compartment syndrome (≥ 25 mmHg) with new organ failure is usually fatal, necessitating surgery (Berry and Fletcher, 2012; Kirkpatrick *et al.*, 2013). Intra-abdominal hypertension occurs in up to 40% of ICU patients (Maddison *et al.*, 2016).

Any interventions that can reduce intra-abdominal hypertension, such as paracentesis, should be initiated. Gross hypertension and abdominal compartment syndrome may necessitate decompressive laparotomy – "open abdomen" – covered by a dressing, but the incision remaining open until underlying hypertension has resolved.

Various devices are marketed to measure intra-abdominal pressure, but bladder devices as part of urinary catheter systems, are used most (De Keulenaer *et al.*, 2009). Ideally, measurement should be taken supine – angles of 30° increase IAP by 4 mmHg, while 45° increases IAP by 9 mmHg (De Keulenaer *et al.*, 2009), although Shuster *et al.* (2010) recommend measuring at 30°.

Artificial livers

Extracorporeal liver support devices (ELSD), such as the molecular adsorbent recirculating system (MARS) and bioartificial livers (BAL), enable people with end-stage chronic liver to survive until transplantation (Rylah and Vercueil, 2010), although their use is almost solely confined to specialist centres. Technology will doubtless advance further, perhaps to permanently implantable devices.

Prognosis

Liver dysfunction is common in ICU patients, but if liver failure develops it is often at a late stage of multi-organ dysfunction syndrome. Outcome of liver failure in ICU patients is often poor, although not hopeless. As with other systems, reversible causes should normally be treated, but families should be made aware of poor prognosis, and multidisciplinary discussions about treatment limitations are often appropriate.

Implications for practice

■ most ICU patients suffer hepatic dysfunction, usually due to hypoperfusion; nurses should actively assess liver function (e.g. clotting, consciousness), documenting their observations;

■ assess neurological state. Deterioration may indicate encephalopathy;

■ gross ascites should be drained;

■ intravenous volume should be optimised;

■ if clotting is prolonged, reassess traumatic aspects of nursing care (e.g. shaving, mouthcare); vitamin K and/or folic acid supplements may be needed;

■ hepatic dysfunction impairs immunity, so infection control is essential to maintain a safe environment;

■ monitor blood sugars frequently and maintain normoglycaemia;

■ electrolytes should be monitored and supplements given – potassium, magnesium and phosphate imbalances often occur;

■ nutrition facilitates recovery;

■ intra-abdominal pressure measurement facilitates early identification of, and treatment for, hepatic compromise;

■ patients are often forgetful, confused and agitated, needing simple and frequently repeated explanations. Conflict should be avoided. Relatives should be reassured that altered personality is caused by the disease, and that patience is needed.

Summary

The liver can be the forgotten vital organ in ICU; other than transplantation centres, few units specialise in hepatic failure, but poor function complicates most pathologies seen in ICU. Liver dysfunction affects many other organs and systems. Once liver failure becomes apparent, prognosis is poor. Extracorporeal liver devices are currently largely confined to specialist liver centres.

Further reading

A number of journals specialise in hepatic and gastrointestinal medicine, such as *Gut*, but articles of use for ICU nurses are more likely to be found in general medical journals, such as McPeake *et al.* (2016). N.I.C.E. (2016c) provides guidance for NAFLD. The European Association for the Study of the Liver (E.A.S.L.) has a useful website with many guidelines, the 2017 acute liver failure guidelines being most relevant for the ICU.

Website

European Association for the Study of the Liver: www.easl.eu.

Clinical scenarios

Julia Smith is 60 years old with a past medical history of alcoholic liver disease. She remains alcohol dependant. She was admitted to ICU with respiratory failure secondary to with gross ascites, bacterial peritonitis and thrombocytopenia. Paracentesis initially removed four litres, three more litres draining subsequently.

Insulin is infused at 10 units/hour; blood glucose is now 8.3 mmol/litre. Blood results include:

INR	2.9
Hb (grams/litre)	9.5
Platelets (10^9/litre)	35
WCC (10^9/litre)	30.6
Neutrophils (10^9/litre)	29.7
Lymphocytes (10^9/litre)	0.5
Monocytes (10^9/litre)	0.5
Urea (mmol/litre)	22.3
Bilirubin (micromol/litre)	223
ALT (units/litre)	34
Alkaline phosphatase (units/litre)	89
Albumin (grams/litre)	28

Arterial blood gas results while mechanically ventilated on FiO_2 of 0.5:

pH	7.25
$PaCO_2$ (kPa)	5.8
(kPa)	12.2
SaO_2 (%)	94.8
Lactate (mmol/litre)	4.9

Q1. What is the significance of Julia's blood results in relation to her liver function and liver damage?

Q2. Four bottles of 100 ml 20% albumin are prescribed to replace ascetic loss. How else might Julia's low albumin level be treated?

Q3. What other treatment strategies may she require? Is she a candidate for transplantation? Include rationales.

Chapter 42

Obstetric admissions to ICU

Contents

Fundamental knowledge

Normal pregnancy, including normal physiological changes

Introduction

Most deliveries are "normal", ICU admission only being needed in 2% of cases in the UK, although incidence is higher elsewhere (Price *et al.*, 2009). Numbers of older mothers, and rates of complications, are increasing (D.O.H., 2010a), resulting in potentially increasing ICU admissions. Overall UK maternal mortality is extremely low, and continuing to fall (9.02 per 100,000 maternities (Knight *et al.*, 2015)), but obstetric patients can be among the sickest in the ICU. This, together with limited literature in ICU texts and journals, and few ICU staff being qualified midwives, can provoke special anxieties among staff. This chapter cites statistics from, and describes care in, First World countries, primarily the UK. For readers elsewhere, priorities and problems may differ significantly.

Antenatal emergencies usually necessitate early delivery or termination of pregnancy, rarely needing ICU admission. Any antenatal ICU admissions are more likely to occur for non-obstetric reasons, such as road traffic accident. Specific obstetric care, if any, depends on foetal age and condition. Antenatal care should optimise conditions for both mother and foetus. Foetal mortality may occur in addition to, or independently of, maternal mortality.

ICU obstetric admissions are usually postnatal and may be for obstetric or non-obstetric reasons. Obstetric reasons are usually:

- hypertensive disorders of pregnancy (e.g. pre-eclampsia, HELLP) and
- postpartum haemorrhage.

Non-obstetric reasons may be for ARDS, sepsis, or other pathologies likely to be familiar to ICU staff. The obstetric population is getting older (McCall *et al.*, 2017), resulting in increased co-morbidities and chronic conditions (Hinton *et al.*, 2015). Many critically ill obstetric patients have co-morbidities, including obesity and mental health problems (Knight *et al.*, 2015).

Medical/nursing care centres on complications, medical treatments supporting failing systems (e.g. mechanical ventilation) and the human care familiar to ICU staff. For example, sepsis, usually from pneumonia, is the most common direct cause of UK maternal deaths (Acosta *et al.*, 2016) and would be managed in the same way as sepsis in other patients (see Chapter 32), so is not discussed further in this chapter. ICU nurses do not need midwifery expertise to care for these pathologies, but midwives should actively be involved in multidisciplinary teams, to provide both psychological reassurance and practical care, such as expressing breast milk, assessing and monitoring uterine contraction, monitoring vaginal discharge, and checking need for anti-rhesus D injections. Midwives also provide valuable links between mother and child while the mother is in ICU.

Normal pregnancy

Normal physiological changes during pregnancy favour foetal growth but place stress on the mother's body, altering many "normal" biochemical/haematological values from nonpregnant levels.

From the first *trimester* (weeks one to 12) the *cardiovascular* system becomes hyperdynamic, with blood volume increasing by about half in healthy mothers (Crozier, 2017). From about 20 weeks' gestational age, aortocaval compression reduces cardiac output by 30–40%, so mothers should not be nursed supine as this may cause hypotension (Maternal Critical Care Working Group, 2011) and so foetal distress. If cardiac reserve is limited, increased cardiac work may precipitate cardiac failure. Increase in erythrocyte numbers does not match increase in blood volume, so causes dilutional *anaemia*, which improves capillary flow.

Onset of labour accelerates *cardiovascular* changes. Cardiac output is variable, but in health increases by up to 50% (Hegewald and Crapo, 2011). Overall, blood pressure normally falls during pregnancy, mainly due to vasodilatation (Valdiviezo *et al.*, 2012). Second-stage labour (contractions and delivery) creates a Valsalva effect, reducing both venous return and cardiac output. For young, healthy hearts, changes should not be problematic, but with pre-existing heart disease these changes could precipitate crises. Uterine contraction during the third stage of labour (delivery of placenta) returns 300–400 ml of blood to systemic circulation, potentially precipitating hypertensive crises.

Maternal hearts are usually robust enough to cope with demands of pregnancy, but cardiac death remains the single main cause of UK indirect maternal deaths (Knight *et al.*, 2015).

Respiratory changes occur for many reasons. Diaphragmatic splinting by the uterus and increased maternal oxygen demand increase risks of maternal hypoxia (Maternal Critical Care Working Group, 2011), so tidal volume typically increases about 10%, and respiratory rate by 15% (Hegewald and Crapo, 2011), increasing PaO_2 and decreasing $PaCO_2$. Renal function normally compensates for respiratory alkalosis to maintain normal pH. Munnur *et al.* (2011) suggest the main cause of obstetric deaths in ICU is ARDS.

Reduced colloid osmotic pressure (dilution), hypertension and vasoconstriction encourage *oedema* formation, including:

- pulmonary oedema (impairing gas exchange);
- airway oedema (obstructing airways);
- cerebral oedema (increasing intracranial pressure).

Airway oedema limits airflow, and complicates intubation (Maternal Critical Care Working Group, 2011), necessitating smaller endotracheal tubes, which increase airway resistance and pressures.

Neurological changes are not normally seen, but cerebral oedema and hypoxia can cause fitting from eclampsia (see below).

Gastrointestinal motility is reduced, contributing to nausea/vomiting, malnutrition and potential acid aspiration ("Mendelsohn's syndrome"). *Liver* disease rarely occurs during pregnancy unless there are pre-existing problems, but impaired function predisposes to immunocompromise, jaundice, coagulopathies, encephalopathy and other neurological complications.

Gestational hyperglycaemia/diabetes is mainly caused by reduced insulin sensitivity, which favours foetal glucose supply (Valdiviezo *et al.*, 2012), but may necessitate insulin supplements during obstetric crises.

Renal changes together with mechanical compression increase risk of urinary tract infection and renal stone formation (Bothamley and Boyle, 2017), which may complicate, but not cause, ICU admission. Acute kidney injury is a relatively common complication (Siribamrungwong and Chinudomwong, 2016).

Impaired *immunity* during the third trimester prevents foetal rejection but increases risk of viral infections.

Obstetric emergencies

While causes of crises may be obstetric in origin, intensive care management focuses largely on systems and problems discussed elsewhere in this book. If antenatal, urgent delivery is paramount, after which the mother is usually transferred to ICU (Robson *et al.*, 2014). Postnatal priorities are usually:

- airway – intubation;
- breathing – mechanical ventilation for respiratory failure/ARDS;
- cardiovascular resuscitation – treating sepsis, fluid resuscitation, haemostasis, normalising electrolytes, haemofiltration for AKI;
- disability – resolving hyperglycaemia and treating any other neurological complications (e.g. hepatic encephalopathy).

(adapted from Liu *et al.*, 2017)

As with all critically ill patients, monitoring and close observation are an essential element of care. Although effects are similar to non-obstetric causes, obstetric pathophysiologies may be less familiar to ICU nurses, so discussion below outlines diseases, specific treatments, and some other pregnancy-related issues.

Hypertensive disorders of pregnancy

Hypertension occurs in 10–15% of pregnancies (Nelson-Piercy, 2015). This can cause various hypertensive disorders.

Pre-eclampsia, probably the most common problem, is hypertension developing after 20 weeks' gestation, together with one or more of new-onset:

- proteinuria;
- other maternal organ dysfunction;
- uteroplacental dysfunction (cell growth restriction).

(Tranquilli *et al.*, 2014).

Pregnancy predisposes to oedema formation, and pulmonary oedema is the main cause of death from pre-eclampsia (Dennis, 2012). Hypertension is usually controlled with hydralazine, reducing diastolic blood pressure by 10–20 mmHg every hour, to reduce maternal and foetal complications (Dennis, 2012), although N.I.C.E. (2010f) also lists labetalol and nifedipine.

Eclampsia is convulsions occurring in a woman with pre-eclampsia (N.I.C.E., 2010f), although eclampsia is not always distinguished from pre-eclampsia – 2013 American College of Gynaecologists definitions of hypertensive disorders of pregnancy list four conditions, including pre-eclampsia, but not eclampsia. Delivery is essential to resolve eclampsia (Dennis, 2012), usually necessitating caesarean section or termination of pregnancy. Fitting should be controlled with magnesium (Dennis, 2012; Robson *et al.*, 2014). Postpartum, there is a risk of stroke (Dennis, 2012). If the mother plans to breastfeed, effects of drugs to the baby should be considered (Dennis, 2012).

Acute fatty liver is a rare condition that is usually life-threatening, necessitating intensive care admission (Liu *et al.*, 2017). Liver failure may cause hepatic encephalopathy (Liu *et al.*, 2017) – see Chapter 41. If liver failure does not resolve, transplantation may be needed (Liu *et al.*, 2017).

HELLP syndrome:

- *Haemolysis*;
- Elevated *Liver* enzymes; and
- Low *Platelets*.

(N.I.C.E., 2010f)

This syndrome causes severe hypertension, coagulopathies and grossly disordered liver function.

Early symptoms are often vague and, so HELLP may become life-threatening before it is diagnosed. Complications include cause:

- disseminated intravascular coagulation;
- abruptia placentae;
- acute kidney injury;
- and other life-threatening problems (Steegers *et al.*, 2010) necessitating ICU admission. HELPP often occurs with pre-eclampsia, so magnesium should be given.

Treatments include urgent delivery of the foetus (induction, caesarean section) (Kulungowski *et al.*, 2009), system support (e.g. mechanical ventilation), and giving clotting factors. The value of steroids is unclear (Dennis, 2012), but N.I.C.E. (2010f) warns against their use.

Haemorrhage

Placental separation leaves a wound of about 300 cm^2 and about 100 severed arteries (McNabb, 2017). Major haemorrhage can therefore easily occur.

To counteract this, third-stage labour normally induces arterial vasoconstriction, with development of a fibrin mesh over the placental site. Incomplete contraction therefore causes major haemorrhage. Bleeding can also occur from genital tract lacerations and coagulopathies. Disseminated intravascular coagulation (DIC – see Chapter 26) may be triggered by pregnancy or its complications.

Postpartum haemorrhage volume is often underestimated (e.g. from loss on sheets) (Mavrides *et al.*, 2016). Prophylactic oxytocics should already have been routinely given (Mavrides *et al.*, 2016), but it is worth checking they have not been forgotten. With haemorrhage, tranexamic acid should be urgently given (WOMAN Trial Collaborators, 2017) and volume replaced.

Thromboembolism

Delivery induces a *pro-coagulant* state, increasing thromboembolism risks (McNabb, 2017). Thromboembolism remains the single main direct cause of obstetric deaths, usually from pulmonary emboli (Knight *et al.*, 2015). Antenatally, oral anticoagulants are contraindicated because they cross the placenta and may cause placental/foetal haemorrhage. All patients should be assessed for thromboprophylaxis (Knight *et al.*, 2015).

Amniotic fluid embolus

This rare condition, sometimes called "anaphylactoid syndrome of pregnancy", is caused by foetal material entering the maternal circulation, where it triggers a gross inflammatory response (Pacheco *et al.*, 2016) – anaphylaxis. Amniotic fluid embolus usually causes:

- respiratory failure;
- shock;
- disseminated intravascular coagulation;
- fitting,

(Sultan *et al.*, 2016)

and may cause cardiac arrest (Pacheco *et al.*, 2016). Treatment therefore focuses on resuscitation:

- intubation and artificial ventilation;
- fluid resuscitation;
- clotting factors; massive transfusion protocols are likely to be activated (Sultan *et al.*, 2016);
- controlling fitting.

If antenatal, the foetus should be urgently delivered (Pacheco *et al.*, 2016). ICU admission is usually postnatal.

Drugs and pregnancy

Additional considerations when giving drugs during pregnancy include:

- antenatal: will they cross the placenta?
- postnatal: are they expressed in breast milk (if breastfeeding)?
- foetal/newborn drug clearance.

Being professionally accountable for each drug given, nurses should withhold drugs and seek advice from their pharmacist if unsure of likely effects. Pharmacists should actively be involved in multidisciplinary teams.

Psychology

Post-traumatic stress disorder frequently occurs in most patients discharged from the ICU, but there can be additional psychological stressors during maternity (Crozier, 2017). Most babies are wanted, so obstetric emergencies can be especially devastating. Miscarriages may create guilt. Other children, usually young, may experience various emotional traumas. Psychological support and care for the mother, partner and family is therefore especially important. Support may be gained from family and friends, chaplains, counselling services, or various support groups.

Bereavement is traumatic, but photographs can become treasured mementoes, which parents may not think to ask for, or take, at the time.

Obstetric emergencies can be psychologically traumatic for staff, most nurses being female, often of similar ages, and possibly planning or raising families of their own.

Prognosis

Most pregnancies are relatively uncomplicated, not requiring critical care. For those needing ICU admission, the robustness of maternal bodies means that most should survive the crisis. Complications occurring during pregnancy, such as cardiovascular disease or gestational diabetes, often indicate increased risks of similar problems in later life (Mol *et al.*, 2016). Health promotion advice should therefore be offered before hospital discharge.

Implications for practice

- ICU admission usually aims to provide respiratory and/or cardiovascular support, so care should follow from problems necessitating admission;
- do not nurse supine; aortocaval compression occludes circulation;
- complications such as hypertension and fitting should be controlled;
- electrolyte imbalances and coagulopathies commonly occur;
- pregnancy causes immunocompromise, so minimise infection risks;

- after the hopes of pregnancy, critical illness can cause devastating stress to patients, partners and family, so psychological needs should be assessed and support provided;
- midwives are valuable members of the team, providing specialist care and advice;
- antenatally, the mother's body should provide an optimal environment for foetal development;
- postnatal obstetric observations should include vaginal examination (amount and type of discharge) and uterine contraction;
- mothers wishing, but currently unable, to breastfeed should be offered opportunities to express breast milk (breast pump); this also relieves breast pain;
- bereavement counselling and care may be needed.

Summary

Pregnancy is a normal physiological function, and most pregnancies occur without serious complications, but life-threatening complications can and do occur, sometimes necessitating ICU admission, usually for cardiovascular or respiratory failure. Antenatal admissions should consider foetal health, but most admissions are postnatal; the precipitating cause (foetus/placenta) having been delivered, system support may be all that is required until homeostasis is restored, although some problems require more aggressive treatments. Interventions used will be familiar to most ICU nurses, but terminology and pathophysiology may differ.

Support groups

- Pre-Eclamptic Toxaemia Society (PETS) 07974 563849;
- Miscarriage Association: 01924 200799;
- Stillbirth and Neonatal Death Society (SANDS): 0808–164–3332; helpline@ sands.org.uk.

Further reading

Triennial reports of maternal mortality provide valuable information and advice; this chapter cites Knight *et al.* (2015), but a report should be published in 2018. The Royal College of Obstetricians and Gynaecologists publishes "Green Top Guidelines" on many topics, which can be downloaded from its website. The two classic midwifery textbooks are *Mayes* (Macdonald and Johnson, 2017) and *Myles* (Marshall and Raynor, 2014). There are a number of midwifery journals, which rarely contain articles of critical illness; critical care nursing journals occasionally contain articles on obstetrics. Articles such as Munnur *et al.* (2011) and Crozier (2017) provides useful systems-based overviews of obstetric admissions to ICU.

Clinical scenarios

Susan Jackson, a 27-year-old primigravida with recently diagnosed pre-eclampsia, is admitted to the ICU following emergency caesarean delivery at 34 weeks' gestation. Susan was progressively hypertensive, oedematous with proteinuria, experienced visual disturbances and epigastric pain. Ms Jackson is mechanically ventilated with intravenous infusions of magnesium and hydralazine. Her temperature is 35.3°C; she has sinus tachycardia of 125 beats/minute; BP is 160/110 mmHg. She is passing about 20 ml/hour urine (pre-pregnant weight was 76 kg), her serum albumin is 24 grams/litre.

Q1. Explain potential causes of Ms Jackson's oliguria including the significance of her proteinuria and hypoalbuminaemia. How should her fluid balance and AKI be managed? Include rationales.

Q2. What other investigations would help identify potential complications of pre-eclampsia? How might you identify whether she develops HELLP?

Q3. What contributions might be useful from other members of the multidisciplinary team? What can midwives offer Ms Jackson, and the team, while she is in the ICU?

Chapter 43

Organ donation

Contents

Fundamental knowledge

Brainstem and cranial nerve function
Immune response

Introduction

Organ transplantation is a treatment for end-stage organ failure, so is potentially life-saving. Despite some recent increases in donation, significant numbers of people continue to die on waiting lists, and numbers of people needing transplants in the UK continue to rise (Mallik *et al.*, 2012). The D.O.H. (2008) report prompted placement of a senior nurse organ donation (SNOD) and clinical lead organ donation (CLOD) in each UK trust to increase donation rates by 50%. Although the target was achieved (N.H.S.B.T., 2013), UK rates continue to lag behind much of Europe (B.M.A., 2012).

Some readers may work in trusts where organs are transplanted; while this chapter briefly includes post-operative care, all ICU patients are potential donors, and possibilities should be explored when any patient dies. Organ donors may also be tissue donors; tissue donation is discussed in Woodrow (2016).

Brainstem death

Limited supply of cadaver organs has encouraged use of live donors (Ikegamin *et al.*, 2008). Living donation rates are increasing (B.M.A., 2012), but this is confined to specialist centres rather than general ICUs.

Otherwise, for organ donation to occur the patient must be dead, without organs having suffered significant ischaemic time. In the UK there are therefore two possible classifications for post-mortem donors:

- brainstem death (BSD);
- donation after circulatory death (DCD – previously called "non-heart-beating" and "donation after cardiac death").

The brainstem contains the vital centres that enable life (respiratory, cardiac, hypothalamus, pituitary gland), so if the brainstem is dead the person cannot survive. Any medical conditions that could prevent brainstem function must be excluded before testing for brainstem death. UK guidance for brainstem death tests is available at https://ficm.ac.uk/sites/default/files/Form%20for%20the%20Diagnosis%20of%20Death%20using%20Neurological%20Criteria%20-%20Full%20Version%20%282014%29.pdf.

Reflexes and responses of each cranial nerves are then tested (individually or in combination). If higher centre responses are absent, brainstem death may be diagnosed. The legal time of death is the first test, although death is not pronounced until confirmed by the second test. Any response from higher centres, however abnormal or limited, prohibits brainstem death diagnosis. Some basal functions may persist (Nair-Collins *et al.*, 2016), and spinal reflex responses ("Lazarus" sign) may appear (Kumar, 2016); although not significant, these may be misinterpreted by relatives or other witnesses as signs of life, so causing anxiety.

Tests should be carried out by two doctors, both of whom have been qualified more than five years and at least one of whom is a consultant (Gardiner and

Manara, 2014), usually the patient's own. Neither doctor making the test should be a member of the transplant team.

If brainstem death cannot be diagnosed, DCD can occur. In theatre, supporting treatments are withdrawn, followed by a "stand-off" time, usually at least five minutes (Algahim and Love, 2015). Provided death occurs, organs may then be retrieved.

The *Human Tissues Act* (1961) established that after death the body becomes the property of the next of kin, giving next of kin the right to refuse donation. Technically, the *Human Tissue Bill* (2004) makes patients' wishes paramount, although patients' wishes continue to be over-ridden by relatives' refusal (B.M.A., 2012). Although next of kin are encouraged to reflect on what the person's wishes were, most people in the UK have not discussed their wishes regarding donation with their family (Webb *et al.*, 2015).

Nursing care

All patients whose life-supporting care is withdrawn should be considered as potential donors. Exclusion criteria for donation are frequently modified, but broadly exclude:

- any disease which may be transplanted;
- any factors that make organs unlikely to be viable.

Each trust should have a SNOD, who may be available to advise likely organs and/or tissues that might be retrieved and can offer advice and information to staff and patients' families. There is always a SNOD on call for the region – check your local number. The NHS Organ Donor Register enables people to record their willingness to be organ donors and can be accessed by NHS staff to check whether patients are on the register. While the majority of the UK population approve of donation, only a (growing) minority are on the register (B.M.A., 2012), or carry cards. So, while being on the donor register indicates patients' wishes, absence from the register should not be interpreted as not wishing to donate.

Donation is co-ordinated nationally by NHS Blood and Transfusion (N.H.S.B.T.). Staff making referrals will need:

- name, date of birth, address, hospital number;
- patient GP details;
- next of kin details, including a contact number;
- brief medical history, including any recent infection, trauma and medication;
- height and weight of patient;
- results of recent blood samples.

Caring for donors and their families can be psychologically stressful. Nurses will usually be involved in discussions with families. Typically, a senior doctor breaks the bad news. If the doctor does not suggest donation, and the patient potentially might be a donor, nurses should raise the possibility. If the next of kin agrees to donation, a SNOD then describes the process, and obtain consent. This is designed to ensure next of kin are informed about the process and anticipated outcome, while risk factors that might make organs or tissues unsuitable are identified. Detailed, often probing, questions at a time of distress and mourning can be difficult but are outweighed by the potentially greater distress of not being given the choice. Nurses will usually accompany the SNOD, both as a witness and to support relatives if needed.

Unlike other terminal care, where death is followed by last offices, diagnosis of brainstem death is followed by optimising organ function for retrieval. This focus on supporting organs for others may seem in conflict with nursing values, where actions should be in patients' best interests, but facilitating patients' wishes to donate *is* in their best interests.

Once transferred to theatre, the SNOD co-ordinates nursing care, including last offices. Death having already been diagnosed, the body is then transferred to the mortuary. If possible, in the UK available donor organs are matched and allocated to UK patients; where this is not possible, they are offered to other European organ sharing organisations. Family, and staff involved in donation, are thanked in writing by the SNOD and informed of how organs are used.

Ethical issues

Transplantation has always maintained a high public profile, ensuring wide-spread discussion of ethical issues. Organ donation relies on public goodwill, so healthcare staff should encourage public awareness.

Organ donation can literally be life-saving; a *moral duty* to facilitate trans-plantation creates dilemmas between whether the onus of duty falls on society or individuals. Traditionally, the UK, like most countries, has had an opt-in system, donation becoming a gift, although since 2015 Wales has had an opt-out system, and at the 2017 Conservative Party Conference Prime Minister Theresa May pledged the government to introduce presumed consent in England (BBC News, 2017).

Organs and tissues are only considered if the offer is unconditional. So, any condition that organs should not be given to recipients with particular diseases or from various social/religious/cultural/ethnic groups will result in transplant services refusing the donation.

No major *religions* absolutely oppose organ donation is principle (Randhawa and Neuberger, 2016), but if the family agrees there may be religion-specific customs to observe. The N.H.S.B.T. produces various information leaflets for major religions, which can valuably be made available both to staff and relatives. The SNOD, and ministers of religions, can often also often provide useful cultural-specific information and support.

Distressed *relatives*, facing inevitable and usually sudden bereavement, may not think to ask about donation. Ormrod et al.'s (2005) small study found that no relatives regretted agreeing to organ donation, but some who refused donation later regretted their decision. Offering donation therefore should be viewed as offering relatives a choice; not offering donation denies that choice. UK refusal rates remain one of the highest in Europe (N.H.S.B.T., 2013). Some relatives may decline donation owing to not wishing to "sacrifice" the body (Sque *et al.*, 2008), although most relatives asked will give consent (N.I.C.E., 2010g). As "time is tissue", possibilities of donation does need to be discussed urgently.

Post-operative care of recipients

Post-operative care of transplant recipients includes aspects needed for any patient who has undergone major surgery, with additional complications created both for supporting grafted organs to function effectively, while preventing infection in patients receiving powerful immunosuppressive drugs. Early extubation is therefore a priority (Glaspole and Williams, 1999). Transplant recipients should be monitored closely for signs of:

- rejection
- electrolyte imbalance
- infection.

Nonfunction. Transplanted organs may fail to ever function. Organ-specific function should be monitored, and if *primary nonfunction* occurs urgent further transplantation is usually organised, if possible. Rejection can occur at any time after transplantation. Hyperacute rejection occurs is relatively rare but occurs within minutes of anastomosis, pre-existing mediators provoking thrombotic occlusion of graft vasculature and irreversible ischaemia. Acute rejection is more common, causing necrosis of individual cells. Chronic rejection can also occur but is likely to be after the patient has been discharged from critical care. Various interventions may support the failing organ, but rejection usually necessitates retransplantation.

Electrolytes. Storage and cooling of organs for transportation usually causes electrolyte imbalance and metabolic acidosis, so homeostasis should be restored. Imbalances, acidosis and reperfusion injury may all cause dysrhythmias. If biochemistry does not stabilise over the first post-operative day, graft failure should be suspected.

Immunosuppressant drugs and multiple invasive lines make patients particularly susceptible to opportunist *infection*. Patients should be monitored for signs of infection.

Pain varies both between individuals and the nature of surgery, but epidural analgesia often provides the most effective cover for patient (Glaspole and Williams, 1999).

Graft versus host disease (GvHD)

When foreign tissue, such as a tissue transplant, enters the body, the immune system initiates a host reaction. Severe cases may cause organ failure or death

(Ferrara *et al.*, 2009). GvHD causes fibrosis, necrosis and necrosis in skin, liver and gut epithelium. Incidence increases with older donors, older recipients, or those with human leukocyte antigen (HLA) mismatch.

Symptoms include:

- skin rashes (typically: face, palms, soles, ears);
- jaundice;
- diarrhoea.

Treatments include corticosteroids and chemotherapy, often with system support.

Implications for practice

- donation should routinely be considered when withdrawing active treatment;
- donation offers families the opportunity to salvage something positive from bereavement;
- SNODs can offer useful support and information at all stages of donation, so should be alerted and involved early;
- any medical conditions that may affect brainstem function must be excluded before brainstem death tests;
- spinal reflexes may occur despite absence of brainstem function; staff and relatives should be warned about these – they are not signs of life;
- in addition to general ICU care, nurses should monitor transplant recipients for signs of:
  - rejection;
  - infection (immunosupression);
  - side effects of immunosupressants and other drugs.

Summary

Transplantation of organs can save lives, while tissue transplantation can improve quality of life, but continuing donor shortage often causes long waiting lists, many patients dying before suitable organs are found. Most organs being retrieved from patients already in the ICU, ICU nurses should promote awareness abo ut transplantation. The usually close rapport with families enables nurses to offer valuable support during crises and discussion.

Useful contacts

- National referral centre – 0800 432 0559;
- National pager – 0800 345 7633;
- Organ Donor Register 0300 123 23 (not 24 hours).

Further reading

Department of Health (2008, 2009) policy documents introduced radical reforms to structures for donation. The B.M.A. (2012) and N.H.S.B.T. (2013) update on progress in the UK. The Academy of Medical Royal Colleges, and their subsidiary UK Donation Ethics Committee, and the British Transplantation Society websites contain many resources, although these are mostly aimed at professionals specialising in donation and transplants.

Clinical scenarios

Mrs Wallace is 50 years old and suffered an out-of-hospital VF arrest. She was successfully resuscitated at the scene, but en route to hospital required further resuscitation and seven defibrillation shocks. She was admitted to the ICU for mechanical ventilation prior to transfer to CT scan the following day. Head scan revealed extensive and diffuse cerebral damage. Her GCS is E1, V1, M1.

Q1. Would Mrs Wallace be considered as a potential organ donor? What other information and actions are required?

Q2. How might permission for Mrs Wallace's organ donation be obtained?

Q3. How can Mrs Wallace's organ function be optimised? What might optimisation affect her care and her family?

Q4. Following brainstem death confirmation, should Mrs Wallace be resuscitated in the event she has a cardiopulmonary arrest? Discuss this with medical and nursing colleagues.

Part IX

Metabolic

Chapter 44

Severe acute pancreatitis

Contents

Fundamental knowledge

Pancreatic anatomy and physiology – endocrine and exocrine functions, Sphincter of Oddi, Ampulla of Vater

Introduction

Pancreatitis is a relatively common disease affecting people of all ages, usually caused by:

- alcoholism, usually in men, median age 51.5 years (Lowe and Sevilla, 2012);
- biliary obstruction, usually in older women; usually from gallstones;
- although only a minority of alcoholics or people with gallstones develop pancreatitis.

Rarer causes include:

- drugs, such thiazide diuretics (Oelschlaeger, 2016);
- animal venoms (rarely seen in the UK);
- idiopathic, such as endoscopy.

Alcohol causes protein in pancreatic enzymes to precipitate, obstructing pancreatic ductules (Hughes, 2004). UK incidence of pancreatitis has doubled in the last 30 years (Baddeley *et al.*, 2011).

Pancreatitis may be acute or chronic. Patients with chronic pancreatitis are seldom admitted to ICUs, so this chapter describes acute pancreatitis. The revised 2012 Atlanta classification for acute pancreatitis is:

- mild: no organ failure;
- moderate severe: transient organ failure (< 48 hours) and/or local or systemic complications;
- severe: persistent organ failure.

(Banks et al., 2013)

Acute severe pancreatitis typically causes:

- severe continuous abdominal pain;
- respiratory failure;
- hypovolaemia and distributive shock (Maheshwari and Subramanian, 2016);
- and other complications, such as acute kidney injury and pyrexia. Severe pancreatitis therefore necessitates ICU admission, but, although progression is often rapid, predicting which patients will progress to severe pancreatitis remains problematic (Tenner *et al.*, 2013).

Overall mortality for pancreatitis is about 5% (Janisch and Gardner, 2016), but about one fifth progress to severe disease (Janisch and Gardner, 2016), which has a mortality of about 15–20% (Johnson *et al.*, 2014). Medical and nursing management focuses on system support to minimise/limit complications (Williams and Williamson, 2010). Priorities of nursing care are listed in Table 44.1.

Pathology

Pancreatic juice, secreted by reflex vagal responses to acidic chyme, enters the duodenum at the Sphincter of Oddi. It is strongly alkaline (pH about 8.0) and includes phospholipidase A, a powerful protein-digesting enzyme. Obstruction to the Ampulla of Vater prevents acid chyme being neutralised, so stimulating continuing release of pancreatic juice. Congestion eventually ruptures pancreatic ductules, releasing pancreatic juice directly into the gland. Autodigestion causes oedema, necrosis and haemorrhage (Sargent, 2006). If fistulae form, pancreatic juice also digests peripancreatic fat.

Damage to cell membranes triggers inflammatory responses:

- capillary leak and oedema, including ascites;
- vasodilatation and hypotension;
- microvascular thromboses;
- further release of cytokines and other mediators,

while adrenal (cortisol) insufficiency impairs anti-inflammatory response (De Waele *et al.*, 2007).

Biomarkers. Serum amylase (normal 30–100 iu/litre) is the most widely used biomarker, often rising to 1000 units/litre within a few hours. Amylase levels do not correlate with severity (Meher *et al.*, 2015). Lipase (normal 0–160 units/litre) is also used (Maheshwari and Subramanian, 2016).

Complications

Acute fluid collections can develop in or near the pancreas. These fluid collections initially lack a wall and are difficult to visualise, but after about four weeks a wall develops, forming a *pancreatic pseudocyst* (Maheshwari and Subramanian, 2016).

5–10% of patients develop necrotising pancreatitis, which may remain sterile or become infected (Banks *et al.*, 2013).

Symptoms

Oedema and distension of the pancreatic capsule, biliary tree obstruction or chemical peritoneal burning by chemicals such as phospholipidase A cause severe acute abdominal *pain*, requiring opioid analgesics such as morphine.

Hypermetabolism is the main cause of *pyrexia*, although infections often occur. Temperature should be monitored. If high, blood cultures should be taken and antipyretics may be needed (see Chapter 8).

Pancreatitis is usually sterile, so prophylactic antibiotics should not be prescribed. But *infection* can occur, especially with necrotic tissue, and increases mortality, so preventing infection is "the most promising . . . treatment" (Uhl *et al.*, 1999, p103).

Common *electrolyte imbalances* include:

- *hyperglycaemia* (Maheshwari and Subramanian, 2016) from impaired insulin secretion, increased glucagon release and circulating antagonists such as catecholamines; blood sugars should be closely monitored; sliding-scale insulin may be prescribed;
- *hypocalcaemia*, mainly due to hypoalbuminaemia; provided ionised calcium remains satisfactory, this should not be treated (Maheshwari and Subramanian, 2016);
- *hypomagnesaemia* is common, especially with alcohol-related pancreatitis.

Respiratory failure, the main cause of death with acute pancreatitis, may be caused by:

- pleural effusions, from autodigestion of lung tissue, especially on the left side;
- atelectasis and *ARDS* (Maheshwari and Subramanian, 2016);
- pulmonary oedema (Maheshwari and Subramanian, 2016);
- reduced lung volume from diaphragmatic splinting, caused by ascites and the grossly distended pancreas,

and often requires artificial ventilation.

Cardiovascular instability is caused if autodigestion provokes sepsis. Gross inflammatory responses cause excessive vasodilatation and capillary leak. Fluid shifts aggravate electrolyte imbalances. Aggressive fluid resuscitation and inotropes are usually needed.

Half of patients with severe pancreatitis develop intra-abdominal hypertension (Jaipuria *et al.*, 2016), which can cause multi-organ failure (see Chapter 41). Hypotension and/or intra-abdominal hypertension often cause *acute kidney injury*, often necessitating haemofiltration.

Direct damage to the *gastrointestinal* system can cause:

- peptic ulceration;
- gastritis;
- translocation of gut bacteria;
- bowel infarction;
- paralytic ileus.

Hypermetabolism increases energy expenditure, necessitating additional nutritional support.

Enteral nutrition is usually possible, and preferable, with pancreatitis (UK Working Party on Acute Pancreatitis, 2005; Al-Omran *et al.*, 2010; Tenner *et al.*, 2013; Blaser *et al.*, 2017). It has been shown to boost immunity (Wang *et al.*, 2013). If enteral feeding is not possible, parenteral nutrition is necessary. Hyperglycaemia often occurs (Maheshwari and Subramanian, 2016), necessitating sliding-scale insulin.

Table 44.1 Priorities of nursing care

- haemodynamic monitoring (ECG, BP, cardiac output studies) – dysrhythmias and hypovolaemia likely
- monitor and support ventilation – probable pulmonary oedema/effusions, diaphragmatic splinting
- pain management – morphine usually needed
- restore normovolaemia – massive fluid shifts; give prescribed fluid resuscitation
- monitor and resolve electrolyte imbalances
- early nutrition, monitor absorption
- thermoregulation – monitor temperature; blood cultures if infection suspected; antipyretics
- monitor urine output – CRRT may be needed
- normoglycaemia – frequent blood glucose monitoring, IVI insulin may be needed

Intra-abdominal haemorrhage often causes bruising or others skin discolouration. "Grey Turner's sign" (bluish-purple discolouration of flanks) or "Cullen's sign" (irregular, bluish-purple discolouration around umbilicus).

Medical treatments

Historically, the treatment of choice was surgery, which is why patients are usually admitted under surgeons. Almost the only remaining indications of surgery are necrotic tissue, which needs urgent surgical debridement, and drainage of collection. Debridement is often through minimally invasive techniques (Maheshwari and Subramanian, 2016), while drainage may be percutaneous. Many drug treatments have been attempted, but cures remain largely evasive (Afghani *et al.*, 2015). Treatment is largely supporting systems and minimising complications:

- artificial ventilation;
- fluids;
- antibiotics if infection is present;
- inotropes;
- renal replacement therapy;
- analgesia;
- nutrition;
- supplements – insulin, electrolytes, micronutrients (magnesium, phosphate), vitamins.

Gallstones should be removed with early endoscopic retrograde cholangiopancreatography (ERCP) (van Santvoort *et al.*, 2009).

Implications for practice

- pain is severe; analgesia (usually opioid) should be provided and its effectiveness assessed;
- large fluids shifts can rapidly cause oedema, including ascites and pulmonary oedema, and hypovolaemia; aggressive fluid resuscitation may prevent organ failure. Arterial blood pressure and fluid balance charts give little indication of intravascular volume;
- respiratory failure remains the main cause of death with acute pancreatitis. Respiratory function should be monitored closely, and atelectasis and pleural effusions treated. Severe respiratory failure often progresses to ARDS;
- Fluid shifts/loss can cause various electrolyte imbalances. Biochemistry should be monitored, and major imbalances rectified;
- blood sugars should be monitored regularly, and insulin regimes followed;
- optimise nutrition, if possible enterally.

Summary

Pancreatitis can cause rapid and severe complications in most other major systems. Severe pancreatitis, seen in ICU, continues to cause high mortality. Current treatment is largely system support to prevent further complications, pain control being a particularly important nursing role.

Further reading

UK national guidelines have not been updated since 2005, although USA guidelines (Tenner *et al.*, 2013) are not significantly different. N.C.E.P.O.D. (2016) provides a useful summary of pancreatitis in the UK.

Clinical scenarios

Myla Vegas is 56 years old and was admitted to the ICU with sudden acute abdominal pain. The pain radiated towards her back and was accompanied by nausea and vomiting. Two years ago she had an ultrasound which detected gallstones. She is 1.6 metres tall and weighs 74 kg. On admission her abdomen was distended.

Other abnormal results from admission assessment include:

Vital signs		Blood serum	
Temperature	38.4°C	Glucose	12 mmol/litre
Respiration	32 per minute	WCC	19.3×10^9/litre
SpO$_2$	88% on FiO$_2$ 0.6	CRP	151 mg/litre
Heart rate	145 bpm	Amylase	1 543 units/litre
3-lead ECG	sinus rhythm, ST elevation	Alkaline phosphatase	250 units/litre
BP	110/60 mmHg	Potassium	3.4 mmol/litre
MAP	77 mmHg	Calcium (total)	1.8 mmol/litre
		Magnesium	0.78 mmol/litre

Q1. With reference to physiology, explain Ms Vegas's results (e.g. why has her temperature and respiratory rate increased, why does she have low potassium with presenting symptoms and diagnosis?)

A CT scan reveals bilateral pleural effusions, basal consolidation, diffuse pancreatic enlargement with peripancreatic fluid and a small amount of fluid around the liver and spleen.

Q2. What is the significance of CT scan results for Ms Vegas? What other complications may occur? How should these be managed?

Q3. How would you manage Ms Vegas's abdominal pain? What aspects of nursing, medical and surgical interventions may contribute to pain, and how can these be minimised?

Chapter 45

Diabetic crises

Contents

Fundamental knowledge

Pancreatic anatomy and physiology, especially production of insulin

Introduction

"Diabetes" means "fountain-like", used to describe the classic symptoms of *polyuria* and *polydipsia*. *Diabetes mellitus* is caused by lack of, or antagonism to, insulin, causing hyperglycaemia, glycosuria (mellitus = honey, from the time when urinalysis was performed by taste), and so osmotic diuresis. *Diabetes insipidus*, from lack of antidiuretic hormone (see Chapter 36), causes polyuria from lack of renal reabsorption of water. This chapter follows the convention of "diabetes" implying diabetes mellitus.

Diabetes mellitus affects more than three million people in the UK (N.I.C.E. 2016d), with many diabetics remaining undiagnosed until a crisis occurs (Audit Commission, 2001). Worldwide, incidence of diabetes continues to increase (N.C.D. Risk Factor Collaboration, 2016; W.H.O., 2016b). It may cause ICU admission but is also one of the commonest co-morbidities.

Insulin, produced by pancreatic beta (β) cells, transports glucose into cells. Lack therefore deprives cells of their main energy sources. Hyperglycaemia causes acute complications, including:

- polyuria, if serum glucose exceeds 11 mmol/litre, the renal reabsorption threshold (Gerich, 2010); glycosuria exerts osmotic force, causing polyuria and so hypovolaemia;
- immunocompromise (reduced oxygen dissociation from haemoglobin, impaired leukocyte migration and increased blood viscosity);
- inflammatory responses from vascular endothelium.

Poorly controlled diabetes can cause/contribute to many diseases:

- cardiovascular disease (e.g. heart failure, stroke);
- chronic kidney disease;
- retinopathy and blindness;
- peripheral neuropathy;
- leg ulcers;
- amputation;
- depression.

(Diabetes UK, 2016)

Even if not acutely life-threatening, complications such as ulcers need nursing care, and, as ulcers are often chronic, advice from specialists such as tissue viability nurses is valuable.

Many patients are diabetic or develop short-term hyperglycaemia in response to stressors of critical illness. But diabetes can also cause crises, necessitating ICU admission. This chapter discusses:

- severe hypoglycaemia;
- diabetic ketoacidosis (DKA);
- hyperosmolar hyperglycaemic state (HHS).

Incidence of severe hypoglycaemia and diabetic ketoacidosis is increasing (D.O.H., 2010b).

The *metabolic syndrome* is also discussed.

There are two different types of diabetes mellitus: type1 and type 2.

Type 1

Previously called "insulin-dependent diabetes mellitus" (IDDM), this is an autoimmune disease (Skyler *et al.*, 2017), which destroys pancreatic beta cells but leaves other pancreatic cells unharmed. This disease typically develops in childhood, the almost total destruction of beta cells usually necessitating life-long insulin therapy. Most type 1 diabetics suffer complications relatively early in life.

Type 2

Previously called "non-insulin-dependent diabetes mellitus" (NIDDM) or "late-onset", type 2 causes most (90% (Diabetes UK, 2016)) cases of diabetes. Typically, this develops in later life (> 65 years (Skyler *et al.*, 2017)), partly from age-related pancreatic decline and often aggravated by obesity (N.I.C.E., 2016d; Skyler *et al.*, 2017). Type 2 is less severe than type 1, as the pancreas has significant remaining function but not always sufficient to cope with demand.

Gestational diabetes, occurring during pregnancy, similarly reflects insulin demand exceeding supply, but usually resolves after childbirth.

Ketones

Glucose is normally the main energy source for cell mitochondria to produce adenosine triphosphate (ATP). Without glucose, cells to resort to metabolism of alternative energy sources, mainly free fatty acids (lyposis). Alternative energy source metabolism is relatively inefficient, producing limited energy but much waste, including ketones. Ketones are filtered by the kidneys, so can be detected on urinalysis. Excessive ketones cause:

- (metabolic) acidosis – ketones form ketoacids;
- osmotic diuresis (Keays, 2014);
- nausea and vomiting (Jerreat, 2010);
- "Kussmaul respiration" – deep, rapid and sighing breaths (Jerreat, 2010);
- a distinctive sickly-sweet smell to breath (in unintubated patients).

Metabolic syndrome

This is a syndrome of inter-related metabolic problems, usually caused by obesity (Kramer *et al.*, 2013), resulting in hyperlipidaemia. High triglyceride levels provoke inflammation, contributing to atherosclerosis, hypertension, and increased risk of myocardial infarction (Skyler *et al.*, 2017). Metabolic syndrome often leads to type 2 diabetes (Skyler *et al.*, 2017) and increases risks of fatty liver disease (E.A.S.L., 2017).

Stress hyperglycaemia

Stress responses usually cause hyperglycaemia by increasing insulin resistance, but transient hyperglycaemia is usually mild, resolves with recovery, is not usually significant and is usually only treated if blood sugar persists above 10 mmol/litre (see Chapter 21).

Severe hypoglycaemia

This may occur if diabetics:

- receive excessive insulin/hypoglycaemics;
- lack sugar and sugar sources;
- develop increased resistance to insulin (e.g. from infection).

Aggressive insulin therapy with inadequate monitoring of blood glucose can cause iatrogenic hypoglycaemia (see Chapter 21). Blood glucose below 1 mmol/litre creates a medical emergency (Keays, 2014), as brain cells rely on constant supplies to survive. Severe hypoglycaemia is treated by giving intravenous glucose, and stabilising acid–base and electrolyte balances. J.B.D.S. (2013a) recommend using 10% or 20% glucose rather than 50%, as the stronger concentration increases risk of extravasation injury. Hypoglycaemia is usually managed in A&E or acute admission wards, but could occur on the ICU, especially if feeds are stopped but insulin infusion continues.

Diabetic ketoacidosis (DKA)

This typically occurs when type 1 diabetics fail to receive sufficient insulin, although can be precipitated by increased insulin resistance, such as from infection (Park, 2007). DKA causes:

- ketonaemia ≥ 3 mmol/litre (× 10 normal); more than ++ on standard urine dipsticks;
- blood glucose > 11 mmol/litre;
- metabolic acidosis: bicarbonate < 15 mmol/litre and/or venous pH < 7.3.
                                                                    (J.B.D.S. 2013b)

Patients may be comatose or acutely confused. Osmotic diuresis from both glycosuria and ketonuria usually causes hypovolaemic shock. Venous statis and hyperosmolality can cause thromboembolism, epilepsy and strokes. DKA usually necessitates ICU admission.

Targets are to each hour:

- reduce blood ketones 0.5 mmol/hour;
- increase venous bicarbonate 3 mmol/hour;
- reduce capillary blood glucose by 3 mmol/hour;
- maintain serum potassium 4–5 mmol/hour.

(J.B.D.S, 2013b)

This necessitates close monitoring of vital signs, blood sugars, fluid balance, electrolytes and neurological state. J.B.D.S (2013b) recommends fixed-rate intravenous insulin infusion (FRIII) of 0.1 units/kilogram, up to a maximum of 15 units/hour. Rapid reduction in blood glucose may cause cerebral oedema. Once blood glucose is < 14 mmol/litre, fluids should be changed to 10% glucose (J.B.D.S, 2013b). Severe acidosis (pH < 7.1) may be treated with bicarbonate infusion, although this is controversial – paradoxically, infusing bicarbonate may exacerbate intracellular acidosis by generating carbon dioxide (Velissaris *et al.*, 2015). Less severe acidosis usually resolves with recovery.

Hyperosmolar hyperglycaemic state (HHS)

(previously called hyperosmolar non-ketotic state – HONKS)

This rare condition is most likely to occur to type 2 diabetics and resembles diabetic ketoacidosis, except that it develops more slowly and ketosis does not occur. Hyperglycaemia causes osmotic diuresis and electrolyte imbalance; as HHS often develops over some days, dehydration is often more severe (Keays, 2014), affecting all fluids compartments, not just the bloodstream. Dehydration increases serum osmolality, which causes neurological complications, including *tonic-clonic seizures*. Rehydration usually resolves HHS, but if hyperglycaemia persists insulin may be needed – J.B.D.S (2012) recommends 0.05 units/kg/hour.

Implications for practice

- diabetes can cause widespread complications and problems throughout the body, so patients should be assessed and treated holistically;
- insulin management should be adjusted with changes in feeding regimes, especially when feeds are stopped;
- UK guidelines (J.B.D.S, 2013b) for managing diabetic ketoacidosis emphasise the primacy of controlling ketoacidosis;
- diabetic ketoacidosis and hyperosmolar hyperglycaemic state should also be treated with aggressive fluid replacement.

Summary

Diabetes affects people of all ages, and incidence is increasing. It may cause or complicate ICU admission. Most diabetics are type 2, although diabetic crises more commonly occur with type 1. Diabetics frequently have co-morbidities and complications.

Useful contact

Diabetes UK, 0345–123–2399.
Wells Lawrence House, 126 Back Church Lane, London E1 1FH.
fax 020–7424–1001.
helpline@diabetes.org.uk.
www.diabetes.org.uk.

Further reading

Many books and journals focus on diabetes, while articles frequently appear in general nursing and medical journals. Less literature focuses on critical care issues. Websites such as Diabetes UK and the American Diabetic Association provide much information, especially for the public, but their focus is not critical care. The Joint British Diabetic Societies (J.B.D.S) publishes guidelines on DKA (2013b) and HHS (2012). Most trusts employ diabetic nurse specialists, who are useful resources for staff as well as patients.

Clinical scenario

Rosemary Davies, a 34-year-old accountant with no previous medical history, was found unconscious and incontinent by her friends. She had been recovering from 'flu, complaining of fever, thirst, tiredness and feeling confused.

Ms Davies was admitted to ICU self-ventilating.

vital signs		laboratory blood results	
respiratory rate	32 breaths/minute	Na⁺	150 mmol/litre
HR	120 beats/minute	K⁺	4.8 mmol/litre
BP	80/60 mmHg	glucose	40 mmol/litre
PPV	17%		
temperature	35.5°C		

ABG showed HCO_3^- 19 mmol/litre with pH 7.15.

Ms Davies is diagnosed as having hyperosmolar hyperglycaemic state (HHS).

Q1. Ms Davies is extremely hyperglycaemic. Identify effects of hyperglycaemia which resulted in her admission, and how this contributes to her tachycardia, hypothermia, unconsciousness.

Q2. Intravenous insulin infusion is commenced. What rate is recommended by the J.B.D.S? What other factors should be considered in correcting hyperglycaemia?

Q3. How is hyperglycaemia managed in your unit/trust? What are potential benefits and limitations of sliding-scale insulin and fixed-rate intravenous insulin infusions? How frequently is blood glucose likely to be checked?

449

Chapter 46

Self-poisoning

Contents

Fundamental knowledge

Neurotransmission synapse
Cell metabolism

Introduction

The UK has one of highest rates of drug overdose in Europe (Clark *et al.*, 2011), causing about 4% of ICU admissions (Clark *et al.*, 2011). Prevalence of alcohol, recreational drugs and opioids is increasing (Clark *et al.*, 2011). Most patients admitted to ICU with deliberate self-harm need only short-term tracheal intubation, few require organ support, and outcome is usually good (Clark *et al.*, 2011). Care focuses on:

- physiological support;
- preventing recurrence of self-harming behaviour (psychiatry);
- dealing with underlying psychopathology.

This chapter focuses on physiological support, as specialist psychological care usually follows ICU discharge. Potential wish to self-harm during ICU stay should be remembered, and so risk factors minimised.

Many drugs and chemicals have potentially harmful/fatal effects if taken in sufficient quantity. The drugs which cause most ill health are nicotine (and the hundreds of other toxins in cigarettes) and alcohol (Mehta, 2016). These are relatively socially acceptable drugs and usually cause insidious rather than sudden changes in health. ICU drug-related admissions are usually either:

- deliberate self-harm, typically involving paracetamol or antidepressants;
- from illicit drugs (e.g. cocaine, "ecstasy") or "legal highs" (e.g. "poppers") taken to achieve pleasure

Some individual drugs are briefly described, followed by discussion of common physiological effects. Self-poisoning with drugs not described often cause similar problems, which will be managed similarly. A challenge for health-care professionals is that changes in illicit drugs, and "legal highs", can be rapid, resulting in limited information about and treatments for them (Patterson *et al.*, 2017). Many wider issues of nursing care discussed in this chapter can be applied to self-poisoning from other drugs, although readers should check applicability before transferring specific aspects.

Antidepressants

People being treated for depression often have access to, or accumulate, large numbers of antidepressant tablets (such as amitriptyline), while suffering from depression places them at high risk of attempting suicide. Increasing prescriptions of antidepressants has caused wider availability, and increased numbers admitted with antidepressant overdose (Berling *et al.*, 2016). Many antidepressants increase ECG PR intervals, potentially causing bradycardia, and prolong QTc, which may trigger ventricular fibrillation.

Paracetamol

Paracetamol (= acetaminophen in USA) remains the most common drug used for self-poisoning in the UK, causing nearly half of all poison admissions to hospitals, and 100–200 deaths each year (Wallace *et al.*, 2003). It is the main cause of hyperacute liver failure (McKinley, 2009), and often also causes acute kidney injury (Gunning, 2009). It is treated with acetylcysteine (Parvolex) (Commission on Human Medicines, 2012; Lancaster *et al.*, 2015), and system support.

Paracetamol is rapidly absorbed, plasma levels peaking within one to two hours of ingestion (Smith, 2007). The toxic threshold for liver damage is 150 mg/kg in adults, although as little as 10–15 grams in 24 hours can cause severe hepatocellular necrosis (Bateman, 2007). Severe overdose usually progresses to hepatic failure, although symptoms may be delayed for two to three days, appearing only after significant, possibly fatal, damage.

Paracetamol overdose is usually impulsive (Turvill *et al.*, 2000; Hawton *et al.*, 2001), so guilt and remorse are likely to become problems for both patients and their families and friends.

Illicit drugs

Paracetamol and antidepressants are usually obtained legally, but "recreational" or "street" drugs are usually obtained, and often produced, illegally. Purity and strength of recreational drugs are often very variable, whether from deliberate dilution (to reduce cost) or chance contamination during non-aseptic illegal manufacture (Bancroft and Reid, 2016). Different tablets may have dissimilar strengths (Schifano *et al.*, 2006), so even users with previous experience of drugs cannot be sure how each dose will affect them (Patterson *et al.*, 2017). Accidental "overdose" occurs easily; individual metabolism and tolerance further influence effect.

Many recreational drugs (such as cocaine and ecstasy) are taken to achieve desired effects or mood, not with intent to self-harm. Usually, the desired effect will be pleasure, through either:

- calming/suppressing/reducing or
- stimulating/increasing

central nervous system function. Drugs which stimulate more often cause acute life-threatening emergencies.

Many drugs taken for pleasure become addictive. They replace endogenous neurotransmitters (especially dopamine), causing a "high" – euphoria, increased libido, and energy. The attractions of many drugs may be seen in clubs; the miseries are more often seen in ICU. "Benefits" fade after a few hours, leaving insufficient endogenous neurotransmitters, so causing a "low" (depression). Drug-users often respond by taking further, often larger, doses, becoming progressively addicted or dependent.

Chemical changes in brain tissue can cause permanent neurological damage; other organs can also suffer acute and chronic harm. Drugs are also frequently mixed, often with alcohol, tobacco and other recreational drugs (D.A.W.N., 2011). Alcohol toxicity can cause various neurological symptoms, including seizures and delirium (Grounds *et al.*, 2014). As drugs are metabolised by the liver, hepatotoxicity frequently occurs (Valente *et al.*, 2016).

If the drug remains in the gut, activated charcoal is usually given. Toxic blood levels may be treated with haemofiltration. If there is an antidote to the drug, that will be started. Otherwise, priorities are system support and psychological care.

Illicit drugs are often transported in body cavities ("body packing"), using plastic bags or condoms, swallowed or inserted into the rectum (Birk *et al.*, 2016). The gut is highly vascular, so, if bags break, drugs are efficiently absorbed. Drug traffickers may be admitted with accidental self-poisoning and, understandably, may be reluctant to admit their continuing rectal drug infusion. Attempts to remove bags may cause further internal spillage (Birk *et al.*, 2016). If there is no indication that drugs have been absorbed, conservative management is safest, but, if bags have ruptured, surgery may be needed (Birk *et al.*, 2016). Progress of intact bags can be monitored with abdominal X-rays and CT scans.

Patients may be drug pushers, regular users or novices experimenting with the drug. They may be in police custody while in hospital or anticipate being arrested when they recover.

Cocaine ("coke") has long been used as a therapeutic analgesic, but also has a long history of recreational use. It is the most commonly used class A drug in England and Wales (Treadwell and Robinson, 2007) and use is increasing (Galvin *et al.*, 2010). Mortality is very high – 60% in Galvin *et al.*'s study, although death is usually from long-term use rather than overdose (Albarran and Cox, 2008). *Crack* is modified cocaine and causes similar symptoms.

Amphetamine sulphate ("speed") has similar effects to cocaine, except they usually last longer. The amphetamine derivative 3–4 methylenedioxymethamphetamine (MDMA, usually called "ecstasy" or "E") is discussed below, but other amphetamines have similar effects. Amphetamines are hepatotoxic (Mokhlesi *et al.*, 2004).

MDMA ("*ecstasy*") is not a new drug, but widespread illicit use is still a recent phenomenon, and increasing (D.A.W.N., 2011). Mortality appears to bear little relation to number of tablets taken, some people surviving considerable numbers while single tablets prove fatal to others. GBH (liquid ecstasy) causes insomnia, anxiety and depression, which often persist for weeks after withdrawal (Winstock and Mitcheson, 2012).

Ketamine ("special K"), an anaesthetic agent and analgesic, is often taken as a cheap alternative to amphetamines, but tolerance develops quickly, resulting in escalation of use (Winstock and Mitcheson, 2012). It can induce nightmare-like hallucinations (Avidan *et al.*, 2017) and provoke schizophrenia. Ketamine is discussed further in Chapter 7.

Legal highs

Many other street drugs are used, and fashion frequently changes. Recent years have seen increasing concerns about "legal highs", drugs that are available legally, although often not for human consumption but in household items such as air fresheners. The most widely legal high is alkyl nitrite ("poppers") (Rewbury *et al.*, 2017). Acutely, nitrate can vasodilate (Ricaurte and McCann, 2005); chronically, it can cause visual impairment from foveal maculopathy (Rewbury *et al.*, 2017). Production being unregulated, contents, and so effects, may vary between brands.

Symptoms

Gross sympathetic system stimulation is especially likely to precipitate cardio-vascular crises (e.g. hypertension, myocardial infarction), and so necessitate admission. But problems may be complicated by impurities in production, mixing with alcohol or other drugs, and the conditions in which the drugs are used – e.g. "clubbing" activities may include vigorous dancing, while costs of drinks may contribute to dehydration and electrolyte imbalances. Care is often complicated by psychological and social problems (Chummun *et al.*, 2010).

Airway/breathing

Smoke from inhaled drugs is far hotter than from cigarettes, potentially causing severe laryngeal oedema, necessitating prophylactic intubation. If consciousness is impaired, patients may have aspirated. Respiratory failure frequently occurs. Multisystem complications often necessitate intubation and artificial ventilation. Drugs such as cocaine can cause status asthmaticus, upper airway obstruction, pulmonary hypertension, barotrauma, and pulmonary oedema (Mokhlesi *et al.*, 2004). Many drugs cause fluid and electrolyte imbalances and trigger inflammatory responses, causing pulmonary oedema (Welsch *et al.*, 2001). Hypercalcaemia may cause trismus (tightening of jaw muscles – "lockjaw") and bruxism (jaw-clenching) (Koesters *et al.*, 2002), which may make oral intubation difficult.

Cardiovascular

Sympathetic nervous system stimulation often causes extreme hypertension and tachycardia. Illicit drug victims are usually young but may have congenital or drug-induced cardiac disease (Ghuran and Nolan, 2000). Intravenous drug abuse ("mainlining") and heavy smoking may have accelerated vascular damage.

Electrolytes and metabolites are often grossly deranged on arrival, including:

- hyperkalaemia;
- hyper/hyponatraemia (Ricaurte and McCann, 2005; Hall and Henry, 2006; Campbell and Rosner, 2008);

■ hypercalcaemia (Brotto and Lee, 2007);
■ hypoglycaemia.

Muscle contraction and hypercapnia often cause lactic acidosis (Waring, 2017).

Hypermetabolism and "serotonin syndrome" often induce malignant hyperpyrexia (Crandall *et al.*, 2002; Ricaurte and McCann, 2005; Hall and Henry, 2006), the cause of most ecstasy-related deaths (Wake, 1995). Ischaemia and rhabdomyolysis may cause acute kidney injury (Campbell and Rosner, 2008) – see Chapter 38. Kidneys should be protected with fluid resuscitation, but haemofiltration is often needed. Kidney injury exacerbates hyperkalaemia.

Disability (neurological)

Immediate neurological complications are likely to be caused by:

■ cerebral vasospasm;
■ intracranial hypertension, causing intracranial bleeding, subarachnoid haemorrhage and strokes (Welsch *et al.*, 2001; Treadwell and Robinson, 2007);
■ hyponatraemic encephalopathy (Hartung *et al.*, 2002);
■ seizures.

Cerebral perfusion and oxygenation should be optimised; antiepileptics may be needed – benzodiazepines can exacerbate cardiac instability. Major tranquillisers should be avoided as they lower seizure threshold, aggravate hypotension and provoke dysrhythmias (MacConnachie, 1997). Treatment for cerebral oedema is discussed in Chapter 36.

Small-scale studies indicate long-term use causes chronic neurological and psychiatric problems (Semple *et al.*, 1999; Reneman *et al.*, 2001), including permanent cognitive impairment (Parrott *et al.*, 1998).

The "low" usually causes generalised fatigue, muscle ache, limited concentration, confusion, anxiety, hypersomnia or insomnia, bizarre and unpleasant dreams, and depression (Chychula and Sciamanna, 2002; Koesters *et al.*, 2002). Survivors often experience frequent and persistent panic attacks ("bad trips"), believing death to be imminent (McGuire *et al.*, 1994).

Patients, relatives and friends often experience guilt about drug use and fear about prosecution. Parents may have been unaware that their children were taking drugs. Drug levels in blood and other specimens will be tested for therapeutic purposes, but there may be legal requirements about saving samples or releasing results to the police or other authorities. Staff should check what samples/information police have a right to demand. Passwords will usually be identified for telephone calls by the police, and often for family members. Many patients, families and friends are anyway likely to fear what staff will tell other authorities.

Healthcare professionals have a duty of care to all patients. But negative attitudes to patients considered as "time-waters", "bed-blockers", immature or "mad" and "sad", may both impair quality of care given and cause further psychological distress to patients and families. Whatever their personal views, nurses caring for victims have the same professional duty of care to them as for other patients (N.M.C., 2015), so should:

- maintain safe environments;
- treat with unconditional positive regard;
- adopt non-judgemental attitudes.

Nurses need to be aware of not only their own attitudes but the attitudes of others, promoting a team approach of unconditional positive regard.

The young age of many illicit drug victims can create uncomfortable reminders for nurses of their own mortality.

Health promotion

Patients admitted with drug overdoses usually recover quickly from their critical illness (Wong, Bellomo *et al.*, 2016). With recovery, health promotion for the patient and other significant people, who may be family or friends, can prevent future crises. With accidental overdose of prescribed medicines, prescriptions should be reviewed and patients should understand the correct dose and any symptoms of over- or under-dose. Those who have deliberately self-harmed have poor longer-term outcomes (Wong, Bellomo *et al.*, 2016), so should be referred for psychiatric support. Users of illicit drugs may also benefit from referral to psychiatric or other support services. Health education can raise awareness of dangers and suggest safer ways to take drugs, so users can make their own informed decisions. Friends and families may need support from specialist agencies, such as support groups or counsellors. When providing information to family and friends, nurses should remember their duty of confidentiality to their patient.

Realisation that drugs are not as safe as they previously thought may make patients and friends receptive to health education, so ICU nurses can provide useful information and contacts. Users often have greater knowledge about recreational drugs than nurses and may have different values and beliefs; adopting moralistic/righteous attitudes may cause alienation. ICU nurses should assess individual needs and offer what support they can but will usually not have specialist knowledge of drugs involved, so should work within their limitations, using specialist services that are available locally. The internet, especially sites such as Toxbase, can provide useful information about drugs.

Implications for practice

- self-poisoning from drugs can affect all major body systems; vital signs should be closely monitored;
- medical management centres around reversing/removing drugs if possible and supporting failing systems;
- Toxbase and the National Poisons Information Service can provide practical information for healthcare staff about drugs causing ICU admission;
- peak effects often occur within hours from ingestion, although wide various occur, partly depending on dose and individual tolerance and metabolism;
- suicide attempts may cause guilt and/or anger among families/friends. Nurses should encourage families to express their needs and emotions but may need to involve counselling or other services. Listening is often more useful (cathartic) than replying to guilt/anger;
- friends and victims may fear sharing information with staff and may experience guilt and fears;
- nurses, and other healthcare professionals, have a duty of care to patients, regardless of the cause of illness;
- nurses should maintain their duty of confidentiality, unless specifically exempted by statute law;
- ICU nurses may be able to offer health information about drugs or support groups;
- psychiatric support should be offered to those who self-harm.

Summary

Self-harm and overdose may necessitate ICU admission. Immediate care necessarily focuses on resuscitation and system support. As well as multisystem physiological problems, not usual for younger people, users (and friends) often experience anxiety or guilt. Care therefore needs to integrate urgent multisystem physiological support with skilful psychological care. Caring for such patients is challenging and can cause distress, but holistic nursing care can contribute significantly to every aspect of recovery.

Support groups

- Families Anonymous: 0207 4984 680, helpline 0845 1200 660, http://-famanon.org.uk;
- Drugline: 01253 311 431, www.druglinelancs.co.uk;
- Turning Point: www.turning-point.co.uk;
- Grove Park, Camberwell, London. 020 7481 7600 (information, but not a helpline).

Further reading

Articles on individual drugs periodically appear in medical, and sometimes nursing, journals; those referenced in the relevant sections of this chapter are likely to be useful for nurses wanting to know more about individual drugs. Information about specific drugs and likely effects from overdoses is available from Toxbase, the national poisons unit (www.toxbase.org).

Clinical scenarios

Lisa Young is 25 years old and was admitted to ICU 10 hours after ingesting 75 amitriptyline (50 mg) tablets. A plasma toxicology screen tested positive for heroin and methadone. Ms Young's urine also tested positive for opioids, benzodiazepine, cocaine and cannabis. Paracetamol and salicylate were not detected. Ms Young is not receiving any sedation; she is agitated and non-compliant with care. She has a urinary catheter but has removed her central venous and arterial cannulae.

Other results:

Glasgow Coma Scale (GCS)	6 (E1, V1, M5)
All limbs flexing spontaneously without any stimuli	
Both pupils are equal, size 2 mm, brisk response to light	
Respiration rate	34 breaths/minute
SpO$_2$	97% on FiO$_2$ of 0.6
Temperature	38.1°C
HR	53 sinus beats/minute
BP	95/68 mmHg
Capillary refill	Three seconds with cool peripheries
Skin feels cool and clammy	
mouth and tongue are dry	
Blood glucose	6.1 mmol/litre
Urine output	20–40 ml/hour

Q1. How will the amitriptyline overdose affect Ms Young's cardio-vascular system? What is the most likely dysrhythmia it will cause? What are likely causes and significance of her urine output and temperature?

Q2. How can Ms Young's risk of seizures and dysrhythmias be reduced? What fluid management would be appropriate? What other strategies might be used to monitor and minimise other complications?

Q3. What are likely long-term effects and outcome of amitriptyline overdose? What advice and support are available for patients like Ms Young in your clinical area? What external agencies might be useful for her?

Part X

Professional

Chapter 47

Transferring critically ill patients

Contents

Fundamental knowledge

Local transfer guidelines
Local transfer equipment

Introduction

Reasons for transferring critically ill patients may be clinical (to specialist centres) or non-clinical (bed shortage). Numbers transferred continue to increase (Fried *et al.*, 2010). Inter-hospital transfer of critically ill patients creates many risks; Cosgrave *et al.*, (2016) suggest that adverse incidents occur in more than half of transfers, although older studies should be treated with caution, owing to relatively less sophisticated transport ventilators and other equipment, as well as more limited monitoring in the not-so-distant past. Kue *et al.* (2011) found that adverse events occurred in fewer than 2% of transfers, although this creates dangers of complacency when potential for far higher rates is present. So transfers should be managed by experienced and reliable nursing and medical staff. Most ICU nurses will therefore assist with transfers moderately frequently during their careers. This chapter provides an overview of how nurses can prepare for safer journeys, using the ABCDE approach.

Transfers within hospitals (e.g. to CT scanning) should create fewer risks but are sometimes given less priority and foresight than external transfers. This chapter largely focuses on external transfers, although many principles apply to internal transfers as well, which should be planned just as carefully.

This chapter focuses on ambulance transfer of Level 3 patients, but many principles apply to transfer by other means (helicopter, air ambulance) and Level 2 patients. Staff involved in aircraft transfer should seek advice before leaving on any special issues and requirement – for example, plane transfers are usually over longer distances, so are more likely to fly at higher altitudes, where differences in atmospheric pressure are more likely to affect equipment. Less equipment and monitoring may be needed for Level 2 patients, although risks should not be underestimated.

Ideally, transfers should be undertaken by specialist transfer teams (Droogh *et al.*, 2015). Dedicated transfer teams improve outcomes (Kue *et al.*, 2011; I.C.S., 2011b), but these are not generally available at present for adults. For children, specialist retrieval teams will usually arrive from the destination paediatric ICU. Some trusts have developed similar transfer teams for adult patients, but many have not. This chapter is for staff working in ICUs where there are not dedicated transfer teams.

Planning

Transfers are stressful for staff involved (Ringdal *et al.*, 2016). Once outside the ICU doors, staff step outside their comfort zone and have to rely on whatever and whoever is at hand or readily contactable. Preparation and planning are therefore important to minimise risks and stressors. While every possible eventuality cannot be predicted, risks should be assessed and safety maintained. Most units have guidelines and equipment for transfer, but it is the individual nurse's responsibility to ensure safety. Allow for the unexpected – ambulances and lifts can break down.

Clarify the precise destination, and how to access it, before leaving. Once arriving at the destination, ambulance crews may be unfamiliar with layout of the hospital and are unlikely to know codes for security doors.

Intubated patients should be accompanied by a nurse and doctor; unintubated patients are usually accompanied only by a nurse. The nurse should have previous experience of transfers (unless gaining the experience by shadowing another). Many trusts provide programmes to prepare staff for transfers, and usually require that only nurses who have completed the programme accompany transfers. The accompanying doctor should be an anaesthetist, in case airway problems occur, but should also have sufficient experience of intensive care to be able to safely manage other problems.

Equipment must be safely secured (I.C.S., 2011b). This is often facilitated by dedicated transfers trolleys, but accompanying staff should ensure safety both before leaving the unit and before commencing any journey. Ensure you are familiar with local equipment and policies for transfer. Everest and Hooper (2014) suggest one third of incidents are equipment-related. Both equipment and medicines should be rationalised so that there is sufficient, without excess. Unnecessary equipment may delay transfers, and access to what is needed. Infusions should be minimised (usually limited to sedatives and vasopressors). Emergency drugs and equipment should be taken. Many units have transfer bags, containing resuscitation drugs, endotracheal tubes and suction equipment, but the transferring nurse should check equipment before leaving the unit, and ensure batteries are sufficiently charged, or sufficient spare batteries are taken. If the patient is ventilated, a portable ventilator is necessary. If possible, this should be attached about an hour before transfer, so that blood gases can be checked in time for any necessary changes to be made, enabling stabilisation of the patient on the ventilator before leaving the unit. With internal transfers, porters are often asked to fetch patients 15–30 minutes before the time of booked procedures. Monitoring will be needed; this should be rationalised so that it is sufficient for safety without being excessive. For some procedures, there may be specific limitations on equipment (e.g. many MRI scanners necessitate excluding most metals – including standard ECG electrodes). Most MRI departments can supply essential equipment suitable for use in the scanner room. Appropriate (usually narrow) alarms limits should be set, as in hospital corridors it may not always be possible to see all equipment continuously, and for radiographical and some other procedures staff usually have to leave the patient, with only a distant view through a window.

Spare drugs may be needed, and the doctor may request specific drugs for transfer. If vasopressors are in progress, dosage may need increasing to counter effects of increased sedation. Equipment should be secured safely; many units have a transfer trolley. Spares should be taken of anything that may be removed (e.g. ECG electrodes in some MRI scanners). For external transfer, patients are often deeply sedated, and sometimes paralysed, so their body should be appropriately protected.

Transfer ambulances are usually well-equipped, but the ambulance may be an unfamiliar environment to both the nurse and doctor, so a member of the ambulance crew should accompany the patient to access whatever is needed.

Family will not usually be able to accompany patients in the ambulance, but if possible parents should accompany children (Masterson and Brenner, 2016; Felmet and Orr, 2017).

Adverse events may range from unfortunate but relatively minor to life-threatening. In Kue *et al.*'s (2011) study, 37% of adverse events caused hypoxia lasting more than five minutes, and a further 37% involved hypotension. Planning priorities should therefore focus on life-threatening risks such as these. Often with limited time to prepare, ABCDE assessment is useful.

Before leaving, clarify what arrangements have been made for staff returning. Ensure you have sufficient money to cover possible expenses on public transport, as planned arrangements for your return might change. A mobile telephone should be available in case of need to contact either the source or destination hospital (I.C.S., 2011b).

Airway

- check the patient's airway is secure and safe;
- check transfer kits contain spare intubation and suction equipment in appropriate sizes;
- if accompanied by an anaesthetist, ensure they can access the patient's airway in the ambulance; if no anaesthetist is transferring the patient, ensure you can access it.

Breathing

- check the portable ventilator;
- establish the patient on the portable ventilator about an hour before transfer, giving time to check blood gases and make appropriate adjustments to settings;
- take spare batteries and sufficient oxygen;
- monitor saturation and end-tidal carbon dioxide (I.C.S., 2011b);
- set appropriate alarm limits;
- position the monitor so you can see it during transfer, and at all times when away from the unit;
- observe respiratory rate and depth;
- if patients are ventilated, oxygen supply, inspired oxygen concentration, ventilator settings and airway pressure should be monitored (I.C.S., 2011b).

Circulation

- ambulance transfer, and more so with aircraft transfer, can negatively affect body function. For example, acceleration exaggerates hypertension and deceleration exaggerates hypotension, so vascular filling should be optimised before leaving the unit (I.C.S., 2011b; Ringdal *et al.*, 2016);

- patients should have at least two cannulae (I.C.S., 2011b);
- ensure sufficient vasopressors and other essential drugs are prepared;
- check resuscitation drugs (usually in a transfer kit);
- ECG, blood pressure (preferably invasive) and temperature should be monitored during transfer (I.C.S., 2011b);
- with some transfers, other equipment (e.g. intra-aortic balloon pump), monitoring and infusions may be indicated.

Disability

- ensure desired levels of analgesia, sedation and paralysis are achieved before leaving the unit;
- ensure sufficient analgesics, sedatives and paralysing agents are prepared.

Exposure

- check lines and limbs are safely secured on transfer to the transport trolley;
- protect any vulnerable parts of the patient's body – e.g. eyes may need a protective cover to prevent corneal abrasions;
- ensure access is available to any cannulae, infusions or other equipment likely to be needed during transfer.

During transport

The law requires that all passengers wear seatbelts; as this includes doctors and nurses, any interventions that necessitate leaving seats also necessitate stopping the vehicle. Before the vehicle starts, ensure monitoring and infusions are visible, and that appropriate access is possible. Each critical care network should have its own documentation for transfer, including observation charts. Frequency and type of observations will usually be at the discretion of the nurse but should be complete enough for early detection of problems, and to withstand scrutiny should actions be brought to court or professional bodies. You may need to request the ambulance to stop, but remember this delays arrival at your destination and prolongs the period of risk.

Should problems, such as breakdown, necessitate leaving the ambulance, high-visibility clothing should be worn. Within hospital buildings, in event of crisis in the corridor, generally it is best to seek help from nearest ward/department, but avoid non-essential delays in reaching destination. In the event of cardiac arrest, 2222 is the national number (remember to state which hospital).

Human factors

People make mistakes, so all aspects of patient safety should recognise potential for human factors to cause harm. While relevant to all topics covered in this book, pressures created through transferring critically ill patients make this an example par excellence. Guidelines and proformas aim to reduce risks. During transfer the nurse and doctor will rely heavily on the ambulance staff, as well as staff at the destination hospital/site, yet will not usually have previously met these people. This makes effective communication especially important. Yet, communication breakdown causes most errors in healthcare (Tschannen *et al.*, 2011). Staff transferring patients should ensure written and verbal (including telephone) communication is clear and concise. Proformas often provide structures for formal handover, but an SBAR (*Situation–Background–Assessment–Response*) structure is also useful.

Implications for practice

- prepare carefully, ensuring adequate supplies without excess;
- be familiar with local equipment, guidelines and documentation;
- assess risks and needs, using an ABCDE approach;
- check all equipment (including emergency drugs, spare airways and suction) and supplies before leaving the unit;
- if using a portable ventilator, commence it early enough to check arterial blood gases before leaving the unit;
- minimise infusions, but take sufficient spare syringes/vials of essential drugs;
- if hypovolaemic, ensure adequate filling before leaving the unit;
- during transfer, maintain essential observations;
- if you have any concerns, alert the doctor/ambulance crew/any other appropriate staff.

Summary

Transfers occur for clinical (patient need) and non-clinical (bed shortage) reasons. All staff will almost inevitably transfer patients, so skills should be developed through accompanying more experienced colleagues on transfer if possible, and attending any local development programmes. Transfer exposes patients to potential risks, but these can be minimised through careful planning. Take sufficient, but not excessive, equipment for the transfer, and ensure sufficient supplies of batteries and oxygen for the journey.

Further reading

The Intensive Care Society (I.C.S., 2011b) provides clear guidance for transporting critically ill (Level 3) patients, much of which is also applicable to Level 2 patients. These guidelines outline training for staff undertaking transfers, so your unit should have access to transfer study days. Staff transferring patients should be familiar with local protocols/guidance/documentation.

Clinical scenarios

Mr Richard Jones was admitted eight days ago with community-acquired pneumonia that failed to respond to any of the antibiotics prescribed during his admission. He has progressively deteriorated and has now developed acute respiratory distress syndrome and acute kidney injury. He is fully ventilated, on 100% oxygen, PEEP 20 cmH$_2$O, and reverse ratio ventilation (1:1). Drug infusions include morphine 10 mg/hour, midazolam 10 mg/hour, atracurium 25 mg/hour, and noradrenaline 0.5 mcg/kg/minute. Prone positioning has been unsuccessfully attempted, and his gases continue to deteriorate. Currently they are:

pH	7.21
PaCO$_2$	8.75
PaO$_2$	7.15
HCO$_3^-$	16.2
SBE	-8.3

He is to be transferred to the regional unit for extracorporeal membrane oxygenation. Transfer time is estimated to be about one hour by emergency ambulance. You will accompany him during transfer.

Q1. List equipment, drugs and personnel that you consider will be needed for safe transfer. Include specific details (e.g. quantities of drugs, qualifications of personnel). Do you know where to locate all of the equipment on your unit?

Q2. Review the transfer proformas/documentation used on your unit. Which parts are and are not applicable to Mr Jones's transfer? What observations would you want to undertake during transfer, and how often would you take these?

Q3. From reading this chapter, what do you think are the six complications most likely to occur during transfer? How would you minimise these risks?

Q4. Reflect on transfers you have experienced, and those you have heard colleagues discuss. What problems occurred? How could you avoid similar problems occurring to you during future transfers?

Chapter 48

Professional perspectives

Contents

Fundamental knowledge

N.M.C. publications
Local hospital and unit policies/
    guidelines/patient group directions

Introduction

Every nurse is accountable for their own practice (N.M.C., 2015), but the ICU often heightens problems due to:

- the critical conditions of patients;
- the differing roles of ICU nurses (see Chapter 1);
- increased technology.

Nurses are often trusted to perform specialised tasks. But enthusiasm to develop skills should be tempered by considerations of safety. This chapter explores issues of what professional practice means, accountability of nurses, professional standards and civil law of negligence, issues affecting all registered nurses.

Professionalism necessitates accepting:

- autonomy
- accountability
- responsibility.

Nursing care should be in patients' best interests. Humans are fallible, so mistakes are inevitable. But risk management seeks to minimise mistakes by altering situations that contribute to error. Nurses should therefore report concerns about actual or potential risks. Where patients are endangered, a clinical incident form should be completed, which will be reviewed by the trust's clinical risk department.

In law, as in life, we are accountable both for what we do (acts) and for what we do not do (omissions). So conscious or unconscious decisions not to act may be called to account.

Professionals are individually accountable for their own practice (N.M.C., 2015), so should continue to develop professionally, updating skills and knowledge. Unfortunately, many employers under-invest in their nursing staff's development, forcing nurses to invest in themselves (Joshua-Amadi, 2002).

Time Out 1

Using a dictionary and other available resources, define accountability and responsibility. How far do the two overlap, or differ? Can one be present without the other? What does the N.M.C. *Code* have to say about them?

Accountability

Dimond (2015) identifies four arenas of professional accountability:

- criminal law;
- civil law;
- employer's contract;
- professional body (N.M.C.),
- adding that accountability between arenas may conflict.

For civil actions in *negligence* to succeed, three conditions must be met:

- a duty of care must exist;
- that duty of care must have been breached;
- resulting harm must have been reasonably foreseeable.

Civil cases failing to establish any one condition on the "balance of probabilities" cannot make a conviction. "Negligence" in different contexts, such as industrial tribunals or the N.M.C.'s Professional Conduct Committee, need not carry these same conditions.

While all four of Dimond's arenas can apply to nurses, conflicts with criminal law are rare. Few laws specifically mention nurses or nursing, so legal accountability and rights of nurses are usually the same as for any other citizen. Any individual suffering harm from another may sue that person through civil law; *negligence* and *assault with battery* are the charges most frequently brought against healthcare staff. Negligence is briefly outlined; nursing accountability through civil law is comprehensively covered in Dimond (2015).

A *duty of care* clearly exists to patients allocated to nurses' care. Breach of that care will usually form the basis of any case. So, any case reaching court almost certainly fulfils the first criterion. The condition least likely to be established is the third. There are two parts to this third condition:

- the breach of care must directly cause harm;
- the harm suffered must have been reasonably foreseeable.

If the *harm* may reasonably have been caused by other factors (judged by the balance of probabilities) links to breach of duty of care cannot be clearly established. Even where harm can be linked to breach of care, it may not be *reasonably foreseeable*: all drugs and treatments have adverse effects, and nurses should be aware of common effects of whatever they give, and recorded allergies of patients, but cannot reasonably know, or be held accountable for, every possible effect. As professional practitioners, nurses are expected to act with autonomy (N.M.C., undated), so decision-making requires sufficient knowledge to evaluate relative benefits and risks from possible actions and omissions ("reasonable" and "sufficient" might be evaluated by the "*Bolam*" test – see glossary). This places an onus on both individual nurses and their employers to maintain relevant knowledge and skills.

The first section, and clause, of the *Code* (N.M.C., 2015) is about prioritising people to "make their care and safety your main concern". Employers pay salaries, so nurses failing to satisfy employers' requirements may find themselves unemployed. Pragmatically, resisting the instructions of employers, managers or senior staff can prove difficult.

Employment contracts and expectations vary; breach of contract can lead to litigation, or more often dismissal. Although this chapter focuses on professional accountability (through the N.M.C.), readers should remember their concurrent accountability to other arenas. Patients, whether conscious or otherwise, have rights; the Mental Capacity Act, and its subsequent development through the Deprivation of Liberty Safeguards (DoLS), is discussed in Woodrow (2016). The law expects healthcare to act in patients' best interests, but sometimes interpreting what best interests are is problematic, especially when conditions or treatments render patients incapable of identifying their own wishes. Traditionally, life-saving treatments have been considered to be in patients' best interests, but the I.C.S. (2017b) states that life-saving treatment is unlawful if patients have capacity and refuse it, or have made an advance directive to this effect. Despite "DO NOT RESUSCITATE" being tattooed clearly on his chest, the team admitting an unknown, unconscious male with multiple co-morbidities to a US hospital initially decided to disregard the tattoo as its legal status was unclear (Holt *et al.*, 2017). Legal dilemmas can be complex, and there is not always time to seek legal guidance. Nurses have a duty to advocate for rights of patients, especially if patients lack capacity to assert their rights for themselves.

Accountability raises two main questions:

- what are the limits of accountability?
- how can conflicts of accountability be reconciled?

Limits of accountability

Individual accountability and professional autonomy may seem desirable ideals, but quality healthcare also relies on multidisciplinary teamwork (Mullally, 2001). Responsibility is inevitably partly shared between disciplines and members of the same discipline. Delegation of particular tasks vary between units and may vary within each unit depending on whoever is best able to perform that task at that time: endotracheal suction may be performed by anaesthetists intubating patients, and later by physiotherapists and nurses.

While only individuals on a professional register have professional accountability (i.e. can be removed from the professional register), in law each mentally competent adult remains legally accountable for their actions. Civil law precedent (*Nettleship v Weston*, 1971) establishes learner/student accountability, despite their inexperience or lack of knowledge (Dimond, 2015). Learners and junior staff may be individually sued if they cause harm, hence the importance of professional indemnity.

Local, national and international guidelines are widely available, including via the internet. Individual and local factors may affect applicability and appropriateness of guidelines to individual patient care. Guidelines, such as those from the National Clinical Institute for Clinical Excellence, are generally reliable, so failure to follow them could result in legal action (Samanta and Samanta, 2004). Apparently, authoritative guidelines can be legally overruled, as shown by *Burke v GMC* (2004), which overruled the 2002 B.M.A. guidelines on withdrawing treatment. Each nurse must individually decide whether (and, if so, how) they should perform tasks.

Conflicts of accountability

Few tasks are ascribed by law to particular professions (Cox, 2010), and the D.O.H. (2006) encourages extension of nursing practice.

In civil law, standards of care expected from qualified nurses are those of the ordinary skilled nurse ("*Bolam* test"). Failure to meet professional standards may also cause removal from the professional register. Where nursing roles are expanded to work previously performed by other professions (e.g. junior doctors), the standards expected are those of the other professions (Caplin-Davies, 1999). So, nurses have a professional duty to ensure they have adequate knowledge and skills to perform tasks they undertake.

Accountability in practice

Patient group directions (PGDs) are legally recognised prescriptions (D.O.H., 2000b), but made for patient groups rather than individual patients. They are agreed locally by relevant professions – usually doctors, nurses and pharmacists. Where both patients and nursing staff fulfil agreed criteria for each direction, nurses can give specified drugs. This facilitates prompt administration and may prevent complications caused by delay.

Complaints are a familiar aspect of contemporary healthcare. They highlight deficiencies in services provided and provide a conduit for public accountability, and may diffuse concerns that would otherwise end in litigation, but have unfortunately encouraged defensive nursing. A significant number of complaints result from failures of communication (Tingle, 2007); ironically, those least ill may complain most, so encouraging diversion of time away from those needing it most. Nurses have a professional duty to prioritise care (acts and omissions) so that actions can be justified.

Litigation consumes millions from the NHS budget – the 2015 NHS Litigation Authority (NHSLA, now renamed NHS Resolution) annual report identified net liabilities of £28.6 million. The 2017 report does not identify net liabilities but does identify a 15% increase in payment costs for clinical payments (NHS Resolution, 2017). Fear of litigation sometimes fosters an ethos of secrecy that conflicts with political rhetoric and professional philosophies of empowerment through providing information. Minimising litigation risks effectively creates substantial income generation but has the added human values of fostering trust between nurses and patients. Vicarious liability (employers being legally liable for actions of their employees, provided employees follow employers' policies (Cox, 2010)) has been made more robust through the Clinical Negligence Scheme for Trusts (CNST).

Record keeping

In addition to recording observations, nursing records should be detailed enough both to provide a basis for immediate care, and to provide information in the event of future enquiries. Records should be factual, as under the Freedom of Information Act (2001) individuals have the right to copies of records about them. Unfortunately, nursing documentation is often poor (Saranto and Kinnunen, 2009). Like any written records, nursing documentation may be used in a court of law; this does not make them "legal documents", but, unlike informal notes, nursing records require clear identification of date, time, patient and nurse. And, if care is not recorded, courts may assume that it was not given.

Implications for practice

- concerns should be reported. Where patient safety is compromised, clinical incident forms should be completed;
- guidelines are useful resources, but are not infallible and do not replace individual accountability;
- each nurse remains individually accountable for their actions;
- nurses should only undertake tasks if competent to do so, refusing any task they do not consider they can safely complete;
- nursing care should be prioritised by patients' best interests;
- each nurse is responsible to ensure adequate and current knowledge for their own practice;
- nurses should be familiar with local policies/procedures/guidelines/standards

Summary

Society's demands, and pace of change, are both likely to continue to increase. ICU nurses often respond positively to challenging and changing work, but enthusiasm should be tempered by considerations of safe practice and how far care meets the holistic needs of each patient. The human and financial costs of professional malpractice can be high for each nurse, employer and patient.

Further reading

Readers should be familiar with N.M.C. publications. Reading codes of other professions can be insightful (e.g. H.C.P.C., G.M.C.). Dimond (2015) remains the key text on nursing and the law, while Cox (2010) provides a useful summary of the issue.

Clinical questions

Q1. Identify areas of accountability and responsibility within the ICU. Reflect on the main areas of accountability in your practice while supervising novice ICU nurses.

Q2. A colleague has failed to attend consecutive mandatory training sessions for over three years, despite being rostered and given study leave. Identify who is accountable when this nurse makes an error in practice. How should this situation be managed to ensure professional accountability and vicarious liability? How far do competencies protect patients and/or nurses? How far do they inhibit care?

Q3. You administer a new trial drug which is currently unlicensed in the UK. The patient suffers associated adverse effects and dies. Who is accountable for the patient's death? What is your accountability in this situation – include factors such as your knowledge of drug administration, awareness of adverse effects, appropriateness of the drug.

Chapter 49

Managing the ICU

Contents

Introduction

Staff who have gained necessary bedside nursing experience and any required educational developments/qualifications may plan managerial experience as part of their professional development, or find one day they are the most senior person on duty (possibly due to sickness of senior staff) and so expected to manage the unit for that shift. This chapter provides a troubleshooting introduction for staff not normally in charge of their units (hence the direct address to readers).

There is noticeably little literature in ICU nursing journals advising staff how to develop management skills. As many staff are unlikely to resource management journals unless undertaking management courses, this consigns development of management skills to the "sitting with Nellie" ethos so antithetical to evidence-based nursing. Evidence and theory for nurse management is often, as here, drawn either from management outside healthcare, or about senior healthcare management, such as lead nurse and team leader roles. When specifically discussing nurse-in-charge of the shift, this chapter uses "shiftleader", reserving "managers" either for more senior managers, or from evidence about senior roles which may also be applicable to shiftleaders.

Time Out 1

Compare previous experience of management (professional or social) with how you have seen others manage the ICU where you work. Note down significant differences. Reflect on why these differences may be necessary. Note what you would do differently, and why.

Starting to manage

Each unit functions slightly differently, depending on its size, location, skill mix, patient groups, local traditions and other factors. Traditions, and so expectations of staff, can help guide shiftleaders, who should not be afraid of drawing on experience and views of others. Previous experiences – professional or social – may be transferable to managing the ICU.

Staff may look to shiftleaders (nurses in charge) for direction. Shiftleaders therefore need sufficient knowledge to provide information. Some information may be factual, some may be local requirements and expectations, but much will be sharing experience and ideas to help others make clinical decisions. There are often no right or wrong answers, just different ways of doing things. This chapter therefore raises issues that different readers may differ over. Options, rather than answers, are usually provided; these issues serve their purpose if they help readers clarify their own values.

A good shiftleader should be visible and accessible to staff, patients and relatives (I.C.S., 2013), enabling other people to do their work. This means providing clinical nursing leadership, supervision and support to teams to optimise safe standards of patient care on each shift (I.C.S., 2013). Drucker (1974) identifies five roles for managers:

- setting objectives;
- organising;
- motivating and communicating;
- measuring targets;
- developing people, including themselves.

Shiftleaders should establish constructive working conditions at the start of each shift, enabling development of staff members' individual strengths and skills while recognising individual needs and limitations. Managers should individually assess and proactively plan and respond to needs for each shift, rather than seek to impose their own agendas on staff.

You may remember most patients from your previous shift; if not, briefly assess patients before taking handover. You may need to walk through your unit to take handover, but if not a brief look at the unit can suggest both the number and dependency of patients. Many units have data sheets providing brief synopses of patients.

Managers rely on their staff to achieve the work, so staff are the shiftleader's most important resource. Staff numbers are important – are there enough staff for patients already on the unit and expected/potential admissions? Staffing levels were discussed in Chapter 1, although the ratios 1:1 for Level 3 patients and 1:2 for Level 2 patients reflect medical acuity rather than nursing workload. But abilities and qualities of staff are also important. "Skill mix" is more than simply counting numbers of staff at each grade. Some staff need more support than others; each has different experience, knowledge and skills to draw on. Most staff will probably be known to you, so scanning the off-duty roster helps your planning; with new or unfamiliar staff (e.g. temporary) you may gain insight into their qualities by asking about their experience and what they feel able and not able to do.

Allocating staff may be guided by managerial structures, such as teams. Specific allocation should consider:

- maintaining patient safety;
- optimising patient treatment, including continuity of care;
- developing and supporting staff.

Larger units, or those with challenging layouts, may need one or more deputy leaders.

Safety during break cover should also be considered: two junior nurses may safely manage adjacent patients when both are present but become unsafe if caring for two patients through covering each other's breaks. Nurse managers remain accountable for their actions; unsafe allocation breaches the *Code* (N.M.C., 2015).

The Health and Safety at Work Act (HM Government, 1974) places specific requirements on managers (and employees) to ensure workplaces are safe; shiftleaders also have wider moral responsibilities for health and safety of their staff and patients. Fire exits should remain clear and accessible at all times and safety and emergency equipment should be in complete and in working order. Emergency equipment varies between units, but may include the resuscitation trolley, intubation trolley and (on cardiothoracic units) thoracotomy pack. Any environmental hazards should be minimised, and where possible removed.

Shiftleaders are responsible for all patients on their unit, even if some responsibilities are devolved to team/area subleaders. Following handover, shiftleaders should visit each patient to make their own assessment, identify needs of each bedside nurse, and pass on any relevant additional information/ expectations. Allow sufficient time for bedside nurses to take individual handovers, complete their own safety checks and make their own patient assessment; seeking information before bedside nurses can fully assimilate it creates stress for the nurse without providing information for shiftleaders. Looking through each patient's notes gives bedside nurses time to complete initial assessment and checks, while giving shiftleaders information that may have been missed in handover. Relevant aspects should then be passed on to the bedside nurse.

Shiftleaders should ensure imminent shifts are adequately covered: check staff numbers and initiate booking of any additional staff required. Numbers of staff needed for each shift may vary with:

- number, location and dependency of patients;
- skill mix of other staff;
- anticipated specific needs, such as transfer or procedures.

Other services (e.g. equipment suppliers/repair) may also need to be contacted.

Shiftleaders may have to assume direct patient care, but this causes role conflict between responsibility to the whole unit as shiftleader and individual responsibility to your patient, and limits your availability to other members of staff. The experience of many nurses in charge who also assume direct patient care is that their patient tends to get neglected. I.C.S. (2013) standards state that shiftleader should be supernumerary. It may be reasonable to allocate two patients to one member of staff; the appropriateness or otherwise of assuming direct patient care necessarily remains an individual decision, based on resources available, and remembering that you remain accountable for whatever decision you make.

Endacott (1999) identifies four key aspects of shift leadership:

- presence (availability);
- information gathering (from bedside nurses);

- supportive involvement (e.g. fetching equipment, checking drugs, reassuring staff);
- direct involvement (taking over from bedside nurses when they are away or unable to cope).

Shiftleaders may also co-ordinate services, contacting other people/departments or liaising with staff on the unit. Shiftleaders should be present during ward rounds so that they are aware of current plans, can contribute to discussion, support staff and co-ordinate activity. Shiftleaders need to maintain clinical skills and credibility; with career progression and increasing management duties, staff may need to identify shifts when they assume direct patient care without unit management responsibilities.

The shiftleader's role can therefore be very demanding. The busyness of most units, together with limited staffing resources, may mean that ideals are not always met; crisis management is often unavoidable. Like bedside nurses, shiftleaders should therefore prioritise their workload, aiming to achieve as much as they reasonably can in the time given. Shiftleaders, like bedside nurses, often work unpaid overtime to complete their work. While the motivation for this is understandable, it is morally questionable and arguably provides an unhealthy example for other staff. Shiftleaders should therefore aim to ensure they, and their staff, leave the unit as near to the end of paid time as reasonably possible.

Morale

Shiftleaders are responsible for enabling others to achieve their work, so should motivate and communicate (Drucker, 1974). Nursing demands high levels of cognitive, affective and psychomotor skills, so the ability of staff to realise their potential is affected by morale. Maintaining staff and unit morale is therefore a management priority (Joshua-Amadi, 2002; Erlen, 2004) – loyal staff are more likely to support shiftleaders during crises. Lack of support is frequently cited as a reason for staff leaving (Hayward et al., 2016).

Historically, management theory often contrasts styles of leadership as authoritarian, laissez-faire and democratic. Democratic or authoritarian leaders use their power and authority to achieve goals and objectives (Firth-Cozens and Mowbray, 2001). The traditional authoritarian ethos of healthcare has arguably been increasingly replaced by promoting democratic involvement and autonomy. For example, "blame" cultures should be replaced by "safety", where mistakes are openly acknowledged ("duty of candour") to enable learning (Hunt, 2016). People make mistakes; increased emphasis on recognising human factors encourages acknowledgement of error through a "no blame culture". Nearly half of errors identified in NAP4 (Cook et al., 2011), the National Audit Project report on airway management, were from human factors These are not new ideas – they surfaced in D.O.H. 2000c, N.P.S.A. 2008, and the Francis (2013) report. Garrouste-Orgeas et al. (2016) suggest that this is seeking "why" rather than "who". Despite the rhetoric, many long-standing problems and pressures limit the effectiveness of cultural change in the NHS (Hignett *et al.*, 2016), and it is questionable how far blame can, or should, be eliminated (Peerally *et al.*, 2017).

Increasing recognition that managers cannot achieve their goals without the assistance of their staff has led to "transformational" leadership to engage and empower staff (Fischer, 2017). Based on work by Bass, Lavoie-Trembla *et al.* (2015) suggest that there are four aspects to transformational leadership:

- idealised influence –acting as role models;
- inspirational motivation – supplying a vision for the team;
- intellectual stimulation – encouraging staff to think creatively;
- individualised consideration – showing concern for needs and feelings of others, providing positive individualised feedback.

Fischer also suggests that leaders can be informal, not necessarily people appointed to management roles, making it compatible with the Humanist philosophy outlined in Chapter 2.

Different styles of management may be appropriate in different situations. For example, authoritarianism is usually the most useful way to manage a cardiac arrest.

Time Out 2

Reflect on the different styles of management you have witnessed and experienced. Make one list of benefits of the style, and another of problems it did or could have caused.

Well-being

People respond to the way they are treated, and this applies as much to staff as patients. Shiftleaders therefore need good interpersonal skills and respect for their staff. They should seek to empower and value their staff. Staff who are actively involved are likely to provide better care, so negotiation is a core management skill. But shiftleaders also have a professional duty to maintain standards. If they observe unsatisfactory practices they should approach staff constructively, identifying why staff are acting that way (rationale, knowledge base), treating incidents as developmental learning opportunities rather than belittling and humiliating experiences for the junior nurse (or possibly shiftleader). If patient safety is compromised, shiftleaders may need to act before discussion.

Breaks from work provide a psychological coping mechanism. European working time regulations are prescriptive about working time, including the right to 20-minute breaks every six hours. Delayed, compromised or missed breaks often cause dissatisfaction, so ensuring smooth (and safe) organisation of breaks for staff is an important managerial duty. Organising break relief varies between units and shifts; where units have a system that works and is familiar to staff, this should be followed. Shiftleaders may need to assume some direct patient responsibilities to cover breaks; this can also provide shiftleaders with valuable opportunities to assess patients, and the nurse's skills and needs. Possible conflicts with managerial duties (above) should be considered, especially if relieving for breaks in inaccessible areas (e.g. side rooms). Shiftleaders should also ensure they have breaks themselves, as (like their staff) they are less likely to be able to function effectively without reasonable breaks.

Ideally, staff should take breaks away from their workspace, but busy shifts may sometimes prevent this. If full breaks cannot be taken, providing refreshments within the clinical area (this task could be delegated) may help staff function safely, and maintain morale. If this creates concerns about infection control or professional appearance, these may be able to be provided away from the immediate bedside. Staff needing breaks are likely to function inefficiently, give less empathy to others and be more difficult to motivate.

When situations are particularly stressful, shiftleaders may be able to support staff by offering additional "stress breaks", making themselves (and other experienced staff) available when necessary, and by acknowledging the stress of the situation.

ICU work is unpredictable; workload sometimes exceeding resources, so shiftleaders and staff should identify priorities, accepting that some lesser priorities are not always achieved. Shiftleaders unable to offer ideal support to staff can still build team rapport and loyalty by acknowledging others' stress.

Extreme stress can result in "burnout", a syndrome causing psychological ill health to the sufferer, increased rates of attrition, and poorer quality of care (Moss *et al.*, 2016). Moss *et al.* suggest that symptoms of burnout include:

Psychological	Physical
frustration	exhaustion/fatigue
anger	insomnia
fear	muscle tension
anxiety	headache
inability to feel happy	GI problems
being unprofessional	
feeling overwhelmed	
disillusionment	
hopelessness	
lack of empathy	
feeling insufficient at work	

Anyone noticing symptoms such as these, whether in themselves, colleagues, or staff they manage, should recognise burnout for what it is and seek ways to support and help the individual.

481

Staffing levels

Staff levels should be individualised to patient/unit needs, although there are recommended minimum staffing levels – see Chapter 1. If shiftleaders consider unit, patient or staff safety is compromised through inadequate staff (or any other problem they are unable to resolve), they should inform senior managers, who have (higher) responsibility for the unit. Concerns should be documented.

During the shift

Shiftleaders who have established mechanisms for staff to work effectively have achieved their most important role, but throughout the remainder of the shift they should ensure the unit continues to run smoothly, solving problems as they occur and providing a resource (knowledge, experience) for and support to more junior staff.

Staff need to feel confidence in their shiftleader. While shiftleaders usually have more experience and knowledge than their staff, each member of staff has the potential to contribute knowledge, experience or values, and shiftleaders should be prepared to learn from, as well as guide and teach, their staff. Like all nurses, shiftleaders should acknowledge limits to their own knowledge and competence (N.M.C., 2015).

Staff need to feel confident that they can approach their shiftleader, so shiftleaders should show positive attitudes and remain accessible, including spending most of their time in the main patient care area.

Shiftleaders are a link between unit nurses and other hospital staff, facilitating active involvement of bedside nurses in ward rounds (Manias and Street, 2001). If medical review of patients does not involve bedside nurses, shiftleaders often become links between medical and nursing staff. Similarly, information to/from other hospital departments or telephone messages from family members are often ciphered through the nurse-in-charge. Promoting interprofessional communication improves care (Rose, 2011).

Shiftleaders may be pressurised to accept patients because there is an empty bed, because there appear to be enough staff or because patients need ICU. Rationing is an unfortunate reality of healthcare, and, when an "ultimate" area such as ICU is involved, pressures cannot always be relieved by admission to other wards. While medical staff must decide whether patients require ICU admission, shiftleaders must decide whether patients can be safely nursed on the unit. This decision includes:

- imminent shifts;
- dependency of patients already on the unit;
- skills of staff available.

Shiftleaders are professionally accountable for decisions about managing nursing on the unit, but faced with coercion or moral blackmail may need considerable skills in assertiveness.

Devolvement of budgets has inevitably led to shiftleaders having both financial authority and responsibilities. At early stages of management experience, these are likely to be deferred to more senior staff, but as you develop your management skills these will increasingly become part of your role. It is therefore valuable to discuss these with your nurse manager/mentor.

Good shiftleaders may inspire loyalty in their staff, but being in charge can isolate shiftleaders from other support mechanisms.

Time Out 3

Using the cues below, jot down plans for your professional development over the next six months. Aims may be clinical, educational and professional. Be realistic, setting sufficient aims to help you develop, but not too many to achieve (six aims is often a reasonable target, but the number and scope vary between individuals). You may wish to share all or part of this with your manager/mentor/colleagues or retain this as a private document in your professional profile. You may wish to divide aims between short-term (a few weeks), medium-term (up to six months) and long-term (after six months), or cover all aims together. Long-term aims will not be achieved fully by your six-month review, but you may have partially progressed towards them. You will probably find setting target dates for achieving aims helpful.

- Over the next six months I would like to achieve (include target times):
- I would like to achieve these because:
- To achieve these I will need (include people and resources):
- I will know I have achieved these aims because (i.e. evaluation):
- Possible problems I anticipate for myself/others:
- Ways to minimise these problems:

Implications for practice

- staff who have met minimum criteria to manage their unit should plan a structure to develop their skills before they find themselves unexpectedly in charge;
- shiftleaders should enable their staff to work safely, efficiently and effectively;
- shiftleaders rely on their staff, so should encourage morale and meet the needs of their staff (professional development, support, breaks);

483

■ shiftleaders should co-ordinate unit activity, so participate in decision-making, both during and between ward rounds;

■ shiftleaders should recognise potential role conflicts and priorities;

■ nurse shiftleaders, like all qualified nurses, are professionally accountable for their decisions and actions.

Summary

This chapter has considered some of the practical issues for ICU nurses who are beginning to develop their management skills. Much has been written elsewhere on wider management issues and theory; nurses developing management careers may need to develop this knowledge further but should first gain practical management skills through structured experiential programmes. Shiftleaders are morally and professionally responsible and accountable for their managerial decisions.

Further reading

Shiftleaders should be familiar with local policies and guidelines. Practising being in charge is probably more valuable than reading about it, especially as little literature on management is written by nurses, and rarely specifically about healthcare. Drucker (e.g. 1974) is an influential management theorist. Literature on nursing management is rarely ICU-specific, but the Intensive Care Society standards (2013) provide comprehensive guidance. The Clinical Human Factors Group has a useful website: www.chfg.org.

Clinical scenario

A patient's next of kin requests a change of nurse, citing a personal characteristic of the nurse which has caused them a loss of confidence.

Q1. As the nurse-in-charge, how would you manage the situation? Justify your actions.

Q2. Reflect on how you would feel if you were the nurse identified. How would you feel if the allocation were changed? How would you feel if expected to continue to care for the patient?

Q3. What implications would there be if the patient lacked capacity or were a child/adolescent?

Chapter 50

Costs of intensive care

Contents

Introduction

Critical illness entails high costs and significant mortality (Crunden, 2010). Mortality and morbidity are higher than with less advanced disease; emotional costs to patients, relatives and staff are also significant. Finite resources, and increasing financial pressures, result in financial costs affecting care – a tyranny of budgets. Costs per patient day in ICU can vary greatly depending on need, but I.C.S. (2015) cites English 2006 averages of £1,647 and Welsh 2012 averages of £1,932 for Level 3 patients. The high financial costs of the ICU inevitably invite scrutiny, such as the introduction of tariffs into the UK's National Health Service, intended to improve quality and productivity (D.O.H., 2009a). Increasing financial pressures are paralleled by increasingly higher public and political expectations. Demand for ICU beds is increasing by about 2.5% each year (Beeknoo and Jones, 2016). For some, healthcare spending is an "unsustainable burden accompanied by waste, overuse, care delays, and other delivery inefficiencies" (Nates *et al.*, 2016), but Dunn *et al.* (2016) consider that the NHS is "buckling under the strain of huge financial and operational pressure". Nursing, and nurses, must therefore assert their financial value in the marketplace of healthcare. While financial costs may have some objectivity, subjectivity surrounds human costs. Having reached the end of this book, nurses developing their ICU careers should be grappling with these questions:

- What price intensive care?
- Are the costs of treating critical illness justifiable from financial, humanitarian and/or moral/ethical perspectives?
- Are the costs of nurses and nursing justifiable?

Spending on health

Workforce accounts for just under half of NHS costs (Dunn *et al.*, 2016), and nurses are the largest single group of workers in health services (Büscher *et al.*, 2009; Buchan *et al.*, 2015). The ICU is labour-intensive and expensive. Successful cures of simpler pathologies (e.g. single organ failure) have created more complex pathologies (e.g. MODS), which increase both cost per patient day and length of stay. Increasingly complex and expensive technology and drugs further strain budgets. ICU budgets may subsidise other departments by providing support services such as Outreach and programmes for high-dependency care. Financial stringencies often encourage budget holders to reduce staff, but this may prove a short-term financial saving with long-term costs. Reducing ICU nurse-to-patient ratios:

- delays weaning from ventilation;
- increases nosocomial infection;
- increase readmission to ICU;
- increases medication errors;
- increase length of ICU patient episodes.

(EfCCNa, 2007)

Treating patients who do not survive costs more than treating patients who do (Vedio *et al.*, 2000), and prolonging dying is cruel. Predicting survival could therefore reduce humanitarian and financial burdens of ICU but raises ethical concerns about reliability and "playing God".

Costs and performance of units, and their staff, is scrutinised closely. Poor-quality critical care may increase financial costs, morbidity and mortality (Davoudian and Blunt, 2009). While external scrutiny is almost inevitable, internal scrutiny can help improve efficiency and effectiveness. There are many ways units can review their effectiveness, including:

- audit;
- mortality and morbidity meetings (Ksouri *et al.*, 2010);
- case review.

Whatever means used, multidisciplinary involvement is beneficial.

While there are pressures on healthcare systems worldwide, the UK spends 9.4% of GDP (gross domestic product) on the NHS, less than is spent on health in the USA or average European Union spending (Beeknoo and Jones, 2016).

Scoring critical illness

There are various scoring systems, mostly developed for medical audit. Audit can help staff learn from experience, and inappropriate admission to ICU can cause excessive and unnecessary human suffering, but applying retrospective audit tools to prospective prediction may create dilemmas. While these tools measure survival in different patient groups, they are poor predictors of outcomes for individual patients, and they often fail to measure morbidity (Ethics Committee of the Society of Critical Care Medicine, 1997; Davoudian and Blunt, 2009). This echoes nursing debate around quality against quantity of life.

The Acute Physiology and Chronic Health Evaluation (*APACHE*) is the most widely used scoring system in ICUs; APACHE II is the version generally used, although a fourth version (Zimmerman *et al.*, 2006) exists – less often used as it is not in the public domain, and so entails costs. It aims to measure/predict mortality. Its design is not too dissimilar to the Waterlow pressure scoring system. Other scoring systems used include:

- SAPS II;
- Health-Related Quality of Life (HRQL);
- Intensive Care National Audit and Research Centre (ICNARC) model.

SAPS II also aims to predict mortality, but Khwannimit and Bhurayanon-tachai (2009) found the customised APACHE II to be more reliable than customised SAPS II. Short-term ICU outcomes are usually measured by survival and discharge, but HRQL scores can measure longer-term morbidity (Lim *et al.*, 2016; McKinley *et al.*, 2016), which has received increasing attention in recent years (see Chapter 3).

Mortality

ICU mortality rates vary, depending on speciality and local factors, but Vincent *et al.*'s (2009) figure of nearly one fifth reflects most reports and probably most units. In the past, statistics generally measured to ICU discharge. N.I.C.E. (2009) suggests that three quarters of ICU patients survive to discharge home, which means that one quarter do not.

Reductions in mortality rates (Hutchins *et al.*, 2009) may reflect improvements in treatments and practice, but may also reflect increasing numbers of patients admitted for Level 2 care. Timely admission to ICU, often facilitated through Critical Care Outreach, can be life-saving. More than half of adverse events occurring within 72 hours of ICU discharge are preventable, involving problems such as poor fluid management (McLaughlin *et al.*, 2007). Improving communication for handover can therefore help reduce morbidity and mortality.

While admission to ICU should be limited to patients who can potentially benefit from it – critically ill patients who have potentially reversible conditions – treatment is not always successful, which risks prolonging death rather than life. When it seems unlikely that conditions can reasonably be reversed, treatment is usually withdrawn to enable dignified death. Most deaths in ICU follow withdrawal of treatment (Meissner *et al.*, 2010), although incidence and practice vary greatly (Azoulay *et al.*, 2009). Experience may suggest interventions are futile, but predictions are based on balancing probabilities rather than absolute certainties; US guidelines recommend describing such interventions as "potentially inappropriate" rather than "futile" (Bosslet *et al.*, 2015). Readers may have occasionally seen "miracle" recoveries, but prolonging suffering for many for the benefit of a small minority is ethically dubious. Decisions to withdraw should therefore be team decisions.

Timmers *et al.* (2011) found that surgical ICU patients had impaired quality of life outcomes, although mortality and morbidity data need to be treated with caution as profiles of diseases, treatments and ICU patients change, and comparing ICU patients with their generational cohorts ignores the fact that people are in hospital because they are ill. More aggressive treatments can often offer older patients more favourable outcomes, but admitting more patients towards the end of their natural life-spans inevitably incurs higher short-term mortality and morbidity. Older data therefore becomes problematic to transfer to current practice, or to compare trends with more recent data.

Morbidity

Quality of life is widely cited, but interpreting quality is subjective. Most ICU patients suffer significant physiological limitations/weakness and psychological problems months after discharge (McKinley *et al.*, 2016). Post-traumatic stress disorder is common following ICU admission (see Chapter 3), only a minority resuming normal work (N.I.C.E., 2009). While antipsychotic drugs may be useful, nurses should also consider all the non-pharmacological approaches (e.g. reducing sensory imbalance – see Chapter 3) that can reduce/prevent post-discharge psychosis.

Prolonged ICU stay (> 48 hours) results in higher mortality (Laupland *et al.*, 2006) and morbidity in survivors (Hofhuis *et al.*, 2008b; Unroe *et al.*, 2010). Prompt ICU discharge therefore appears beneficial. But discharge during the night increases mortality and morbidity (Yang *et al.*, 2016), perhaps due to discharge being premature, or perhaps due to limited assessment and monitoring on wards overnight (I.C.S., 2015). If nurses are to be advocates for their patients (Williams *et al.*, 2016), they should voice concerns whenever they consider discharge to be premature.

Handover, and especially handover documentation, from ICU to ward staff can reduce adverse events following ICU discharge (Chaboyer *et al.*, 2008). Chaboyer found the three main adverse events were:

- healthcare-associated infection/sepsis;
- accident or injury;
- other complications (e.g. deep-vein thrombosis, pulmonary oedema, myocardial infarction).

While critical illness incurs some mortality and morbidity, avoidable mortality and morbidity does occur, and can be reduced by multidisciplinary review/audit/case conferences (Ksouri *et al.*, 2010), which provide an opportunity to learn from experience and change practices.

Bed occupancy

In the UK many adult ICUs average 80–85% bed occupancy, which given the peaks and troughs inevitably results in frequent 100% bed occupancy (Beeknoo and Jones, 2016). This places pressures of staff, especially if the numbers of beds actually on the unit exceed numbers of funded beds. It also increases risks of infection and errors. In part, problems reflect reduction of beds within hospitals, resulting in delayed discharges from ICU. Beeknoo and Jones (2016) call for more flexible use of resources by creating larger, centralised ICUs. To meet demand, ICUs sometimes create extra beds in auxiliary areas such as theatre recovery, but this creates risks for patients and staff that should be documented through incident reporting.

Litigation

When harm is suffered, people usually have a legal right to compensation. While the morality of this is understandable, and generally laudable, escalation of litigation costs in the NHS is expensive, diverting much-needed resources from clinical care and engendering a culture of defensive practice. More than one quarter of ICU-related litigation costs between 1995 and 2012 involved positioning, skincare and nursing standards (Pascall *et al.*, 2015).

Nursing

Within the relatively few decades intensive care units have existed, nursing and nursing roles have changed dramatically. Nurses have adopted increasingly complex technical skills, especially in areas such as the ICU. New roles have developed, such as advanced practitioners. While such roles emerge from aims to reduce costs while improving quality (W.H.O., 2009), and individual motivation may be more important than formal roles/titles for improving quality of nursing care, new roles do provide opportunities for nurses to develop nursing practice, and to justify the costs of nursing. Individually, nurses should proactively constantly seek to improve their own practice. Collectively, nurses should seek to advance the value of nursing within their own area of practice. Continuing expansion of roles is likely, and probably desirable, although must be tempered if they risk compromising individuals' health (e.g. sickness, "burnout") and quality of care. The last two decades have seen accumulating evidence that ensuring adequate numbers of nurses reduces patient mortality (e.g. Needleman *et al.*, 2011; Aiken *et al.*, 2014).

Implications for practice

- costs involve both financial and human aspects; human costs are subjective, including debatable issues such as quality of life, but are fundamentally central to nursing values;
- medical outcome scoring systems are available, but predictive reliability for individuals is debated, so rationing by scoring systems is ethically questionable;
- post-discharge follow-up can reduce psychological costs for patients and identify areas of nursing practice needing development. Critical Care Outreach teams can often provide units with valuable insights from former patients;
- multidisciplinary case conferences, audit and/or mortality and morbidity meetings provide a valuable means to learn from avoidable mortality/morbidity, and to change practices;
- nurses and nursing are valuable within ICU; quality nursing can reduce financial, emotional, mortality and morbidity costs of critical illness.

Summary

This final chapter has revisited issues raised at the start of this book:

- What fundamentally are we doing for our patients?
- What should we be doing?
- And how should we be doing it?

There are many possible answers to these questions; discussion in other chapters should have developed readers' awareness of these in everyday practice.

As professionals, ICU nurses need to evaluate both financial and humanitarian costs of intensive care to determine its ultimate value. Too often, it seems as though healthcare is resourced down to a price rather than up to a standard. Lack of strategic planning in the UK (Marangozo *et al.*, 2016), together with a chronically grossly underfunded and bureaucratic NHS, can provoke local enthusiasm to cut costs through false economies. In 2015/16 NHS provider deficits reached an all-time high of £2.45 billion (Kings Fund, 2016). Cheapest is not always best, and nurse advocacy may include resisting inappropriate and dangerous decisions at all levels. Attempts to equate financial with humanitarian (morbidity) costs may help nurses justify their value, but also create the danger that (to adapt Oscar Wilde) we know the price of everything but the value of nothing.

Further reading

N.I.C.E. (2009) provides valuable insights into and guidance about rehabilitation after critical illness. In the wake of demise of the Liverpool Care Pathway, a number of national reports, such as C.Q.C. (2016), have promoted humane perspectives. Professional groups such as the Intensive Care Society publish documents about many aspects of the ICU, their 2015 guidelines being a key document.

Clinical questions

Q1. List the positive benefits of the critical care process and categorise these into:

a) benefits to patients;
b) benefits to friends and family;
c) benefits to health practitioners;
d) benefits to society and the public.

Q2. What data does your unit have about costs? Audit staff/ICNARC co-ordinators may be able to provide specific information regarding staff costs, treatments, disposables, and resources. What recruitment costs were incurred over the last 12 months? What is the local cost for study leave/mandatory training and temporary staff?

Q3. List practical strategies, which can be implemented by ICU nurses, to improve quality of life for ICU patients following discharge both from the unit and the hospital. What resources does your unit, including Critical Care Outreach, have for supporting patients after discharge? Include any advice sheets and intranet resources.

Glossary

abdominal compartment syndrome IAP ≥ 20 mmHg + organ failure not previously present

allograft transplant tissue from the same species (e.g. cadaver heart valves)

anabolism building up

anacrotic notch abnormal notch occurring on arterial blood pressure traces before the main pressure peak

anion negatively charged ion

anthropometry measurement of body weight using relationships between height, weight and size

anxiolysis removing ("breakdown" of) anxiety

arterial tonometry a non-invasive means of continuously measuring arterial pressure

atelectasis collapse of alveoli

autologous from the same individual (e.g. autologous blood = patients' own blood)

autologous transfusion transfusion of patients' own blood

balloon tamponade inflation of balloon-tipped catheters (e.g. Minnesota tube) places direct pressure on bleeding points, so can stop internal bleeding in the same way nurses use digital pressure to stop bleeding after arterial lines are removed

barotrauma damage to alveoli from excessively high (peak) airway pressure

Beta (β) lactam class of antibiotics (e.g. ceftazidime, penicillin)

blepharitis inflammation of eyelash follicles and sebaceous glands

Böhr effect carbon dioxide and hydrogen reduce affinity of oxygen for haemoglobin, so acidosis increases dissociation

***Bolam* test**   case law precedent establishing that practitioners were not guilty of negligence if their practice conformed to that of a reasonable body of opinion held by practitioners skilled in the area of question

bradycardia   heart rate below 60 beats per minute

bruxia   jaw-clenching

calorie (cal, c)   amount of heat needed to raise one gram of water 1°C at atmospheric pressure (= small calorie)

Calorie (Cal, C)   amount of heat needed to raise one kilogram of water 1°C at atmospheric pressure (= large calorie, kilocalorie)

capillary occlusion pressure   the pressure at which capillary flow will be prevented, resulting in ischaemia, anaerobic metabolism and (eventually) infarction of tissue (e.g. pressure sore formation)

catabolism   breaking down

cation   positively charged ion

chemotaxis   movement of cell/organism to/from chemical substance

chronotrope   (*chronos* = time) affecting heart rate. Positive chronotropes (e.g. atropine) increase heart rate. Negative chronotropes (e.g. beta-blockers) reduce heart rate. Inotropes are usually also chronotropic

circadian rhythm   the "body clock", an endogenous rhythm around the day. Normal circadian rhythm lasts about 24 hours, but abnormal rhythms can take longer or shorter. Circadian rhythm affects various endogenous hormone levels, so disturbed circadian rhythm results in various abnormal body responses (e.g. wakefulness at night)

coagulopathies   disorders (pathologies) of clotting, such as DIC, sickle cell anaemia

colloid osmotic pressure   the osmotic pressure created by large molecules (e.g. proteins) that retain plasma in the intravascular space. Fluids with high colloid osmotic pressures therefore assist return of extravascular fluid (oedema) into the bloodstream

commensal   endogenous bacteria helping normal human functions

complements   plasma proteins (produced in the liver), which facilitate phagocytosis

coning   see tentorial herniation

Cori cycle   glycolysis in contracting muscles produces lactate, which the liver normally converts back into glucose, enabling further glycolysis-induced lactate

CABG   coronary artery bypass grafts

creatine kinase (CK)   enzyme release with skeletal and cardiac muscle injury. Pathology Harmony normal ranges 40–320 (male) and 25–200 (female) units/litre

Cullen's sign   irregular, bluish-purple discolouration around umbilicus

cytokines   chemical mediators of inflammatory and immune processes, including tumour necrosis factor alpha (TNFα) and interleukins

daltons (Da)   molecular weight

D-dimer   fibrinolysis product used to measure clotting

dead space   the space between air/gas mix and alveoli; physiological adult dead space is about 150 ml; on ventilators dead space extends from the Y connector to alveoli

depolarisation   reduction of membrane potential to a less negative value

dialysate   fluid used for dialysis

dialysis   movement of solutes through semipermeable membranes by a concentration gradient, so greater differences in concentrations result in faster movement

dicrotic notch   the notch normally seen on downstrokes of arterial waveforms, representing closure of the aortic valve, which causes transient slight increases in pressure

diffuse axonal injury   widespread injury caused by shearing forces, usually from rotational acceleration (e.g. road traffic accidents)

diffusion   movement of molecules from an area of higher concentration to an area of lower concentration

eicosanoids   fatty acid

ejection fraction   stroke volume as a fraction of ventricular blood volume. Normal left ventricular ejection fraction is > 50% or more, but dysfunctional ventricles (e.g. myocardial infarction) eject less. Figures inversely indicate extent of myocardial damage

endogenous   inside the person

endoleak   continued blood flow through aneurysm sac around repair/stent

erythropoiesis   production of erythrocytes (red blood cells)

exogenous   from outside the person

flow monitoring   monitoring of cardiovascular flow, previously called "cardiac output studies"

Frank–Starling law   the force exerted during each heartbeat is directly proportional to the length or degree of myocardial fibre stretch; so increasing fibre length (e.g. with positive inotropes) increases stroke volume

free radicals   atoms with one or more unpaired electron in their outer orbit; this makes them inherently unstable, so they react readily with other molecules to pair the free electron

glycolysis   breakdown of glucose

glycosides   carbohydrates that when hydrolysed produce a sugar and a non-sugar. Digoxin is a cardiac glycoside

glycosuria   sugar in urine; blood sugar is filtered by the kidney, but normally is all reabsorbed. When blood sugar exceeds 11 mmol/litre, renal tubules are unable to reabsorb all the sugar (Gerich. 2010). As glucose creates high osmotic pressure, the tubules also reabsorb less water, resulting in polyuria

gravid   pregnancy (e.g. primigravida = first pregnancy)

Grey Turner's sign   bluish-purple discolouration of flanks, indicated acute haemorrhagic pancreatitis

Haldane effect   a rise in oxyhaemoglobin shifts the carbon dioxide dissociation curve to right

half-life   time taken a chemical to lose half of its active effect

Hertz   SI unit of frequency, = one cycle/second

heterotopic   graft into different site

hyper-   high

hypercalcaemia   high serum calcium (normal whole blood level: 2.2–2.6 mmol/litre; normal ionised level 1.0–1.5 mmol/litre – see Chapter 21)

hyperchloraemia   high blood chloride (normal = 95–108 mmol/litre)

hyperglycaemia   high serum glucose

hyperkalaemia   high serum potassium (normal serum levels are 3.5–5.3 mmol/litre)

hypernatraemia   high serum sodium (normal: 133–146 mmol/litre)

hypo-   low

hysteresis   literally, the difference between two phenomena; medically, usually refers to lung differences between inspiration and expiration (pressure/volume curve), where passive elastic recoil allows greater volume in relation to airway pressure during expiration than during inspiration; so manipulating I:E ratio also manipulates mean airway pressure

interleukin   see Chapter 24

isothermic saturation boundary   where 100% relative humidity is reached at 37°C; normally (in adults) just below the carina

joule   a unit to measure energy (= 10^7 ergs or 1 watt second)

keratitis   inflammation of the cornea

keratopathy   non-inflammatory corneal disease

kilocalorie   amount of heat needed to raise one kilogram of water 1°C at atmospheric pressure (= Calorie, C)

kiloDaltons   1000 daltons (Da) = 1 kDa; a unit of molecular weight

kilojoule   1000 joules

Krebs' cycle   (citric acid cycle) a chain of intracellular chemical reactions to metabolise fat for energy. Krebs' cycle is efficient at energy (adenosine triphosphate) production, but produces metabolic wastes (acids, ketones, carbon dioxide, water). See Chapter 9

Kussmaul respiration   deep, rapid, sighing type of breath, caused by ketones, so associated with diabetic ketoacidosis

leukotriene   released by leukocytes; increases capillary "leak"

lipolysis   breakdown of fat

Marfan's syndrome   hereditary connective tissue disorder; symptoms include elongation of limbs and aortic aneurysms

microcirculation   capillaries

millimole   unit for measuring chemicals; 1 mole = relative atomic mass in grams of each element

mitochondria   (single: mitochondrion) organelles within cytoplasm that produce cell energy by glycolysis (combustion of glucose with oxygen); often called the "powerhouse" of the cell

monoclonal antibodies   antibodies (B leukocytes) that have been cloned (in a laboratory) from a single genetic strand, so each monoclonal antibody is identical and specific to a particular antigen

myocytes   cardiac muscle cells

neuromuscular blockade   (chemical) paralysis

nitric oxide   endogenous vasodilator

nosocomial infection   an infection acquired in hospital (technically, at least 22 hours following admission)

oncotic   osmotic pressure of colloids in solution

orthotropic   tissue graft being placed in its normal anatomical position

osmolarity   number of dissolved particles per litre of solution

osmosis   movement of a pure solute (e.g. water) through semipermeable membrane, the membrane being impermeable to the solute, but permeable to solvent

osmosis   passage of water through semipermeable membranes from an area of low to an area of high solute concentration

ototoxic   toxic to the ear (oto = ear); damage is caused to the eighth cranial nerve or the organs of hearing and balance. Many drugs (e.g. gentamicin, furosemide) can be ototoxic

oxygen radicals   either single oxygen atoms (O, rather than O_2) or superoxide radicals (e.g. O_3). One or more unbound oxygen atoms results in high reactivity, causing tissue damage

para   birth (e.g. primapara = first birth)

paracentesis   drainage of ascites

parity   number of pregnancies (including stillbirths/miscarriages) reaching 20 weeks' gestation

paroxysm   sudden; paroxysmal atrial tachycardia is atrial tachycardia that appears (and often disappears) suddenly

permissive hypercapnia   tolerating abnormally high arterial carbon dioxide tensions (pCO_2) to enable smaller tidal volumes, and so limit/avoid barotrauma and volutrauma

petechial   flecks of blood in skin caused by capillary bleeds

pleth   see plethysmograph

plethysmograph   instrument for measuring changes in blood volume

polydipsia   excessive thirst

post coronary arrest syndrome   cardiogenic and vasodilatory shock, leading to multi-organ dysfunction

prostacyclin (PGI$_2$)   an active arachidonic acid metabolite; inhibits angiotensin-mediated vasoconstriction, stimulates renin release, inhibits platelet aggregation (so used for anticoagulation)

protease inhibitors   protease is an essential enzyme for viral replication, so protease inhibitors prevent viral replication

prothrombin time   a test to measure clotting; normal prothrombin time is 11–12.5 seconds; prolonged prothrombin time indicates deficiency in one or more clotting factors

pruritis   itch

reactive oxygen species   unstable oxygen molecules, with one or more unpaired electron in their outer orbit; this makes them inherently unstable, so they react readily with other molecules to pair the free electron

repolarisation   restoration of cell to its resting potential

rescue therapy   (often controversial) treatment used when conventional treatments have failed

saturated fatty acid   fats with univalent bonds joining all atoms; valency determines hydrogen binding capacity of molecules, so saturated fatty acids contribute to hypercholestrolaemia and cardiovascular (especially coronary) disease. Most animal fats are saturated

septal myomectomy   open-heart surgery to treat severe hypertrophic obstructive cardiomyopathy (HOCM)

shunt   "shunting" describes a conduit between two body compartments. In respiratory medicine this usually describes movement of blood from venous to arterial circulation without effective ventilation, typically from intra-pulmonary problems, such as ARDS, but can also be caused by an atrial-septal defect allowing blood to pass between the atria without entering the pulmonary circulation. "Shunt" can also be used to describe an abnormal conduit directly joining an artery to a vein, such as an arteriovenous shunt used for haemodialysis access, or a drain inserted to remove excess fluid (e.g. an intraventricular shunt to drain CSF from the ventricles of the brain, and so relieve intracranial hypertension)

sigh breath   an occasional, especially large breath

solvent drag (convection)   movement of fluid by osmotic pressures from solutes moving across a semipermeable membrane

somatotrophin   growth hormone

Starling's Law   (of the heart) see Frank–Starling law

tentorial herniation   brainstem forced into spinal column from raised intra-cranial pressure ("coning")

tonic-clonic seizures   generalised fitting

transmembrane pressure   the pressure across a membrane. Where artificial technologies replicate capillary function, such as the "artificial kidneys" used for haemofiltration, excessive pressure may rupture the necessarily delicate membrane. Being artificial, damage is permanent and irreparable. As the surface area of the filter becomes progressively engorged with clots, filtrate is forced through a smaller area, increasing transmembrane pressure. Measuring transmembrane pressure should identify impending rupture of the artificial kidney. Stopping filters before maximum transmembrane pressure is reached enabled blood in the circuit to be safely returned to the patient. See manufacturers' instructions for maximum transmembrane pressures of individual models

trimester   pregnancy is divided into three trimesters: trimester 1 = up to week 12; trimester 2 = weeks 13–28; trimester 3 = week 29 to delivery

tunica intima   inner layer of blood vessel wall

ultrafiltration   removal of fluid through a membrane under pressure

volutrauma   high lung volumes (in relation to space available) can cause sheering damage to lung tissue; the concept is similar to barotrauma. Volutrauma is sometimes spelled "volotrauma"

von Willebrand factor   an extrinsic (tissue-dependent) clotting factor

References

Abbas, A.K., Lichtman, A.H., Pillai, S. 2015. *Cellular and Molecular Immunology.* 8th edition. Philadelphia. Elsevier Saunders.

Abdulla, A., Bone, M., Adams, N., *et al.* 2013. Evidence-based clinical practice guidelines on management of pain in older people. *Age and Ageing.* 42 (2): 151–153.

Acosta, C.D., Harrison, D.A., Rowan, K., *et al.* 2016. Maternal morbidity and mortality from severe sepsis: a national cohort study. *BMJ Open.* 6 (8): e012323. doi:10.1136/bmjopen-2016012323.

Adembri, C., Kastamoniti, E., Bertolozzi, I., *et al.* 2004. Pulmonary injury follows systemic inflammatory reaction in infrarenal aortic surgery. *Critical Care Medicine.* 32 (5): 1170–1177.

Adhikari, N.K., Dellinger, R.P., Lundin, S., *et al.* 2014. Inhaled nitric oxide does not reduce mortality in patients with acute respiratory distress syndrome regardless of severity: systematic review and meta-analysis. *Critical Care Medicine.* 42 (2): 404–412.

Adhikari, N.K.J., Fowler, R.A., Bhagwanjee, S., Rubenfeld, G.D. 2010. Critical care and the global burden of critical illness in adults. *Lancet.* 376 (9749): 1339–1346.

Afghani, E., Pandol, S.J., Shimosegawa, T., *et al.* 2015. Acute pancreatitis – progress and challenges: a report on an international symposium. *Pancreas.* 44 (8): 1195–1210.

Agarwai, M., Cottam, S. 2009. Laboratory tests in hepatic failure. *Anaesthesia and Intensive Care Medicine.* 10 (7): 326–327.

Agewall, S., Beltrame, J.F., Reynolds, H.R., *et al.*, on behalf of the WG on Cardiovascular Pharmacotherapy. 2016. ESC working group position paper on myocardial infarction with non-obstructive coronary arteries. *European Heart Journal.* 38 (3): 143–153.

Aggarwal, V., Singh, R., Singh, J.B., *et al.* 2017. Outcomes of mechanically ventilated critically ill geriatric patients in Intensive Care Unit. *Journal of Clinical and Diagnostic Research.* 11 (7): OC01-OC03.

Ahlers, S.M., van der Veen, A., van Dijk, M., *et al.* 2010. The use of the Behaviour Pain Scale to assess pain in conscious sedated patients. *Anesthesia & Analgesia.* 110 (1): 127–133.

Ahmed, S., Murugan, R. 2013. Dexmedetomidine use in the ICU. Are we there yet? *Critical Care.* 17 (3): 342–347.

Ahuja, C.S., Wilson, J.R., Nori, S., *et al.* 2017. Traumatic spinal cord injury. *Nature Reviews Disease Primers.* 3: 17018.

Aiken, L.H., Sloane, D., Griffiths, P., *et al.* for the RN4CAST Consortium. 2016. Nursing skill mix in European hospitals: cross-sectional study of the association with mortality, patient ratings, and quality of care. *BMJ Quality & Safety.* Published online 15 November 2016. doi:10.1136/bmjqs-2016005567.

Aiken, L.H., Sloane, D.M., Bruyneel, L., *et al.* RN4CAST consortium. 2014. Nurse staffing and education and hospital mortality in nine European countries: a retrospective observational study. *Lancet.* 383 (9931): 1824–1830.

Aïssaoui, Y., Zeggwagh, A.A., Zekraoui, A., *et al.* 2005. Validation of a Behavioral Pain Scale in critically ill, sedated, and mechanically ventilated patients. *Anesthesia & Analgesia.* 101 (5): 1470–1476.

Åkerman, E., Granberg-Axéll, A., Ersson, A., *et al*. I. 2010. Use and practice of patient diaries in Swedish intensive care units: a national survey. *Nursing in Critical Care*. 15 (1): 26–33.

Alansari, M.A., Hijazi, M.H., Maghrabi, K.A. 2015. Making a difference in eye care of the critically ill patient. *Journal of Intensive Care Medicine*. 30 (6): 311–317.

Alasad, J., Ahmad, M. 2005. Communication with critically ill patients. *JAN*. 50 (4): 356–362.

Albarran, J.W., Cox, H. 2008. Assessing and managing the patient with chest pain due to cardiac syndrome X, cocaine misuse and herpes zoster. *In* Albarran, J., Tagney, J. (eds) *Chest Pain: Advanced Assessment and Management Skills*. Oxford. Blackwell. 234–255.

Alexander, J.H., Smith, P.K. 2016. Coronary-artery bypass grafting. *New England Journal of Medicine*. 374 (20): 1954–1964.

Algahim, M.F., Love, R.B. 2015. Donation after circulatory death: the current state and technical approaches to organ procurement. *Current Opinion in Organ Transplantation*. 20 (2): 127–132.

Allegranzi, B., Gayet-Ageron, A., *et al*. 2013. Global implementation of WHO's multimodal strategy for improvement of hand hygiene: a quasi-experimental study. *Lancet Infectious Diseases*. 13 (10): 843–851.

Allen, S. 2005. Prevention and control of infection in the ICU. *Current Anaesthesia & Critical Care*. 16 (5): 191–199.

Allen, S.J., Martinez, E.G., Gregorio, G.V., Dans, L.F. 2010. Probiotics for treating acute infectious diarrhoea. *Cochrane Database of Systematic Reviews*, Issue 11. Art. No.: CD003048. doi:10.1002/14651858.CD003048.pub3.

Allingstrup, M., Wetterslev, J., Ravn, F.B., *et al*. 2016. Antithrombin III for critically ill patients. *Cochrane Database of Systematic Reviews*, Issue 2. Art. No.: CD005370. doi:10.1002/14651858.CD005370.pub3.

Allison, A. 1994. High frequency jet ventilation – where are we now? *Care of the Critically Ill*. 10 (3): 122–124.

Almerud, S., Alapack, R.J., Fridlund, B., Ekebergh, M. 2007. Of vigilance and invisibility – being a patient in technologically intense environments. *Nursing in Critical Care*. 12 (3): 151–158.

Alobaidi, R., Basu, R.K., Goldstein, S.L., Bagshaw, S.M. 2015. Sepsis-associated Acute Kidney Injury. *Seminars in Nephrology*. 35 (1): 2–11.

Al-Omran, M., Albalawi, Z.H., Tashkandi, M.F., Al-Ansary, L.A. 2010. Enteral versus parenteral nutrition for acute pancreatitis. *Cochrane Database of Systematic Reviews*, Issue 1. Art. No.: CD002837. doi:10.1002/14651858.CD002837.pub2.

Alshayeb, H.M., Showkat, A., Babar, F., *et al*. 2011. Severe hypernatremia correction rate and mortality in hospitalized patients. *The American Journal of the Medical Sciences*. 341 (5): 356–360.

Alway, A., Halm, M.A., Shilhanek, M., St. Pierre, J. 2013. Do earplugs and eye masks affect sleep and delirium outcomes in the critically ill? *American Journal of Critical Care*. 22 (4): 357–360.

Amato, M.B., Meade, M.O., Slutsky, A.S., *et al*. 2015. Driving pressure and survival in the acute respiratory distress syndrome. *New England Journal of Medicine*. 372 (8): 747–755.

American College of Obstetricians and Gynecologists, Task Force on Hypertension in Pregnancy. 2013. Hypertension in pregnancy. *Obstetric Gynecology*. 122 (5): 1122–1131.

Amide, C. 2017. Nervous system alterations. *In* Sole, M.L., Klein, D.G., Moseley, M.J. (eds). *Introduction to Critical Care Nursing*. 7th edition. St Louis, MO. Elsevier. 342–389.

Andrew, C.M. 1998. Optimizing the human experience: nursing the families of people who die in intensive care. *Intensive and Critical Care Nursing*. 14 (2): 59–65.

Andrews, P.J.D. 2015. Hypothermia for intracranial hypertension after traumatic brain injury. *New England Journal of Medicine*. 373 (25): 2403–2412.

Andriolo, B.N.G., Andriolo, R.B., Saconato, H., *et al*. 2015. Early versus late tracheostomy for critically ill patients. *Cochrane Database of Systematic Reviews*, Issue 1. Art. No.: CD007271. doi:10.1002/14651858.CD007271.pub3.

Annane, D. 2016. What is the evidence for harm of neuromuscular blockade and corticosteroid use in the intensive care unit? *Seminars in Respiratory and Critical Care Medicine*. 37 (1): 51–56.

Annane, D., Bellisant, E., Bollaert, P.-E., *et al*. 2009. Corticosteroids in the treatment of severe sepsis and septic shock in adults. *JAMA*. 301 (12): 2362–2375.

Annane, D., Sharshar, T. 2015. Cognitive decline after sepsis. *Lancet Respiratory Medicine*. 3 (1): 61–69.

Annecke, T., Fischer, J., Hartmann, H., Tschoep, J., Rehm, M., Conzen, P., Sommerhoff, C.P., Becker, B.F. 2011. Shedding of the coronary endothelial glycocalyx: effects of hypoxia/reoxygenation vs ischaemia/reperfusion. *British Journal of Anaesthesia*. 107 (5): 679–686.

Ansen, T.C., van Bommel, J., Mulder, P.G., *et al*. 2009. Prognostic value of blood lactate levels: does the clinical diagnosis at admission matter? *Trauma*. 66 (2): 377–385.

Anthony, D., Papanikolaou, P., Parboteeah, S., Saleh, M. 2010. Do risk assessment scales for pressure ulcers work? *Journal of Tissue Viability*. 19 (4): 132–136.

Anthony, D., Parboteeah, S., Salen, M., Papnikolaou, P. 2008. Norton, Waterlow and Braden scores: a review of the literature and a comparison between the scores and clinical judgement. *Journal of Clinical Nursing*. 17 (5): 646–653.

Antman, E.M., Hand, M., Armstrong, P.W., *et al*. 2008. 2007 focused update on the ACC/AHA 2004 guidelines for the management of patients with ST-elevation myocardial infarction: a report of the American College of Cardiology/American Heart Association Task Force on Practice Guidelines. *Journal of the American College of Cardiology*. 151 (2): 210–247.

Antonio, N., Jensen, L. 2014. Improving clinical practice in the management of elderly patients hospitalized with antimicrobial resistant organisms. *Journal of Nursing Education and Practice*. 4 (8): 107–114.

Appleton, R., Kinsella, J. 2012. Intensive care unit-acquired weakness. *Continuing Education in Anaesthesia, Critical Care and Pain*. 12 (2): 62–66.

Arbour, C., Gélinas, C., Michaud, C. 2011. Impact of the implementation of the Critical-Care Pain Observation Tool (CPOT) on pain management and clinical outcomes in mechanically ventilated trauma intensive care unit patients: A pilot study. *Journal of Trauma Nursing*. 18 (1): 52–60.

ARDS Definition Task Force, Ranieri, V.M., Rubenfeld, G.D., Thompson, B.T., *et al*. 2012. Acute respiratory distress syndrome: the Berlin Definition. *JAMA*. 307 (23): 2526–2533.

ARDSNet. 2008. NIH NHLBI ARDS Clinical Network Mechanical Ventilation Protocol Summary. www.ardsnet.org/files/ventilator_protocol_2008–07.pdf downloaded 16 October 2016.

Argettant. 2013. *Package Leaflet: Information for the User. Noradrenaine (Norepinephrine) 1 mg/ml concentrate for solution for infusion*. Lyon, France. Argettant.

Arroyo-Novoa, C.M., Figueroa-Ramos, M.I., Puntillo, K.A., *et al*. 2008. Pain related to tracheal suctioning in awake acutely and critically ill adults: a descriptive study. *Intensive and Critical Care Nursing*. 24 (1): 20–27.

Asadian, S., Khatony, A., Moradi, G., Abdi, A., Rezaei, M. 2016. Accuracy and precision of four common peripheral temperature measurement methods in intensive care patients. *Medical Devices (Auckland)*. 9: 301–308.

Asakura, H. 2014. Classifying types of disseminated intravascular coagulation: clinical and animal models. *Journal of Intensive Care*. 2: 20.

Asfar, P., Meziani, F., Hamel, J.-F., the SEPSISPAM Investigators. 2014. High versus low blood-pressure target in patients with septic shock. *New England Journal of Medicine*. 370 (17): 1583–1593.

Ash, D. 2005. Sustaining safe and acceptable bowel care in spinal cord injured patients. *Nursing Standard*. 20 (8): 55–64.

Ashraf, A., Conil, J.M., Georges, B., *et al*. 2008. Relation between ventilatory pressures and intra-abdominal pressure. *Critical Care*. 12 (supplement 2): P324.

Ashworth, P. 1980. *Care to Communicate*. London. Royal College of Nursing.

Atia, A.M., Abdel-Rahma, K.A. 2016. Traumatic brain injury: treatment with mild prolonged hypothermia. *Journal of Anesthesia & Clinical Research*. 7: 7 doi:10.4172/2155–6148. 1000645.

Audit Commission. 2001. *Testing Times*. London. Audit Commission.

Augustine, G., Augustine, S. 2017, April. Accurate Non-Invasive Temperature Monitoring Device. In *Proceedings of the 2017 Design of Medical Devices Conference* (pp. V001T11A015–V001T11A015), 10–13 April 2017, Minneapolis, MN, DMD2017-3476.

Auld, F., Maschauer, E.L., Morrison, I., *et al.* 2017. Evidence for the efficacy of melatonin in the treatment of primary adult sleep disorders. *Sleep Medicine Reviews*. 34: 10–22.

Australian and New Zealand Intensive Care Society Clinical Trials Group. 2000. Low-dose dopamine in patients with early renal dysfunction: a placebo-controlled randomised trial. *Lancet*. 356 (9248): 2139–2143.

Avidan, M.S., Maybrier, H.R., Abdallah, A.B., *et al.*, on behalf of the PODCAST Research Group. 2017. Intraoperative ketamine for prevention of postoperative delirium or pain after major surgery in older adults: an international, multicentre, double-blind, randomised clinical trial. *Lancet*. 390 (10091): 267–275.

Avidan, M.S., Zhang, L., Burnside, B.A., *et al.* 2008. Anesthesia awareness and the Bispectral Index. *New England Journal of Medicine*. 358 (11): 1097–1108.

Awdish, R.L.A. 2017. A view from the edge – creating a culture of caring. *New England Journal of Medicine*. 376 (1): 7–9.

Ayello, E., Braden, B. 2002. How and why to do pressure ulcer risk assessment. *Advances in Skin & Wound Care*. 15 (3): 125–131.

Ayhan, H., Tastan, S., Iyigun, E., *et al.* 2015. Normal saline instillation before tracheal suctioning: "What does the evidence say? What do the nurses think?": multimethod study. *Journal of Critical Care*. 30 (4): 762–767.

Azar, G., Love, R., Choe, E. Flint, L, Steinberg, S. 1996. Neither dopamine nor dobutamine reverses the depression in mesenteric blood flow caused by positive end-expiratory pressure. *Journal of Trauma*. 40 (5): 679–685.

Azoulay, É., Metnitz, B., Sprung, C.L., *et al.*, SAPS 3 Investigators. 2009. End-of-life practices in 282 intensive care units: data from the SAPS 3 database. *Intensive Care Medicine*. 35 (4): 623–630.

B.A.C.C.N. 2012. *Position Statement on Visiting in Adult Critical Care Units in the United Kingdom*. Newcastle-upon-Tyne. British Association of Critical Care Nurses.

Bachir, N.M., Larson, A.M. 2012. Adult liver transplantation in the United States. *American Journal of the Medical Sciences*. 343 (6): 462–469.

Badacsony, A., Goldhill, A., Waldmann, C., Goldhill, D.R. 2007. A prospective observational study of ICU patient position and frequency of turning. *Journal of the Intensive Care Society*. 8 (2): 26.

Baddeley, R.N.B., Skipworth, J.R.A., Pereira, S.P. 2011. Acute pancreatitis. *Medicine*. 39 (2): 108–115.

Bagherian, B., Sabzevari, S., Mirzaei, T., Ravary, A. 2017. Meaning of caring from critical care nurses' perspective: a phenomenological study. *Journal of Intensive and Critical Care*. 3 (3): 33.

Bahouth, M.N. 2018. Patient management: nervous system. *In* Morton, P.G., Fontaine, D.K. (eds). *Critical Care Nursing: A Holistic Approach*. 11th edition. Philadelphia. Wolters Kluwer. 660–674.

Bai, M., Zhou, M., He, L., Ma, F., Li, Y., Yu, Y., Wang, P., Li, L., King, R., Zhao, L., Sun, S. 2015. Citrate versus heparin anticoagulation for continuous renal replacement therapy: an updated meta-analysis of RCTs. *Intensive Care Medicine*. 41 (12): 2098–2110.

Baid, H. 2009. A critical review of auscultating bowel sounds. *BJN*. 18 (18): 1125–1129.

Bailey, A., Leditschke, I., Ranse, J., Grove, K. 2008. Impact of a pandemic triage tool on intensive care admission. *Critical Care*. 12 (supplement 2): P349.

Bailey, D., Jackson, L., White, D. 2004. HBO therapy: beyond the bends. *RN*. 27 (9): 31–35.

Baiyda, D.K., Agarwal, A., Khaana, P., Arora, M.K. 2011. Pregabalin in acute and chronic pain. *Journal of Anaesthesiology Clinical Pharmacology*. 27 (3): 307–314.

Bajwa, S.J.S., Haldar, R. 2015. Clinical challenges of endocrinological origin in neurocritical care practice. *Neurotransmitter* 2.

Baker, A., Richardson, D., Craig, G. 2012. Extracorporeal carbon dioxide removal ($ECCO_2R$) in respiratory failure: an overview, and where next? *Journal of the Intensive Care Society*. 13 (3): 232–237.

Baker, M., Harbottle, L. 2014. Parenteral nutrition. *In* Gandy, J. (ed.). *Manual of Dietetic Practice*. 5th edition. Oxford. Wiley Blackwell. 357–364.

Bancroft, A., Reid, P.S. 2016. Concepts of illicit drug quality among darknet market users: purity, embodied experience, craft and chemical knowledge. *International Journal of Drug Policy*. 35: 42–49.

Banks, P.A., Bollen, T.L., Dervenis, C., *et al.*, Acute Pancreatitis Classification Working Group. 2013. Classification of acute pancreatitis—2012: revision of the Atlanta classification and definitions by international consensus. *Gut*. 62 (1): 102–111.

Baranoski, S., Ayello, E.A., Levine, J.M., *et al.* 2012. Skin: an essential organ. *In* Baronoski, S., Ayello, E.A. (eds). *Wound Care Essentials*. Philadelphia. Wolters Kluwer. 52–81.

Barbier, F., Coquet, I., Legrief, S., *et al.* 2009. Etiologies and outcome of acute respiratory failure in HIV-infected patients. *Intensive Care Medicine*. 35 (10): 1678–1686.

Barone, J.E. 2009. Fever: fact and fiction. *Journal of Trauma*. 67 (2): 406–409.

Barr, J., Fraser, G.L., Puntillo, K., *et al.* 2013. Clinical practice guidelines for the management of pain, agitation, and delirium in adult patients in the Intensive Care Unit. *Critical Care Medicine*. 41 (1): 263–306.

Barratt, J. 2007. What to do with patients with abnormal dipstick urinalysis. *Medicine*. 35 (7): 365–367.

Barrett, K.E., Barman, S.M., Boitano, S., Brooks, H.L. 2016. *Ganong's Review of Medical Physiology*. 25th edition. New York. McGraw Hill Education Lange.

Basner, M., Babisch, W., Davis, A., *et al.* 2014. Auditory and non-auditory effects of noise on health. *Lancet*. 383 (9925): 1325–1332.

Bassetti, M., Welte, T., Wunderink, R.G. 2016. Treatment of gram-negative pneumonia in the critical care setting. Is the beta-lactam antibiotic backbone broken beyond repair? *Critical Care*. 20 (19).

Bateman, D.N. 2007. Poisoning: focus on paracetamol. *Journal of the Royal College of Physicians of Edinburgh*. 37 (4): 332–334.

Bath, M.F., Saratzis, A., Saedon, M., *et al.* 2017. Patients with small abdominal aortic aneurysm are at significant risk of cardiovascular events and this risk is not addressed sufficiently. *European Journal of Vascular and Endovascular Surgery*. 53 (2): 255–260.

Batterink, J., Cessford, T.A., Taylor, R.A.I. 2015. Pharmacological interventions for the acute management of hyperkalaemia in adults. *Cochrane Database of Systematic Reviews*, Issue 10. Art. No.: CD010344. doi:10.1002/14651858.CD010344.pub2.

Baxter. 2015. Plasma-Lyte 148 (pH 7.4) solution for infusion. Summary of product characteristics. Thetford. Baxter Healthcare.

Baxter, B.T. 2004. Could medical intervention work for aortic aneurysms? *American Journal of Surgery*. 188 (6): 628–632.

Bayer, O., Reinhart, K., Sakr, Y., *et al.* 2011. Renal effects of synthetic colloids and crystalloids in patients with severe sepsis: a prospective sequential comparison. *Critical Care Medicine*. 39 (6): 1335–1342.

BBC News. 2017. www.bbc.co.uk/news/av/uk-wales-politics-41499932/theresa-may-pledges-presumed-consent-on-organ-donation-in-england accessed 21 December 2017.

B.C.S.H. 2012. *Guidelines on the Diagnosis and Management of Thrombocytopenic Purpura and other Thrombotic Microangiopathies*. London. British Committee for Standards in Haematology.

Becker, B.F., Chappell, D., Jacob, M. 2010. Endothelial glycocalyx and coronary vascular permeability: the fringe benefit. *Basic Respirology & Cardiology*. 105 (6): 687–701.

Beeknoo, N., Jones, R. 2016. Achieving economy of scale in critical care, planning information necessary to support the choice of bed numbers. *British Journal of Medical Research*. 17 (9): 1–15.

Behrendt, C.E. 2000. Acute respiratory failure in the United States. *Chest*. 118 (4): 1100–1105.

Bein, T., Grasso, S., Moerer, O., *et al.* 2016. The standard of care of patients with ARDS: ventilatory settings and rescue therapies for refractory hypoxemia. *Intensive Care Medicine*. 42 (5): 699–711.

Bein, T., Weber-Carstens, S., Goldmann, A., *et al.* 2013. Lower tidal volume strategy (approximately 3 ml/kg) combined with extracorporeal CO_2 removal versus "conventional" protective ventilation (6 ml/kg) in severe ARDS: the prospective randomized Xtravent-study. *Intensive Care Medicine*. 39 (5): 847–849.

Bell, L. 2008. Evaluation of and caring for patients with pressure ulcers. *American Journal of Critical Care*. 17 (4): 348.

Bell, M., SWING, Granath, F., Schön, S., *et al.* 2007. Continuous renal replacement therapy is associated with less chronic renal failure than intermittent haemodialysis after acute renal failure. *Intensive Care Medicine*. 33 (5): 773–780.

Bellapart, J., Boots, R. 2012. Potential use of melatonin in sleep and delirium in the critically ill. *British Journal of Anaesthesia*. 108 (4): 572–580.

Belletti, A., Benedetto, U., Biondi-Zoccai, G., *et al.* 2017. The effect of vasoactive drugs on mortality in patients with severe sepsis and septic shock. A network meta-analysis of randomized trials. *Journal of Critical Care*. 37: 91–98.

Bellomo, R., Hegarty, C., Story, D., Ho, L., Bailey, M. 2012. Association between a chloride-liberal vs chloride-restrictive intravenous fluid administration strategy and kidney injury in critically ill adults. *JAMA*. 308 (15): 1566–1572.

Benner, P., Sutphen, M., Leonard-Kahn, V., Day, L. 2008. Formation and everyday ethical comportment. *American Journal of Critical Care*. 17 (5): 473–476.

Bénony, H., Daloz, L., Bungener, C., *et al.* 2002. Emotional factors and subjective quality of life in subjects with spinal cord injuries. *American Journal of Physical Medicine and Rehabilitation*. 81 (6): 437–445.

Berbara, H., Mair, S., Beitz, A., *et al.* 2014. Pulmonary vascular permeability index and global end-diastolic volume: are the data consistent in patients with femoral venous access for trans-pulmonary thermodilution: a prospective observational study. *BMC Anesthesiology*. 14: 81.

Bercu, Z.L., Fischman, A.M., Kim, E., *et al.* 2015. TIPS for Refractory Ascites: a 6-year single-center experience with expanded polytetrafluoroethylene–covered stent-grafts. *American Journal of Radiology*. 204 (3): 654–661.

Berden, A., Göçeroğlu, A., Jayne, D., *et al.* 2012. Diagnosis and management of ANCA associated vasculitis. *BMJ*. 343 (7840): 40–44.

Bergbom, I., Askwall, A. 2000. The nearest and dearest: a lifeline for ICU patients. *Intensive and Critical Care Nursing*. 16 (6): 384–395.

Bergstrom, N., Braden, B.J., Laguzza, A., Holman, V. 1987. The Braden Scale for Predicting Pressure Sore Risk. *Nursing Research*. 36 (4): 205–210.

Berkelmans, G.H., van Workum, F., Weijs, T.J., *et al.* 2017. The feeding route after esophagectomy: a review of literature. *Journal of Thoracic Disease*. 9 (supplement 8): S785.

Berling, I., Buckley, N.A., Isbister, G.K. 2016. The antipsychotic story: changes in prescriptions and overdose without better safety. *British Journal of Clinical Pharmacology*. 82 (1): 249–254.

Bernal, W., Auzinger, G., Dhawan, A., Wendon, J. 2010. Acute liver failure. *Lancet*. 376 (9736): 190–201.

Bernard, S.A., Buist, M. 2003. Induced hypothermia in critical care medicine: a review. *Critical Care Medicine*. 31 (7): 2041–2051.

Berry, A.M., Davidson, P.M., Masters, J., Rolls, K. 2007. Systematic literature review of oral hygiene practices for intensive care patients receiving mechanical ventilation. *American Journal of Critical Care*. 16 (5): 552–562.

Berry, N., Fletcher, S. 2012. Abdominal compartment syndrome. *Continuing Education in Anaesthesia, Critical Care & Pain*. 12 (3): 110–116.

Berthomier, T., Mansour, A., Bressollette, L., Le Roy, F., Mottier, D. 2016. Venous blood clot structure characterization using scattering operator. *2016 2nd International Conference on Frontiers of Signal Processing (ICFSP)*. Warsaw. pp. 73–80.

Betts, J., Betts, P., Sage, I. 1999. *Leah Betts: The Legacy of Ecstasy*. London. Robson.

Bharadwaj, S., Ginoya, S., Tandon, P., *et al.* 2016. Malnutrition: laboratory markers vs nutritional assessment. *Gastroenterology Report*. 4 (4): 272–280.

Bhatraju, P., Crawford, J., Hall, M., Lang, J.D. 2015. Inhaled nitric oxide: current clinical concepts. *Nitric Oxide*. 50: 114–128.

Biedrzycka, A., Lango, R. 2016. Tissue oximetry in anaesthesia and intensive care. *Anaesthesiology Intensive Therapy*. 48: 41–48.

Bijur, P.E., Shah, P.D., Esses, D. 2016. Temperature measurement in the adult Emergency Department. Oral, tympanic membrane and temporal artery temperatures versus rectal temperature. *Emergency Medicine Journal*. 33 (12): 843–847.

Bilotta, F., Caramia, R., Paoloni, F.P., *et al.* 2009. Safety and efficacy of intensive insulin therapy in critical neurosurgical patients. *Anesthesiology.* 110 (3): 456–458.

Birchley, G., Gooberman-Hill, R., Deans, Z., *et al.* 2017. "Best interests" in paediatric intensive care: an empirical ethics study. *Archives of Disease in Childhood.* 102 (10): 930–935.

Bird, J. 2003. Selection of pain measurement tools. *Nursing Standard.* 18 (13): 33–39.

Birk, M., Bauerfeind, P., Deprez, P.H., *et al.* 2016. Removal of foreign bodies in the upper gastro-intestinal tract in adults: European Society of Gastrointestinal Endoscopy (ESGE) Clinical Guideline. *Endoscopy.* 48 (5): 489–496.

Birn, H., Christensen, E. 2006. Renal albumin absorption in physiology and pathology. *Kidney International.* 69 (3): 440–449.

Bisson, J., Younker, J. 2006. Correcting arterial blood gases for temperature: (when) is it clinically significant? *Nursing in Critical Care.* 11 (5): 232–238.

Bjovatn, B., Dale, S., Hogstad-Erikstein, R., *et al.* 2012. Self-reported sleep and health among Norwegian hospital nurses in intensive care units. *Nursing in Critical Care.* 17 (4): 180–188.

Black, J.B. 2016. *An Integrative Review Focusing on Accuracy and Reliability of Clinical Thermometers.* Walden Dissertations and Doctoral Studies. Walden University, USA.

Blackburn, F., Bookless, B. 2002. Valve disorders. *In* Hatchett, R., Thompson, D. (eds). *Cardiac Nursing: a comprehensive guide.* Edinburgh. Churchill Livingstone. 260–286.

Blackwell, C.W., Guido-Sanz, F. 2016. Diagnosing HIV infection in adult patients in the Intensive Care Unit. *Journal of the Association of Nurses in AIDS Care.* 27 (6): 864–869.

Blackwood, B., Wilson-Barnett, J., Trinder, J. 2004. Protocolized weaning from mechanical ventilation: ICU physicians' views. *Journal of Advanced Nursing.* 48 (1): 26–34.

Blanch, L., Villagra, A., Sales, B., *et al.* 2015. Asynchronies during mechanical ventilation are associated with mortality. *Intensive Care Medicine.* 41 (4): 633–641.

Blaser, A.R., Starkopf, J., Alhazzani, W., *et al.* 2017. Early enteral nutrition in critically ill patients: ESICM clinical practice guidelines. *Intensive Care Medicine.* 43 (3): 380–398.

Blenkharn, A., Faughnan, S., Morgan, A. 2002. Developing a pain assessment tool for use by nurses in an adult intensive care unit. *Intensive and Critical Care Nursing.* 18 (6): 332–341.

Blot, S.I., Serra, M.L., Koulenti, D., *et al.*, EU-VAP/CAP Study Group. 2011. Patient to nurse ratio and risk of ventilator-associated pneumonia in critically ill patients. *American Journal of Critical Care.* 20 (1):e1-e9; doi:10.4037/ajcc2011555. http://ajcc.aacnjournals.org/content/19/6.toc. downloaded 2 January 2011.

Blume, C., Lechinger, J., Santhi, N., *et al.* 2017. Significance of circadian rhythms in severely brain-injured patients A clue to consciousness? *Neurology.* 88: Published online 19 April 2017. doi:10.1212/WNL.0000000000003942.

Blumenthal, I. 2001. Carbon monoxide poisoning. *Journal of the Royal Society of Medicine.* 94 (6): 270–272.

B.M.A. 2012. *Building on Progress: Where Next for Organ Donation Policy in the UK?* London. British Medical Association.

B.N.F. 2017. *British National Formulary.* http://bnf.nice.org.uk/ Last updated 30 November 2017. Accessed 28 December 2017.

Bodenham, A., Babu, S., Bennett, J., *et al.* 2016. Safe vascular access 2016. *Anaesthesia.* 71 (5): 573–585.

Boehringer Ingelheim. 2015. *Professional Leaflet. Catapres Amoules 150 microgram in 1 ml Solution for Injection.* Barcelona. Boehringer Ingelheim,

Boles, J.-M., Bion, J., Connors, A., *et al.* 2007. Weaning from mechanical ventilation, *European Respiratory Journal* 29 (5): 1033–1055.

Bombardier, C.H., Fann, J.R., Temkin, N.R., *et al.* 2010. Rates of major depressive disorder and clinical outcomes following traumatic brain injury. *JAMA.* 303 (19): 1938–1945.

Boral, B.M., Williams, D.J., Boral, L.I. 2016. Disseminated intravascular coagulation. *American Journal of Clinical Pathology.* 146 (6): 670–680.

Bosslet, G.T., Pope, T.M., Rubenfeld, G.D., *et al.*, on behalf of The American Thoracic Society ad hoc Committee on Futile and Potentially Inappropriate Treatment. 2015. An Official ATS/AACN/ACCP/ESICM/SCCM Policy Statement: Responding to Requests for Potentially Inappropriate Treatments in Intensive Care Units. *American Journal of Respiratory and Critical Care Medicine.* 191 (11): 1318–1330.

Bothamley, J., Boyle, M. 2017. Hypertensive and medical disorders in pregnancy. *In* Macdonald, S., Johnson G.J. (eds). *Mayes' Midwifery: A Textbook for Midwives*. 15th edition. Edinburgh. Elsevier. 914–945.

Bouju, P., Tadié, J.M., Barbarot, N., *et al.* 2017. Clinical assessment and train-of-four measurements in critically ill patients treated with recommended doses of cisatracurium or atracurium for neuromuscular blockade: a prospective descriptive study. *Annals of Intensive Care.* 7 (1): 10.

Boumendil, A., Maury, E., Reinhard, I., *et al.* 2004. Prognosis of patients aged 80 years and over admitted in medical intensive care unit. *Intensive Care Medicine.* 30 (4): 647–654.

Bourdages, M., Bigras, J.-L., Farrell, C.A., *et al.* 2010. Cardiac arrhythmias associated with severe traumatic brain injury and hypothermia therapy. *Pediatric Critical Care Medicine.* 11 (3): 439–441.

Bourke, S.J., Burns, G.P. 2015. *Respiratory Medicine Lecture Notes.* 9th edition. Chichester. Wiley Blackwell.

Bowsher, J., Boyle, S., Griffiths, J. 1999. Oral care. *Nursing Standard.* 13 (37): 31.

Braden, B.J. 2012. The Braden Scale for predicting pressure sore risk: reflections after 25 years. *Advances in Skin & Wound Care.* 26 (2): 61.

Bradley, C. 2001. Crystalloid, colloid or small volume resuscitation? *Intensive and Critical Care Nursing.* 17 (5): 304–306.

Braithwaite, B., Cheshire, N.J., Greenhalgh, R.M., *et al.* 2015. Endovascular strategy or open repair for ruptured abdominal aortic aneurysm: one-year outcomes from the IMPROVE randomized trial. *European Heart Journal.* 36 (31): 2061–2069.

Branson, R.D. 2005. The role of ventilator graphs when setting dual-control modes. *Respiratory Care.* 50 (2): 187–201.

Brauser, D. 2010. Critically ill patients with H1N1 often have acute kidney injury, failure. *National Kidney Foundation (NKF) 2010 Spring Clinical Meetings*: Abstract 31. Presented 14 April 2010.

Bray, K., Hill, K., Robson, W., *et al.* 2004. British Association of Critical Care Nurses position statement on the use of restraint in adult critical care units. *Nursing in Critical Care.* 9 (5): 199–212.

Bray, K., Wren, I., Baldwin, A., *et al.* 2009. *BACCN Standards for Staffing in Critical Care.* Newcastle-upon-Tyne. BACCN.

Brenner, B., Corbridge, T., Kazzi, A. 2009. Intubation and mechanical ventilation of the asthmatic patient in respiratory failure. *Proceedings of the American Thoracic Society.* 6 (4): 371–379.

Briegel, I., Dolch, M., Irlbeck, M., *et al.* 2013. Quality of results of therapy of acute respiratory failure: changes over a period of two decades. *Anaesthesist.* 62 (4): 261–270.

Briel, M., Meade, M., Mercat, A., *et al.* 2010. Higher vs lower positive end-expiratory pressure in patients with acute lung injury and acute respiratory distress syndrome: systematic review and meta-analysis. *JAMA.* 303 (9): 865–873.

Brignall, K.A., Davidson, A.C. 2009. Weaning from mechanical ventilation: art or science? *Care of the Critically Ill.* 25 (1): 22–28.

Brims, F.J.H., Davies, M.G., Elia, A., Griffiths M.J.D. 2004. The effects of pleural fluid drainage on oxygenation in mechanically ventilated patients after cardiac surgery. *Thorax.* 59 (ii40): S129.

Brochard, L., Abroug, F., Brenner, M., *et al.*, TS/ERS/ESICM/SCCM/SRLF Ad Hoc Committee on Acute Renal Failure. 2010. An official ATS/ERS/ESICM/SCCM/SRLF statement: prevention and management of acute renal failure in the ICU patient. *American Journal of Respiratory and Critical Care Medicine.* 181 (10): 1128–1155.

Brogan, T.V., Thiagarajan, R.R., Rycus, P.T., Bartlett, R.H., Bratton, S.L. 2009. Extracorporeal membrane oxygenation in adults with severe respiratory failure: a multi-center database. *Intensive Care Medicine.* 35 (12): 2105–2114.

Brott, T.G., Hobson, R.W., Howard, G., *et al.*, CREST Investigators. 2010. Stenting versus endarterectomy for treatment of carotid-artery stenosis. *NEJM.* 363 (1): 11–23.

Brotto, V., Lee, G. 2007. Substance abuse and its implications for the critical care nurse. *Intensive & Critical Care Nursing.* 23 (2): 64–70.

B.T.S. 2002. Non-invasive ventilation in acute respiratory failure. *Thorax.* 57 (3): 192–211.

B.T.S. 2017. BTS guideline for oxygen use in adults in healthcare and emergency settings. *Thorax*. 72 (supplement 1): i1–i90.

Buchan, J., Twigg, D., Dussault, G., Duffield, C., Stone, P.W. 2015. Policies to sustain the nursing workforce: an international perspective. *International Nursing Review*. 62 (2): 162–170.

Buendgens, L., Bruensing, J., Matthes, M., *et al*. 2014. Administration of proton pump inhibitors in critically ill medical patients is associated with increased risk of developing Clostridium difficile–associated diarrhea. *Journal of Critical Care*. 29 (4): 696-e11.

Builic, D., Bennett, M., Shehabi, Y. 2014. Delirium in the intensive care unit and long–term cognitive and psychosocial functioning: literature review. *Australian Journal of Advanced Nursing*. 33 (1): 44–52.

Burchiel, K.J., Hsu, F.P. 2001. Pain and spasticity after spinal cord injury: mechanisms and treatment. *Spine*. 26 (24S): S146-S160.

Burkhart, C.S., Siegemund, M., Steiner, L.A. 2010. Cerebral perfusion in sepsis. *Critical Care*. 14: 215.

Burns, K.E.A., Adhikari, N.K.J., Keenan, S.P., Meade, M. 2009. Use of non-invasive ventilation to wean critically ill adults off invasive ventilation: meta-analysis and systematic review. *BMJ*. 339 (7706): 1305–1308.

Burry, L., Rose, L., McCullagh, I.J., *et al*. 2014. Daily sedation interruption versus no daily sedation interruption for critically ill adult patients requiring invasive mechanical ventilation. *Cochrane Database of Systematic Reviews*, Issue 7. Art. No.: CD009176. doi:10.1002/14651858.CD009176.pub2.

Büscher, A., Sivertsen, B., White, J. 2009. *Nurses and Midwives: A Force for Health*. Copenhagen. WHO Regional Office for Europe.

Byrne, A.L., Bennett, M., Chatterji, R., *et al*. 2014. Peripheral venous and arterial blood gas analysis in adults: are they comparable? A systematic review and meta-analysis. *Respirology*. 19 (2): 168–175.

Cahill, N.E., Dhaliwal, R., Day, A.G., Jiang, X., Heyland, D.K. 2010. Nutrition therapy in the critical care setting: what is "best achievable" practice? An international multicenter observational study. *Critical Care Medicine*. 38 (2): 395–401.

Caironi, P., Carlesso, E., Cressoni, M., *et al*. 2015. Lung recruitability is better estimated according to the Berlin definition of acute respiratory distress syndrome at standard 5 cm H2O rather than higher positive end-expiratory pressure: a retrospective cohort study. *Critical Care Medicine*. 43 (4): 781–790.

Calás, T., Wilkin, M., Oliphant, C.M. 2016. Naloxone: an opportunity for another chance. *Journal for Nurse Practitioners*. 2016; 12 (3): 154–160.

Calzia, E., Stahl, W. 2004. The place of helium in the management of severe acute respiratory failure. *International Journal of Intensive Care*. 11 (2): 65–69.

Câmara, V.G.N., de Medeiros Araújo, J.N., de Lima Fernandes, A.P.N., *et al*. 2016. Methods for detection of dry eye in critically ill patients: an integrative review. *International Archives of Medicine*. 9 (58): 1–10.

Camm, A.J., Lip, G.Y.H., De Caterina, R., *et al*. 2012. 2012 focused update of the ESC Guidelines for the management of atrial fibrillation. *European Heart Journal*. 33 (21): 2719–2747.

Campbell, B., Richley, D., Ross, C., Eggett, C.J. 2017. Clinical guidelines by consensus: recording a standard 12-lead electrocardiogram. An approved method by the Society for Cardiological Science and Technology (SCST). Available at: www.scst.org.uk/resources/SCST_ECG_Recording_Guidelines_2017 accessed 6 December 2017.

Campbell, G.A., Rosner, M.H. 2008. The agony of ecstasy: MDMA (3,4-Methylenedioxy-methamphetamine) and the kidney. *Clinical Journal of the American Society of Nephrology*. 3 (6): 1852–1860.

Caplin-Davies, P.J. 1999. Doctor-nurse substitution: the workforce equation. *Journal of Nursing Management*. 7 (2): 71–79.

Cardim, D., Robba, C., Bohdanowicz, M., *et al*. 2016. Non-invasive monitoring of intracranial pressure using transcranial doppler ultrasonography: is it possible? *Neurocritical Care*. 25 (3): 473–491.

Carney, D., DiRocco, J., Nieman, G. 2005. Dynamic alveolar mechanics and ventilator-induced lung injury. *Critical Care Medicine*. 33 (supplement 3): S122-S128.

Carney, N., O'Reilly, C., Ullman, J.S., *et al*. 2016. *Guidelines for the Management of Severe Traumatic Brain Injury*. 4th edition. Brain Trauma Foundation. USA.

Caroff, D.A., Li, L., Muscedere, J., Klompas, M. 2016. Subglottic secretion drainage and objective outcomes: a systematic review and meta-analysis. *Critical Care Medicine*. 44 (4): 830–840.

Carrell, T.W.G., Wolfe, J.H.N. 2005. Non-cardiac vascular disease. *Heart*. 91 (2): 265–270.

Carson, J.L., Guyatt, G., Heddle, N.M., *et al*. 2016. Clinical practice guidelines from the AABB: red blood cell transfusion thresholds and storage. *JAMA*. 316 (9): 2025–2035.

Carter, S. 2009. Renewing pride in teaching: Using theory to advance nursing scholarship. *Nurse Education in Practice*. 9 (2): 119–126.

Caserta, R.A., Marra, A.R., Durão, M.S., *et al*. 2012. A program for sustained improvement in preventing ventilator associated pneumonia in an intensive care setting. *BMC Infectious Diseases*. 12 (234).

Castagno, C., Varetto, G., Quaglino, S., *et al*. 2016. Acute kidney injury after open and endo-vascular elective repair for infrarenal abdominal aortic aneurysms. *Journal of Vascular Surgery*. 64 (4): 928–933.

Cataland, S.R., Wu, H.M. 2014. How I treat: the clinical differentiation and initial treatment of adult patients with atypical hemolytic uremic syndrome. *Blood*. 123 (16): 2478–2484.

Cavaliere, F., Antonelli, M., Arcangeli, A., *et al*. 2002. Effects of acid-base abnormalities on blood capacity of transporting CO_2: adverse effect of metabolic acidosis. *Intensive Care Medicine*. 28 (5): 609–615.

Cavolli, R., Kaya, K., Aslan, A., Emiroglu, O., Erturk, S., Korkmaz, O., Oguz, M., Tasoz, R., Ozyurda, U. 2008. Does sodium nitroprusside decrease the incidence of atrial fibrillation after myocardial revascularisation? *Circulation*. 118 (5): 476–481.

C.D.C. 2013. *Antibiotic Resistance Threats in the United States, 2013*. Atlanta, Georgia. Centers for Disease Control and Prevention.

Cepeda, J.A., Cooper, B., Hails, J., *et al*. 2005. Isolation of patients in single rooms or cohorts to reduce spread of *MRSa* in intensive-care units: prospective two-centre study. *Lancet*. 365 (9456): 295–304.

Chaboyer, W., Thalib, L., Foster, M., *et al*. 2008. Predictors of adverse events in patients after discharge from the intensive care unit. *American Journal of Critical Care*. 17 (3): 255–263.

Chan, M., Yusuf, E., Giulieri, S., *et al*. 2016. A retrospective study of deep sternal wound infections: clinical and microbiological characteristics, treatment, and risk factors for complications. *Diagnostic Microbiology and Infectious Disease*. 84 (3): 261–265.

Chandrashekhar, Y., Westaby, S., Narula, J. 2009. Mitral stenosis. *Lancet*. 374 (9697): 1213–1300.

Chaney, J.C., Derdak, S. 2002. Minimally invasive hemodynamic monitoring for the intensivist: current and emerging technology. *Critical Care Medicine*. 30 (10): 2338–2345.

Chang, L.-Y., Wang, K.-W.K., Chao, Y.-F. 2008. Influence of physical restraint on unplanned extubation of adult intensive care patients: a case-control study. *American Journal of Critical Care*. 17 (5): 408–415.

Chanques, G., Payen, J.-F., Mercier, G., *et al*. 2009. Assessing pain in non-intubated critically ill patients unable to self-report: an adaptation of the Behavioral Pain Scale. *Intensive Care Medicine*. 35 (12): 2060–2067.

Charlton, M., Thompson, J.P. 2016. Drugs affecting the autonomic nervous system. *Anaesthesia & Intensive Care Medicine*. 17 (11): 575–580.

Chassard, D., Bruguerolle, B. 2004. Chronobiology and anesthesia. *Anesthesiology*. 100 (2): 413–427.

Checketts, M.R., Alladi, R., Ferguson, K., *et al*. 2015. Recommendations for standards of monitoring during anaesthesia and recovery 2015: Association of Anaesthetists of Great Britain and Ireland. *Anaesthesia*. 71 (1): 85–93.

Chen, H.L., Cao, Y.J., Shen, W.Q., Zhu, B. 2017. Construct validity of the Braden scale for pressure ulcer assessment in acute care: a structural equation modeling approach. *Ostomy/Wound Management*. 63 (2): 38–41.

Chen, J.M.H., Heran, B.S., Perez, M.I., Wright, J.M. 2010. Blood pressure lowering efficacy of beta-blockers as second-line therapy for primary hypertension. *Cochrane Database of Systematic Reviews*, Issue 1. Art No: CD007185. doi:10.1002/14651858.CD007185.pub2.

Chen, J.W., Gombart, Z.J., Rogers, S., *et al.* 2011. Pupillary reactivity as an early indicator of increased intracranial pressure: the introduction of the Neurological Pupil Index. *Surgical Neurology International*. 2: 82. doi:10.4103/2152–7806.82248.

Chen, S.L., Li, J.P., Li, L.F., Zeng, T., He, X. 2016. Elevated preoperative serum alanine amino-transferase/aspartate aminotransferase (ALT/AST) ratio is associated with better prognosis in patients undergoing curative treatment for gastric adenocarcinoma. *International Journal of Molecular Sciences*. 17 (6): 911.

Chesnut, R.M., Temkin, N., Carney, N., *et al.* 2012. A trial of intracranial-pressure monitoring in traumatic brain injury. *New England Journal of Medicine*. 366 (26): 2471–2481.

Chevalier, P., Scridon, A. 2011. Genetic bases for atrio-ventricular block-induced torsades de pointes. *E-journal of Cardiology Practice*. 10 (8).

Chey, W.D., Leontiadis, G.I., Howden, C.W., Moss, S.F. 2017. ACG Clinical guideline: treatment of *helicobacter pylori* infection. *The American Journal of Gastroenterology*. 112 (2): 212–238.

Cho, S.-H., Hwang, J.H., Kim, J. 2008. Nurse staffing and patient mortality in intensive care units. *Nursing Research*. 57 (5): 322–330.

Cholley, P., Thouverez, M., Floret, N., *et al.* 2008. The role of water fittings in intensive care rooms as reservoirs for the colonization of patients with *Pseudomonas aeruginosa*. *Intensive Care Medicine*. 34 (8): 1428–1433.

Choudhury, A.H., Cox, E.F., Francis, S.T., Lobo, D.N. 2012. A randomized, controlled, double-blind crossover study on the effects of 2-L infusions of 0.9% saline and Plasma-Lyte 148 on renal blood flow velocity and renal cortical tissue perfusion in healthy volunteers. *Annals of Surgery*. 256 (1): 18–24.

Choudhury, A.H., Cox, E.F., Francis, S.T., Lobo, D.N. 2014. A randomized, controlled, double-blind crossover study on the effects of 1-l infusions of 6% hydroxyethyl starch suspended in 0.9% saline (Voluven) and a Balanced Solution (Plasma Volume Redibag) on blood volume, renal blood flow velocity, and renal cortical tissue perfusion in healthy volunteer. *Annals of Surgery*. 259 (5): 881–887.

Chowdhury, S.R., Lawton, T., Akram, A., *et al.* 2017. Citrate versus non-citrate anticoagulation in continuous renal replacement therapy: results following a change in local critical care pro-tocol. *Journal of the Intensive Care Society*. 18 (1): 47–51.

Chowell, G., Bertozzi, S.M., Colchero, M.A., *et al.* 2009. Severe respiratory disease concurrent with the circulation of H1N1 influenza. *New England Journal of Medicine*. 361 (7): 674–679.

Christensen, V.L., Holm, A.M., Kongerud, J., *et al.* 2016. Occurrence, characteristics, and pre-dictors of pain in patients with chronic obstructive pulmonary disease. *Pain Management Nursing*. 17 (2): 107–118.

Chrousos, G.P. 2009. Stress and disorders of the stress system. *Nature Reviews Endocrinology*. 5 (7): 374–381.

Chumbley, G. 2011. Use of ketamine in uncontrolled acute and procedural pain. *Nursing Standard*. 25 (15–17): 35–37.

Chummun, H., Tilley, V., Ibe, J. 2010. 3,4-methylenedioxyamfetamine (ecstasy) use reduces cognition. *British Journal of Nursing*. 19 (2): 94–100.

Chychula, N.M., Sciamanna, C. 2002. Help substance abusers attain and sustain abstinence. *The Nurse Practitioner*. 27 (11) 30–47.

Clark, D., Murray, D.B., Ray, D. 2011. Epidemiology and outcomes of patients admitted to critical care after self-poisoning. *Journal of the Intensive Care Society*. 12 (4): 268–273.

Clarke, G. 1993. Mouthcare and the hospitalised patient. *British Journal of Nursing*. 2 (4): 225–227.

Clay, A.S., Behina, M., Brown, K.K. 2001. Mitochondrial disease. *Chest*. 120 (2): 634–648.

Clay, M. 2002. Assessing oral health in older people. *Nursing Older People*. 14 (8): 31–32.

Cockett, A. 2010. Cardiac disease. *In* Cockett, A., Day, H. (eds). 2010. *Children's High Dependency Nursing*. Chichester. Wiley-Blackwell. 93–124.

Cockett, A., Day, H. (eds). 2010. *Children's High Dependency Nursing*. Chichester. Wiley-Blackwell.

Coeytaux, R.R., Williams, J.W., Gray, R.N., Wang, A. 2010. Percutaneous heart-valve replace-ment for aortic stenosis: state of the evidence. *Annals of Internal Medicine*. 153 (5): 314–324.

Cogo, P.E., Poole, D., Codazzi, D., *et al.* 2010. Outcomes of children admitted to adult intensive care units in Italy between 2003–2007. *Intensive Care Medicine.* 36 (8): 1403–1409.

Coia, J.E., Duckworth, G.J., Edwards, D.I., *et al.*, Joint Working Party of the British Society of Antimicrobial Chemotherapy, the Hospital Infection Society, and the Infection Control Nurses Association. 2006. Guidelines for the control and prevention of meticillin-resistant *Staphylococcus aureus* (MRSA) in healthcare facilities. *Journal of Hospital Infections.* 63S: S1-S44.

Coleman, S., Gorecki, C., Nelson, E.A., Closs, S.J., Defloor, T., Halfens, R., Farrin, A., Brown, J., Schoonhoven, L., Nixon, J. 2013. Patient risk factors for pressure ulcer development: systematic review. *International Journal of Nursing Studies.* 50 (7): 974–1003.

Collins, B.R., O'Brien, L. 2015. Prevention and management of constipation in adults. *Nursing Standard.* 29 (32): 49–58.

Comfort, A. 1977. *A Good Age.* London. Mitchell Beazey.

Commission on Human Medicines. 2012. Paracetamol overdose: new guidance on use of intravenous acetylcysteine (letter, dated 3 September). Secretary of Commission, S. Singh, Floor 4.T 151 Buckingham Palace Road, Victoria, London SW1W 9SZ.

Compton, F., Bojarski, C., Siegmund, B., van der Giet, M. 2014. Use of a nutrition support protocol to increase enteral nutrition delivery in critically ill patients. *American Journal of Critical Care.* 23 (5): 396–403.

Constantin, J.M., Momon, A., Mantz, J., *et al.* 2016. Efficacy and safety of sedation with dexmedetomidine in critical care patients: a meta-analysis of randomized controlled trials. *Anaesthesia Critical Care & Pain Medicine.* 35 (1): 7–15.

Conti, C.R. 2011. Is hyperoxic ventilation important to treat acute coronary syndromes such as myocardial infarction? *Clinical Cardiology.* 34 (3): 132–133.

Cook, T., Woodall, N., Frerk, C. 2011. *Major Complications of Airway Management in the United Kingdom.* London. The Royal College of Anaesthetists.

Cooper, D.J., Higgins, A.M., Nichol, A.D. 2014. Lactic acidosis. *In* Bersten, A.D., Soni, N. (eds). *Intensive Care Manual.* 7th edition. Edinburgh. Butterworth-Heinemann Elsevier. 158–164.

Cooper, N., Forrest, K., Cramp, P. 2006. *Essential Guide to Acute Care.* 2nd edition. London. BMJ Books.

Corley, A., Caruana, L., Barnett, A., *et al.* 2011. Oxygen delivery through high-flow nasal cannulae increases end-expiratory volume and reduces respiratory rate in post-cardiac surgical patients. *British Journal of Anaesthesia.* 107 (6): 998–1004.

Corne, J., Kumaran, M. 2016. *Chest X-ray Made Easy.* 4th edition. Edinburgh. Elsevier.

Cortés, D.O., Bonor, A.R., Vincent, J.L. 2014. Isotonic crystalloid solutions: a structured review of the literature. *British Journal of Anaesthesia.* 112 (6): 968–981.

Cosgrave, D., Chandler, J., Bates, J. 2016. How do I transport the critically ill patient? *In* Deutschman, C.S., Neligan, P.J. (eds). *Evidence-Based Practice of Critical Care.* 2nd edition. Philadelphia. Elsevier.

Coté, C.J., Goldstein, A., Fuchsman, W.H., Hoaglin, D.C. 1988. The effect of nail polish on pulse oximetry. *Anesthesia & Analgesia.* 67 (7): 683–686.

Cotter, G., Moshkovitz, Y., Kaluski, E., *et al.* 2004. Accurate, noninvasive continuous monitoring of cardiac output by whole-body electrical bioimpedance. *Chest.* 125 (4): 1431–1440.

Courtney, M.D., Edwards, H.E., Chang, A.M., *et al.* 2011. A randomised controlled trial to prevent hospital readmissions and loss of functional ability in high risk older adults: a study protocol. *BMC Health Service Research.* 11: 202.

Cox, C. 2010. Legal responsibility and accountability. *Nursing Management.* 17 (3): 18–20.

C.Q.C. 2012. *The State of Health Care and Adult Social Care in England.* London. Care Quality Commission.

C.Q.C. 2016. *A Different Ending. Addressing Inequalities in End of Life Care.* Newcastle upon Tyne. Care Quality Commission.

Craig, T., Mathieu, S. 2017. CANDLE: the critical analysis of the nocturnal distribution of light exposure – a prospective pilot study quantifying the nocturnal light intensity on a critical care unit. *Journal of the Intensive Care Society.* Article first published online: 13 December 2017. p.1751143717748095.

Crandall, C.G., Vongpatanasin, W., Victor, R.G. 2002. Mechanism of cocaine-induced hyperthermia in humans. *Annals of Internal Medicine*. 136 (11): 785–791.

Crawford, D., Greene, N., Wentworth, S. 2005. *Thermometer Review: UK Market Survey*. Medicines and Healthcare products Regulatory Agency Evaluation 04144. London. M.H.R.A.

Creagh-Brown, B.C., James, D.A., Jackson, S.H. 2005. The use of the Tempa.Dot thermometer in routine clinical practice. *Age and Ageing*. 34 (3): 297–299.

Cree, C. 2003. Acquired brain injury: acute management. *Nursing Standard*. 18 (11): 45–54.

Crisp, N., Chen, L. 2014. Global supply of health professionals. *New England Journal of Medicine*. 370 (10): 950–957.

Crocker, C. 2009. Weaning from ventilation – current state of the science and art. *Nursing in Critical Care*. 14 (4): 185–190.

Crozier, T.M.E. 2017. General care of the pregnant patient in the intensive care unit. *Seminars in Respiratory and Critical Care Medicine*. 38 (2): 208–217.

Crunden, E. 2010. A reflection from the other side of the bed – an account of what it is like to be a patient and a relative in an intensive care unit. *Intensive and Critical Care Nursing*. 26 (1): 18–23.

Cruz, F.F., Rocco, P.R.M., Pelosi, P. 2017. Anti-inflammatory properties of anaesthetic agents. *Critical Care*. 21: 67.

Curley, G.F., Laffey, J.G. 2014. Acidosis in the critically ill – balancing risks and benefits to optimize outcome. *Critical Care*. 18: 129. doi:10.1186/cc13815.

Curley, M.A.Q., Wypij, D., Watson, S., *et al.*, for the RESTORE Study Investigators and the Pediatric Acute Lung Injury and Sepsis Investigators (PALISI) Network. 2012. Protocolized sedation vs usual care in pediatric patients mechanically ventilated for acute respiratory failure: a randomized clinical trial. *JAMA*. 308 (19): 1985–1992. doi:10.1001/jama. 2012. 13872.

Cuthbertson, B.H., Rattray, J., Campbell, M.K., *et al.* 2009. The PRaCTICal study of nurse-led intensive care follow-up programmes for improving long-term outcomes from critical illness: a pragmatic randomised controlled trial. *BMJ*. 339 (7728): 106.

Damas, P., Frippiat, F., Ancion, A., *et al.* 2015. Prevention of ventilator-associated pneumonia and ventilator-associated conditions. A randomized controlled trial with subglottic secretion suctioning. *Critical Care Medicine*. 43 (1): 22–30.

Damuth, E., Mitchell, J.A., Bartock, J.L., *et al.* 2015. Long-term survival of critically ill patients treated with prolonged mechanical ventilation: a systematic review and meta-analysis. *Lancet Respiratory Medicine*. 3 (7): 544–553.

Daneman, N., Sarwar, S., Fowler, R.A., Cuthbertson, B.H., SuDDICU Canadian Study Group. 2013. Effect of selective decontamination of antimicrobial resistance in intensive care units: a systematic review and meta-analysis. *Lancet Infectious Diseases*. 13 (4): 328–341.

Daneshmandi, M., Neiseh, F., SadeghiShermeh, M., Ebadi, A. 2012. Effect of eye mask on sleep quality in patients with acute coronary syndrome. *Journal of Caring Sciences*. 1 (3): 135–143.

Darouiche, R. 2006. Spinal epidural abscess. *New England Journal of Medicine*. 355 (19): 2012–2020.

Dasgupta, S., Das, S., Chawan, N.S., Hazra, A. 2015. Nosocomial infections in the intensive care unit: incidence, risk factors, outcome and associated pathogens in a public tertiary teaching hospital of Eastern India. *Indian Journal of Critical Care Medicine*. 19 (1): 14–20.

Dautzenberg, M.J.D., Wekesa, A.N., Gniadkowski, M., *et al.*, on behalf of the Mastering Hospital Antimicrobial Resistance in Europe Work Package 3 Study Team. 2015. The association between colonization with carbapenemase-producing *enterobacteriaceae* and overall ICU mortality: an observational cohort study. *Critical Care Medicine*. 43 (6): 1170–1177.

Davenport, A., Stevens, P. 2008. *Clinical Practice Guidelines: Acute Kidney Injury*. 4th edition. London. UK Renal Association.

Davidson, J.E., Aslakson, R.A., Long, A.C., *et al.* 2017. Guidelines for family-centered care in the neonatal, pediatric, and adult ICU. *Critical Care Medicine*. 45 (1): 103–128.

Davies, S.W., Leonard, K.L., Falls Jr., R.K., *et al.* 2015. Lung protective ventilation (ARDSNet) versus APRV: ventilatory management in a combined model of acute lung and brain injury. *Journal of Trauma and Acute Care Surgery*. 78 (2): 240–251.

Davis, M.D., Walsh, B.K., Sittig, S.E., Restrepo, R.D. 2013. AARC Clinical Practice Guideline: blood gas analysis and hemoximetry: 2013. *Respiratory Care*. 58 (10): 1694–1703.

Davoudian, P., Blunt, M. 2009. Outcome from intensive care and measuring performance. *Surgery*. 27 (5): 212–215.

D.A.W.N. 2011. Emergency Department Visits Involving Ecstasy. The Drugs Abuse Warning Network. The DAWN Report. 24 March. Center for Behavioral Health Statistics and Quality, Substance Abuse and Mental Health Services Administration (SAMHSA), USA.

Dawson, D. 2005. Development of a new eye care guideline for critically ill patients. *Intensive and Critical Care Nursing*. 21 (2): 118–122.

De Backer, D., Biston P., Devriendt J., *et al*. 2010. Comparison of dopamine and norepinephrine in the treatment of shock. *New England Journal of Medicine*. 362 (9): 779–789.

De Barbieri, I., Frigo, A.C., Zampieron, A. 2009. Quick change versus double pump while changing the infusion of inotropes: an experimental study. *Nursing in Critical Care*. 14 (4): 200–206.

de Beauvoir, S. 1970. *Old Age*. London. Penguin.

de Carvalho, F.P.B., Simpson, C.A., de Oliveira, L.C., *et al*. 2016. Pressure injuries: predisposing conditions and risk factors in adult ICU. *International Archives of Medicine*. 9 (159): 1–8.

de Chambrun, M.P., Bréchot, N., Lebreton, G., *et al*. 2016. Venoarterial extracorporeal membrane oxygenation for refractory cardiogenic shock post-cardiac arrest. *Intensive Care Medicine*. 42 (12): 1999–2007.

de Jong, E., van Oers, J.A., Beishuizen, A., *et al*. 2016. Efficacy and safety of procalcitonin guidance in reducing the duration of antibiotic treatment in critically ill patients: a randomised, controlled, open-label trial. *Lancet*. 16 (7): 819–827.

De Keulenaer, B.L., De Waele, J.J., Powell, B., Malbrain, M.L.N.G. 2009. What is normal intra-abdominal pressure and how is it affected by positioning, body mass and positive end-expiratory pressure? *Intensive Care Medicine*. 35 (6): 969–976.

de Oliveira, C., Watt, R., Hamer, M. 2010. Toothbrushing, inflammation, and risk of cardio-vascular disease: results from Scottish Health Survey. *BMJ*. 340 (7761): 1400.

De Santis, V., Singer, M. 2015. Tissue oxygen tension monitoring of organ perfusion: rationale, methodologies, and literature review. *British Journal of Anaesthesia*. 115 (3): 357–365.

De Waele, J.J., Hoste, E.A.J., Baert, D., *et al*. 2007. Relative adrenal insufficiency in patients with severe acute pancreatitis. *Intensive Care Medicine*. 33 (10): 1754–1760.

Deeny, P. 2005. Care of older people in critical care: the hidden side of the moon. *Intensive and Critical Care Nursing*. 21 (6): 325–327.

Del Sorbo, L., Cypel, M., Fan, E. 2014. Extracorporeal life support for adults with severe acute respiratory failure. *Lancet Respiratory Medicine*. 2 (2): 154–164.

Delaney, A. 2016. Physiology of body fluids. *In* Webb, A., Angus, D.C., Finger, S., Gattinoni, L., Singer, M.P.M. (eds) *Oxford Textbook of Critical Care*. 2nd edition. Oxford. Oxford University Press. 304–307.

Delisle, S., Ouellet, P., Bellemare, P., *et al*. 2011. Sleep quality in mechanically ventilated patients: comparison between NAVA and PSV modes. *Annals of Intensive Care*. 1 (1): 42.

Dellinger, R.P., Levy, M.M, Rhodes, A., *et al*., Surviving Sepsis Campaign Guidelines Committee including the Pediatric Subgroup. 2013. Surviving Sepsis Campaign: international guidelines for management of severe sepsis and septic shock. *Critical Care Medicine*. 41 (2): 580–637.

Demirel, S., Cumurcu, T., Fırat, P., *et al*. 2014. Effective management of exposure keratopathy developed in intensive care units: the impact of an evidence based eye care education pro-gramme. *Intensive and Critical Care Nursing*. 30 (1): 38–44.

den Uil, C.A., Galli, G., Jewbali, L.S., *et al*. 2017. First-line support by intra-aortic balloon pump in non-ischaemic cardiogenic shock in the era of modern ventricular assist devices. *Cardiology*. 138: 1–8.

Deng, Y., Luo, L., Hu, Y., Fang, K., Liu, J. 2016. Clinical practice guidelines for the management of neuropathic pain. A systematic review. *BMC Anesthesiology*. 16 (12).

Dennis, A.T. 2012. Management of pre-eclampsia: issues for anaesthetists. *Anaesthesia*. 67 (9): 1009–1020.

Dennis, M., Kadri, A., Coffey, J. 2012. Depression in older people in the general hospital: a systematic review of screening instruments. *Age and Ageing*. 41: 148–154.

Dernaika, T.A., Keddissi, J.I., Kinasewitz, G.T. 2009. Update on ARDS: beyond the low tidal volume. *American Journal of the Medical Sciences*. 337 (5): 360–367.

Deroy, R. 2000. Crystalloids or colloids for fluid resuscitation – is that the question? *Current Anaesthesia and Critical Care*. 11 (1): 20–26.

Devlin, J.W., Fong, J.J., Howard, E.P., *et al.* 2008. Assessment of delirium in the intensive care unit: nursing practices and perceptions. *American Journal of Critical Care*. 17 (6): 555–565.

Devlin, M. 2000. The nutritional needs of the older person. *Professional Nurse*. 16 (3): 951–955.

Dewhurst, A., Rawlins, T. 2009. Percutaneous valve replacement and repair in the adult: techniques and anaesthetic considerations. *Current Anaesthesia & Critical Care*. 20 (4): 155–159.

Dhar, A.K., Barton, D.A. 2016. Depression and the link with cardiovascular disease. *Frontiers in Psychiatry*. 7: article 33.

Dheda, K., Gumbo, T., Gandhi, N.R., *et al.* 2014. Global control of tuberculosis: from extensively drug-resistant to untreatable tuberculosis. *Lancet Respiratory Medicine*. 2 (4): 321–338.

Dhillon, R., Clark, J. 2009. Infection in the intensive care unit (ICU). *Current Anaesthesia & Critical Care*. 20 (4): 175–182.

Di Mario, C., Dudek, D., Piscione, F., *et al.*, CARESS-in-AMI (Combined Abcixmab RE-erplase Stent Study in Acute Myocardial Infection) Investigators. 2008. Immediate angioplasty versus standard therapy with rescue angioplasty after thrombolysis in the Combined Abcixmab RE-erplase Stent Study in Acute Myocardial Infection (CARESS-in-AMI): an open, prospective, randomised, multicentre trial. *Lancet*. 371 (9612): 559–568.

Di Mussi, R., Spadaro, S., Mirabella, L., *et al.* 2016. Impact of prolonged assisted ventilation on diaphragmatic efficiency: NAVA *versus* PSV. *Critical Care*. 20: 1.

Diabetes UK. 2016. *Facts and Stats*. https://diabetes-resources-production.s3-eu-west-1.amazonaws.com/diabetes-storage/migration/pdf/DiabetesUK_Facts_Stats_Oct16.pdf accessed 27 September 2017.

Diabetes UK. 2017. www.diabetes.org.uk/guide-to-diabetes/managing-your-diabetes/testing accessed 26 December 2017.

Dickson, S.J., Batson, S., Copas, A.J., *et al.* 2007. Survival of HIV-infected patients in the intensive care unit in the era of highly active antiretroviral therapy. *Thorax*. 62 (11): 964–968.

Dimond, B. 2015. *Legal Aspects of Nursing*. 7th edition. Harlow. Pearson.

Dind, A., Allahwala, U., Asrress, K.N., *et al.* 2017. Contemporary management of ST-elevation myocardial infarction. *Heart Lung and Circulation*. 26: 114–121.

Dive, A., Foret, F., Jamart, J., *et al.* 2000. Effects of dopamine on gastrointestinal motility during critical illness. *Intensive Care Medicine*. 26 (7): 901–907.

D.O.H. 1997. *A Bridge to the Future – Nursing Standards, Education and Workforce Planning in Paediatric Intensive Care*. London. HMSO.

D.O.H. 2000a. *Comprehensive Critical Care – A Review of Adult Critical Care Services*. London. Department of Health.

D.O.H. 2000b. *Health Services Circular HSC 2000/26*. London. Department of Health.

D.O.H. 2000c. *An Organisation with a Memory*. London. Department of Health.

D.O.H. 2001. *National Service Framework for Older People*. London. Department of Health.

D.O.H. 2006. *Modernising Nursing Careers*. London. Department of Health.

D.O.H. 2007. *High Impact Intervention 1: Central Venous Care Bundle*. London. Department of Health.

D.O.H. 2008a. *National Infarct Angioplasty Project*. London. Department of Health.

D.O.H. 2008b. *Organs for Transplants*. London. Department of Health.

D.O.H. 2009a. *NHS 2010–2015: from Good to Great. Preventative, People-Centred, Productive*. London. Department of Health.

D.O.H. 2009b. *New H1N1v Influenza: Current Situation and Next Steps*. Letter, dated 2 July 2009 (Gateway ref: 12167).

D.O.H. 2010a. *Midwifery 2010. Delivering Expectations*. London. Department of Health.

D.O.H. 2010b. *Six Years On: Delivering the Diabetes National Service Framework*. London. Department of Health.

D.O.H. 2016. *The UK: Your Partner for Patient Safety*. Published 17 March 2016. www.gov.uk/government/publications/the-uk-your-partner-for-patient-safety/the-uk-your-partner-for-patient-safety downloaded 10 January 2017.

Donaldson, L.J., Panesar, S.S., Darzi, A. 2014. Patient-safety-related hospital deaths in England: thematic analysis of incidents reported to a national database, 2010–2012. *PLoS ONE.* http://dx.doi.org/10.1371/journal.pmed.1001667.

Donnelly, M.C., Hayes, P.C., Simpson, K.J. 2016. The changing face of liver transplantation for acute liver failure: assessment of current status and implications for future practice. *Liver Transplantation.* 22 (4): 527–535.

Dougherty, L., Lister, S. (eds). 2015. *The Royal Marsden Hospital Manual of Clinical Nursing Procedures.* 9th edition. Oxford. Wiley-Blackwell. 418–532.

Doyle, J.F., Schortgen, F. 2016. Should we treat pyrexia? And how do we do it? *Critical Care.* 20: 303.

Drahnak, D.M., Custer, N. 2015. Prone positioning of patients with Acute Respiratory Distress Syndrome. *Critical Care Nurse.* 35 (6): 29–37.

Drakulovic, M.B., Torres, A., Bauer, T.T., *et al.* 1999. Supine body position as a risk factor for nosocomial pneumonia in mechanically ventilated patients: a randomised trial. *Lancet.* 354 (9193): 1851–1858.

Droogh, J.M., Smit, M., Absalom, A.R., Ligtenberg, J.J.M., Zijlstra, J.G. 2015. Transferring the critically ill patient: are we there yet? *Critical Care.* 19 (1): 62.

Drucker, P.F. 1974. *Management.* London. Butterworth-Heinemann.

Dua, K., Banerjee, A. 2010. Guillain-Barré syndrome: a review. *British Journal of Hospital Medicine.* 71 (9): 495–498.

Dumas, R.P., Martin, N.D. 2016. What's new in critical illness and injury science? Important considerations for work of breathing during tracheostomy weaning and decannulation. *International Journal of Critical Illness and Injuries Science.* 6 (3): 95–97.

Dunn, P., McKenna, H., Murray, R. 2016. *Deficits in the NHS 2016.* London. The King's Fund.

Durrington, H.J. 2017. Light intensity on Intensive Care Units – a short review. *Journal of Intensive and Critical Care.* 3 (2): 23.

Easby, D., Dalrymple, P. 2009. Monitoring arterial, central and pulmonary capillary wedge pressure. *Anaesthesia and Intensive Care Medicine.* 10 (1): 38–44.

E.A.S.L. (European Association for the Study of the Liver). 2017. EASL Clinical Practice Guideline on the management of acute (fulminant) hepatic failure. *Journal of Hepatology.* 66 (5): 1047–1081.

Eastwood, G.M., Tanaka, A., Espinoza, E.D.V., *et al.* 2016. Conservative oxygen therapy in mechanically ventilated patients following cardiac arrest: a retrospective nested cohort study. *Resuscitation.* 101: 108–114.

Echols, J., Friedman, B., Mullins, R.F., Still, J.M. Jr. 2004. Initial experience with a new system for the control and containment of fecal output for the protection of patients in a large burn centre. *Chest.* 126 (supplement 4): 862S.

Edwards, S. 2017. Reflecting differently. New dimensions: reflection-before-action and reflection-beyond-action. *International Practice Development Journal.* 7 (1).

Eeles, E.M.P., Hubbard, R.E., White, S.V., *et al.* 2010. Hospital use, institutionalisation and mortality associated with delirium. *Age and Ageing.* 39 (4): 470–475.

EfCCNa. 2007. *Position Statement on Workforce Requirements within European Critical Care Nursing.* Amsterdam. The European Federation of Critical Care Nursing Associations.

EfCCNa. 2012. *Position Statement on Nurses' Role in Weaning from Ventilation.* Amsterdam. The European Federation of Critical Care Nursing Associations.

EfCCNa. 2017. *Results from a Questionnaire Exploring Critical Care Nursing Practice Issue.* Amsterdam. European Federation of Critical Care Nursing Associations.

Ehlenbach, W.J., Hough, C.L., Crane, P.K., Haneuse, S.J.P.A., Carson, S.S., Curtis, J.R., Larson, E.B. 2010. Association between acute care and critical illness hospitalization and cognitive function in older adults. *JAMA.* 303 (8): 763–770.

El-Ansary, D., Adams, R., Torns, L., Elkins M. 2000. Sternal instability following coronary artery bypass grafting. *Physiotherapy Theory and Practice.* 16 (1): 27–33.

Eliopoulos, C. 2013. *Gerontological Nursing.* 8th edition. Philadelphia. Wolters Kluwer Lippincott Williams & Wilkins.

Elliott, R, McKinley S, Cistulli P, Fien M. 2013. Characterisation of sleep in intensive care using 24-hour polysomnography: an observational study. *Critical Care.* 17: R46.

Elliott, R., McKinley, S., Fox, V. 2008. Quality improvement program to reduce the prevalence of pressure ulcers in an intensive care unit. *American Journal of Critical Care*. 17 (4): 328–334.

El-Rabbany, M., Zaghlol, N., Bhandari, M., Azarpazhooh, A. 2015. Prophylactic oral health procedures to prevent hospital-acquired and ventilator-associated pneumonia: a systematic review. *International Journal of Nursing Studies*. 52 (1): 452–464.

E.L.S.O. 2017. *Guidelines for Cardiopulmonary Extracorporeal Life Support*. August 2017. version 1.4. Ann Arbor, MI. Extracorporeal Life Support Organization.

Ely, E.W., Truman, B., Shintani, A., *et al*. 2003. Monitoring sedation status over time in ICU patients: reliability and validity of the Richmond Agitation-Sedation Scale (RASS). *JAMA*. 289 (22): 2983–2991.

Endacott, R. 1999. Role of the allocated nurse and shift leader in the intensive care unit: findings of an ethnographic study. *Intensive and Critical Care Nursing*. 15 (1): 10–18.

Engström, M., Schött, U., Romner, B., Reinstrup, P. 2006. Acidosis impairs the coagulation: a thromboelastographic study. *Journal of Trauma*. 61 (3): 624–628.

Eriksson, T., Lindahl, B., Bergbom, I. 2010. Visits in an intensive care unit – an observational hermeneutic study. *Intensive & Critical Care Nursing*. 26 (1): 51–57.

Erlen, J.A. 2004. Wanted – nurses. *Orthopaedic Nursing*. 23 (4): 289–292.

Estcourt, L.J., Birchall, J., Allard, S., *et al*., on behalf of the British Committee for Standards in Haematology. 2017. Guidelines for the use of platelet transfusions. *British Journal of Haematology*. 176 (3): 365–394.

E.S.V.S. 2017. Management of descending thoracic aorta diseases. Clinical practice guidelines of the European Society for Vascular Surgery (ESVS). *European Journal of Vascular and Endovascular Surgery*. 53 (1): 4–52.

Ethics Committee of the Society of Critical Care Medicine. 1997. Consensus statement of the Society of Critical Care Medicine's Ethics Committee regarding futile and other possible inadvisable treatments. *Critical Care Medicine*. 25 (5): 887–891.

Everest, E., Hooper, M.R. 2014. Transport of the critically ill. *In* Bersten, A.D., Soni, N. (eds). *Intensive Care Manual*. 7th edition. Edinburgh. Butterworth-Heinemann Elsevier. 26–37.

Eves, N.D., Ford, G.T. 2007. Helium-oxygen: a versatile therapy to "lighten the load" of chronic obstructive pulmonary disease (COPD). *Respiratory Medicine: COPD Update*. 3 (3): 87–94.

Facchin, F., Fan, E. 2015. Airway pressure release ventilation and high-frequency oscillatory ventilation: potential strategies to treat severe hypoxemia and prevent ventilator-induced lung injury. *Respiratory Care*. 60 (10): 1509–1521.

Facioli, A.M., Amorim, F.F., de Almeida, K.J.Q. 2012. A model for humanization in critical care. *Permanente Journal*. 16 (4): 75–77.

Fagnoul, D., Combes, A., De Backer, D. 2014. Extracorporeal cardiopulmonary resuscitation. *Current Opinion in Critical Care*. 20 (3): 259–265.

Fajardo-Dolci, G., Gutierrez-Vega, R., Arboleya-Casanova, H., *et al*. 2010. Clinical characteristics of fatalities due to influenza A (H1N1) virus in Mexico. *Thorax*. 65 (6): 505–509.

Fallis, W.M. 2005. The effect of urine flow rate on urinary bladder temperature in critically ill adults. *Heart & Lung*. 34 (3): 209–216.

Fanelli, V., Vlachou, A., Ghannadian, S., *et al*. 2013. Acute respiratory distress syndrome: new definition, current and future therapeutic options. *Journal of Thoracic Disease*. 5 (3): 326–334.

Farfel, J.M., Franca, S.A., Sima, M. do C., *et al*. 2009. Age, invasive ventilatory support and outcomes in elderly patients admitted to intensive care units. *Age and Ageing*. 38 (5): 515–520.

Farley, A., McLafferty, E. 2008. Nursing management of the patient with hypothermia. *Nursing Standard*. 22 (17): 43–46.

Faulds, M., Meekings, T. 2013. Temperature management in critically ill patients. *Continuing Education in Anaesthesia, Critical Care & Pain*. 13 (3): 75–79.

Fearnhead, N.S. 2011. Acute lower gastrointestinal bleeding. *Medicine*. 39 (2): 101–104.

Feil, N. 1993. *The Validation Breakthrough*. Baltimore, MD. Health Professionals Press.

Feldheiser, A., Pavlova, V., Bonomo, T., *et al*. 2013. Balanced crystalloid compared with balanced colloid solution using a goal-directed haemodynamic algorithm. *British Journal of Anaesthesia*. 110 (2): 231–240.

Felmet, K., Orr, R. 2017. Transport of the critically ill child. *In* Watson, R.S., Thompson, A. (eds) *Pediatric Intensive Care*. New York. Oxford University Press. 23–31.

517

Ferguson, N.D., Cook, D.J., Guyatt, G.H., *et al.*, the OSCILLATE Trial Investigators and the Canadian Critical Care Trials Group. 2013. High-frequency oscillation in early acute respiratory distress syndrome. *New England Journal of Medicine.* 368 (9): 795–805.

Fernández-Barat, L., Ferrer, M., De Rosa, F., Gabarrús, A., Esperatti, M., Terraneo, S., Rinaudo, M., Bassi, G.L, Torres, A. 2017. Intensive care unit-acquired pneumonia due to *Pseudomonas aeruginosa* with and without multidrug resistance. *Journal of Infection.* 74 (2): 142–152.

Ferrara, J.L.M., Levine, J.E., Reddy, P., Holler, E. 2009. Graft-versus-host disease. *Lancet.* 373 (9674): 1550–1561.

Ferrer, M., Sellarés, J., Valencia, M., *et al.* 2009. Non-invasive ventilation after extubation in hypercapnic patients with chronic respiratory disorders: randomised controlled trial. *Lancet.* 374 (9695): 1082–1088.

Figuerosa-Ramos, M.I., Arroyo-Novoa, C.M., Lee, K.A., Padilla, G., Puntillo, K.A. 2009. Sleep and delirium in ICU patients: a review of mechanisms and manifestations. *Intensive Care Medicine.* 35 (5): 781–795.

Firth, M., Prather, C.M. 2002. Gastrointestinal motility problems in the elderly patient. *Gastroenterology.* 122 (6): 1688–1700.

Firth-Cozens, J., Mowbray, D. 2001. Leadership and the quality of care. *Quality in Health Care.* 10 (supplement II): ii3–ii7.

Fischer, S.A. 2017. Developing nurses' transformational leadership skills. *Nursing Standard.* 31 (51): 54–61.

Fisher, S., Walsh, G., Cross, N. 2002. Nursing management of the cardiac surgical patient. *In* Hatchett, R., Thompson, D. (eds) *Cardiac Nursing: A Comprehensive Guide.* Edinburgh. Churchill Livingstone. 426–461.

Flaatten, H., De Lange, D.W., Morandi, A., *et al.* 2017. The impact of frailty on ICU and 30-day mortality and the level of care in very elderly patients (≥ 80 years). *Intensive Care Medicine.* doi:10.1007/s00134–017–4940–8.

Focà, E., Magro, P., Motta, D., *et al.* 2016. Screening for neurocognitive impairment in HIV-infected individuals at first contact after HIV diagnosis: the experience of a large clinical center in northern Italy. *International Journal of Molecular Sciences.* 17 (4): 434.

Fogarty, A., Lingford-Hughes, A. 2004. Addiction and substance misuse. *Medicine.* 32 (7): 29–33.

Ford, P.N.R., Thomas, I., Cook, T.M., Whitley, E., Peden, C.J. 2007. Determinants of outcome in critically ill octogenarians after surgery: an observational study. *BJA.* 99 (6): 824–829.

Forrest, E.H. 2009. The management of alcoholic hepatitis. *British Journal of Hospital Medicine* 70 (12): 680–684.

Forsyth, R.J., Wolny, S., Rodrigues, B. 2010. Routine intracranial pressure monitoring in acute coma. *Cochrane Database of Systematic Reviews,* Issue 2. Art. No.: CD002043. doi:10.1002/14651858.CD002043.pub2.

Foster, J. 2016. The health challenges behind alcohol. *Nursing in Practice.* 93.

Foxall, F. 2008. *Arterial Blood Gas Analysis.* Keswick. M&K Update.

Francis, R. 2013. *Report of the Mid Saffordshire NHS Foundation Trust Public Enquiry.* London. The Stationery Office.

Frank, A., Bonney, M., Bonney, S., *et al.* 2012. Myocardial ischemia reperfusion injury – from basic science to clinical bedside. *Seminars in Cardiothoracic & Vascular Anesthesia.* 16 (3): 123–132.

Freedberg, D.E., Salmasian, H., Cohen, B., *et al.* 2016. Receipt of antibiotics in hospitalized patients and risk for *Clostridium difficile* infection in subsequent patients who occupy the same bed. *JAMA Internal Medicine.* x Published online 10 October 2016. doi:10.1001/jamainternmed.2016.6193.

Fried, M.J., Bruce, J., Colquhoun, R., Smith, G. 2010. Inter-hospital transfers of acutely ill adults in Scotland. *Anaesthesia.* 65 (2): 136–144.

Fuller, B.M., Mohr, N.M., Skrupky, L., Fowler, S., Kollef, M.H., Carpente, C.R. 2015. The use of inhaled prostaglandins in patients with ARDS: a systematic review and meta-analysis. *Chest.* 147 (6): 1510–1522.

Gaasbeek, A., Meinders, E. 2005. Hypophosphatemia: an update on its etiology and treatment. *American Journal of Medicine.* 118 (10): 1094–1101.

Gacouin, A., Camus, C., Gros, A., *et al*. 2010. Constipation in long-term ventilated patients: associated factors and impact on intensive care unit outcomes. *Critical Care Medicine*. 38 (10): 1933–1938.

Gaeeni, M., Farahani, M.A., Seyedfatemi, N., Mohammadi, N. 2015. Informational support to family members of intensive care unit patients: the perspectives of families and nurses. *Global Journal of Health Science*. 7 (2): 8–19.

Gaffney, A.M., Widhurt, S.M., Annich, G.M., Radomski, M.W. 2010. Extracorporeal life support. *BMJ*. 341 (7780): 982–986.

Gagné, R.M. 1975. *Essentials of Learning for Instruction*. New York. Holt, Reinhart & Winston.

Gagné, R.M. 1985. *The Condition of Learning and Theory Instruction*. London. Holt, Reinhart & Winston.

Gajic, O., Rana, R., Winters, J.L., *et al*. 2007. Transfusion-related acute lung injury in the critically ill. *American Journal of Respiratory and Critical Care Medicine*. 176 (9): 886–891.

Gall, H., Sommer, N., Milger, K., *et al*. 2016. Survival with sildenafil and inhaled iloprost in a cohort with pulmonary hypertension: an observational study. *BMC Pulmonary Medicine*. 16 (1): 5.

Gallagher, R., McKinley, S. 2009. Anxiety, depression and perceived control in patients having coronary artery bypass grafts. *Journal of Advanced Nursing*. 65 (11): 2386–2396.

Gallando García, M.B., Gallardo, P.F., Cabra Bellido, M.J., Sánchez, G.P., Bondía Navaro, J.A. 2012. Alternativas Terapéuticas a las transfusions de sangre en pacientes graves. *Revista de Hemattologia*. 13 (4): 153–164.

Gallop, K.H., Kerr, C.E.P., Nixon, A., *et al*. 2015. A qualitative investigation of patients' and caregivers' experiences of severe sepsis. *Critical Care Medicine*. 43 (2): 296–307.

Galvin, S., Campbell, M., Marsh, B., O'Brien, B. 2010. Cocaine-related admissions to an intensive care unit: a five-year study of incidence and outcomes. *Anaesthesia*. 65 (2): 163–166.

Gammon, J., Morgan-Samuel, H., Gould, D. 2008. A review of the evidence for suboptimal compliance of healthcare practitioners to standard/universal infection control precautions. *Journal of Clinical Nursing*. 17 (2): 157–168.

Gandhi, N.R., Nunn, P., Dheda, K., *et al*. 2010. Multidrug-resistant and extensively drug-resistant tuberculosis: a threat to global control of tuberculosis. *Lancet*. 375 (9728): 1830–1843.

Gandy, J. (ed.). 2014. *Manual of Dietetic Practice*. 5th edition. Oxford. Wiley Blackwell.

Ganz, F.D. 2012. Sleep and immune function. *Critical Care Nursing*. 32 (2): e19-e25.

Garcia-Tsao, G., Bosch, J. 2015. Varices and variceal hemorrhage in cirrhosis. a new view of an old problem. *Clinical Gastroenterology and Hepatology*. 13 (12): 2109–2117.

Gardiner, D., Manara, A. 2014. *Form for the Diagnosis of Death using Neurological Criteria*. London. Faculty of Intensive Care Medicine.

Garrouste-Orgeas, M., Flaatten, H., Moreno, R. 2016. Understanding medical errors and adverse events in ICU patients. *Intensive Care Medicine*. 42 (1): 107–109.

Garrouste-Orgeas, M., Coquet, I., Perier, A., *et al*. 2012. Impact of an intensive care unit diary of psychological distress in patients and relatives. *Critical Care Medicine*. 40 (7): 2033–2040.

Garvey, G., Belligan, G. 2009. MRSA: isolation could do more harm than good. *In* Ridley, S. (ed.). *Critical Care Focus 16: Infection*. London. Intensive Care Society. 73–89.

Gasper, E.A., McEwing, G., Richardson, J. 2016. *Oxford Handbook of Children and Young People's Nursing*. Oxford. Oxford University Press.

Gattinoni, L., Quintel, M. 2016. How ARDS should be treated. *Critical Care*. 20: 86.

Gaudry, S., Hajage, D., Schortgen, F., *et al*., for the AKIKI Study Group. 2016. Initiation strategies for Renal-Replacement Therapy in the Intensive Care Unit. *The New England Journal of Medicine*. 375 (2): 122–133.

Gazendam, J.A., Van Dongen, H.P., Grant, D.A., *et al*. 2013. Altered circadian rhythmicity in patients in the ICU. *Chest*. 144 (2): 483–489.

Geeraerts, T., Merceron, S., Benhamou, D., Vigué, B., Duranteau, J. 2008. Non-invasive assessment of intracranial pressure using ocular sonography in neurocritical care patients. *Intensive Care Medicine*. 34 (11): 2062–2067.

Geijer, J.R., Hultgren, N.E., Evanoff, N.G., *et al*. 2016. Comparison of brachial dilatory responses to hypercapnia and reactive hyperemia. *Physiological Measurement*. 37 (3): 380.

Gélinas, C., Chanques, G., Puntillo, K. 2014. In pursuit of pain: recent advances and future directions in pain assessment in the ICU. *Intensive Care Medicine*. 40 (7): 1009–1014.

Gélinas, C., Fillion, L., Puntillo, K.A., Viens, C., Fortier, M. 2006. Validation of the Critical-Care Pain Observation Tool in adult patients. *American Journal of Critical Care*. 15 (4): 420–427.

Gerich, J.E. 2010. Role of the kidney in normal glucose homeostasis and in the hyperglycaemia of diabetes mellitus: therapeutic implications. *Diabetic Medicine*. 27 (2): 136–142.

Gerschman, R., Gilbert, D.L., Nye, S.W., Dwyer, P., Fenn, W.O. 1954. Oxygen poisoning and X-irradiation – a mechanism in common. *Science*. 119: 623–626.

Ghashut, R.A., McMillan, D.C., Kinsella, J., *et al*. 2016. The effect of the systemic inflammatory response on plasma zinc and selenium adjusted for albumin. *Clinical Nutrition*. 35 (2): 381–387.

Ghuran, A., Nolan, J. 2000. Recreational drug misuse: issues for the cardiologist. *Heart*. 83 (6): 627–633.

Giannini, E.G., Testa, R., Savarin, V. 2005. Liver enzyme alteration: a guide for clinicians. *Canadian Medical Association Journal*. 172 (3): 367–379.

Gibbison, B., Sheikh, A., McShane, P., Haddow, C., Soar, J. 2012. Anaphylaxis admissions to UK critical care units between 2005 and 2009. *Anaesthesia*. 67 (8): 833–838.

Gibson, A.J., Davis, F.M. 2010. Hyperbaric oxygen therapy in the treatment of post cardiac surgical strokes – a case series and review of the literature. *Anesthesia and Intensive Care*. 38 (1): 175–184.

Gillies, D., Todd, D.A., Foster, J.P., Batuwitage, B.T. 2017. Heat and moisture exchangers versus heated humidifiers for mechanically ventilated adults and children. *Cochrane Database of Systematic Reviews*, Issue 9. Art. No.: CD004711. doi:10.1002/14651858.CD004711.pub3.

Girard, T.D., Alhazzani, W., Kress, J.P., *et al*. 2017. An official American Thoracic Society/ American College of Chest Physicians clinical practice guideline: liberation from mechanical ventilation in critically ill adults. Rehabilitation protocols, ventilator liberation protocols, and cuff leak tests. *American Journal of Respiratory and Critical Care Medicine*. 195 (1): 120–133.

Glaspole, I.N., Williams, T.J. 1999. Lung transplantation. *Medicine*. 27 (11): 146–148.

Glauser, T., Shinnar, S., Gloss, D., 2016. Evidence-Based Guideline: Treatment of Convulsive Status Epilepticus in Children and Adults: Report of the Guideline Committee of the American Epilepsy Society. *Epilepsy Currents*. 16 (1): 48–61.

Gluud, L.L., Vilstrup, H., Morgan, M.Y. 2016. Non-absorbable disaccharides versus placebo/no intervention and lactulose versus lactitol for the prevention and treatment of hepatic encephalopathy in people with cirrhosis. *Cochrane Database of Systematic Reviews*, Issue 4. Art. No.: CD003044. doi:10.1002/14651858.CD003044.pub3.

Goffman, E. 1963. *Stigma*. London. Penguin.

Gok, F., Kilicasan, A., Yosunkaya, A. 2015. Ultrasound-guided nasogastric feeding tube placement in critical care patients. *Nutrition in Clinical Practice*. 30 (22): 257–260.

Goldberg, D.S., Forde, K.A., Carbonari, D.M., *et al*. 2016. Population-representative incidence of drug-induced acute liver failure based on an analysis of an integrated healthcare system. *Gastroenterology*. 148 (7): 1353–1361.e3.

Goldhill, D.R., Badacsonyi, A., Goldhill, A.A., Waldmann, C. 2008. A prospective observational study of ICU patient position and frequency of turning. *Anaesthesia*. 63 (5): 509–515.

Golding, R., Taylor, D., Gardner, H., Wilkinson, J.N. 2016. Targeted temperature management in intensive care – do we let nature take its course? *Journal of the Intensive Care Society*. 17 (2): 154–159.

Gomes, E.C., Silva, A.N., Oliveira, M.R. 2012. Oxidants, antioxidants, and the beneficial roles of exercise-induced production of reactive species. *Oxidative Medicine and Cellular Longevity*. Volume 2012, Article ID 756132.

Goodnough, L.T., Schrier, S.L. 2014. Evaluation and management of anemia in the elderly. *American Journal of Hematology*. 89 (1): 88–96.

Gopal, S., Jayakumar, D., Nelson, P.N. 2009. Meta-analysis on the effect of dopexamine on in-hospital mortality. *Anaesthesia*. 64 (6): 589–594.

Gordon, A.C., Perkins, G.D., Singer, M., *et al*. 2016. Levosimendan for the prevention of acute organ dysfunction in sepsis. *New England Journal of Medicine*. 375 (17): 1638–1648.

Gould, D. 2008. Enterococcal infection. *Nursing Standard*. 22 (27): 40–43.

Gould, D. 2012. Skin flora: implications for nursing. *Nursing Standard*. 26 (33): 48–56.

Goulding, G. 2014. Unrecognised carotid arterial cannulation: prevention and management. *Anaesthesia & Intensive Care*. 42 (6): 696–699.

Goyal, A., Spertus, J.A., Gosch, K., Venkitachalam, L., Jones, P.G., Van den Berghe, G., Kosiborod, M. 2012. Serum potassium levels and mortality in acute myocardial infarction. *JAMA*. 307 (2): 157–164.

Grap, M.J., Munro, C.L., Ashtiani, B., Bryant, S. 2003. Oral care interventions in critical care: frequency and documentation. *American Journal of Critical Care*. 12 (2): 113–118.

Grap, M.J., Munro, C.L., Hamilton, V.A., Elswick, R.K., Sessler, C.N., Ward, K.R. 2011. Early, single chlorhexidine application reduces ventilator-associated pneumonia in trauma patients. *Heart & Lung*. 40: e115–122.

Greaves, L.C., Reeve, A.K., Taylor, R.W., Turnbull, D.M. 2012. Mitochondrial DNA and disease. *Journal of Pathology*. 226 (2): 274–286.

Grebenik, C.R., Sinclair, M.E. 2003. Which inotrope? *Current Paediatrics*. 13 (1): 6–11.

Green, S.M. 2011. Cheerio, Laddie! Bidding farewell to the Glasgow Coma Scale. *Annals of Emergency Medicine*. 58 (5): 427–430.

Greenhalgh, J., Hockenhull, J., Rao, N., *et al*. 2010. Drug-eluting stents versus bare metal stents for angina or acute coronary syndromes. *Cochrane Database of Systematic Reviews*, Issue 5. Art. No.: CD004587. doi:10.1002/14651858.CD004587.pub2.

Greenhawt, M., Turner, P.J., Kelso, J.M. 2018. Administration of influenza vaccines to egg allergic recipients: a practice parameter update 2017. *Annals of Allergy, Asthma and Immunology*. 120 (1): 49–52.

Greenlee, M., Wingo, C.S., McDonough, A.A., *et al*. 2009. Narrative review: evolving concepts in potassium homeostasis and hypokalaemia. *Annals of Internal Medicine*. 150 (9): 619–625.

Grice, E.A., Segre, J.A. 2011. The skin microbiome. *Nature Reviews Microbiology*. 9 (4): 244–253.

Grounds, M., Snelson, C., Whitehouse, T., *et al*. 2014. *Intensive Care Society Review of Best Practice for Analgesia and Sedation in the Critical Care*. London. Intensive Care Society.

Gucyetmez, B., Atalan, H.K. 2016. C Reactive Protein and hemogram parameters for the non-sepsis systemic inflammatory response syndrome and sepsis: what do they mean? *PLoS ONE* 11 (2): e0148699. doi:10.1371/journal. pone.0148699.

Guenter, P.A., Settle, R.G., Perlmutter, S., *et al*. 1991. Tube feeding-related diarrhoea in acutely ill patients. *Journal of Parenteral and Enteral Nutrition*. 15 (3): 277–280.

Guérin, C., Reignier, J., Richard, J.-C., *et al*., for the PROSEVA Study Group. 2013. Prone positioning in Severe Acute Respiratory Distress Syndrome. *The New England Journal of Medicine*. 368 (23): 2159–2168.

Guest, M. 2017. Patient transfer from the intensive care unit to a general ward. *Nursing Standard*. 32 (10): 45–51.

Güneş, Ü.Y., Zaybak, A. 2008. Does the body temperature change in older people? *Journal of Clinical Nursing*. 17 (17): 2284–2287.

Gunn, S.R., Early, B.J., Zenati, M.S., Ochoa, J.B. 2009. Use of a nasal bridle prevents accidental nasoenteral feeding tube removal. *JPEN*. 33 (1): 50–54.

Gunning, K. 2009. Hepatic failure. *Anaesthesia and Intensive Care Medicine*. 10 (3): 124–126.

Gupta, A. 2015. Biofilm quantification and comparative analysis of MIC (minimum inhibitory concentration) & MBIC (minimum biofilm inhibitory concentration) value for different antibiotics against *E. coli*. *International Journal of Current Microbiology and Applied Sciences*. 4 (2): 198–224.

Gupta, N.P., Mullamalla, U.R., Velappan, P., *et al*. 2015. Why is an IABP not the answer to cardiogenic shock after percutaneous coronary intervention? Is it that noradrenaline helps, especially by improving the RV function in addition to LV function? A view point. *Journal of Vascular Medicine and Surgery*. 3 (5): 220. doi:10.4172/2329-6925.1000220.

Gupta, R.K., Nikkar-Esfahani, A., Jamjoom, D.Z.A. 2010. Spontaneous intracerebral haemorrhage: a clinical review. *British Journal of Hospital Medicine*. 71 (9): 499–506.

Guzman-Castello, M., Ahmadi-Abhari, S., Bandosz, P., *et al*. 2017. Forecasted trends in disability and life expectancy in England and Wales up to 2025: a modelling study. *Lancet Public Health*. 2 (7): E309–313.

Haddad, S.H., Arabi, Y.M. 2012. Critical care management of severe traumatic brain injury in adults. *Scandinavian Journal of Trauma, Resuscitation and Emergency Medicine*. 20 (1): 12.

Hahn, R.G. 2014. Should anaesthetists stop infusing isotonic saline? *British Journal of Anaesthesia*. 112 (1): 4–6.

Hahn, R.G., Lyons, G. 2016. The half-life of infusion fluids. An educational review. *European Journal of Anaesthesiology*. 33 (7): 475–482.

Haitsma, J.J., Lachmann, B. 2002. Partial liquid ventilation in acute respiratory distress syndrome. *In* Evans, T.W., Griffiths, M.J.D., Keogh, B.F. (eds) *ARDS*. Sheffield. European Respiratory Society Journals. 208–219.

Hall, A.P., Henry, J.A. 2006. Acute toxic effects of "Ecstasy" (MDMA) and related compounds: overview of pathophysiology and clinical management. *British Journal of Anaesthesia*. 96 (6): 678–685.

Hall, J., Horsley, M. 2007. Diagnosis and management of patients with *Clostridium-difficile*-associated diarrhoea. *Nursing Standard*. 21 (46): 49–56.

Hall, J.E. 2016. *Guyton and Hall. Textbook of Medical Physiology*. 13th edition. Philadelphia. Elsevier.

Hall, M.M., Rajasekaran, S., Thomsen, T.W., Peterson, A.R. 2016. Lactate: friend or foe? *PM&R*. 8: S8-S15.

Hampton, J.R. 2013a. *The ECG made Easy*. 8th edition. Edinburgh. Churchill Livingstone Elsevier.

Hampton, J.R. 2013b. *The ECG in Practice*. 6th edition. Edinburgh. Churchill Livingstone Elsevier.

Hampton, J.R. 2013c. *150 ECG Problems*. 4th edition. Edinburgh. Churchill Livingstone Elsevier.

Hans-Geurts, I.J.M., Hop, W.C.J., Kok, N.F.M., *et al.* 2007. Randomized clinical trial of the impact of early enteral feeding on postoperative ileus and recovery. *British Journal of Surgery*. 94 (5): 555–561.

Happ, M.B., Baumann, B.M., Sawicki, J., *et al.* 2010. SPEACS-2: Intensive Care Unit "Communication Rounds" with speech language pathology. *Geriatric Nursing*. 31 (3): 170–177.

Harbath, S., Sax, H., Gastmeier, P. 2003. The preventable proportion of nosocomial infections: an overview of published reports. *Journal of Hospital Infection*. 54 (4): 258–266.

Harcombe, C. 2004. Nursing patients with ARDS in the prone position. *Nursing Standard*. 18 (19): 33–39.

Hare, M., McGowan, S., Wynaden, D., *et al.* 2008. Nurses' descriptions of changes in cognitive function in the acute care setting. *Australian Journal of Advanced Nursing*. 26 (1), 21–25.

Harioka, T., Matsukawa, T., Ozaki, M., *et al.* 2000. "Deep-forehead" temperature correlates well with blood temperature. *Canadian Journal of Anaesthesia*. 47 (10): 980–983.

Harris, P.D., Barnes, R. 2008. The uses of helium and xenon in current clinical practice. *Anaesthesia*. 63 (3): 284–293.

Hartog, C.S., Bauer, M., Reinhart, K. 2011. The efficacy and safety of colloid resuscitation in the critically ill. *Anesthesia & Analgesia*. 112 (1): 156–164.

Hartog, C.S., Rothaug, J., Goettermann, A., *et al.* 2010. Room for improvement: nurses' and physicians' views of a post-operative pain management program. *Acta Anaesthesiologica Scandinavica*. 54 (3): 277–283.

Hartung, T.K., Schofield, E., Short, A.I., *et al.* 2002. Hyponatraemic states following 3,4-methylenedioxymethamphetamine (MDMA, "ecstasy") ingestion. *QJM*. 95 (7): 431–437.

Harvey, M.A., Davidson, J.E. 2016. Postintensive Care Syndrome: right care, right now . . . and later. *Critical Care Medicine*. 44 (2): 381–385.

Harvey, S., Harrison, D.A., Singer, M., *et al.*, PAC-Man study collaboration. 2005. Assessment of the clinical effectiveness of pulmonary artery catheters in management of patients in intensive care (PAC-Man): a randomised controlled trial. *Lancet*. 366 (9484): 472–477.

Hawton, K., Townsend, E., Deeks, J., *et al.* 2001. Effects of legislation restricting pack size of paracetamol and salicylate on self poisoning in the United Kingdom: before and after study. *BMJ*. 322 (7296): 1203–1207.

Hayes, N., Ball, J. 2012. Achieving safe staffing for older people in hospital. *Nursing Older People*. 24 (4): 20–24.

Hayward, D., Bungay, V., Wolff, A.C., MacDonald, V. 2016. A qualitative study of experienced nurses' voluntary turnover: learning from their perspectives. *Journal of Clinical Nursing*. 25 (9–10): 1336–1345.

Hayward, J. 1975. *Information: A Prescription against Pain*. London. Royal College of Nursing.

Heart Protection Study Collaborative Group. 2012. Effects on 11-year mortality and morbidity of lowering LDL cholesterol with simvastatin for about 5 years in 20536 high-risk individuals: a randomised controlled trial. *Lancet*. 378 (9808): 2013–2020.

Hébert, P.C., Wells, G., Blajchman, M.A. *et al.*, Transfusion Requirements Investigators for the Canadian Critical Care Trials Group. 1999. A multicenter randomized, controlled clinical trial of transfusion requirements in critical care. *New England Journal of Medicine*. 340 (6): 409–417.

Hedges, C., Redeker, N.S. 2008. Comparison of sleep and mood in patients after on-pump and off-pump coronary artery bypass surgery. *American Journal of Critical Care*. 17 (2): 133–141.

Hegewald, M.J., Crapo, R.O. 2011. Respiratory physiology in pregnancy. *Clinics in Chest Medicine*. 32 (1): 1–13.

Heintz, B.H., Halilovic, J., Christensen, C.L. 2010. Vancomycin-resistant enterococcal urinary tract infections. *Pharmacotherapy*. 30 (11): 1136–1149.

Hellyer, T.P., Ewan, V., Wilson, P., Simpson, A.J. 2016. The Intensive Care Society recommended bundle of interventions for the prevention of ventilator-associated pneumonia. *Journal of the Intensive Care Society*. 17 (3): 238–243.

Heming, N., Mazeraud, A., Verdonk, F., *et al.* 2017. Neuro-anatomy of sepsis-associated encephalopathy. *Critical Care*. 21: 65.

Henderson-Smart, D.J., Cools, F., Bhuta, T., Offringa, M. 2007. Elective high frequency oscillatory ventilation versus conventional ventilation for acute pulmonary dysfunction in preterm infants. *Cochrane Database of Systematic Reviews*, Issue 3. Art. No.: CD000104. doi:10.1002/14651858.CD000104.pub2.

Hendricks-Thomas, J., Patterson, E. 1995. A sharing in critical thought by nursing faculty. *Journal of Advanced Nursing*. 22 (3): 594–599.

Hennessey, I.A.M., Japp, A.G. 2016. *Arterial Blood Gases Made Easy*. 2nd edition. Edinburgh. Elsevier.

Henricson, M, Berglund, A.-L., Määttä, S., Ekman, R., Segesten, K. 2008. The outcome of tactile touch on oxytocin in intensive care patients: a randomised controlled trial. *Journal of Clinical Nursing*. 17 (19): 2624–2633.

Henricson, M., Segesten, K., Berglund, A.-L., Määttä S. 2009. Enjoying tactile touch and gaining hope when being cared for in intensive care – a phenomenological hermeneutical study. *Intensive & Critical Care Nursing*. 25 (6): 323–331.

Hermanides, J., Hollmann, M.W., Stevens, M.F., Lirk, P. 2012. Failed epidural: causes and management. *British Journal of Anaesthesia*. 109 (2): 144–154.

Hermans, G., Van den Berghe, G. 2015. Clinical review: intensive care unit acquired weakness. *Critical Care*. 19: 274.

Herridge, M.S., Moss, M., Hough, C.L., *et al.* 2016. Recovery and outcomes after the acute respiratory distress syndrome (ARDS) in patients and their family caregivers. *Intensive Care Medicine*. 42 (5): 725–738.

Hess, D.R. 2002. Mechanical ventilation strategies: what's new and what's worth keeping? *Respiratory Care*. 47 (9): 1007–1017.

Hetzel, G.R., Schmitz, M., Wissing, H., *et al.* 2011. Regional citrate versus systemic heparin for anticoagulation in critically ill patients on continuous venovenous haemofiltration: a prospective randomized multicentre trial. *Nephrology, Dialysis, Transplantation*. 26 (1): 232–239.

Hevener, S., Rickabaugh, B., Marsh, T. 2016. Using a decision wheel to reduce use of restraints in a medical-surgical Intensive Care Unit. *American Journal of Critical Care*. 25 (6): 479–486.

Hickey, J.V. (ed.). 2014. *Neurological and Neurosurgical Nursing*. 7th edition. Philadelphia. Wolters Kluwer Lippincott Williams & Wilkins.

Higgins, C. 2013. *Understanding Laboratory Investigations*. 3rd edition. Oxford. Wiley-Blackwell.

Hignett, S., Lang, A., Pickup, L., *et al.* 2016. More holes than cheese. What prevents the delivery of effective, high quality and safe health care in England? *Ergonomics*. doi:10.1080/00140139.2016.1245446.

Hillas, G., Vassilakopoulos, T., Plantza, P., *et al.* 2010. C-reactive protein and procalcitonin as predictors of survival and septic shock in ventilator-associated pneumonia. *European Respiratory Journal*. 35 (4): 805–811.

Hine, K. 2007. The use of physical restraint in critical care. *Nursing in Critical Care.* 12 (1): 6–11.

Hinkelbein, J., Genzwuerker, H.V. 2008. Fingernail polish does not influence pulse oximetry to a clinically relevant dimension. *Intensive & Critical Care Nursing.* 24 (1): 4–5.

Hinton, L., Locock, L., Knight, M. 2015. Maternal critical care: what can we learn from patient experience? A qualitative study. *BMJ Open.* 5 (4): e006676. doi:10.1136/bmjopen-2014006676.

HM Government. 1974. Health and Safety at Work Act. www.legislation.gov.uk/ukpga/1974/37 accessed 10 October 2017.

Ho, A.M.-H., Lee, A., Karmakar, M.K., Dion, P.W., Chung, D.C., Contardi, L.H. 2003. Heliox vs air-oxygen mixtures for the treatment of patients with acute asthma. *Chest.* 123 (3): 882–890.

Ho, K.M. 2016. Pitfalls in haemodynamic monitoring in the postoperative and critical care setting. *Anaesthesia & Intensive Care.* 44: 1.

Ho, K.M., Power, B.M. 2010. Benefits and risks of furosemide in acute kidney injury. *Anaesthesia.* 65 (3): 283–293.

Hodd, J., Doyle, A., Carter, J., *et al.* 2010. Extubation in intensive care units in the UK: an online survey. *Nursing in Critical Care.* 15 (6): 281–284.

Hofhuis, J.G., Spronk, P.E., van Stel, H.F., *et al.* 2008a. Experiences of critically ill patients in the ICU. *Intensive and Critical Care Nursing.* 24 (5): 300–313.

Hofhuis, J.G.M., Spronk, P.E., van Stel, H.F., *et al.* 2008b. The impact of critical illness of perceived health-related quality of life during ICU treatment, hospital stay and after hospital discharge. *Chest.* 233 (2): 377–385.

Hogan, H., Healey, F., Neale, G., *et al.* 2012. Preventable deaths due to problems in English acute hospitals: a retrospective case record review study. *BMJ Quality & Safety.* 21 (9): 737–745.

Holloway, T., Penson, J. 1987. Nursing education as social control. *Nurse Education Today.* 7 (5): 235–241.

Holm-Knudsen, R.J., Rasmussen, L.S. 2009. Paediatric airway management: basic aspect. *Acta Anaesthesiologica Scandinavica.* 53 (1): 1–9.

Holt, G.E., Sarmento, B., Kett, D., Goodman, K.W. 2017. An unconscious patient with a DNR tattoo. *New England Journal of Medicine.* 377 (22): 2192–2193.

Hopkins, P.M. 2008. Malignant hyperthermia. *Current Anaesthesia & Critical Care.* 19 (1): 22–33.

Hopper, A.B., Vilke, G.M., Castillo, E.M., *et al.* 2015. Ketamine use for acute agitation in the emergency department. *The Journal of Emergency Medicine.* 48.(6): 712–719.

Hopson, A.S.M., Greenstein, A. 2007. Intravenous infusions in hyperbaric chambers: effect of compression on syringe function. *Anaesthesia.* 62 (6): 602–604.

Hoste, E.A., Bagshaw, S.M., Bellomo, R., *et al.* 2015. Epidemiology of acute kidney injury in critically ill patients: the multinational AKI-EPI study. *Intensive Care Medicine.* 41 (8): 1411–1423.

Houghton, A.R., Gray, D. 2014. *Making Sense of the ECG.* 4th edition. Boca Raton, Florida. CRG Press; Taylor & Francis.

Htun, A.T. 2015. Perioperative fluid therapy. *International Journal of Healthcare Sciences.* 3 (2): 514–521.

Huang, L., Quartin, A., Jones, D., Havlir, D.V. 2006. Intensive care of patients with HIV infection. *New England Journal of Medicine.* 355 (2): 173–181.

Hubbard, R.E., Lyons, R.A., Woodhouse, K.W., *et al.* 2003. Absence of ageism in access to critical care: a cross-sectional study. *Age and Ageing.* 32 (4): 382–387.

Hughes, E. 2004. Understanding the care of patients with acute pancreatitis. *Nursing Standard.* 18 (18): 45–52.

Hulatt, I. 2014. Restraint is a last resort, use it rarely and wisely. *Nursing Standard.* 28 (31): 22–23.

Hung, M., Vuylsteke, A., Valchanov, K. 2012. Extracorporeal membrane oxygenation: coming to an ICU near you. *Journal of the Intensive Care Society.* 13 (1): 31–38.

Hunningher, A., Smith, M. 2006. Update on the management of severe head injury in adults. *Care of the Critically Ill.* 22 (5): 124–129.

Hunt, B.J., Allard, S., Keeling, D., *et al.*, on behalf of the British Committee for Standards in Haematology. 2015. A practical guideline for the haematological management of major haemorrhage. *British Journal of Haematology.* 170 (6): 788–803.

Hunt, J. 2016. Speech to the Global Patient Safety Summit. London, 9–10 March 2016.

Hunter, J., Quarterman, C., Waseem, M., Wills, A. 2011. Diagnosis and management of nectrotizing fasciitis. *Hospital Medicine*. 72 (7): 391–395.

Hunter, J.D. 2002. Rhabdomyolysis. *Care of the Critically Ill*. 18 (2): 52–55.

Hunter, J.D. 2012. Ventilator associated pneumonia. *BMJ*. 341 (7859): 41–44.

Hunter, J.D., Doddi, M. 2010. Sepsis and the heart. *BJA*. 104 (1): 3–11.

Huskins, W.C., Huckabee, C.M., O'Grady, N.P., *et al.*, STAR*ICU Trial Investigators. 2011. Intervention to reduce transmission of resistant bacteria in intensive care. *New England Journal of Medicine*. 364 (15): 407–418.

Hutchins, A., Durand, M.A., Grieve, R., *et al.* 2009. Evaluation of modernisation of adult critical care services in England: time series and cost effectiveness analysis. *BMJ*. 339 (7730): 1130.

Ibeh, N.I., Dirisu, J., Uteh, U.E., Ibeh, I.N. 2012. Bacterial neonatal septicaemia "aetiological agents and prevalence in a third world country". *Novel Science International Journal of Medical Science*. 1 (4): 85–91.

I.C.N. 2012. *The ICN Code of Ethics for Nurses*. Geneva. International Council of Nurses.

I.C.S. 2009a. *Statement on the Use of Unlicensed Medicines or Licensed Medicines for Unlicensed Uses in Critically Ill Patients*. London. Intensive Care Society.

I.C.S. 2009b. *Standards and Recommendations for the Provision of Renal Replacement Therapy on Intensive Care Units in the United Kingdom*. London. Intensive Care Society.

I.C.S. 2011a. *Standards for Capnography in Critical Care (revision)*. London: Intensive Care Society. (In 2016 an update was published, confirming the validity of the 2011 standards)

I.C.S. 2011b. *Guidelines for the Transport of the Critically Ill Adult*. 3rd edition. London. Intensive Care Society.

I.C.S. 2013. *Core Standards for Intensive Care Unit*. London. Intensive Care Society/Faculty of Intensive Care Medicine.

I.C.S. 2014. *Standards for the Care of Adult Patients with a Temporary Tracheostomy*. London. Intensive Care Society.

I.C.S. 2015. *Guidelines for the Provision of Intensive Care Service*. London. Intensive Care Society.

I.C.S. 2017a. *Medication Concentrations in Critical Care Areas* version 2.2. London. Intensive Care Society.

I.C.S. 2017b. *ICS / FICM Guidance on MCA / DoL*. February 2017. London. Intensive Care Society.

Iggulden, H. 2006. *Care of the Neurological Patient*. Oxford. Blackwell.

Ikegamin, T., Takeromi, A., Soejima, Y., *et al.* 2008. Living donor liver transplantation for acute liver failure: a 10-year experience in a single centre. *Journal of the American College of Surgeons*. 206 (3): 412–418.

Ilies, C., Bauer, M., Berg, P., *et al.* 2012. Investigation of the agreement of a continuous non-invasive arterial pressure device in comparison with invasive radial artery measurement. *British Journal of Anaesthesia*. 108 (2): 202–210.

Imanaka, H., Takeuchi, M., Tachibana, K., *et al.* 2010. Effects of open lung approach policy on mechanical ventilation duration in postoperative patients with chronic thromboembolism with pulmonary hypertension: a case-matched study. *Anesthesia and Intensive Care*. 38 (3): 461–466.

International Carotid Stenting Study Investigators. 2010. Carotid artery stenting compared with endarterectomy in patients with symptomatic carotid stenosis (International Carotid Stenting Study): an interim analysis of a randomised controlled trial. *Lancet*. 375 (9719): 985–997.

International Council of Nurses. 2006. *The ICN Code of Ethics for Nurses*. Geneva. International Council of Nurses.

Iotti, G.A., Polito, A., Belliato, M., *et al.* 2010. Adaptive support ventilation versus conventional ventilation for total ventilatory support in acute respiratory failure. *Intensive Care Medicine*. 36 (8): 1371–1379.

Iverson, E., Celious, A., Kennedy, C.R., *et al.* 2014. Factors affecting stress experienced by surrogate decision-makers for critically ill patients: implications for nursing practice. *Intensive and Critical Care Nursing*. 30 (2): 77–85.

Iwashyna, J.T., Ely, E.W., Smith, D.M., Langa, K.M. 2010. Long-term cognitive impairment and functional disability among survivors of severe sepsis. *JAMA*. 304 (16): 1787–1794.

Jabusch, K.M., Lewthwaite, B.J., Mandzuk, L.L., *et al.* 2015. The pain experience of inpatients in a teaching hospital. Revisiting a strategic priority. *Pain Management Nursing.* 16 (1): 69–76.

Jack, L., Voyer, F., Courtney, M., Venkatesh, B. 2010. Probiotics and diarrhoea management in enterally tube fed critically ill patients – what is the evidence. *Intensive and Critical Care Nursing.* 26 (6): 314–326.

Jackson, J., Ey, W., Morey, M., *et al.* 2012. Cognitive and physical rehabilitation of intensive care unit survivors: results of the RETURN randomized controlled pilot investigation. *Critical Care Medicine.* 40 (4): 1088–1097.

Jaipuria, J., Bhandari, V., Chawla, A.S., Singh, M. 2016. Intra-abdominal pressure: time ripe to revise management guidelines of acute pancreatitis? *World Journal of Gastrointestinal Pathophysiology.* 15; 7 (1): 186–196.

Jalloh, I., Helmy, A., Shannon, R.J., *et al.* 2013. Lactate uptake by the injured human brain: evidence from an arteriovenous gradient and cerebral microdialysis study. *Journal of Neurotrauma.* 30 (12): 2031–2037.

James, P., Hanna, S. 2014. Upper airway obstruction in children. *In* Bersten, A.D., Soni, N. (eds). *Intensive Care Manual.* 7th edition. Edinburgh. Butterworth-Heinemann Elsevier. 1076–1084.

Janisch, N.H., Gardner, T.B. 2016. Advances in management of acute pancreatitis. *Gastroenterology Clinics of North America.* 45 (1): 1–8.

J.B.D.S. 2012. *The Management of the Hyperosmolar Hyperglycaemic State (HHS) in Adults with Diabetes.* London. Joint British Diabetes Societies.

J.B.D.S. 2013a. *The Hospital Management of Hypoglycaemia in Adults with Diabetes Mellitus.* Revised edition. London. Joint British Diabetes Societies.

J.B.D.S. 2013b. *The Management of Diabetic Ketoacidosis in Adults.* 2nd edition. London. Joint British Diabetes Societies.

Jefferies, S., Weatherall, M., Young, P., Beasley, R. 2011. A systematic review of the accuracy of peripheral thermometry in estimating core temperatures among febrile critically ill patients. *Critical Care and Resuscitation.* 13 (3): 194–199.

Jellinger, P.D., Handelsman, Y., Rosenblit, P.D., *et al.* 2017. American Association of Clinical Endocrinologists and American College of Endocrinology guidelines for management of dyslipidemia and prevention of cardiovascular disease. *Endocrine Practice.* 23 (supplement 2): 1–87.

Jenkins, I.A., Playfor, S.D., Bevan, C., *et al.* 2007. Current United Kingdom sedation practice in pediatric intensive care. *Pediatric Anesthesia,* 17 (1): 675–683.

Jerreat, L. 2010. Managing diabetic ketoacidosis. *Nursing Standard.* 24 (34): 49–55.

Jevon, P., Ewens, B. 2012. *Monitoring the Critically Ill Patient.* 3rd edition. Chichester. Blackwell.

Joannidis, M., Druml, W., Forni, L.G. *et al.* 2010. Prevention of acute kidney injury and protection of renal function in the intensive care unit. *Intensive Care Medicine.* 36 (3): 392–411.

Joannidis, M., Druml, W., Forni, L.G., *et al.* 2017. Prevention of acute kidney injury and protection of renal function in the intensive care unit: update 2017. *Intensive Care Medicine.* 43 (6): 730–749.

Joffe, A.M., Hallman, M., Gélinas, C., *et al.* 2013. Evaluation and treatment of pain in critically ill adults. *Seminars in Respiratory and Critical Care Medicine.* 34 (2): 189–200.

Johnson, C.D., Besselink, M.G., Carter, R. 2014. Acute pancreatitis. *BMJ.* 349 doi:http://dx.doi.org/10.1136/bmj.g4859.

Jones, C., Bäckman, C., Capuzzo, M., *et al.*, RACHEL group. 2010. Intensive care diaries reduce new onset post-traumatic stress disorder following critical illness: a randomised, controlled trial. *Critical Care.* 14: R168.

Jones, C.V. 2004. The importance of oral hygiene in nutritional support. *In* White, R. (ed.) *Trends in Oral Health Care.* Dinton. Quay Books. 72–83.

Jonkman, A.H., Jansen, D., Heunks, L.M.A. 2017. Novel insights in ICU-acquired respiratory muscle function: implications for clinical care. *Critical Care.* 21: 64.

Joshua-Amadi, M. 2002. Recruitment and retention. *Journal of Nursing Management.* 9 (8): 17–21.

Jowett, N.I., Thompson, D.R. 2007. *Comprehensive Coronary Care.* 4th edition. Edinburgh. Baillière Tindall.

Jubran, A. 2015. Pulse oximetry. *Critical Care*. 19: 272.

Jubran, A., Grant, B.J.B., Duffner, L.A., *et al.* 2013. Effect of pressure support vs unassisted breathing through a tracheostomy collar on weaning duration in patients requiring prolonged mechanical ventilation. A randomized trial. *JAMA*. 309 (7): 671–677.

Jung, S., Kim, H., Yang, H. 2008. The effects of temperature monitoring methods and thermal management methods during spinal surgery. *Anesthesiology*. 109: A1133.

Juurlink, D.N., Buckley, N.A., Stanbrook, M.B., *et al.* 2005. Hyperbaric oxygen for carbon monoxide poisoning. *Cochrane Database Systematic review*. 1:CD002041.

Kacmarek, R.M., Wiedemann, H.P., Lavin, P.T., *et al.* 2006. Partial liquid ventilation in adult patients with acute respiratory distress syndrome. *American Journal of Respiratory & Critical Care Medicine*. 173 (8): 882–889.

Kaier, T.E., Twerenbold, R., Puelacher, C., *et al.* 2017. Direct comparison of cardiac myosin-binding protein C with cardiac troponins for the early diagnosis of acute myocardial infarction. *Circulation*. 10.1161/CIRCULATIONAHA.117.028084.

Kakkar, A.K., Cimminiello, C., Goldhaber, S.Z., *et al.*, LIFENOX Investigators. 2011. Low-molecular weight heparin and mortality in acutely ill medical patients. *New England Journal of Medicine*. 365 (26): 2463–2472.

Kallet, R.H, Matthay, M.A. 2013. Hyperoxic acute lung injury. *Respiratory Care*. 58 (1): 123–141.

Kalucka, J., Bierhansl, L., Wielockx, B., *et al.* 2017. Interaction of endothelial cells with macrophages – linking molecular and metabolic signalling. *European Journal of Physiology*. 469 (3–4): 473–483.

Kamdar, B.B., Huang, M., Dinglas, V.D., *et al.* 2017. Joblessness and lost earnings after ARDS in a 1-year national multicenter study. *American Journal of Respiratory & Critical Care Medicine*. 196 (8): 1012–1020.

Kamdar, B.B., Needham, D.M., Collop, N.A. 2012. Sleep deprivation in critical illness: its role in physical and psychological recovery. *Journal of Intensive Care Medicine*. 27 (2): 97–111.

Kamel, H., Navi, B.B., Nakagawa, K., *et al.* 2011. Hypertonic saline versus mannitol for the treatment of elevated intracranial pressure: a meta-analysis of randomized clinical trials. *Critical Care Medicine*. 39 (3): 554–559.

Kanagasundaram, S. 2007. Renal replacement therapy in acute kidney injury: an overview. *British Journal of Hospital Medicine*. 68 (6): 292–297.

Kapoor, A., Dharel, N., Sanyal, J. 2016. Endoscopic diagnosis and therapy in gastro-esopageal variceal bleeding. *Gastrointestinal Endoscopy Clinics of North America*. 25 (3): 491–507.

Karch, J., Molkentin, J.D. 2015. Regulated necrotic cell death: the passive aggressive side of Bax and Bak. *Circulatory Research*. 116 (11): 1800–1809.

Karlsson, C., Tisell, A., Engström, Å., Andershed, B. 2011. Family members' satisfaction with critical care: a pilot study. *Nursing in Critical Care*. 16 (1): 11–18.

Kass, J.E. 2003. Heliox redux. *Chest*. 123 (3): 673–676.

Kaussen, T., Srinivasan, P.K., Afify, M., *et al.* 2012. Influence of two different levels of intra-abdominal hypertension on bacterial translocation in a porcine model. *Annals of Intensive Care*. 2 (supplement 1): S17.

K.D.I.G.O. 2012. Clinical Practice Guideline for Acute Kidney Injury. *Kidney International*. 2 (supplement 1): 1–138.

Keays, R. 2014. Diabetic emergencies. *In* Bersten, A.D., Soni, N. (eds). *Intensive Care Manual*. 7th edition. Edinburgh. Butterworth-Heinemann. 629–636.

Keeling, D., Baglin, T., Tait, C., *et al.*, British Committee for Standards in Haematology. 2011. Guidelines on oral anticoagulation with warfarin. 4th edition. *British Journal of Haematology*. 154 (3): 311–324.

Kelly, C.P., LaMont, J.T. 2008. *Clostridium difficile* – more difficult than ever. *New England Journal of Medicine*. 359 (18): 1932–1940.

Kelly, T., Timmis, S., Twelvetree, T. 2010. Review of the evidence to support oral hygiene in stroke patients. *Nursing Standard*. 24 (37): 35–38.

Keogh, B.F., Cordingley, J.J. 2002. Current invasive ventilatory strategies in acute respiratory distress syndrome. *In* Evans, T.W., Griffiths, M.J.D., Keogh, B.F. (eds) *ARDS*. Sheffield. European Respiratory Society Journals. 161–180.

Kessler, C. 2009. Glycaemic control in hospital: how tight should it be? *Nursing*. 39 (11): 38–43.

Khalaila, R., Zbidat, W., Anwar, K., *et al*. 2011. Communication difficulties and psychoemotional distress in patients receiving mechanical ventilation. *American Journal of Critical Care*. 20 (6): 470–479.

Khamnuan, P., Chongruksut, W., Jearwattanakanok, K., *et al*. 2015. Necrotizing fasciitis: risk factors of mortality. *Risk Management and Healthcare Policy*. 8: 1–7.

Khitan, Z.J., Malhotra, D., Raj, D.S., Tzamaloukas, A.H., Shapiro, J.I. 2015. Alkali therapy in lactic acidosis. *Marshall Journal of Medicine*. 1 (1): Article 6.

Khwannimit, B., Bhurayanontachai, R. 2009. The performance of customised APACHE II and SAPS II in predicting mortality of mixed critically ill patients in a Thai medical intensive care unit. *Anaesthesia and Intensive Care*. 37 (5): 784–790.

Kings Fund. 2016. *Sustainability and Transformation Plans in the NHS*. London. The King's Fund.

Kirkpatrick, A.W., Roberts, D.J., De Waele, J., *et al*. 2013. Intra-abdominal hypertension and the abdominal compartment syndrome: updated consensus definitions and clinical practice guidelines from the World Society of the Abdominal Compartment Syndrome. *Intensive Care Medicine*. 39 (7): 1190–1206.

Kite, K., Pearson, L. 1995. A rationale for mouth care: the integration of theory with practice. *Intensive and Critical Care Nursing*. 11 (2): 71–76.

Klek, S., Forbes, A., Gabe, S., *et al*. 2016. Management of acute intestinal failure: a position paper from the European Society for Clinical Nutrition and Metabolism (ESPEN) Special Interest Group. *Clinical Nutrition*. 35 (6): 1209–1218.

Klompas, M., Speck, K., Howell, M.D., *et al*. 2014. Reappraisal of routine oral care with chlorhexidine gluconate for patients receiving mechanical ventilation: systematic review and meta-analysis. *JAMA Internal Medicine*. 174 (5): 751–761.

Klouwenberg, P.M.C.K., Zaal, I.J., Spitoni, C., *et al*. 2014. The attributable mortality of delirium in critically ill patients: prospective cohort study. *BMJ*. 349: g6652.

Knaus, W.A., Draper, E.A., Wagner, D.P., Zimmerman, J.E. 1985. APACHE II: a severity of disease classification system. *Critical Care Medicine*. 13 (10): 818–829.

Knight, A.R., Fry, L.E., Clancy, R.L., Pierce, J.D. 2011. Understanding the effects of oxygen administration in haemorrhagic shock. *Nursing in Critical Care*. 16 (1): 28–33.

Knight, M., Tuffnell, D., Kenyon, S., *et al*. 2015. *Saving Lives, Improving Mothers' Care*. Oxford. National Perinatal Epidemiology Unit.

Knoll, M., Lautenschlaeger, C., Borneff-Lipp, M. 2010. The impact of workload on hygiene compliance in nursing. *British Journal of Nursing*. 19 (16): S18–S22.

Koesters, S.C., Rogers, P.D., Rajasingham, C.R. 2002. MDMA ("ecstasy") and other "club drugs". The new epidemic. *The Pediatric Clinics of North America*. 49 (2): 415–433.

Kogos, S.C. Jr, Richards, J.S., Banos, J., *et al*. 2005. A descriptive study of pain and quality of life following Guillain-Barre Syndrome: one year later. *Journal of Clinical Psychology in Medical Settings*. 12 (2): 111–116.

Kollisch-Singule, M., Emr, B., Jain, S.V., *et al*. 2015. The effects of airway pressure release ventilation on respiratory mechanics in extrapulmonary lung injury. *Intensive Care Medicine Experimental*. 3: 35.

Kotani, T., Katayama, S., Fukuda, S. *et al*. 2016. Pressure-controlled inverse ratio ventilation as a rescue therapy for severe acute respiratory distress syndrome. *SpringerPlus*. 5: 716.

Kottner, J., Lichterfeld, A., Blume-Peytavi, U. 2013. Maintaining skin integrity in the aged. *The British Journal of Dermatology*. 169 (3): 528–542.

Krajcova, A., Waldauf, P., Andel, M., Duska, F. 2015. Propofol infusion syndrome: a structured review of experimental studies and 153 published case reports. *Critical Care*. 19 (1): 398.

Krajewski, M.L., Raghunathan, K., Paluszkiewicz, S.M., *et al*. 2015. Meta-analysis of high- versus low-chloride content in perioperative and critical care fluid resuscitation. *British Journal of Surgery*. 102 (1): 24–36.

Kramer, C.K., Zinman, B., Retnakaran, R. 2013. Are metabolically healthy overweight and obesity benign conditions? A systematic review and meta-analysis *Annals of Internal Medicine*. 159 (11): 758–769.

Kraut, J.A., Madias, N.E. 2014. Lactic acidosis. *New England Journal of Medicine*. 37 (24): 2309–2319.

Krishnan, J.A., Moore, D., Robeson, C., *et al.* 2004. A prospective, controlled trial of a protocol-based strategy to discontinue mechanical ventilation. *American Journal of Respiratory and Critical Care Medicine*. 169 (6): 673–678.

Krotsetis, S., Richards, K.C., Behncke, A., Köpke, S. 2017. The reliability of the German version of the Richards Campbell sleep questionnaire. *Nursing in Critical Care*. 22 (4): 247–252.

Ksouri, H., Balanant, P.-Y., Tadié, J.-M., *et al.* 2010. Impact of morbidity and mortality conferences on analysis of mortality and critical events in intensive care practice. *American Journal of Critical Care*. 19 (2): 135–145.

Kudchadkar, S.R., Yaster, M., Punjabi, N.M. 2014. Sedation, sleep promotion, and delirium screening practices in the care of mechanically ventilated children: a wake-up call for the pediatric critical care community. *Critical Care Medicine*. 42 (7): 1592–1600.

Kue, R., Brown, P., Ness, C., Scheulen, J. 2011. Adverse clinical events during intrahospital transport by a specialized team: a preliminary report. *American Journal of Critical Care*. 20 (2): 153–164.

Kuffler, D.P. 2012. Maximizing neuroprotection: where do we stand? *Therapeutics and Clinical Risk Management*. 8 (1): 185–194.

Kulungowski, A.M., Kashuk, J.L., Moore, E.E., *et al.* 2009. Hemolysis, elevated liver enzymes, and low platelets syndrome: when is surgical help needed? *American Journal of Surgery*. 198 (6): 916–920.

Kumar, A., Ellis, P., Arabi, Y., Roberts, D., *et al.*, Cooperative Antimicrobial Therapy of septic Shock Database Research group. 2009. Initiation of inappropriate antimicrobial therapy results in a fivefold reduction of survival in human septic shock. *Chest*. 136 (5): 1237–1248.

Kumar, A., Roberts, D., Wood, K.E., *et al.* 2006. Duration of hypotension before initiation of effective antimicrobial therapy is the critical determinant of survival in human septic shock. *Critical Care Medicine*. 34 (6): 1589–1596.

Kumar, L. 2016. Brain death and care of the organ donor. *Journal of Anaesthesiology, Clinical Pharmacology*. 32 (2): 146–152.

Kusahara, D.M., Friedlander, L.T., Peterlini, M.A.S., Pedreira, M.L.G. 2012. Oral care and oropharyngeal and tracheal colonization by Gram-negative pathogens in children. *Nursing in Critical Care*. 17 (3): 115–122.

Kushimoto, S., Taira, Y., Kitazawa, Y., *et al.*, Study Group PP. 2012. The clinical usefulness of extravascular lung water and pulmonary vascular permeability index to diagnose and characterize pulmonary edema: a prospective multicenter study on the quantitative differential diagnostic definition for acute lung injury/acute respiratory distress syndrome. *Critical Care*. 16: R232. 10.1186/cc11898.

Kuwabara, S., Yuki, N. 2013. Axonal Guillain-Barré syndrome: concepts and controversies. *Lancet Neurology*. 12 (12): 1180–1188.

Kwong, J.C., Vasa, P.P., Campitelli, M.A., *et al.* 2013. Risk of Guillain-Barré syndrome after seasonal influenza vaccination and influenza health-care encounters: a self-controlled study. *Lancet Infectious Diseases*. 13 (9): 769–776.

LaBrecque, D.R., Abbas, Z., Anania, F., *et al.* 2014. World Gastroenterology Organisation global guidelines: nonalcoholic fatty liver disease and nonalcoholic steatohepatitis. *Journal of Clinical Gastroenterology*. 48 (6): 467–473.

Lai, T.-S., Wang, C.-Y., Pan, S.-C., *et al.*, on behalf of the National Taiwan University Hospital Study Group on Acute Renal Failure (NSARF). 2013. Risk of developing severe sepsis after acute kidney injury. A population-based cohort study. *Critical Care*. 17 (5).

Lam, S.W., Strickland, R. 2014. Thermal disorders. *In* Bersten, A.D., Soni, N. (eds). *Intensive Care Manual*. 7th edition. Edinburgh. Butterworth-Heinemann. 829–843.

Lamia, B., Kim, H.K., Hefner, A., *et al.* 2008. How accurate are different arterial pressure-derived estimates of cardiac output and stroke volume variation measures in critically ill patients? *Critical Care*. 12 (supplement 2): P100.

Lampariello, S., Clement, M., Aralihond, A.P., *et al.* 2010. Stabilisation of critically ill children at the district general hospital prior to intensive care retrieval: a snapshot of current practice. *Archives of Diseases in Childhood*. 95 (8): 681–685.

Lamy, A., Devereaux, P.J., Prabhakaran, D., *et al.*, CORONARY Investigators. 2012. Off-pump or on-pump coronary-artery bypass grafting at 30 days. *New England Journal of Medicine.* 366 (16): 1489–1497.

Lancaster, E.M., Hiatt, J.R., Zarrinpa, A. 2015. Acetaminophen hepatotoxicity: an updated review. *Archives of Toxicology.* 89 (2): 193–199.

Landis, E.M. 1930. Micro-injection studies of capillary blood pressure in human skin. *Heart.* 15: 209–228.

Lange, N.R., Kozlowski, J.K., Gust, R., *et al.* 2000. Effect of partial liquid ventilation on pulmonary vascular permeability and edema after experimental acute lung injury. *American Journal of Respiratory and Critical Care Medicine.* 162 (1): 271–277.

Lanone, S., Taillé, C., Boczkowski, J., Aubier, M. 2005. Diaphragmatic fatigue during sepsis and septic shock. *Intensive Care Medicine.* 31 (12): 1611–1617.

Lapinsky, S.E., Granton, J.I. 2004. Critical care lessons from severe acute respiratory syndrome. *Current Opinion in Critical Care.* 10 (1): 53–58.

Larson, E.L., Cohen, B., Ross, B., Behta, M. 2010. Isolation precautions for methicillin-resistant *Staphylococcus aureus*: electronic surveillance to monitor adherence. *American Journal of Critical Care.* 19 (1): 16–26.

Larsson, E., Vishnevskaya, L., Kalin, B., *et al.* 2011. High frequency of thoracic aneurysms in patients with abdominal aortic aneurysms. *Annals of Surgery.* 253 (1): 180–184.

Laskou, M., Katsiari, M., Mainas, E., *et al.* 2008. ICU patients: does age make any difference? *Critical Care.* 12 (supplement 2): P496.

Laupland, K.B., Kirkpatrick, A.W., Kortbeek, J.B., Zuege, D.J. 2006. Long-term mortality outcome associated with prolonged admission to the ICU. *Chest.* 129 (4): 954–959.

Lavoie-Tremblay, M., Fernet, C., Lavigne, G.L., Austin, S. 2015. Transformational and abusive leadership practices: impacts on novice nurses, quality of care and intention to leave. *Journal of Advanced Nursing.* 72 (3): 582–592.

Lawes, E.G. 2003. Hidden hazards and dangers associated with the use of HME/filters in breathing circuits. Their effect on toxic metabolite production, pulse oximetry and airway resistance. *BJA.* 91 (2): 249–264.

Lawn, S.D., Zumla, A.I. 2011. Tuberculosis. *Lancet.* 378 (9785): 57–72.

Lawson, N., Thompson, K., Saunders, G., *et al.* 2010. Sound intensity and noise evaluation in a critical care unit. *American Journal of Critical Care.* 19 (6): e88-e98. doi:10.4037/ajcc2010180. http://ajcc.aacnjournals.org/content/19/6.toc downloaded 2 January 2011.

Leadingham, C. 2014. *Maintaining the Vision in the Intensive Care Unit.* Wright State University CORE Scholar. Doctor of Nursing Practice Program Projects. College of Nursing and Health Student Publications. http://corescholar.libraries.wright.edu/nursing_dnp/1 accessed 10 January 2017.

Leddy, R., Wilkinson, J.M. 2015. Endotracheal suctioning practices of nurses and respiratory therapists: how well do they align with clinical practice guidelines? *Canadian Journal of Respiratory Therapy.* 51 (3): 60–64.

Ledwith, M.B., Bloom, S., Maloney-Wilensky, E., *et al.* 2010. Effect of body position on cerebral oxygenation and physiologic parameters in patients with acute neurological conditions. *Journal of Neuroscience Nursing.* 42 (5): 280–287.

Lee Char, S.J., Evans, L.R., Malvar, G.L., White, D.B. 2010. A randomised trial of two methods to disclose prognosis to surrogate decision makers in Intensive Care Units. *American Journal of Respiratory and Critical Care Medicine.* 182 (7): 905–909.

Lee, B.H., Inui, D., Suh, G.Y., *et al.* 2012. Association of body temperature and antipyretic treatments with mortality of critically ill patients with and without sepsis: multi-centered prospective observational study. *Critical Care.* 16 (1): R33.

Lee, G., Twerenbold, R., Tanglay, Y., *et al.* 2016. Clinical benefit of high-sensitivity cardiac Troponin I in the detection of exercise-induced myocardial ischemia. *American Heart Journal.* 173 (1): 8–17.

Lerolle, N., Trinquart, L., Bornstain, C., *et al.* 2010. Increased intensity of treatment and decreased mortality in elderly patients in an intensive care unit over a decade. *Critical Care Medicine.* 38 (1): 59–64.

Levett, D., Bennett, M.H., Millar, I. 2015. Adjunctive hyperbaric oxygen for necrotizing fasciitis. *Cochrane Database of Systematic Reviews*, Issue 1. Art. No.: CD007937. doi:10.1002/14651 858.CD007937.pub2.

Levi, M., Toh, C.H., Thachil, J., Watson, H.G. 2009. Guidelines for the diagnosis and management of disseminated intravascular coagulation. *British Journal of Haematology*. 145 (1): 24–33.

Lewis, S.J., Heaton, K.W. 1997. Stool form scale as a useful guide to intestinal transit time. *Scandinavian Journal of Gastroenterology*. 32 (9): 920–924.

Li, H., Manwani, B., Len, S.X. 2011. Frailty, inflammation, and immunity. *Aging and Disease*. 2 (6): 466–473.

Li, N., Li, H., Yu, R., *et al*. 2016. A prospective study of blood glucose detection using arterial blood gas analysis and peripheral glucometry after cardiac surgery with cardiopulmonary bypass: accuracy and influences. *International Journal of Clinical and Experimental Medicine*. 9 (7): 13070–13078.

Liaw, P., Ito, T., Iba, T., *et al*. 2016. DAMP and DIC: the role of extracellular DNA and DNA-binding proteins in the pathogenesis of DIC. *Blood Reviews*. 30 (4): 257–261.

Lichtman, J.H., Froelicher, E.S., Blumenthal, J.A., *et al*., the American Heart Association Statistics Committee of the Council on Epidemiology and Prevention and the Council on Cardiovascular and Stroke Nursing. 2014. Depression as a risk factor for poor prognosis among patients with acute coronary syndrome: systematic review and recommendations: a scientific statement from the American Heart Association. *Circulation*. 129 (12): 1350–1369.

Light, R.W., Rogers, J.T., Moyers, J.P., *et al*. 2002. Prevalence and clinical course of pleural effusions at 30 days after coronary artery and cardiac surgery. *American Journal of Respiratory and Critical Care Medicine*. 166 (12): 1567–1571.

Lilja, F., Mani, K., Wanhainen, A. 2017. Editor's Choice–Trend-break in abdominal aortic aneurysm repair with decreasing surgical workload. *European Journal of Vascular and Endovascular Surgery*. 5 3 (6): 811–819.

Lim, S.-M., Webb, S.A. 2005. Nosocomial bacterial infections in Intensive Care Units. I: organisms and mechanisms of antibiotic resistance. *Anaesthesia*. 60 (9): 887–902.

Lim, W.C., Black, N., Lamping, D., *et al*. 2016. Conceptualizing and measuring health-related quality of life in critical care. *Journal of Critical Care*. 31 (1): 183–193.

Lindberg, G., Hamid, S.S., Malfertheiner, P., *et al*. 2011. World Gastroenterology Organisation Global Guideline. Constipation—a global perspective. *Journal of Clinical Gastroenterology*. 45 (6): 483–487.

Lindén, V.B., Lidegran, M.K., Frise, G., *et al*. 2009. ECMO in ARDS: a long-term follow-up study regarding pulmonary morphology and function and health-related quality of life. *Acta Anaesthesiologica Scandinavica*. 53 (4): 489–495.

Ling, J.M., Klimaj, S., Toulouse, T., Mayer, A.R. 2013. A prospective study of gray matter injuries in mild traumatic brain injury. *Neurology*. 81 (24): 2121–2127.

Litman, R.S., Griggs, S.M., Dowling, J.J., Riazi, S. 2018. Malignant hyperthermia susceptibility and related diseases. *Anesthesiology*. 128 (1): 159–167.

Liu, J., Ghaziani, T.T., Wolf, J.L. 2017. Acute fatty liver disease of pregnancy: updates in pathogenesis, diagnosis, and management. *American Journal of Gastroenterology*. 112 (6): 838–846.

Liu, L.L., Aldrich, M., Shimabukuro, D.W., *et al*. 2010. Rescue therapies for acute hypoxemic respiratory failure. *Anesthesia & Analgesia*. 111 (3): 693–702.

Liwu, A. 1990. Oral hygiene in intubated patients. *Australian Journal of Advanced Nursing*. 7 (2): 4–7.

Llewellyn, L. 2007. Changing inotrope infusions: which technique is best? *Nursing Times*. 103 (8): 30–31.

Lloyd, D.G., Ma, D., Vizcaychipi, M.P. 2012. Cognitive decline after anaesthesia and critical care. *Continuing Education in Anaesthesia, Critical Care & Pain*. 12 (3): 105–109.

Loveday, H.P., Wilson, J.A., Pratt, R.J., *et al*. 2014. epic3: national evidence-based guidelines for preventing healthcare-associated infections in NHS hospitals in England. *Journal of Hospital Infection*. 86 (supplement 1): S1–S70.

Lovich-Sapola, J., Smith, C.E., Brandt, C.P. 2015. Postoperative pain control. *Surgical Clinics of North America*. 95: 301–308.

Lowe, M.E., Sevilla, W.A. 2012. Nutritional advice for prevention of acute pancreatitis: review of current opinion. *Nutrition and Dietary supplements.* 4: 71–81.

Lower, J. 2003. Using pain to assess neurologic response. *Nursing.* 33 (6): 56–57.

Luckhaupt, S.E. 2012. Short sleep duration among workers. United States, 2010. *Morbidity & Mortality Weekly Report.* 61 (16): 281–285.

Luetz, A., Heymann, A., Radtke, F.M., *et al.* 2010. Different assessment tools for intensive care unit delirium: which score to use? *Critical Care Medicine.* 38 (2): 409–418.

Lumb, A.B. 2017. *Nunn's Applied Respiratory Physiology.* 8th edition. Edinburgh. Elsevier.

Maben, J. 2009. Splendid isolation? The pros and cons of single rooms for the NHS. *Nursing Management.* 16 (2): 18–19.

MacConnachie, A.M. 1997. Ecstasy poisoning. *Intensive and Critical Care Nursing.* 13 (6): 365–366.

Macdonald, S., Johnson G. (eds). 2017. *Mayes' Midwifery: A Textbook for Midwives.* 15th edition. Edinburgh. Elsevier.

Macias, C.A., Rosengart, M.R., Puyana, J.-C., *et al.* 2009. The effects of trauma centre care, admission volume, and surgical volume on paralysis after traumatic spinal cord injury. *Annals of Surgery.* 249 (1): 10–17.

Macintyre, P., Schug, S.S. 2014. *Acute Pain Management: A Practical Guide.* 4th edition. Boca Raton, FL. CRC Press Taylor & Francis.

Macintyre, P.E., Schug, S.A., Scott, D.A., *et al.*, Acute Pain Management Scientific Evidence Working Group of the Australian and New Zealand College of Anaesthetists and Faculty of Pain Medicine. 2010. *Acute Pain Management: Scientific Evidence.* 3rd edition. Melbourne. Australian and New Zealand College of Anaesthetists, Faculty of Pain Medicine.

MacLaren, R., Reynolds, P.M., Allen, R.R. 2014. Histamine-2 receptor antagonists vs proton pump inhibitors on gastrointestinal tract hemorrhage and infectious complications in the intensive care unit. *JAMA Internal Medicine.* 174 (4): 564–574.

Macnaughton, P.D. 2006. New ventilators for the ICU – usefulness of lung performance reporting. *British Journal of Anaesthesia.* 97 (1): 57–63.

Maczulak, A. 2010. *Allies and Enemies: How the World Depends on Bacteria.* Upper Saddle River, NJ. FT Press. Pearson Education.

Maddison, L., Starkopf, J., Blaser, A.R. 2016. Mild to moderate intra-abdominal hypertension: does it matter? *World Journal of Critical Care Medicine.* 5 (1): 96–102.

Maggiore, S.M., Idone, F.A., Vaschetto, R., *et al.* 2014. Nasal High-Flow versus Venturi mask oxygen therapy after extubation. Effects on oxygenation, comfort, and clinical outcome. *American Journal of Respiratory Critical Care Medicine.* 190 (3): 282–288.

Magill, S.S., Edwards, J.R., Bamberg, W., *et al.*, for the Emerging Infections Program Healthcare-Associated Infections and Antimicrobial Use Prevalence Survey Team. 2014. Multistate point-prevalence survey of health care–associated infections. *New England Journal of Medicine.* 370 (13): 1198–1208.

Maheshwari, R., Subramanian, R.M. 2016. Severe acute pancreatitis and necrotizing pancreatitis. *Critical Care Clinics.* 32 (2): 279–290.

Maitland, K., Kiguli, S., Opoka, R.O., *et al.*, FEAST Trial Group. 2011. Mortality after fluid bolus in African children with severe infection. *New England Journal of Medicine.* 364 (26): 2483–2495.

Malhotra, A., Drazen, J.M. 2013. High-frequency oscillatory ventilation on shaky ground. *New England Journal of Medicine.* 368 (9): 863–865.

Malietzis, G., Johns, N., Al-Hassi, H.O., *et al.* 2016. Low muscularity and myosteatosis is related to the host systemic inflammatory response in patients undergoing surgery for colorectal cancer. *Annals of Surgery.* 263 (2): 320–325.

Mallik, M., Callaghan, C.J., Hope, M., *et al.* 2012. Comparison of liver transplantation outcomes from adult split liver and circulatory death donor. *British Journal of Surgery.* 99 (6): 839–847.

Mandelstam, M. 2007. *Betraying the NHS.* London. Jessica Kingsley.

Manias, E., Street, A. 2001. Nurse-Doctor interactions during critical care ward rounds. *Journal of Clinical Nursing.* 10 (4): 442–450.

Manley, K., McCormac, B. 2008. Person-centred care. *Nursing Management.* 15 (8): 12–13.

Manning, L., Hirakawa, Y., Arima, H., *et al.*, for the INTERACT2 investigators. 2014. Blood pressure variability and outcome after acute intracerebral haemorrhage: a post-hoc analysis of INTERACT2, a randomised controlled trial. *Lancet Neurology.* 13 (4): 364–373.

Manocha, S., Walley, K.R., Russell, J.A. 2003. Severe acute respiratory distress syndrome (SARS): a critical care perspective. *Critical Care Medicine.* 31 (11): 2684–2692.

Marangozo, R., Williams, M., Buchan, J. 2016. *The Labour Market for Nurses in the UK and Its Relationship to the Demand for, and Supply of, International Nurses in the NHS.* Brighton. Institute for Employment Studies.

March, A. 2005. A review of respiratory management in spinal cord injury. *Journal of Orthopaedic Nursing.* 9 (1): 19–26.

March, K.S., Hickey, J.V. 2014. Intracranial hypertension: theory and management of increased intracranial pressure. *In* Hickey, J.V. (ed.). *Neurological and Neurosurgical Nursing.* 7th edition. Philadelphia. Wolters Kluwer Lippincott Williams and Wilkins. 266–299.

Margarey, J.M., McCutcheon, H.H. 2005. "Fishing with the dead" – recall of memories from ICI. *Intensive & Critical Care Nursing.* 21 (6): 344–354.

Marieb, E.N., Hoehn, K. 2016. *Human Anatomy and Physiology.* 10th edition. Harlow. Pearson Educational.

Marik, P.E. 2002. Low-dose dopamine: a systematic review. *Intensive Care Medicine.* 28 (7): 877–883.

Marik, P.E., Bellomo, R. 2016. Fluid responsiveness: an evolution of our understanding. *British Journal of Anaesthesia.* 112 (4): 617–620.

Marik, P.E., Cavallazzi, R. 2013. Does the central venous pressure predict fluid responsiveness? An updated meta-analysis. *Critical Care Medicine.* 41 (7): 1774–1781.

Marik, P.E., Lemson, J. 2014. Fluid responsiveness: an evolution of our understanding. *British Journal of Anaesthesia.* 112 (4): 617–620.

Marik, P.E., Young, A., Sibole, S., Levitov, A. 2012. The effect of APRV ventilation on ICP and cerebral hemodynamics. *Neurocritical Care.* 17 (2): 219–223.

Marini, J.J. 2015. Does high-pressure, high-frequency oscillation shake the foundations of lung protection? *Intensive Care Medicine.* 41 (12): 2210–2212.

Marret, E., Remy, C., Bonnet, F., Postoperative Pain Forum Group. 2007. Meta-analysis of epidural analgesia *versus* parenteral opioid analgesia after colorectal surgery. *British Journal of Surgery.* 94 (6): 665–673.

Marshall, A.P., West, S.H. 2003. Gastric tonometry and enteral nutrition: a possible conflict in critical care nursing practice. *American Journal of Critical Care.* 12 (4): 349–356.

Marshall, K., Raynor, M. (eds). 2014. *Myles Textbook for Midwives.* Edinburgh. Baillière Tindall Elsevier.

Mårtensson, J., Bellomo, R. 2015. Are all fluids bad for the kidney? *Current Opinion in Critical Care.* 21 (4): 292–301.

Martinez, G., Vuylsteke, A. 2012. Extracorporeal membrane oxygenation in adults. *Continuing Education in Anaesthesia, Critical Care & Pain.* 12 (2): 57–61.

Maslow, A.H. 1954/1987. *Motivation and Personality.* 3rd edition. New York. Harper & Row.

Maslow, A.H. 1971. *The Farthest Reaches of Human Nature.* London. Penguin.

Masterson, K., Brenner, M. 2016. "Don't put the parent out": parents' perspectives of being present during an inter-hospital transfer. *Journal of Clinical Nursing.* 25 (9–10): 1301–1307.

Maternal Critical Care Working Group. 2011. *Providing Equity of Critical and Maternity Care for the Critically Ill Pregnant or Recently Pregnant Woman.* London. The Royal College of Anaesthetists.

Maund, E., McDaid, C., Rice, S., *et al.* 2011. Paracetamol and selective and non-selective non-steroidal anti-inflammatory drugs for the reduction in morphine-related side-effects after major surgery: a systematic review. *British Journal of Anaesthesia.* 106 (3): 292–297.

Maunder, T. 1997. Principles and practice of managing difficult behaviour situations in intensive care. *Intensive and Critical Care Nursing.* 13 (2): 108–110.

Mavrides, E., Allard, S., Chandraharan, E., *et al.*, on behalf of the Royal College of Obstetricians and Gynaecologists. 2016. Green Top Guide 52: prevention and management of postpartum haemorrhage. *BJOG: An International Journal of Obstetrics & Gynaecology.* 124: e106–e149.

May, K. 2009. The pathophysiology and causes of raised intracranial pressure. *British Journal of Nursing*. 18 (15): 911–914.

Maybauer, D.M., Talke, P.O., Westphal, M., *et al.* 2006. Positive-end expiratory pressure ventilation increases extravascular lung water due to a decrease in lung lymph flow. *Anaesthesia and Intensive Care*. 34 (3): 329–333.

McCaffery, M., Pasero, C. 1999. *Pain Clinical Manual*. 2nd edition. St Louis, MO. Mosby.

McCall, S.J., Nair, M., Knight, M. 2017. Factors associated with maternal mortality at advanced maternal age: a population-based case–control study. *BJOG: An International Journal of Obstetrics & Gynaecology*. 124 (8): 1225–1233.

McCarthy, K. 2015. *Pseudomonas aeruginosa*: evolution of antimicrobial resistance and implications for therapy. *Seminars in Respiratory and Critical Care Medicine*. 36 (1): 44–55.

McClave, S.A., Taylor, B.E., Martindale, R.G., *et al.*, Society of Critical Care Medicine, American Society for Parenteral and Enteral Nutrition. 2016. Guidelines for the provision and assessment of nutrition support therapy in the adult critically ill patient: Society of Critical Care Medicine (SCCM) and American Society for Parenteral and Enteral Nutrition (A.S.P.E.N.). *Journal of Parenteral and Enteral Nutrition*. 40 (2): 159–211.

McCormack, V., Tolhurst-Cleaver, S. 2017. Acute Respiratory Distress Syndrome. *BJA Education*. 17 (5): 161–165.

McCoy, R.G., Lipska, K.J., Yao, X., *et al.* 2016. Intensive treatment and severe hypoglycemia among adults with type 2 diabetes. *JAMA Internal Medicine*. Published online 6 June 2016. doi:10.1001/jamainternmed. 2016. 2275.

McCusker, J., Cole, M.G., Voyer, P., *et al.* 2011. Prevalence and incidence of delirium in long-term care. *International Journal of Geriatric Psychology*. 26 (11): 1152–1161.

McGrath, M. 2008. The challenges of caring in a technological environment: critical care nurses' experiences. *Journal of Clinical Nursing*. 17 (8): 1096–1004.

McGuire, P.K., Cope, H., Fahy, T.A. 1994. Diversity of psychopathy associated with use of 3,4-methylenedioxymethamphetamine ("ecstasy"). *British Journal of Psychiatry*. 165 (3): 391–395.

McIntyre, P.B., O'Brien, K.L., Greenwood, B., van de Beek, D. 2012. Effects of vaccines on bacterial meningitis worldwide. *Lancet*. 379 (9854): 1073–1711.

McKeever, T.M., Hearson, G., Housley, G., *et al.* 2016. Using venous blood gas analysis in the assessment of COPD exacerbations. *Thorax*. 71 (3): 210–215.

McKinley, M. 2009. Acute liver failure. *Nursing*. 39 (3): 38–44.

McKinley, S., Coote, K., Stein-Parbury, J. 2003. Development and testing of a Faces Scale for the assessment of anxiety in critically ill patients. *Journal of Advanced Nursing*. 41 (1): 73–79.

McKinley, S., Fien, M., Elliott, R., Elliott, D. 2016. Health-related quality of life and associated factors in intensive care unit survivors 6 months after discharge. *American Journal of Critical Care*. 25 (1): 52–58.

McLaughlin, N., Leslie, G.D., Williams, T.A., Dobb, G.J. 2007. Examining the occurrence of adverse events within 72 hours of discharge from the intensive care unit. *Anaesthesia & Intensive Care*. 35 (4): 486–493.

McMahon, S., Koltzenburg, M., Tracey, I., Turk, D.C. 2013. *Wall & Melzack's Textbook of Pain*. 6th edition. Philadelphia. Elsevier Saunders.

McNabb, M. 2017. Physiological changes from late pregnancy until the onset of lactation: from nesting to suckling-lactation and parent-infant attachment. *In* Macdonald, S., Johnson G.J. (eds). *Mayes' Midwifery: A Textbook for Midwives*. 15th edition. Edinburgh. Elsevier. 562–585.

McNarry, A.F., Patel, A. 2017. The evolution of airway management–new concepts and conflicts with traditional practice. *British Journal of Anaesthesia*. 119 (supplement 1): i154–i166.

McNicol, E.D., Ferguson, M.C., Hudcova, J. 2015. Patient controlled opioid analgesia versus non-patient controlled opioid analgesia for postoperative pain (Review). *Cochrane Database of Systematic Reviews*, Issue 6. Art. No.: CD003348. doi:10.1002/14651858.CD003348.pub3.

McPeake, J., Forrest, E., Quasim, T., Kinsella, J., O'Neill, A. 2016. Health and social consequences of an alcohol-related admission to critical care: a qualitative study. *BMJ Open*. 6 (4): p.e009944.

McWilliam, S., Riordan, A. 2010. How to use: C-reactive protein. *Archives of Disease in Childhood Education & Practice.* 95 (2): 55–58.

Mebazaa, A., Nieminen, M.S., Packer, M., *et al.* SURVIVE Investigators. 2007. Levosimendan vs dobutamine for patients with acute decompensated heart failure. *JAMA.* 297 (17): 1883–1891.

Meher, S., Mishra, T.S., Sasmal, P.K., *et al.* 2015. Role of biomarkers in diagnosis and prognostic evaluation of acute pancreatitis. *Journal of Biomarkers.* doi.org/10.1155/2015/519534.

Mehta, A.J. 2016. Alcoholism and critical illness: a review. *World Journal of Critical Care Medicine.* 5 (1): 27.

Meierkord, H., Boon, P., Engelsen, B., *et al.* 2010. EFNS guideline on the management of status epilepticus in adults. *European Journal of Neurology.* 17 (3): 348–355.

Meissner, A., Genga, K.R., Studart, F.S., *et al.* 2010. Epidemiology of and factors associated with end-of-life decisions in a surgical intensive care unit. *Critical Care Medicine.* 38 (4): 1060–1068.

Mela, E.K., Drimtzias, E.G., Christofidou, M.K., *et al.* 2010. Ocular surface bacterial colonisation in sedated intensive care unit patients. *Anesthesia and Intensive Care.* 38 (1): 190–193.

Melzack, R., Wall, P. 1988. *The Challenge of Pain.* 2nd edition. London. Penguin.

Memişoğulları, R., Yüksel, H., Yıldırım, H.A., Yavuz, Ö. 2010. Performance characteristics of dipstick and microscopic urinalysis for diagnosis of urinary tract infection. *European Journal of General Medicine.* 7 (2).

Meng, J., Hu, M., Lai, Z., *et al.* 2016. Levosimendan versus dobutamine in myocardial injury patients with septic shock: a randomized controlled trial. *Medical Science Monitor.* 22: 1486–1496.

Meyer, J., Sturdy, D. 2004. Exploring the future of gerontological nursing outcomes. *Journal of Clinical Nursing.* 13 (6b) (*International Journal of Older People Nursing*): 128–134.

M.H.R.A. 2014. Intravenous dantrolene. *Drug Safety Update.* 7 (12): A2.

Mick, D.J., Ackerman, M.H. 2004. Critical care nursing for older adults: pathophysiological and functional considerations. *Nursing Clinics of North America.* 39 (3): 473–493.

Miller, E., Hoschler, K., Stanford, E., *et al.* 2010. Incidence of 2009 pandemic influenza A H1N1 infection in England: a cross-sectional serological study. *Lancet.* 375 (9720): 1100–1108.

Miller, R.F., Allen, E., Copas, A., *et al.* 2006. Improved survival for HIV infected patients with severe *Pneumocystis jirovecii* pneumonia is independent of highly active antiviral therapy. *Thorax.* 61 (8): 716–721.

Mina, M.J., Klugman, K.P. 2014. The role of influenza in the severity and transmission of respiratory bacterial disease. *Lancet Respiratory Medicine.* 2 (9): 750–763,

Mirrakhimov, A.E., Voore, P., Halytskyy, O., *et al.* 2015. Propofol infusion syndrome in adults: a clinical update. *Critical Care Research and Practice.* 2015.

Mo, Y., Zimmermann, A.E. 2013. Role of dexmedetomidine for the prevention and treatment of delirium in intensive care unit patients. *Annals of Pharmacotherapy.* 47 (6): 869–876.

Moerer, O., Beck, J., Brander, L., *et al.* 2008. Subject-ventilator synchrony during neural versus pneumatically triggered non-invasive helmet ventilation. *Intensive Care Medicine.* 34 (9): 1615–1623.

Mokhlesi, B., Garimella, P.S., Joffe, A., Velho, V. 2004. Street drug abuse leading to critical illness. *Intensive Care Medicine.* 30 (8): 1526–1536.

Mol, B.W.J., Roberts, C.T., Thangaratinam, S., *et al.* 2016. Pre-eclampsia, *Lancet.* 387 (10022): 999–1011.

Moler, F.W., Silverstein, F.S., Holubkov, R., THAPCA Trial Investigators. 2015. Therapeutic hypothermia after out-of-hospital cardiac arrest in children. *New England Journal of Medicine.* 372 (20): 1898–1908.

Møller, C.H., Penninga, L., Wetterslev, J., *et al.* 2012. Off-pump versus on-pump coronary artery bypass grafting for ischaemic heart disease. *Cochrane Database of Systematic Reviews,* Issue 3. Art. No.: CD007224. doi:10.1002/14651858.CD007224.pub2.

Molyneux, A.J., Birks, J., Clarke, A., *et al.* 20154. The durability of endovascular coiling versus neurosurgical clipping of ruptured cerebral aneurysms: 18 year follow-up of the UK cohort of the International Subarachnoid Aneurysm Trial (ISAT). *Lancet.* 385 (9969): 691–697.

Monaco, F., Drummond, G.B., Ramsay, P., *et al.* 2010. Do simple ventilation and gas exchange measurements predict early successful weaning from respiratory support in unselected general intensive care patients? *British Journal of Anaesthesia.* 105 (3): 326–333.

Monte-Verde, D., Nosanchuk, J.S. 2016. The sensitivity and specificity of nitrite testing for bacteriuria. *Laboratory Medicine*. 12 (12): 755–757.

Moore, I., Bhat, R., Hoenich, N., *et al.* 2009. A microbiological survey of bicarbonate-based replacement circuits in continuous veno-venous haemofiltration. *Critical Care Medicine*. 37 (2): 496–500.

Moore, Z.E.H., Cowman, S. 2014 Risk assessment tools for the prevention of pressure ulcers. *Cochrane Database of Systematic Reviews*, Issue 2. Art. No.: CD006471. doi:10.1002/14651 858.CD006471.pub3.

Moos, S.I., Nagan, G., de Weijert, R.S., *et al.* 2014. Patients at risk for contrast-induced nephropathy and mid-term effects after contrast administration: a prospective cohort study. *The Netherlands Journal of Medicine*. 72 (7): 363–371.

Morange, S., Roch, A., for the ACURASYS Study Investigators. 2010. Neuromuscular blockers in early acute respiratory distress syndrome. *The New England Journal of Medicine*. 363 (12): 1107–1116.

Morens, D.M., Taubenberger, J.K., Harvey, H.A, Memoli, M.J. 2010. The 1918 influenza pandemic: lessons for 2009 and the future. *Critical Care Medicine*. 38 (supplement 4): e10.

Moss, M., Good, V.S., Gozal, D., *et al.* 2016. An official critical care societies collaborative statement—burnout syndrome in critical care health-care professionals: a call for action. *Chest*. 150 (1): 17–26.

Mullally, S. 2001. Future clinical role of nurses in the United Kingdom. *Postgraduate Medical Journal*. 77 (907): 337–339.

Munnur, U., Bandi, V., Guntupalli, K.K. 2011. Management principles of the critically ill obstetric patient. *Clinics in Chest Medicine*. 32 (1): 53–60.

Munoz-Price, L.S., Weinstein, R.A. 2008. Acinetobacter infection. *New England Journal of Medicine*. 358 (12): 1271–1281.

Munro, C.L., Grap, M.J., Jones, D.J., *et al.* 2009. Chlorhexidine, toothbrushing, and preventing ventilator-associated pneumonia in critically ill adults. *American Journal of Critical Care*. 18 (5): 428–437.

Murdoch, J., Larsen, D. 2004. Assessing pain in cognitively impaired older adults. *Nursing Standard*. 18 (38): 33–39.

Murphy, P.J., Marriage, S.C., Davis, P.J. (eds). 2009. *Case Studies in Pediatric Critical Care*. Cambridge. Cambridge University Press.

Murphy, T., Robinson, S. 2006. Renal failure and its treatment. *Anaesthesia and Intensive Care Medicine*. 7 (7): 247–252.

Murray, M.J., DeBlock, H., Erstad, B., *et al.* 2016. Clinical practice guidelines for sustained neuromuscular blockade in the adult critically ill patient. *Critical Care Medicine*. 44 (11): 2079–2013.

Murray, P.R., Rosenthal, K.S., Pfaller, M.A. 2009. *Medical Microbiology*. 6th edition. St Louis, MO. Mosby.

Muscedere, J., Rewa, O., McKechnie, K., *et al.* 2011. Subglottic secretion drainage for the prevention of ventilator-associated pneumonia: a systematic review and meta-analysis. *Critical Care Medicine*. 39 (8): 1985–1991.

Musters, C. 2010. Managing patients without their consent: a guide to recent legislation. *British Journal of Hospital Medicine*. 71 (2): 87–90.

Myburgh, J.A. 2014. Fluid resuscitation in acute medicine: what is the current situation? *Journal of Internal Medicine*. 277 (1): 56–68.

Mythen, M.G. 2015. Does gastric tonometry-guided therapy reduce total mortality in critically ill patients? *Critical Care*. 19: 172.

Nachamkin, I., Shadomy, S.V., Moran, A.P., *et al.* 2008. Anti-ganglioside antibody induction by swine (A/NJ/1976/H1N1) and other influenza vaccines: insights into vaccine-associated Guillain-Barré Syndrome. *The Journal of Infectious Diseases*. 198 (2): 226–233.

Nag, S., Kapadia, A., Stewart, D.J. 2011. Review: molecular pathogenesis of blood–brain barrier breakdown in acute brain injury. *Neuropathology and Applied Neurobiology*. 37 (1) 3–23.

Naidu, K.S.B., Govender, P., Ada, J.K. 2015. Biomedical applications and toxicity of nanosilver: a review. *Medical Technology SA*. 29 (2): 13–19.

Nair-Collins, M., Northrup, J., Olcese, J. 2016. Hypothalamic–pituitary function in brain death: a review. *Journal of Intensive Care Medicine.* 31 (1): 41–50.

Nakashima, R., Hifumi, T., Kawakita, K., *et al.* 2017. Critical care management focused on optimizing brain function after cardiac arrest. *Circulation Journal.* 81 (4): 427–439.

Nates, J.L., Nunnally, M., Kleinpell, R., *et al.* 2016. A framework to enhance clinical operations, development of institutional policies, and further research. *Critical Care Medicine.* 44 (8): 1553–1602.

National Collaborating Centre for Women's and Children's Health. 2013. *Feverish Illness in Children: Assessment and Initial Management in Children Younger than 5 Years.* London. National Institute for Clinical Excellence/ Royal College of Paediatrics and Child Health/Royal College of Obstetricians and Gynaecologists.

National Heart, Lung, and Blood Institute Acute Respiratory Distress Syndrome (ARDS) Clinical Trials Network. 2006. Comparison of two fluid-management strategies in acute lung injury. *The New England Journal of Medicine.* 354 (24): 2564–2575.

Natriuretic Peptides Studies Collaboration. 2016. Natriuretic peptides and integrated risk assessment for cardiovascular disease: an individual-participant-data meta-analysis. *Lancet Diabetes and Endocrinology.* 4 (1): 840–849.

Navalesia, P., Longhini, F. 2015. Neurally adjusted ventilatory assist. *Current Opinion in Critical Care.* 21 (1): 58–64.

Naylor, A.R. 2009. Optimal medical therapy during carotid endarterectomy: a personal view. *Acta Chirurgica Belgica.* 109 (3): 285–291.

N.C.D. Risk Factor Collaboration. 2016. Worldwide trends in diabetes since 1980: a pooled analysis of 751 population-based studies with 4·4 million participants. *Lancet.* 387 (10027): 1513–1530.

N.C.E.P.O.D. 2009. *An Acute Problem.* London. National Confidential Enquiry into Patient Outcome and Death.

N.C.E.P.O.D. 2010a. *A Mixed Bag.* London. National Confidential Enquiry into Patient Outcome and Death.

N.C.E.P.O.D. 2010b. *An Age Old Problem.* London. National Confidential Enquiry into Patient Outcome and Death.

N.C.E.P.O.D. 2014. *On the Right Trach?* London. National Confidential Enquiry into Patient Outcome and Death.

N.C.E.P.O.D. 2015a. *Just Say Sepsis! A Review of the Process of Care Received by Patients with Sepsis.* London. National Confidential Enquiry into Patient Outcome and Death.

N.C.E.P.O.D. 2015b. *Time to Get Control? A Review of the Care Received by Patients Who Had a Severe Gastrointestinal Haemorrhage.* London. National Confidential Enquiry into Patient Outcome and Death.

N.C.E.P.O.D. 2016. *Treat the Cause: A Review of the Quality of Care Povided to Patients Treated for Acute Pancreatitis.* London. National Confidential Enquiry into Patient Outcome and Death.

Nebout, S., Pirracchio, R. 2012. Should we monitor ScVO2 in critically ill patients? *Cardiology Research and Practice.* doi:10.1155/2012/370697.

Nee, P.A., Bailey, D.J., Todd, V., *et al.* 2016. Critical care in the emergency department: acute kidney injury. *Emergency Medicine Journal.* 33 (5): 361–365.

Needham, D.M., Colantuoni, E., Mendez-Tellez, P.A., *et al.* 2012. Lung protective mechanical ventilation and two-year survival in patients with acute lung injury: prospective cohort study. *BMJ.* 344 (7854): 16.

Needham, D.M., Yang, T., Dinglas, V.D., *et al.* 2015. Timing of low tidal volume ventilation and intensive care unit mortality in acute respiratory distress syndrome. A prospective cohort study. *American Journal of Respiratory and Critical Care Medicine.* 191 (2): 177–185.

Needleman, J., Buerhaus, P., Pankratz, S., *et al.* 2011. Nurse staffing and inpatient hospital mortality. *New England Journal of Medicine.* 364 (11): 1037–1045.

Nelson-Piercy, C. 2015. *Handbook of Obstetric Medicine.* 5th edition. Boca Raton, FL. CRC Press, Taylor and Francis Group.

Newton, J.N., Briggs, A.D.M., Murray, C.J.L., *et al.* 2015. Changes in health in England, with analysis by English regions and areas of deprivation, 1990–2013: a systematic analysis for the Global Burden of Disease Study 2013. *Lancet*. 386 (10010): 2257–2574.

N.H.S.B.T. 2013. *Taking Organ Transplantation to 2020*. Liverpool. NHS Blood & Transplant.

NHS England. 2013. Placement devices for nasogastric tube insertion DO NOT replace initial position checks. *Patient Safety Alert*. NHS/PSA/W/2013/001.

NHS England. 2014. *Improving Outcomes for Patients with Sepsis*. London. NHS England.

NHS England. 2016. *Pandemic Influenza*. London. NHS England.

NHS Estates. 2003. *Facilities for Critical Care. HBN 57*. Norwich. The Stationery Office.

NHS Improvement. 2016. *The Adult Patient Who Is Deteriorating: Sharing Learning from Literature, Incident Reports and Root Cause Analysis Investigations*. London. NHS Improvement.

NHS Litigation Authority. 2015. *Report and Accounts 2013/14*. London. NHS Litigation Authority.

NHS Resolution. 2017. *Annual Report and Accounts 2016/17*. London. NHS Resolution.

N.I.C.E. 2006. *Nutrition Support in Adults*. London. National Institute for Clinical Excellence.

N.I.C.E. 2008. *Laparoscopic Repair of Abdominal Aortic Aneurysm*. London. National Institute for Clinical Excellence.

N.I.C.E. 2009. *Rehabilitation after Critical Illness*. London. National Institute for Clinical Excellence.

N.I.C.E. 2010a. *Delirium. Diagnosis, Prevention and Management*. London. National Institute for Clinical Excellence.

N.I.C.E. 2010b. *Neuropathic Pain. Clinical Guideline 96*. London. National Institute for Clinical Excellence.

N.I.C.E. 2010c. *Meningitis (Bacterial) and Meningococcal Meningitis (Bacterial) and Meningococcal Septicaemia in Under 16s: Recognition, Diagnosis and Management Diagnosis and Management*. London. National Institute for Clinical Excellence. (updated 2015, update due 2018)

N.I.C.E. 2010d. *Venous Thromboembolism: Reducing the Risk for Patients in Hospital*. London. National Institute for Clinical Excellence. (updated 2015)

N.I.C.E. 2010e. *Chest Pain of Recent Onset. Clinical Guideline 95*. London. National Institute for Clinical Excellence.

N.I.C.E. 2010f. *Hypertension in Pregnancy: Diagnosis and Management. Clinical Guideline 107*. London. National Institute for Clinical Excellence.

N.I.C.E. 2010g. *Organ Donation for Transplants Draft Scope for Consultation*. London. National Institute for Clinical Excellence.

N.I.C.E. 2011. *Therapeutic Hypothermia Following Cardiac Arrest. Interventional Procedure Guidance 386*. London. National Institute for Clinical Excellence.

N.I.C.E. 2012a. *Epilepsies: Diagnosis and Management*. London. National Institute for Clinical Excellence.

N.I.C.E. 2012b updated 2016. *Acute Upper Gastrointestinal Bleeding in Over 16s: Management. Clinical Guideline 141*. London. National Institute for Clinical Excellence (update available online at www.nice.org.uk/guidance/cg141/chapter/ 1-guidanc, last accessed 3 July 2017).

N.I.C.E./National Collaborating Centre for Cancer. 2012. *Neutropenic Sepsis: Prevention and Management of Neutropenic Sepsis in Cancer Patients*. London. National Institute for Clinical Excellence.

N.I.C.E. 2013a. *Myocardial Infarction with ST-Segment Elevation: Acute Management*. London. National Institute for Clinical Excellence.

N.I.C.E. 2013b. *Acute Kidney Injury. Prevention, Detection and Management of Acute Kidney Injury Up to the Point of Renal Replacement Therapy. N.I.C.E. Clinical Guideline 169*. London. National Institute for Clinical Excellence.

N.I.C.E. 2013c. *Intravenous Fluid Therapy in Adults in Hospital. N.I.C.E. Clinical Guideline 174*. London. National Institute for Clinical Excellence (updated May 2017).

N.I.C.E. 2014a. *Acute Heart Failure: Diagnosing and Managing Acute Heart Failure in Adults. Clinical Guideline 187*. London. National Institute for Clinical Excellence.

N.I.C.E. 2014b. *Head Injury: Triage, Assessment, Investigation and Early Management of Head Injury in Children, Young People and Adults*. London. National Institute for Clinical Excellence (updated 2017).

N.I.C.E. 2016a. *Sepsis: Recognition, Diagnosis and Early Management. N.I.C.E. Guideline 51.* London. National Institute for Clinical Excellence.

N.I.C.E. 2016b. *CytoSorb Therapy for Sepsis. Medtech Innovation Briefing.* Published 29 November 2016 http://nice.org.uk/guidance/mib87.

N.I.C.E. 2016c. *Non-Alcoholic Fatty Liver Disease (NAFLD): Assessment and Management.* London. National Institute for Clinical Excellence.

N.I.C.E. 2016d. *Type 2 Diabetes in Adults: Management.* London. National Institute for Clinical Excellence.

NICE-SUGAR Study investigators. 2009. Intensive versus conventional glucose control in critically ill patients. *New England Journal of Medicine.* 360 (130): 1283–1297.

Nichani, R., McGrath, B., Owen, T., *et al.*, Association of North Western Intensive Care Units collaborative (ANWICU kNoWLeDGe) hypothermia registry. 2012. Cooling practices and outcome following therapeutic hypothermia for cardiac arrest. *Journal of the Intensive Care Society.* 11 (2): 102–106.

Nicholls, S.J., Wang, Z., Koeth, R., *et al.* 2007. Metabolic profiling of arginine and nitric oxide pathways predicts hemodynamic abnormalities and mortality in patients with cardiogenic shock after acute myocardial infarction. *Circulation.* 116 (20): 2315–2324.

Nielsen, A.H., Angel, S. 2016. Relatives perception of writing diaries for critically ill. A phenomenological hermeneutical study. *Nursing in Critical Care.* 21 (6): 351–357.

Nielsen, N., Wetterslev, J., Cronberg, T., *et al.*, for the TTM Trial Investigators. 2013. Targeted temperature management at 33°C versus 36°C after cardiac arrest. *New England Journal of Medicine.* 369 (23): 2197–2206.

Niemi, T.T., Suojaranta-Ylinen, R.T., *et al.* 2006. Gelatin and hydroxyethyl starch, but not albumin, impair hemostasis after cardiac surgery. *Anesthesia & Analgesia.* 102 (4): 998–1006.

Nightingale, F. 1859/1980. *Notes on Nursing: What It Is, and What It Is Not.* Edinburgh. Churchill Livingstone.

Nijs, N., Toppets, A., Defloor, T., *et al.* 2009. Incidence and risk factors for pressure ulcers in the intensive care unit. *Journal of Clinical Nursing.* 18 (9): 1258–1266.

Nilles, K.M., Subramanian, R.M. 2012. Intensive care management of patients prior to liver transplantation. *In* Abdeldayem, H. (ed.). *Liver Transplantation – basic Issues.* Rijeka, Croatia. InTech. 321–331.

Nilsson, O., Hultgren, R., Letterstål, A. 2017. Perceived learning needs of patients with abdominal aortic aneurysm. *Journal of Vascular Nursing.* 35 (1): 4–11.

Nitzan, M., Romem, A., Koppel, R. 2014. Pulse oximetry: fundamentals and technology update. *Medical Devices (Auckland).* 7: 231–239.

Niven, D.J., Gaudet, J.E., Laupland, K.B., *et al.* 2015. Accuracy of peripheral thermometers for estimating temperature: a systematic review and meta-analysis. *Annals of Internal Medicine.* 163 (10): 768–777.

Niven, D.J, Laupland, K.B. 2016. Pyrexia: aetiology in the ICU. *Critical Care.* 20 (1): 247.

Niven, D.J, Laupland, K.B. 2013. Pharmacotherapy of fever control among hospitalized adult patients. *Expert Opinion on Pharmacotherapy.* 14 (6): 735–745.

Niven, D.J., Stelfox, H.T., Laupland, K.B. 2013. Antipyretic therapy in febrile critically ill adults: a systematic review and meta-analysis. *Journal of Critical Care.* 28 (3): 303–310.

N.M.C. 2009. Position statement: working during a surge in the swine flu pandemic. www.nmc-uk.org/aarticleprint.aspx?ArticleID=3897 accessed 19 October 2009.

N.M.C. 2015 *The Code: Professional Standards of Practice and Behaviour for Nurses and Midwives.* London. Nursing and Midwifery Council.

N.M.C. (undated, possibly 2017). *Enabling Professionalism in Nursing and Midwifery Practice.* London. Nursing and Midwifery Council.

Nolan, J.P., Kelley, F.E. 2011. Airway challenges in critical care. *Anaesthesia.* 66 (supplement 2): 81–92.

Nolan, J.P., Soar, J., Cariou, A., *et al.* 2015. European Resuscitation Council and European Society of Intensive Care Medicine 2015 guidelines for post-resuscitation care. *Intensive Care Medicine.* 41 (12): 2039–2056.

Norfolk, D. 2013. *Handbook of Transfusion Medicine*. 5th edition. Norwich. The Stationery Office.

N.P.S.A. 2002. *Patient Safety Alert. Ref PSA 01*. London. National Patient Safety Agency.

N.P.S.A. 2004a. *Achieving Our Aims. Evaluating the Results of the Pilot Cleanyourhands Campaign*. London. National Patient Safety Agency.

N.P.S.A. 2004b. *Bowel Care for Patients with Established Spinal Cord Lesions*. 15 September. London. National Patient Safety Agency.

N.P.S.A. 2008. *A Compendium of Patient Safety in Practice*. London. National Patient Safety Agency.

N.P.S.A. 2010. *Design for Patient Safety*. London. National Patient Safety Agency.

Nyirenda, M., Tang, J.I., Padfield, P.L., Seckl, J.R. 2009. Hyperkalaemia. *BMJ*. 339 (7728): 1019–1024.

O'Brien, I.D., Shacklock, E., Middleditch, A., Bigham, C. 2016. Inaccuracies in calculating predicted body weight and its impact on safe ventilator settings. *Journal of the Intensive Care Society*. 17 (3): 191–195.

O'Brien, J.M. Jr., Aberegg, S.K., Ali, N.A., *et al*. 2009. Results from the national sepsis practice survey: predictions about mortality and morbidity and recommendations for limitation of care orders. *Critical Care*. 13: R96. doi:10.1186/cc7926.

O'Brien, J.M. Jr, Aberegg, S.K., Ali, N.A., *et al*. 2009. Results from the national sepsis practice survey: predictions about mortality and morbidity and recommendations for limitation of care orders. *Critical Care*. 13: R96. doi:10.1186/cc7926.

O'Brien, J.M. Jr., Lu, B., Ali, N.A., *et al*. 2007. Alcohol dependence is independently associated with sepsis, septic shock, and hospital mortality among adult intensive care unit patients. *Critical Care Medicine*. 35 (2) 345–350.

O'Connor, M., Bucknall, T., Manias, E. 2010. International variations in outcomes from sedation protocol research: where are we at and where do we go from here? *Intensive & Critical Care Nursing*. 26 (4): 189–195.

O'Connor, T.M., O'Halloran, D.J., Shanahan, F. 2000. The stress response and the hypothalamic-pituitary-adrenal axis: from molecule to melancholia. *QJM*. 93 (6): 323–333.

O'Grady, N.P., Barie, P.S., Bartlett, J.G., *et al*. 2008. Guidelines for evaluation of new fever in critically ill adult patients: 2008 update from the American College of Critical Care Medicine and the Infectious Diseases Society of America. *Critical Care Medicine*. 36 (4): 1330–1349.

O'Neal, J.B., Shaw, A.D., Billings, F.T. 2016. Acute kidney injury following cardiac surgery: current understanding and future directions. *Critical Care*. 20: 187.

O'Neill, L.J., Carter, D.E. 1998. Adult/elderly care nursing. The implications of head injury for family relationships. *British Journal of Nursing*. 7 (14): 842–846.

O'Reilly, M. 2003. Oral care of the critically ill: a review of the literature and guidelines for practice. *Australian Critical Care*. 16 (3): 101–109.

O'Shea, P. 1997. Altered consciousness and stroke. *In* Goldhill, D.R., Withington, P.S. (eds). *Textbook of Intensive Care*. London. Chapman & Hall. 495–502.

Oddo, M., Crippa, I.A., Mehta, S., *et al*. 2016. Optimizing sedation in patients with acute brain injury. *Critical Care*. 20: 128.

Oelschlaeger, L.M. 2016. Drug-induced acute pancreatitis and hydrochlorothiazide: investigating the link. *MOJ Public Health*. 4 (2): 00075.

Oh, E.G., Lee, W.H., Yoo, J.S., *et al*. 2009. Factors related to incidence of eye disorders in Korean patients at intensive care units. *Journal of Clinical Nursing*. 18 (1): 29–35.

Olson, D., Stutzman, S., Saju, C., Wilson, M., Zhao, W., Aiyagar, V. 2016. Interrater reliability of pupillary assessments. *Neurocritical Care*. 24 (2): 251–257.

Onishi, A., St Ange, K., Dordick, J.S., Linhardt, R.J. 2016. Heparin and anticoagulation. *Frontiers in Bioscience, Landmark*. 21: 1372–1392.

Oostdijk, E.A.N., de Smet, A.M.G.A., Blok, H.E.M., *et al*. 2010. Ecological effects of selective decontamination on resistant gram-negative bacterial colonization. *American Journal of Respiratory and Critical Care Medicine*. 181 (5): 452–457.

Ormerod, C., Farrer, K., Lal, S. 2010. Refeeding syndrome: a clinical review. *British Journal of Hospital Medicine*. 71 (12): 686–690.

Ormrod, J.A., Ryder, T., Chadwick, R.J., Bonner, S.M. 2005. Experiences of families when a relative is diagnosed brain stem dead: understanding of death, observation of brain stem death testing and attitudes to organ donation. *Anaesthesia*. 60 (10): 1002–1008.

Osler, M., Mårtensson, S., Wium-Andersen, I.K., *et al.* 2016. Depression after first hospital admission for acute coronary syndrome: a study of time of onset and impact on survival. *American Journal of Epidemiology*. 55 (5): 1991–1997.

Ouellet, M.-C., Beaulieu-Bonneaux, S., Morinx, C.M. 2015. Sleep-wake disturbances after traumatic brain injury. *Lancet Neurology*. 14 (7): 746–757.

Outhoff, K. 2016. Evidence of the safety and efficacy of statins: review. *Professional Nursing Today*. 20 (1): 15–17.

Pacheco, L.D., Saade, G., Hankins, G.D., Clark, S.L., Society for Maternal-Fetal Medicine (SMFM). 2016. Amniotic fluid embolism: diagnosis and management. *American Journal of Obstetrics and Gynecology*. 215 (2): B16-B24.

Padilla, C.F. 2014. Most important needs of family members of critical patients in light of the critical care family needs inventory. *Investigación y Educación en Enfermería*. 32 (2): 306–316.

Page, V. 2010. Management of delirium in the intensive care unit. *British Journal of Hospital Medicine*. 71 (7): 372–376.

Page, V.J., Ely, E.W., Gates, S., *et al.* 2013. Effect of intravenous haloperidol on the duration of delirium and coma in critically ill patients (Hope-ICU): a randomised, double-blind, placebo-controlled trial. *Lancet Respiratory Medicine*. 1 (7): 515–523.

Paiva, J.-A., Pereira, J.M., Tabah, A., *et al.* 2016. Characteristics and risk factors for 28-day mortality of hospital acquired fungemias in ICUs. *Critical Care*. 20 (53).

Palevsky, E.M. 2009. Intensity of continuous renal replacement therapy in acute kidney injury. *Seminars in Dialysis*. 22 (2): 151–154.

Pallet, N. 2017. The diagnosis-wide landscape of hospital-acquired AKI. *Clinical Journal of the American Society of Nephrology*. CJN.10981016.

Pandharipande, P.P., Girard, T.D., Jackson, J.C., *et al.*, for the BRAIN-ICU Study Investigators. 2013. Long-term cognitive impairment after critical illness. *New England Journal of Medicine*. 369 (14): 1306–1316.

Paratz, J., Ntoumenopoulos, G. 2014. Detection of secretion retention in the ventilated patient. *Current Respiratory Medicine Review*. 10 (3): 151–157.

Parienti, J.J., Mongardon, N., Mégarbane, B., *et al.*, 3SITES Study Group. 2015. Intravascular complications of central venous catheterization by insertion site. *New England Journal of Medicine*. 373 (13): 1220–1229.

Parikh, M., Webb, S.T. 2012. Cations: potassium, calcium, and magnesium. *Continuing Education in Anaesthesia, Critical Care & Pain*. 12 (4): 195–198.

Park, C. 2007. Diabetic ketoacidosis. *Journal of the Royal College of Physicians of Edinburgh*. 37 (1): 40–43.

Park, S.Y., Kim, H.J., Yoo, K.H., *et al.* 2015. The efficacy and safety of prone positioning in adult patients with acute respiratory distress syndrome: a meta-analysis of randomized controlled trials. *Journal of Thoracic Disease*. 7 (3): 356–367.

Parrott, A.C., Lees, A., Garnham, N.J., *et al.* 1998. Cognitive performance in recreational users of MDMA or "ecstasy": evidence for memory deficits. *Journal of Psychopharmacology*. 12 (1): 79–83.

Parry, N., Evans, I., Southall, P. 2010. "What's the potassium?" *Journal of the Intensive Care Society*. 11 (2): 146.

Pascall, E., Trehane, S.-J., Georgiou, A., Cook, T.M. 2015. Litigation associated with intensive care unit treatment in England: an analysis of NHSLA data 1995–2012. *British Journal of Anaesthesia*. 115 (4): 601–607.

Patel, A.S., Burnard, K.G. 2009. Cardiovascular haemodynamics and shock. *Surgery*. 27 (11): 459–464.

Patel, R., Sweeting, M.J., Powell, J.T., Greenhalgh, J.M., for the EVAR trial investigators. 2016. Endovascular versus open repair of abdominal aortic aneurysm in 15-years' follow-up of the UK endovascular aneurysm repair trial 1 (EVAR trial 1): a randomised controlled trial. *Lancet*. 388 (10058): 2366–2374.

Patterson, Z.R., Young, M.M., Vaccarino, F.J. 2017. Novel psychoactive substances: what educators need to know. *Clinical Pharmacology & Therapeutics*. 101 (2): 173–175.

Patton, H., Misel, M., Gish, R.G. 2012. Acute liver failure in adults: an evidence-based management protocol for clinicians. *Gastroenterology & Hepatology*. 8 (3): 161–212.

Payen, J.-F., Bru, O., Bosson, J.-L., *et al*. 2001. Assessing pain in critically ill sedated patients by using a behavioral pain scale. *Critical Care Medicine*. 29 (12): 2258–2263.

Peake, J., Peiffer, J.J., Abbiss, C.R., *et al*. 2008. Body temperature and its effect on leukocyte mobilization, cytokines and markers of neutrophil activation during and after exercise. *European Journal of Applied Physiology*. 102 (4): 391–401.

Peek, G., Mugford, M., Tiruvoipati, R., *et al*., CESAR trial collaboration. 2009. Efficacy and economic assessment of conventional ventilator support versus extracorporeal membrane oxygenation for severe adult respiratory failure (CESAR): a multicentre randomised controlled trial. *Lancet*. 374 (9698): 1351–1363.

Peerally, M.F., Carr, S., Waring, J., Dixon-Woods, M. 2017. The problem with root cause analysis. *BMJ Quality & Safety*. 26 (5): 417–422.

Pender, L.R., Frazier, S.K. 2005. The relationship between dermal pressure ulcers, oxygenation and perfusion in mechanically ventilated patients. *Intensive and Critical Care Nursing*. 21 (1): 29–38.

Pépin, J., Valiquette, L., Cossette, B. 2005. Mortality attributable to nosocomial *Clostridium difficile*–associated disease during an epidemic caused by a hypervirulent strain in Quebec. *Canadian Medical Association Journal*. 173 (9): 1037–1042.

Perazella, M.A. 2012. Drug use and nephrotoxicity in the Intensive Care Unit. *Kidney International*. 81 (12): 1172–1178.

Pereira, K., Carrion, A.F., Martin, P., *et al*. 2015. Current diagnosis and management of post-transjugular intrahepatic portosystemic shunt refractory hepatic encephalopathy. *Liver International*. 35 (12): 2487–2494.

Perel, A., Pizov, R., Cotev, S. 2014. Respiratory variations in the arterial pressure during mechanical ventilation reflect volume status and fluid responsiveness. *Intensive Care Medicine*. 40 (6): 798–807.

Perel, P., Roberts, I., Ker, K. 2013. Colloids versus crystalloids for fluid resuscitation in critically ill patients. *Cochrane Database of Systematic Reviews*, Issue 2. Art. No.: CD000567. doi:10.1002/14651858.CD000567.pub6.

Perez-Padilla, R., de la Rosa-Zamboni, D., de Leon, S.P., *et al*., INER Working Group on Influenza. 2009. Pneumonia and respiratory failure from swine-origin influenza A (H1N1) in Mexico. *New England Journal of Medicine*. 361 (7): 680–689.

Perner, A., Haase, N., Wiis, J., *et al*. 2010. Central venous oxygen saturation for the diagnosis of low cardiac output in septic shock patients. *Acta Anaesthesiologica Scandinavica*. 54: 98–102.

Perrotti, A., Mariet, A.S., Durst, C., *et al*. 2016. Relationship between depression and health-related quality of life in patients undergoing coronary artery bypass grafting: a MOTIV-CABG substudy. *Quality of Life Research*. 25 (6): 1433–1440.

Petrovsky, N., Ettinger, U., Hill, A., *et al*. 2014. Sleep deprivation disrupts prepulse inhibition and induces psychosis-like symptoms in healthy humans. *The Journal of Neuroscience*. 34 (27): 9134–9140.

Petrucci, N., De Feo, C. 2013. Lung protective ventilation strategy for the acute respiratory distress syndrome. *Cochrane Database of Systematic Reviews*, Issue 2. Art. No.: CD003844. doi:10.1002/14651858.CD003844.pub4.

Petter, A.H., Chiolero, R.L., Cassina, T., *et al*. 2003. Automatic "respirator/weaning" with adaptive support ventilation, the effect on duration of endotracheal intubation and patient management. *Anesthesia & Analgesia*. 97 (6): 1743–1750.

Picone, D.S., Schultz, M.G., Otahal, P., *et al*. 2017. Accuracy of cuff-measured blood pressure: systematic reviews and meta-analyses. *Journal of the American College of Cardiology*. 70 (5): 572–586.

P.I.C.S. 2015a. *Standards for the Care of Critically Ill Children*. 5th edition. London. Paediatric Intensive Care Society.

P.I.C.S. 2015b. *Quality Standards for the Care of Critically Ill Children*. London. Paediatric Intensive Care Society.

Pilbeam, S.P. 2006. Ventilator Graphics. *In* Pilbeam, S.P., Cairo, J.M. (eds). *Mechanical Ventilation: Physiological and Clinical Applications.* 4th edition. St Louis, MO. Mosby Elsevier. 177–204.

Pinsky, M.R. 2014. Functional hemodynamic monitoring. *Current Opinion in Critical Care.* 20 (3): 288–293.

Pisani, M.A. 2009. Considerations in caring for the critically ill older patients. *Intensive Care Medicine.* 24 (2): 83–95.

Pitkin, A., Scott, R., Salmon, J. 1997. Hyperbaric oxygen therapy in intensive care. *British Journal of Intensive Care.* 7 (3): 107–113.

Pitt, T. 2007. Management of antimicrobial-resistant *Acinitobacter* in hospitals. *Nursing Standard.* 21 (35): 51–56.

Pleym, H., Wahba, A., Videm, V., Asberg, A., Lydersen, S., Bjella, L., Dale, O., Stenseth, R. 2006. Increased fibrinolysis and platelet activation in elderly patients undergoing coronary bypass surgery. *Anesthesia & Analgesia.* 102 (3): 660–667.

Pneumatikos, I.A., Dragoumanis, C.K., Bouros, D.E. 2009. Ventilator-associated pneumonia of endotracheal tube-associated pneumonia? *Anesthesiology.* 10 (3): 673–680.

Polderman, K.H., Girbes, A.R.J. 2002. Central venous catheter use. Part 1: mechanical complications. *Intensive Care Medicine.* 28 (1): 1–17.

Ponikowski, P., Voors, A.A., Anker, S.D., *et al.* 2016. 2016 ESC guidelines for the diagnosis and treatment of acute and chronic heart failure. The Task Force for the diagnosis and treatment of acute and chronic heart failure of the European Society of Cardiology (ESC) developed with the special contribution of the Heart Failure Association (HFA) of the ESC. *European Heart Journal.* 37 (27): 2129–2200.

Potijk, M.R., Janszky, I., Reijneveld, S.A., Falkstedt, D. 2016. Risk of coronary heart disease in men with poor emotional control: a prospective study. *Psychosomatic Medicine.* 78 (1): 60–67.

Powell, K., Davis, L., Morris, A.M., Chi, A., Bensley, M.R., Huang, L. 2009. Survival for patients with HIV admitted to the ICU continues to improve in the current era of combination antiretroviral therapy. *Chest.* 135 (1): 11–17.

Powell, T. 2004. *Head Injury: A Practical Guide.* 2nd edition. Bicester. Speechmark.

Powell-Tuck, J., Gosling, P., Lobo, D.N., *et al.* 2008/2011. *British Consensus Guidelines on Intravenous Fluid Therapy for Adult Surgical Patients. GIFTASUP.* London. BAPEN, Association for Clinical Biochemistry, Association of Surgeons of Great Britain and Ireland, Society of Academic and Research Surgery, Renal Association, Intensive Care Society.

Power, B. 2014. Acute cardiac syndromes, investigations and interventions. *In* Bersten, A.D., Soni, N. (eds). *Intensive Care Manual.* 7th edition. Edinburgh. Butterworth-Heinemann. 167–190.

Prasad, A., Hermann, J. 2011. Myocardial infarction due to percutaneous coronary intervention. *New England Journal of Medicine.* 364 (5): 453–464.

Preiser, J.-C., Devos, P., Ruiz-Santana, S., *et al.* 2009. A prospective randomised multi-centre controlled trial on tight glycaemic control by intensive insulin therapy in adult intensive care units: the Glucontrol study. *Intensive Care Medicine.* 35 (10): 1738–1748.

Preiser, J-C., van Zanten, A.R.H., Berger, M.M., *et al.* 2015. Metabolic and nutritional support of critically ill patients: consensus and controversies. *Critical Care.* 19: 35.

Preston, S.D., Southall, A.R., Neil, M., Das, S.K. 2008. Geriatric surgery is about diseases not age. *Journal of the Royal Society of Medicine.* 101: 409–415.

Price, A.M., Plowright, C., Makowski, A., Misztal, B. 2008. Using a high-flow respiratory system (Vapotherm) within a high dependency setting. *Nursing in Critical Care.* 13 (6): 298–303.

Price, J., Magruder, J.T., Young, A., *et al.* 2016. Long-term outcomes of aortic root operations for Marfan syndrome: a comparison of Bentall versus aortic valve-sparing procedures. *The Journal of Thoracic and Cardiovascular Surgery,* 151 (2): 330–338.

Price, J.R., Cole, K., Bexley, A., *et al.,* the Modernising Medical Microbiology informatics group. 2017. Transmission of *Staphylococcus aureus* between health-care workers, the environment, and patients in an intensive care unit: a longitudinal cohort study based on whole-genome sequencing. *Lancet Infectious Diseases.* 17 (2): 207–214.

Price, L.C., Germain, S., Wuncoll, D., Nelson-Piercy, C. 2009. Management of the critically ill obstetric patient. *Obstetrics, Gynaecology and Reproductive Medicine.* 19 (12): 350–358.

Price, R., Maclennan, G., Glen, J. 2014. Selective digestive or oropharyngeal decontamination and topical oropharyngeal chlorhexidine for prevention of death in general intensive care: systematic review and network meta-analysis. *BMJ*. 348: g2197 doi:10.1136/bmj.g2197.

Priori, S.G., Blomström-Lundqvist, C., Mazzanti, A., *et al.*, The Task Force for the Management of Patients with Ventricular Arrhythmias and the Prevention of Sudden Cardiac Death of the European Society of Cardiology (ESC). 2015. 2015 ESC Guidelines for the management of patients with ventricular arrhythmias and the prevention of sudden cardiac death. *European Heart Journal*. 36 (11): 2793–2867.

Public Health England. 2016a. *Tuberculosis in England 2016 Report*. London. Public Health England.

Public Health England. 2016b. *HIV Diagnoses, Late Diagnoses and Numbers Accessing Treatment and Care. 2016 Report*. London. Public Health England.

Public Health England. 2017. *Seasonal Influenza: Guidance for Adult Critical Care Units*. Version 1.0, July 2017. London. Public Health England.

Puchakayala, M.R. 2006. Descending thoracic aortic aneurysms. *Continuing Education in Anaesthesia, Critical Care & Pain*. 6 (2): 54–59.

Pulak, L.M., Jensen, L. 2016. Sleep in the Intensive Care Unit. *Intensive Care Medicine*. 31 (1): 14–23.

Pulsion Medical Systems. 2008. *Get the Complete Picture . . . Advanced Haemodynamic Monitoring*. Munich. Pulsion Medical Systems AG.

Puntillo, K.A., Arai, S., Cohen, N.H., *et al.* 2010. Symptoms experienced by intensive care unit patients at high risk of dying. *Critical Care Medicine*. 38 (11): 2155–2160.

Pyxaras, S.A., Hunziker, L., Chieffo, A., *et al.* 2016. Long-term clinical outcomes after percutaneous coronary intervention versus coronary artery bypass grafting for acute coronary syndrome from the DELTA registry: a multicentre registry evaluating percutaneous coronary intervention versus coronary artery bypass grafting for left main treatment. *EuroIntervention*. 12: e623–e631.

Rajaratnam, S.M.W., Arendt, J. 2001. Health in a 24 hour society. *Lancet*. 3581 (9286): 999–1005.

Rajpaul, K., Acton, C. 2016. Using heel protectors for the prevention of hospital-acquired pressure ulcer. *British Journal of Nursing*. 25 (6): Tissue Viability Supplement.

Ramnarayan, P., Thiru, K., Paslow, R.C., *et al.* 2010. Effect of specialist retrieval teams on outcomes in children admitted to paediatric intensive care units in England and Wales: a retrospective cohort study. *Lancet*. 376 (9742): 698–704.

Ramsay, M.A., Savege, T.M., Simpson, B.R., Goodwin, R. 1974. Controlled sedation with alpha-xalone-alphadolone. *BMJ*. 2 (920): 656–659.

Ramsay, P., Huby, G., Thompson, A., Walsh, T. 2014. Intensive care survivors' experience of ward-based care. Meleis' theory of nursing transitions and role development among critical care outreach services. *Journal of Clinical Nursing*. 23 (5–6): 605–615.

Randhawa, G., Neuberger, J. 2016. Role of religion in organ donation—development of the United Kingdom Faith and Organ Donation Action Plan. *Transplantation Proceedings*. 48 (3): 689–694.

Rang, H.P., Dale, M.M., Ritter, J.M., Flower, R.J. 2007. *Pharmacology*. 6th edition. Edinburgh. Churchill Livingstone Elsevier.

Rankin, J. 2006. Godzilla in the corridor: the Ontario SARS crisis in historical perspective. *Intensive & Critical Care Nursing*. 22 (3): 130–137.

Rathbun, S.W., Whitsett, T.L., Vesely, S.K., Raskob, G.E. 2004. Clinical utility of D-dimer in patients with suspected pulmonary embolism and nondiagnostic lung scans or negative CT findings. *Chest*. 125 (3): 851–855.

Rattenbury, N., Mooney, G., Bowen, J. 1999. Oral assessment and care for inpatients. *Nursing Times*. 95 (49): 52–53.

R.C.N. 2008. *Bowel Care, including Digital Rectal Examination and Manual Removal of Faeces*. London. Royal College of Nursing.

R.C.N. 2016. *Positive and Proactive Care*. London. Royal College of Nursing.

R.C.N. 2016. *Standards for Infusion Therapy*. 4th edition. London. Royal College of Nursing.

R.C.O.G. 2007. *Green Top Guide 28: Thromboembolic Disease in Pregnancy and the Puerperium: Acute Management*. London. Royal College of Obstetricians and Gynaecologists.

R.C.P. 2008. *Nov-Invasive Ventilation in Chronic Obstructive Pulmonary Disease: Management of Acute Type 2 Respiratory Failure*. London. Royal College of Physicians.

R.C.P.C.H. 2015. *The Management of Children and Young People with an Acute Decrease in Level of Consciousness*. London. Royal College of Paediatrics and Child Health.

Reding, M.T., Cooper, D.L. 2012. Barriers to effective diagnosis and management of a bleeding patient with undiagnosed bleeding disorder across multiple specialties: results of a quantitative case-based survey. *Journal of Multidisciplinary Healthcare*. 5: 277–287.

Reilly, D.E. 1980. *Behavioural Objectives – Evaluation in Nursing*. New York. Appleton Century Crofts.

Reinhart, K., Perner, A., Sprung, C.L., *et al*. 2012. Consensus statement of the ESICM task force on colloid volume therapy in critically ill patients. *Intensive Care Medicine*. 38 (3): 368–383.

Reisner-Senelar, L. 2011. The birth of intensive care medicine: Bjorn Ibsen's records. *Intensive Care Medicine*. 37 (7): 1084–1086.

Reitsma, S., Slaaf, D.W., Vink, H., *et al*. 2007. The endothelial glycocalyx: composition, functions, and visualization. *European Journal of Physiology*. 454 (3): 345–359.

Rello, J., Koulenti, D., Blot, S., *et al*. 2007. Oral care practices in intensive care units: a survey of 59 European ICUs. *Intensive Care Medicine*. 33 (6): 1066–1070.

Rello, J., Lisboa, T., Koulenti, D. 2014. Respiratory infections in patients undergoing mechanical ventilation. *Lancet Respiratory Medicine*. 2 (9): 764–767.

Rello, J., Rouby, J.J., Sole-Lleonart, C., *et al*. 2017. Key conceptional considerations on nebulization of antimicrobial agents to mechanically ventilated patients: a consensus statement from the European Society of Clinical Microbiology and Infectious Diseases. *Clinical Microbiology and Infection*. 23 (9) 640–646.

Renal Replacement Therapy Investigators. 2009. High intensity continuous renal replacement therapy does not improve mortality in critically ill patients. *New England Journal of Medicine*. 361 (17): 1627–1638.

Reneman, L., Booij, J., de Bruin, K., *et al*. 2001. Effects of dose, sex and long-term abstention from use on toxic effects of MDMA (ecstasy) on brain serotonin levels. *Lancet*. 358 (9296): 1864–1869.

Renton, M.C., Snowden, C.P. 2005. Dopexamine and its role in the protection of hepatospanchnic and renal perfusion in high-risk surgical and critically ill patients. *British Journal of Anaesthesia*. 94 (4): 459–467.

Resuscitation Council (UK). 2015. *Resuscitation Guidelines*. London. Resuscitation Council.

Retter, A., Wyncoll, D., Pearse, R., *et al*., British Committee for Standards in Haematology. 2012. Guidelines on the management of anaemia and red cell transfusion in adult critically ill patients. *British Journal of Haematology*, 160 (4): 445–464.

Rewbury, R., Hughes, E., Purbrick, R., *et al*. 2017. Poppers: legal highs with questionable contents? *British Journal of Ophthalmology*. 101 (11): 1530–1534.

Rhodes, A., Evans, L.E., Alhazzani, W., *et al*. 2017. Surviving Sepsis Campaign: International Guidelines for Management of Sepsis and Septic Shock: 2016. *Critical Care Medicine*. 45 (3): 486–552.

Riambau, V., Böckler, D., Brunkwall, J., *et al*. 2017. Editor's choice–management of descending thoracic aorta diseases. *European Journal of Vascular and Endovascular Surgery*. 53 (1): 4–52.

Ricaurte, G.A., McCann, U.D. 2005. Recognition and management of complications of new recreational drug use. *Lancet*. 365 (9477): 2137–2145.

Richardson, A., Carter, R. 2017. Falls in critical care: a local review to identify incidence and risk. *Nursing in Critical Care*. 22 (5): 270–275.

Richardson, J.D., Cocanour, C.S., Kern, J.A., *et al*. 2004. Perioperative risk assessment in elderly and high-risk patients. *Journal of the American College of Surgeons*. 199 (1): 133–146.

Rijkenberg, S., Stilma, W., Endeman, H., *et al*. 2015. Pain measurement in mechanically ventilated critically ill patients: behavioral pain scale versus critical-care pain observation tool. *Journal of Critical Care*. 30 (1): 167–172.

Riker, R.R., Fraser, G.L., Simmons, L.E., Wilkins, M.L. 2001. Validating the Sedation-Agitation Scale with the Bispectral Index and Visual Analog Scale in adult ICU patients after cardiac surgery. *Intensive Care Medicine*. 27 (5): 853–858.

545

Riley, B., de Beer, T. 2014. Acute cerebrovascular complications. *In* Bersten, A.D., Soni, N. (eds). *Intensive Care Manual*. 7th edition. Edinburgh. Butterworth-Heinemann Elsevier. 568–579.

Rimmer, E., Houston, B.L., Kumar, A., *et al*. 2014. The efficacy and safety of plasma exchange in patients with sepsis and septic shock: a systematic review and meta-analysis. *Critical Care*. 18 (6): 699.

Ringdal, M., Chaboyer, W., Stomberg, M.W. 2016. Intrahospital transports of critically ill patients: critical care nurses' perceptions. *Nursing in Critical Care*. 21 (3): 178–184.

Robson, S.E., Marshall, J.E., Doughty, R., McLean, M. 2014. Medical conditions of significance to midwifery practice. *In* Marshall, J.E., Raynor, M.D. (eds). *Myles Textbook for Midwives*. 16th edition. Edinburgh. Saunders Elsevier. 243–286.

Rodden, A.M., Spicer, L., Diaz, V.A., Steyer, T.E. 2007. Does fingernail polish affect pulse oximeter readings? *Intensive and Critical Care Nursing*. 23 (1): 51–55.

Rogers, C.R. 1951. *Client-Centred Therapy*. London. Constable.

Rogers, C.R. 1967. *On Becoming a Person*. London. Constable.

Rogers, C.R. 1983. *Freedom to Learn for the 80s*. New York. Merrill.

Romyn, D.M. 2001. Disavowal of the behaviorist paradigm in nursing education: what makes it so difficult to unseat? *Advances in Nursing Science*. 23 (3): 1–10.

Roper, N., Logan, W., Tierney, A. 1996. *The Elements of Nursing*. 4th edition. Edinburgh. Churchill Livingstone.

Ropper, A.H. 2012. Hyperosmolar therapy for raised intracranial pressure. *New England Journal of Medicine*. 367 (8): 746–752.

Ros, C., McNeill, L., Bennett, P. 2009. Review: nurses can improve patient nutrition in intensive care. *Journal of Clinical Nursing*. 18 (17): 2406–2415.

Rose, L. 2011. Interprofessional collaboration in the ICU: how to define? *Nursing in Critical Care*. 16 (1): 5–10.

Rose, L., Baldwin, I., Crawford, T., Parke, R. 2010. Semirecumbent positioning in ventilator-dependent patients: a multicenter, observational study. *American Journal of Critical Care*. 19: e100–e108. doi:10.4037/ajcc2010783.

Rose, L., Blackwood, B., Burns, S.M., *et al*. 2011. International perspectives on the influence of structure and process of weaning from mechanical ventilation. *American Journal of Critical Care*. 20: e10–e18.

Rose, L., Schultz, M.J., Cardwell, C.R., *et al*. 2013. Automated versus non-automated weaning for reducing the duration of mechanical ventilation for critically ill adults and children. *Cochrane Database of Systematic Reviews*, Issue 6. Art. No.: CD009235. doi:10.1002/14651858.CD009235.pub2.

Rosenberger, S.R., Von Rueden, K.T., Des Champs, E.S. 2018. Shock, systemic inflammatory response syndrome, and multiple organ dysfunction syndrome. *In* Morton, P.G., Fontaine, D.K. (eds). *Critical Care Nursing: A Holistic Approach*. 11th edition. Philadelphia. Wolters Kluwer. 1049–1070.

Ross, N., Eynon, C.A. 2005. Intracranial pressure monitoring. *Current Anaesthesia and Critical Care*. 16 (5): 255–261.

Ruiz, I.A., Squair, J.W., Phillips, A.A., *et al*. 2017. Incidence and natural progression of neurogenic shock following traumatic spinal cord injury. *Journal of Neurotrauma*. 35 (3): 461–466.

Russell, R.R., McAuley, D. 2009. Management of non-accidental injury on the pediatric intensive care unit. *In* Murphy, P.J., Marriage, S.C., Davis, P.J. (eds). *Case Studies in Pediatric Critical Care*. Cambridge. Cambridge University Press. 155–161.

Rylah, B., Vercueil, A. 2010. Intensive therapy of the patient with liver disease. *British Journal of Hospital Medicine*. 71 (7): 377–381.

Sabol, V.K., York, A.S. 2018a. Patient management: gastrointestinal system. *In* Morton, P.G., Fontaine, D.K. (eds). *Critical Care Nursing: A Holistic Approach*. 11th edition. Philadelphia. Wolters Kluwer. 782–797.

Sabol, V.K., York, A.S. 2018b. Common gastrointestinal disorders. *In* Morton, P.G., Fontaine, D.K. (eds). *Critical Care Nursing: A Holistic Approach*. 11th edition. Philadelphia. Wolters Kluwer. 916–954.

Sacks, O. 1990. *Awakenings*. revised edition. London. Picador.

Saidi, M., Brett, S. 2009. Pandemic influenza: clinical epidemiology. *In* Ridley, S. (ed.). *Critical Care Focus 16: Infection*. London. Intensive Care Society. 117–134.

Salluh, J.I., Wang, H., Schneider, E.B., *et al.* 2015. Outcome of delirium in critically ill patients: systematic review and meta-analysis. *BMJ* 2015; 350 doi:http://dx.doi.org/10.1136/bmj.h2538.

Samanta, A., Samanta, J. 2004. NICE guideline and law: clinical governance implications for trusts. *Clinical Governance*. 9 (4): 212–215.

Samraj, R.S., Nicolas, L. 2015. Near infrared spectroscopy (NIRS) derived tissue oxygenation in critical illness. *Clinical and Investigative Medicine*. 38 (5): E285-E295.

Samuelson, K.A.M., Lundberg, D., Fridlund, B. 2007. Stressful experiences in relation to depth of sedation in mechanically ventilated patients. *Nursing in Critical Care*. 12 (2): 93–104.

Sanada, H., Sugama, J., Thigpen, B., *et al.* 2006. A new instrument for predicting pressure ulcer risk in an intensive care unit. *Journal of Tissue Viability*. 16 (3): 21–26.

Sanfilippo, F., Santonocito, C., Veenith, T., *et al.* 2014. The role of neuromuscular blockade in patients with traumatic brain injury: a systematic review. *Neurocritical Care*. 22 (2): 325–334.

Saranto, K., Kinnunen, U.-M. 2009. Evaluating nursing documentation – research designs and methods: systematic review. *Journal of Advanced Nursing*. 65 (3): 464–476.

Sargent, S. 2006. Pathophysiology, diagnosis and management of acute pancreatitis. *British Journal of Nursing*. 15 (18): 999–1005.

Sarhan, H.A., El-Garhy, O.H., Ali, M.A., Youssef, N.A. 2016. The efficacy of nebulized magnesium sulfate alone and in combination with salbutamol in acute asthma. *Drug Design, Development and Therapy*. 10: 1927–1933. doi:10. 2147/DDDT.S103147.

Sarvimaki, A., Sanderlin Benko, S. 2001. Values and evaluation in health care. *Journal of Nursing Management*. 9 (3): 129–137.

Saugel, B., Meidert, A.S., Langwieser, N., *et al.* 2014. An autocalibrating algorithm for non-invasive cardiac output determination based on the analysis of an arterial pressure waveform recorded with radial artery applanation tonometry: a proof of concept pilot analysis. *Journal of Clinical Monitoring and Computing*. 28 (4): 357–362.

Saw, M.M., Chandler, B., Ho, K.M. 2012. Benefits and risks of using gelatin solution as a plasma expander for perioperative and critically ill patients: a meta-analysis. *Anaesthesia & Intensive Care*. 40 (1): 17–32.

Sayar, S., Turget, S., Doğan, H., *et al.* 2009. Incidence of pressure ulcers in intensive care unit patients at risk according to the Waterlow scale and factors influencing the development of pressure sores. *Journal of Clinical Nursing*. 18 (5): 765–774.

Schairer, J.R., Keteyian, S.J. 2016. Pathophysiology and causes of cardiac tamponade. *In* Webb, A., Angus, D.C., Finger, S., Gattinoni, L., Singer, M.P.M. (eds). *Oxford Textbook of Critical Care*. 2nd edition. Oxford. Oxford University Press. 780–783.

Scheer, F.A.J.L., Shea, S.A. 2014. Human circadian system causes a morning peak in prothrombotic plasminogen activator inhibitor-1 (PAI-1) independent of the sleep/wake cycle. *Blood*. 123 (4): 590–593.

Scheinkestel, C.D., Bailey, M., Myles, P.S., *et al.* 1999. Hyperbaric or normobaric oxygen for acute carbon monoxide poisoning: a randomised controlled clinical trial. *Medical Journal of Australia*. 170 (5): 203–210.

Schifano, F., Corkery, J., Deluca, P., Oyefeso, A., Ghodse, A.H. 2006. Ecstasy (MDMA, MDA, MDEA, MBDB) consumption, seizures, related offences, prices, dosage levels and deaths in the UK (1994–2003). *Journal of Psychopharmacology*. 20 (3): 456–463.

Schläpfer, J., Wellens, H.J. 2017. Computer-interpreted electrocardiograms: benefits and limitations. *Journal of the American College of Cardiology*. 70 (9): 1183–1192.

Schmidt, M., Hodgson, C., Combes, A. 2013. Extracorporeal gas exchange for acute respiratory failure in adults: a systematic review. *Critical Care*. 19: 99.

Schmidt, M., Stewart, C., Bailey, M., *et al.* 2014. Mechanical ventilation management during extracorporeal membrane oxygenation for acute respiratory distress syndrome: a retrospective international multicenter study. *Critical Care Medicine*. 43 (3): 654–664.

Schneemilch, C.E., Bachmann, H., Ulrich, A., *et al.* 2006. Clonidine decreases stress response in patients undergoing carotid endartrectomy under regional anesthesia: a prospective, randomized, double-blinded, placebo-controlled study. *Anesthesia & Analgesia*. 103 (2): 297–302.

Schuetz, P., Müeller, B. 2016. Procalcitonin in critically ill patients: time to change guidelines and antibiotic use in practice. *Lancet.* 16 (7): 758–760.

Schweickert, W.D., Pohlman, M.C., Pohlman, A.S., *et al.* 2009. Early physical and occupational therapy in mechanically ventilated, critically ill patients: a randomised controlled trial. *Lancet.* 373 (9678): 1874–1882.

Scott, E.M., Leaper, D.J., Clark, M. 2001. Effects of warming therapy on pressure ulcers – a randomised trial. *AORN.* 73 (5): 921–938.

Scrase, W., Tranter, S. 2011. Improving evidence-based care for patients with pyrexia. *Nursing Standard.* 25 (29): 37–41.

Sedwick, M.B., Lance-Smith, M., Reeder, S.J., Nardi, J. 2012. Using evidence-based practice to prevent ventilator-associated pneumonia. *Critical Care Nurse.* 32 (4): 41–50.

Seligman, M.E.P. 1975. *Helplessness: On Depression, Development and Death.* New York. W.H. Freeman.

Semple, D.N., Ebmeier, K.P., Glabus, M.F., *et al.* 1999. Reducing *in vivo* binding to the serotonin transporter in the cerebral cortex of MDMA ("ecstasy") users. *British Journal of Psychiatry.* 175 (July): 63–69.

Serpa Neto, A., Cardoso, S.O., Manetta, J.A., *et al.* 2012. Association between use of lung-protective ventilation with lower tidal volumes and clinical outcomes among patients without acute respiratory distress syndrome: a meta-analysis. *JAMA.* 308 (9): 1651–1659.

Sertaridou, E., Papaioannou, V., Kolios, G., Pneumatikos, I. 2015. Gut failure in critical care: old school versus new school. *Annals of Gastroenterology.* 28 (3): 309–322.

Sessler, D.I. 2008. Temperature monitoring and perioperative thermoregulation. *Anesthesiology.* 109 (2): 318–338.

Sever, M.S., Vanholder, R., Lameire, N. 2006. Management of crush related injuries after disasters. *New England Journal of Medicine.* 354 (10): 1052–1063.

Sevransky, J.E., Checkley, W., Herrera, P., *et al.* 2015. Protocols and hospital mortality in critically ill patients: The United States Critical Illness and Injury Trials Group Critical Illness Outcomes Study. *Critical Care Medicine.* 43 (10): 2076–2084.

Seymour, C.W., Liu, V.X., Iwashyna, T.J., *et al.* 2016. Assessment of clinical criteria for sepsis for the Third International Consensus Definitions for Sepsis and Septic Shock (Sepsis-3). *JAMA.* 315 (8): 762–774.

Shaheen, B., Bakir, M., Jain, S. 2014. Corneal nerves in health and disease. *Survey of Ophthalmology.* 59 (3): 263–285.

Shahina, E.S.M., Dassena, T., Halfens, R.J.G. 2009. Incidence, prevention and treatment of pressure ulcers in intensive care patients: a longitudinal study. *International Journal of Nursing Studies.* 46 (4): 413–421.

Shaikh, N., Mehesry, T., Hussain, G., *et al.* 2016. Use of steroid for extubation failure due to stridor in surgical intensive care patients. *International Journal of Critical Care and Emergency Medicine.* 2: 013.

Shanks, G.D., MacKenzie, A., Waller, M., Brundage, J.F. 2011. Low but highly variable mortality among nurses and physicians during the influenza pandemic of 1918–1919. *Influenza and Other Respiratory Viruses.* 5 (3): 213–219.

Shannon-Lowe, J., Matheson, N.J., Cooke, F.J., Aliyu, S.H. 2010. Prevention and medical management of *Clostridium difficile* infection. *BMJ.* 340 (7747): 605–662.

Sharif, H, Hou, S. 2017. Autonomic dysreflexia: a cardiovascular disorder following spinal cord injury. *Neural Regeneration Research.* 12 (9): 1390.

Sharma, P., Dasgupta, I., Barua, S. 2015. Effect of nail polish colour on pulse oximetry reading. *International Journal of Advanced Research.* 3 (8): 596–600.

Sharp, L.S., Rozycki, G.S., Feliciano, D.V. 2004. Rhabdomyolysis and secondary renal failure in critically ill surgical patients. *American Journal of Surgery.* 188 (6): 801–806.

Sharp, S., McAllister, M., Broadbent, M. 2015. The vital blend of clinical competence and compassion: How patients experience person-centred care. *Contemporary Nurse.* doi:10.1080/10376178. 2015.1020981.

Shaw, A.D., Raghunathan, K., Peyerl, F.W., *et al.* 2014. Association between intravenous chloride load during resuscitation and in-hospital mortality among patients with SIRS. *Intensive Care Medicine.* 40 (12): 1897–1905.

Shehabi, Y., Bellomo, R., Reade, M., *et al.* 2012. Sedation Practice in Intensive Care Evaluation (SPICE) Study Group and the ANZICS CTG: Early intensive care sedation predicts long-term mortality in mechanically ventilated critically ill patients. *American Journal of Respiratory and Critical Care Medicine.* 186 (8): 724–731.

Sheikh, A, Hurwitz, B., van Schayck, C.P., *et al.* 2012. Antibiotics versus placebo for acute bacterial conjunctivitis. *Cochrane Database of Systematic Reviews*, Issue 9. Art. No.: CD001211. doi:10.1002/14651858.CD001211.pub3.

Shekar, K., Gregory, S.D., Fraser, J.F. 2016. Mechanical circulatory support in the new era: an overview. *Critical Care.* 20 (66).

Shiao, J., Koh, D., Lo, L.-H., *et al.* 2007. Factors predicting nurses' consideration of leaving their job during the SARS outbreak. *Nursing Ethics.* 14 (1): 5–17.

Shuhaiber, J.H., Hur, K., Gibbons, R. 2010. The influence of preoperative use of ventricular assist devices on survival after heart transplantation: propensity score matched analysis. *BMJ.* 340 (7742): 354.

Shuster, M.H., Haines, T., Sekula, L.K., *et al.* 2010. Reliability of intrabladder pressure measurement in intensive care. *American Journal of Critical Care.* 19 (1): 29–39.

Siddiqui, A., Behrendt, R., Lafluer, M., Craft, S. 2013. A continuous bedside pressure mapping system for prevention of pressure ulcer development in the medical ICU: a retrospective analysis. *Wounds.* 25 (12): 333–339.

Simons, F.E.R., Ardusso, L.R.F., Bilò, M.B., *et al.*, World Allergy Organization. 2011. World Allergy Organization guidelines for the assessment and management of anaphylaxis. *WAO Journal.* 4 (1): 13–37.

Simons, K.J., Simons, E.R. 2010. Epinephrine and its use in anaphylaxis: current issues. *Current Opinion in Allergy and Clinical Immunology.* 10 (4): 354–361.

Sinan, M., Ertan, N.Z., Mirasoglu, B., *et al.* 2016. Acute and long-term effects of hyperbaric oxygen therapy on hemorheological parameters in patients with various disorders. *Clinical Hemorheology and Microcirculation.* 62 (1): 79–88.

Singer, M., Deutschman, C.S., Seymour, C.W., *et al.* 2016. The Third International Consensus Definitions for Sepsis and Septic Shock (Sepsis-3). *JAMA.* 315 (8): 775–787.

Singer, P., Berger, M., Van den Berghe, G., *et al.* 2009. ESPEN guidelines on parenteral nutrition: intensive care. *Clinical Nutrition.* 28 (4): 387–400.

Singh, A., Laribi, S., Teerlink, J.R., Mebazaa, A. 2017. Agents with vasodilator properties in acute heart failure. *European Heart Journal.* 38 (5): 317–325.

Singh, B., Hanson, A.C., Alhurani, R.S., *et al.* 2013. Trends in the incidence and outcomes of disseminated intravascular coagulation in critically ill patients (2004–2010): a population-based study. *Chest.* 143 (5): 1235–1242.

Sipahi, I., Akay, M.H., Dagdelen, S., *et al.* 2014. Coronary Artery Bypass Grafting vs Percutaneous Coronary Intervention and long-term mortality and morbidity in multivessel disease: meta-analysis of randomized clinical trials of the arterial grafting and stenting era. *JAMA Internal Medicine.* 174 (2): 223–230.

Sireesha, S., Prasad, B.S., Suresh, J. 2018. Comparison of nebulized Salbutamol versus Adrenaline in the treatment of wheeze associated respiratory tract infection. *International Journal of Contemporary Pediatrics.* 5 (1): 169–172.

Siribamrungwong, M., Chinudomwong, P. 2016. Relation between acute kidney injury and pregnancy-related factors. *Journal of Acute Disease.* 5 (1): 22–28.

Skeie, G.O., Apostolski, S., Evoli, A., *et al.* 2010. Guidelines for treatment of autoimmune neuro-muscular transmission disorders. *European Journal of Neurology.* 17: 893–902.

Skinner, B.F. 1971. *Beyond Freedom and Dignity.* London. Penguin.

Skyler, J.S., Bakris, G.L., Bonifacio, E., *et al.* 2017. Differentiation of diabetes by pathophysiology, natural history, and prognosis. *Diabetes.* 66 (2): 241–255.

Slutsky, A.S. 2015. History of mechanical ventilation: from Vesalius to ventilator-induced lung injury. *American Journal of Respiratory and Critical Care Medicine.* 191 (10): 1106–1115.

Slutsky, A.S., Ranieri, V.M. 2013. Ventilator-induced lung injury. *New England Journal of Medicine.* 369 (22): 2126–2136.

Smith, A., Taylor, C. 2005. Analysis of blood gases and acid-base balance. *Surgery.* 23 (6): 194–198.

Smith, D.H. 2007. Managing acute acetaminophen toxicity. *Nursing.* 37 (1): 58–63.

Smith, M., Meyfroidt, G. 2017. Critical illness: the brain is always in the line of fire. *Intensive Care Medicine*: 1–4.

Soares, M., Esteves, S. 2016. Significantly prolonged neuromuscular blockade after a single dose of rocuronium. *European Journal of Anaesthesiology*. 33: 1–2.

Sole, M.L., Bennett, M., Ashworth, S. 2015. Clinical indicators for endotracheal suctioning in adult patients receiving mechanical ventilation. *American Journal of Critical Care*. 24 (4): 318–324.

Sontag, S. 1989. *AIDS and its Metaphors*. London. Penguin.

Sood, P., Paul, G., Puri, S. 2010. Interpretation of arterial blood gas. *Indian Journal of Critical Care Medicine*. 14 (2): 57–64.

Sookoian, S., Castaño, G.O., Scian, R., *et al.* 2016. Serum aminotransferases in nonalcoholic fatty liver disease are a signature of liver metabolic perturbations at the amino acid and Krebs cycle level. *The American Journal of Clinical Nutrition*. 103 (2): 422–434.

Sourial, M., Chahine, E.B., Ishak, M. 2014. Update on the management of *Clostridium difficile* infection. *US Pharmacist*. 39 (12): 50–54.

Spasovski, G., Vanholder, R., Allolio, B., *et al.*, on behalf of the Hyponatraemia Guideline Development Group. 2014. Clinical practice guideline on diagnosis and treatment of hyponatraemia. *European Journal of Endocrinology*. 170: G1–G47.

Spitzer, A.T., Sims, K.M. 2016. A comparison of the impact of cuffed versus uncuffed endotracheal tubes on the incidence of tracheal tube exchange and on post-extubation airway morbidity in pediatric patient undergoing general anesthesia: a systematic review protocol. *JBI Database of Systematic Reviews and Implementation Reports*, 10–17.

Sprung, C.L., Cohen, R., Adini, B. 2010. Recommendations and standard operating procedures for intensive care unit and hospital preparations for an influenza epidemic or mass disaster. *Intensive Care Medicine*. supplement 1.

Sque, M., Long, T., Payne, S., Allardyce, D. 2008. Why relatives do not donate organs for transplants: "sacrifice" or "gift of life"? *Journal of Advanced Nursing*. 61 (2): 134–144.

Squizzato, A., Hunt, B.J., Kinaswitz, B.G., *et al.* 2016. Supportive management strategies for disseminated intravascular coagulation. *Thrombosis and Haemostasis*. 115 (5): 896–904.

Sridhar, S., Botbol, Y., Macian, F., Cuervol, A.M. 2012. Autophagy and disease: always two sides to a problem. *Journal of Pathology*. 226 (1): 255–273.

Stafford, A., Haverland, A., Bridges, E. 2014. Noise in the ICU. *American Journal of Nursing*. 114 (5): 57–63.

Starling, E. 1896. On the absorption of fluid from the connective tissue spaces. *Journal of Physiology*. 19 (4): 312–326.

Stasseno, P., Di Tommaso, L., Monaco, M., *et al.* 2009. Aortic valve replacement. *Journal of the American College of Cardiology*. 54 (20): 1862–1868.

Stather, P.W., Sidloff, D., Dattani, N., *et al.* 2013. Systematic review and meta-analysis of the early and late outcomes of open and endovascular repair of abdominal aortic aneurysm. *British Journal of Surgery*. 100 (7): 863–872.

Steegers, E.A.P., van Dadelszen, P., Duvekot, J.J., Pijnenborg, R. 2010. Pre-eclampsia. *Lancet*. 376 (9741): 631–644.

Steggall, M.J. 2007. Urine samples and urinalysis. *Nursing Standard*. 22 (14–16): 42–45.

Stein, R.A. 2009. Lessons from outbreaks of H1N1 influenza. *Annals of Internal Medicine*. 151 (1): 59–62.

Steingrub, J.S., Lagu, T., Rothberg, M.B., *et al.* 2014. Treatment with neuromuscular blocking agents and the risk of in-hospital mortality among mechanically ventilated patients with severe sepsis. *Critical Care Medicine*. 42 (1): 90–96.

Steinhubl, S.R., Bhaat, D.L., Brennan, D.M., *et al.*, CHARISMA investigators. 2009. Aspirin to prevent cardiovascular disease: the association of aspirin dose and clopidogrel with thrombosis and bleeding. *Annals of Internal Medicine*. 150 (6): 379–386.

Steptoe, A., Kivimäki, M. 2012. Stress and cardiovascular disease. *Nature Reviews Cardiology*. 9: 360–370.

Sterns, R.H., Silver, S.M. 2016. Complications and management of hyponatremia. *Current Opinion in Nephrology and Hypertension*. 25 (2): 114–119.

Stevens, D.L., Bryant, A.E. 2017. Necrotizing soft-tissue infections. *New England Journal of Medicine.* 377 (23): 2253–2265.

Stewart, N.I., Gunning, K., Cuthbertson, B.H., UK Intensive Care Society. 2012. Regionalisation of intensive care and extra-corporeal membrane oxygenation services in the UK: beliefs about the evidence, benefits and harm. *Journal of the Intensive Care Society.* 13 (3): 244–250.

Stokes, T., Shaw, E.J., Juarez-Garcia, A., *et al.* 2004. *Clinical Guidelines and Evidence Review for the Epilepsies: Diagnosis and Management in Adults and Children in Primary and Secondary Care.* London. Royal College of General Practitioners.

Storey, M., Jordan, S. 2008. An overview of the immune system. *Nursing Standard.* 23 (15–17): 47–56.

Stremler, R., Haddad, S., Pullenayegum, E., Parshuram, C. 2017. Psychological outcomes in parents of critically ill hospitalized children. *Journal of Pediatric Nursing.* 34 (1): 36–43.

Strøm, T., Martinussen, T., Toft, P. 2010. A protocol of no sedation for critically ill patients receiving mechanical ventilation: a randomised trial. *Lancet.* 375 (9713): 475–480.

Sturgess, D.J. 2014. Haemodynamic monitoring. *In* Bersten, A.D., Soni, N. (eds). *Intensive Care Manual.* 7th edition. Edinburgh. Butterworth-Heinemann Elsevier. 122–137.

Su, X., Meng, Z.-T., Wu, X.-H., *et al.* 2016. Dexmedetomidine for prevention of delirium in elderly patients after non-cardiac surgery: a randomised, double-blind, placebo-controlled trial. *Lancet.* 388 (10054): 1893–1902.

Suarez, J.I., Tarr, R.W., Selman, W.R. 2006. Aneurysmal subarachnoid haemorrhage. *New England Journal of Medicine.* 354 (4): 387–396.

Sud, S., Friedrich, J.O., Taccone, P., *et al.* 2010. Prone ventilation reduces mortality in patients with acute respiratory failure and severe hypoxaemia: systematic review and meta-analysis. *Intensive Care Medicine.* 36 (4): 585–599.

Sud, S., Sud, M., Friedrich, J.O., *et al.* 2010. High frequency oscillation in patients with acute lung injury and acute respiratory distress syndrome (ARDS): systematic review and meta-analysis. *BMJ.* 340 (7759): 1290.

Sultan, P., Seligman, K., Carvalho, B. 2016. Amniotic fluid embolism: update and review. *Current Opinion in Anesthesiology.* 29 (3): 288–296.

Sung, J.J.Y. 2010. Peptic ulcer bleeding: an expedition of 20 years from 1989–2009. *Journal of Gastroenterology and Hepatology.* 25 (2): 229–233.

Sung, J.J.Y. 2014. Acute gastrointestinal bleeding. *In* Bersten, A.D., Soni, N. (eds). *Intensive Care Manual.* 7th edition. Edinburgh. Butterworth-Heinemann. 488–494.

Suraweera, D., Sundaram, V., Saab, S. 2016. Evaluation and management of hepatic encephalopathy: current status and future directions. *Gut and Liver.* 10 (4): 509–519.

Svensson, M.-L., Lindberg, L. 2012. The use of propofol sedation in a paediatric intensive care unit. *Nursing in Critical Care.* 17 (4): 198–203.

Szaflarski, N.L. 1996. Preanalytic error associated with blood gas/pH measurement. *Critical Care Nurse.* 16 (3): 89–100.

Szura, M., Pasternak, A. 2015. Upper non-variceal gastrointestinal bleeding – review the effectiveness of endoscopic hemostasis methods. *World Journal of Gastrointestinal Endoscopy.* 7 (13): 1088–1095.

Taccone, P., Pesenti, A., Latini, R., *et al.*, Prone-Supine II Study Group. 2009. Prone positioning in patients with moderate and severe acute respiratory distress syndrome. A randomized controlled trial. *JAMA.* 302 (18): 1977–1984.

Tambyraja, A.L., Chalmers, R.T.A. 2009. Aortic aneurysms. *Surgery.* 27 (8): 342–345.

Tane, N., Okuda, N., Imanaka, H., Nishimura, M. 2015. Neurally adjusted ventilatory assist improves patient-ventilator synchrony in a patient with tetanus and unstable diaphragmatic electrical activity. *Respiratory Care.* 60 (4): e76-e79.

Tasaka, C.L., Duby, J.J., Pandya, K., *et al.* 2016. Inadequate sedation during therapeutic paralysis: use of bispectral index in critically ill patients. *Drugs – Real World Outcomes.* 3 (2): 201–208. doi:10.1007/s40801-016-0076-3.

Task Force on the Diagnosis and Management of Acute Pulmonary Embolism of the European Society of Cardiology (Torbicki, A., Perrier, A., Konstantintinides, S., Agnelli, G., Galiè, N., Pruszczyk, P., Bengel, F., Brady, A.J.B., Ferreira, D., Janssens, U., Klepetko, W., Mayer, E.,

Remy-Jardin, M., Bassand, J-P). 2008. Guidelines on the diagnosis and management of acute pulmonary embolism. *European Heart Journal*. 29 (18): 2276–2315.

Task Force for the Management of Atrial Fibrillation of the European Society of Cardiology (ESC). 2010a. Guidelines for the management of atrial fibrillation. *European Heart Journal*. 31 (19): 2369–2429.

Task Force on Myocardial Revascularization of the European Society of Cardiology (ESC) and the European Association for Cardio-Thoracic Surgery (EACTS). 2010b. Guidelines on myocardial revascularization. *European Heart Journal*. 31 (20): 2501–2555.

Task Force for the Management of Acute Coronary Syndromes (ACS) in Patients Presenting without persistent ST-Segment Elevation of the European Society of Cardiology (ESC). 2011. ESC Guidelines for the management of acute coronary syndromes in patients presenting without persistent ST-segment elevation. *European Heart Journal*. 32 (23): 2999–3054.

Task Force for the Management of Arterial Hypertension of the European Society of Hypertension (ESH) and of the European Society of Cardiology (ESC). 2013. 2013 ESH/ESC Guidelines for the management of arterial hypertension. *European Heart Journal*. 34 (28): 2159–2219.

Task Force for the Diagnosis and Management of Pericardial Diseases of the European Society of Cardiology (ESC). 2015. 2015 ESC Guidelines for the diagnosis and management of pericardial disease. *European Heart Journal*. 36 (42): 2921–2964.

Task Force for the Diagnosis and Treatment of Acute and Chronic Heart Failure of the European Society of Cardiology (ESC). 2016a. 2016 ESC Guidelines for the diagnosis and treatment of acute and chronic heart failure. *European Heart Journal*. 37 (27): 2129–2200.

Task Force for the Management of Atrial Fibrillation of the European Society of Cardiology (ESC). 2016b. 2016 ESC Guidelines for the management of atrial fibrillation developed in collaboration with EACT. *European Heart Journal*. 37 (38): 2893–2962.

Task Force for the Management of Acute Coronary Syndromes in Patients Presenting without Persistent ST-Segment Elevation of the European Society of Cardiology (ESC) (Roffi, M., Patrono, C., Collet, J.P., Mueller, C., Valgimigli, M., Andreotti, F., Bax, J.J., Borger, M.A., Brotons, C., Chew, D.P., Gencer, B., Hasenfuss, G., Kjeldsen, K., Lancellotti, P., Landmesser, U., Mehilli, J., Mukherjee, D., Storey, R.F., Windecker, S.). 2016c. 2015 ESC Guidelines for the Management of Acute Coronary Syndromes in Patients Presenting without Persistent ST-Segment Elevation. *European Heart Journal*. 37: 267–315.

Tassaux, D., Gainnier, M., Battisti, A., Jolliet, P. 2005. Helium-oxygen decreases inspiratory effort and work of breathing during pressure support in intubated patients with chronic obstructive pulmonary disease. *Intensive Care Medicine*. 31 (11): 1501–1507.

Tayyib, N., Coyer, F. 2016. Effectiveness of pressure ulcer prevention strategies for adult patients in intensive care units: a systematic review protocol. *JBI Database of Systematic Reviews and Implementation Reports*. 13 (6): 432–444.

TEAM Study Investigators. 2015. Early mobilization and recovery in mechanically ventilated patients in the ICU: a bi-national, multi-centre, prospective cohort study. *Critical Care*. 19 (1): 81.

Teasdale, G. 2014. Forty years on: updating the Glasgow Coma Scale. *Nursing Times*. 110 (42): 12–16.

Teasdale, G., Jennett, B. 1974. Assessment of coma and impaired consciousness. *Lancet*. ii (7872): 81–83.

Teman, N.R., Thomas, J., Bryner, B.S., *et al.* 2015. Inhaled nitric oxide to improve oxygenation for safe critical care transport of adults with severe hypoxemia. *American Journal of Critical Care*. 24 (2): 110–117.

Tenner, S., Baillie, J., DeWitt, J., Vege, S.S. 2013. American College of Gastroenterology Guideline: management of acute pancreatitis. *The American Journal of Gastroenterology*. 108 (9): 1400–1415.

Terekeci, H., Kucukardali, Y., Top, C., *et al.* 2009. Risk assessment study of the pressure ulcers in intensive care unit patients. *European Journal of Internal Medicine*. 20 (4): 394–397.

Terrio, H., Brenner, L.A., Irvins, B.J., *et al.* 2009. Preliminary findings regarding prevalence and sequelae in a US Army brigade combat team. *Journal of Head Trauma & Rehabilitation*. 24 (1): 14–23.

Thacker, V., Patel, K. 2017. Recent advances in pharmacotherapy of acute coronary syndrome. *International Journal of Basic & Clinical Pharmacology*. 5 (5): 1695–1703.

Thajudeen, A., Stecker, E.C., Shehata, M., *et al.* 2012. Arrhythmias after heart transplantation: mechanisms and management. *Journal of the American Heart Association*. 1 (2): e001461.

Than, N.N., Newsome, P.N. 2015. A concise review of non-alcoholic fatty liver disease. *Atherosclerosis*. 239 (1): 192–202.

The Australia and New Zealand Extracorporeal Membrane Oxygenation (ANZ EMO) Influenza investigators. 2009. Extracorporeal membrane oxygenation for 2009 influenza A (H1N1) acute respiratory distress syndrome. *JAMA*. 302 (17): 1888–1895.

The United Kingdom EVAR Trial Investigators. 2010. Endovascular versus open repair of abdominal aortic aneurysm. *New England Journal of Medicine*. 362 (20): 1863–1871.

Thiele, H., Zeymer, U., Neumann, F.-J., *et al.*, IABP-SHOCK II Trial Investigators. 2013. Intra-aortic balloon counterpulsation in acute myocardial infarction complicated by cardiogenic shock (IABP-SHOCK II): final 12 month results of a randomised, open-label trial. *Lancet*. 382 (9905): 1638–1645.

Thiele, R.H., Isbell, J.M., Rosner, M.H. 2015. AKI associated with cardiac surgery. *Clinical Journal of the American Society of Nephrology*. 10 (3): 500–514.

Thomas, A.N., Taylor, R.J. 2012. Review of patient safety incidents reported from critical care units in North-West England in 2009 and 2010. *Anaesthesia*. 67 (7): 706–713.

Thomas, N. (ed.). 2014. *Renal Nursing*. 4th edition. Oxford. Wiley-Blackwell.

Thomas, P., Lynch, K., Mason, A., *et al.* 2014. In-hospital and post-discharge mortality in the extreme elderly admitted to intensive care. *Journal of the Intensive Care Society*. 15 (1): 48–52.

Thumbikat, P., Hussain, N., McClelland, M.R. 2009. Acute spinal cord injury. *Surgery*. 27 (7): 280–286.

Thygesen, K., Alpert, J.S., Jaffe, A.S., *et al.*, Joint ESC/ACCF/AHA/WHF Task Force for the Universal Definition of Myocardial Infarction. 2012. Third universal definition of myocardial infarction. *European Heart Journal*. 33 (20): 2551–2567.

Timmers, T.K., Verhofstad, M.H.J., Moons, K.G.M., *et al.* 2011. Long-term quality of life after surgical intensive care admission. *Archives of Surgery*. 146 (4): 412–418.

Tingle, J. 2007. Recurring themes in NHS complaints. *British Journal of Nursing*. 16 (5): 265.

Tirlapur, N., Puthucheary, Z.A., Cooper, J.A., *et al.* 2016. Diarrhoea in the critically ill is common, associated with poor outcome, and rarely due to *Clostridium difficile*. *Scientific Reports*. 6.

Tiruvoipati, R., Botha, J.A., Pilcher, D., Bailey, M. 2013. Carbon dioxide clearance in critical care. *Anaesthesia and Intensive Care*. 41 (2): 157–162.

Tobin, M.J., Laghi, F., Jurban, A. 2010. Ventilator-induced respiratory muscle weakness. *Annals of Internal Medicine*. 153 (4): 240–245.

Tonelli, M., Riella, M. 2014. Chronic kidney disease and the aging population. *Nephrology Dialysis Transplantation*. 29 (2): 221–224.

Torres, A., Ewig, S., Lode, H., Carlet, J., European HAP Working Group. 2009. Defining, treating and preventing hospital acquired pneumonia: European perspective. *Intensive Care Medicine*. 35 (1): 9–29.

Townsend, N., Wickramasinghe, K., Bhatnagar, P., *et al.* 2012. *Coronary Heart Disease Statistics 2012 edition*. London. British Heart Foundation.

Trachsel, D., McCrindle, B.W., Nakagawa, S., Bohn, D. 2005. Oxygenation index predicts outcome in children with acute hypoxemic respiratory failure. *American Journal of Respiratory and Critical Care Medicine*. 172 (2) 206–211.

Tramm, R., Ilic, D., Davies, A.R., *et al.* 2015. Extracorporeal membrane oxygenation for critically ill adults. *Cochrane Database of Systematic Reviews*. Issue 1. Art. No.: CD010381. doi:10.1002/14651858.CD010381.pub2.

Tranquilli, A.L., Dekker, G., Magee, L., *et al.* 2014. The classification, diagnosis and management of the hypertensive disorders of pregnancy: a revised statement from the ISSHP. *Pregnancy Hypertension: An International Journal of Women's Cardiovascular Health*. 4 (2): 97–104.

Traynor, M. 2009. Humanism and its critiques in nursing research literature. *Journal of Advanced Nursing*. 65 (7): 1560–1567.

Treadwell, S.D., Robinson, T.G. 2007. Cocaine use and stroke. *Postgraduate Medical Journal.* 83 (980): 389–394.

Treger, R., Pirouz, S., Kamangar, N., Corry, D. 2010. Agreement between central venous and arterial blood gas measurements in the Intensive Care Unit. *Clinical Journal of the American Society of Nephrologists.* 5 (3): 390–394.

Treloar, D.M. 1995. Use of a clinical assessment tool for orally intubated patients. *American Journal of Critical Care.* 4 (5): 355–360.

Tremper, K.K. 2002. Perfluorochemical "red blood cell substitutes": the continued search for an indication. *Anesthesiology.* 97 (6): 1333–1334.

Tripathi, D., Stanley, A.J., Hayes, P.C., *et al.* 2015. UK guidelines on the management of variceal haemorrhage in cirrhotic patients. *Gut.* 64 (11): 1680–1704.

Truche, A.-S., Darmon, M., Bailly, S., *et al.* 2016. Continuous renal replacement therapy versus intermittent hemodialysis in intensive care patients: impact on mortality and renal recovery. *Intensive Care Medicine.* 42 (9): 1408–1417.

Truijen, J., van Lieshout, J.J., Wesselink, W.A., Westerhof, B.E. 2012. Noninvasive continuous hemodynamic monitoring. *Journal of Clinical Monitoring and Computing.* 26 (2): 267–278.

Tschannen, D., Keenan, G., Aebersold, M., *et al.* 2011. Implications of nurse-physician relations: report of a successful intervention. *Nursing Economics.* 29 (3): 127–135.

Tujios, S.R., Hynan, L.S., Vazquez, M.A., *et al.*, Acute Liver Failure Study Group. 2015. Risk factors and outcomes of acute kidney injury in patients with acute liver failure. *Clinical Gastroenterology and Hepatology.* 13 (2): 352–359.

Tumbarello, M., De Pascale, G., Trecarichi, E.M., *et al.* 2013. Clinical outcomes of *Pseudomonas aeruginosa* pneumonia in intensive care unit patients. *Intensive Care Medicine.* 39 (4): 682–692.

Turnbull, B. 2008. High-flow humidified oxygen therapy used to alleviate respiratory distress. *British Journal of Nursing.* 17 (19): 1226–1230.

Turner-Cobb, J.M., Smith, P.C., Ramchandani, P., *et al.* 2016. The acute psychobiological impact of the intensive care experience on relatives. *Psychology, Health & Medicine.* 21 (1): 20–26.

Turvill, J.L., Burroughs, A.K., Moore, K.P. 2000. Change in occurrence of paracetamol overdose in UK after introduction of blister packs. *Lancet.* 355 (9220): 2048–2049.

Tzeng, H.-M., Yin, C.-Y. 2012. Physical restraint use rate and total fall and injurious fall rates: an exploratory study in two US acute care hospitals. *Open Journal of Nursing.* 2: 170–175.

Uhl, W., Buchler, M.W., Malfertheiner, P., *et al.*, German Pancreatitis Study Group. 1999. A randomised, double-blind, multicentre trial of octreotide in moderate to severe acute pancreatitis. *Gut.* 45 (1): 97–104.

UK Working Party on Acute Pancreatitis. 2005. UK guidelines for the management of acute pancreatitis. *Gut.* 54: supplement III.

Ullman, A.J., Aitken, L.M., Rattray, J., *et al.* 2014. Diaries for recovery from critical illness. *Cochrane Database of Systematic Reviews*, Issue 12. Art. No.: CD010468. doi:10.1002/14651858.CD010468.pub2.

Ungar, A., Rivasi, G., Rafanelli, M., *et al.* 2016. Safety and tolerability of Tilt Testing and Carotid Sinus Massage in the octogenarians. *Age and Ageing.* 45 (2): 242–248.

Unroe, M., Mahn, J.M., Carson, S.S., *et al.* 2010. One-year trajectories of care and resource utilization for recipients of prolonged mechanical ventilation. *Annals of Internal Medicine.* 153 (3): 167–175.

Unverzagt, S., Wachsmuth, L., Hirsch, K., *et al.* 2014. Inotropic agents and vasodilator strategies for acute myocardial infarction complicated by cardiogenic shock or low cardiac output syndrome. *Cochrane Database of Systematic Reviews*, Issue 1. Art. No.: CD009669. doi:10.1002/14651858.CD009669.pub2.

Urbano, L.A., Oddo, M. 2012. Therapeutic hypothermia for traumatic brain injury. *Current Neurology and Neuroscience Reports.* 12: 580–591.

VA/NIH acute kidney injury trial network. 2008. Intensity of renal support in critically ill patients with acute kidney injury. *NEJM.* 359 (1): 7–20.

Valdiviezo, C., Garovic, V.D., Ouyang, P. 2012. Preeclampsia and hypertensive disease in pregnancy: their contributions to cardiovascular risk. *Clinical Cardiology.* 35 (3): 160–165.

Valente, M.J., Araújo, A.M., Bastos, M.D.L., *et al.* 2016. Editor's highlight: characterization of hepatotoxicity mechanisms triggered by designer cathinone drugs (β-Keto amphetamines). *Toxicological Sciences.* 153 (1): 89–102.

Valgimigli, M., Gagnor, A., Calabró, P., *et al.*, for the MATRIX Investigators. 2015. Radial versus femoral access in patients with acute coronary syndromes undergoing invasive management: a randomised multicentre trial. *Lancet.* 385 (9986): 2465–2476.

Valiathan, R., Ashman, M., Asthana, D. 2016. Effects of ageing on the immune system: infants to elderly. *Scandinavian Journal of Immunology.* 83 (4): 255–266.

Vamos, M., Erath, J.W., Hohnloser, S.H. 2015. Digoxin-associated mortality: a systematic review and meta-analysis of the literature. *European Heart Journal.* 36 (28): 1831–1838.

Van Den Berghe, G., Wouters, P., Weekers, F., *et al.* 2001. Intensive insulin therapy in critically ill patients. *New England Journal of Medicine.* 345 (19): 1359–1367.

Van den Berghe, G., de Zegher, F. 1996. Anterior pituitary function during critical illness and dopamine treatment. *Critical Care Medicine.* 24 (9): 1580–1590.

van Harten, A.E., Scheeren, T.W.L., Absalom, A.R. 2012. A review of postoperative cognitive dysfunction and neuroinflammation associated with cardiac surgery and anaesthesia. *Anaesthesia.* 67 (3): 280–293.

van Nunen, L.X., Noc, M., Kapur, N.K., *et al.* 2016. Usefulness of intra-aortic balloon pump counterpulsation. *The American Journal of Cardiology,* 117 (3): 469–476.

van Santvoort, H., Besselink, M.G., de Vries, A.C., *et al.*, Dutch Acute Pancreatitis Study Group. 2009. Early endoscopic retrograde cholangiopancreatography in predicted severe acute biliary pancreatitis: a prospective multicenter study. *Annals of Surgery.* 250 (1): 68–75.

van Welzen, M., Carey, T. 2002. Autonomic dysreflexia: guidelines for practice. *Connect.* 2 (1): 13–21.

VanGilder, C., Amlung, S., Harrison, P., Meyer, S. 2009. Results of the 2008–2009 International Pressure Ulcer Prevalence Survey and a 3-year, acute care, unit-specific analysis. *Ostomy Wound Management.* 55 (11): 39–45.

Vanhoutte, P.M. 2002. Ageing and endothelial dysfunction. *European Heart Journal.* 4 (supplement A): A8-A17.

Vanmassenhove, J., Kielstein, J., Jörres, A., Van Biesen, W. 2017. Management of patients at risk of acute kidney injury. *Lancet.* 389 (10084): 2139 – 2151.

Vargas, M., Chiumello, D., Sutherasan, Y., *et al.* 2017. Heat and moisture exchangers (HMEs) and heated humidifiers (HHs) in adult critically ill patients: a systematic review, meta-analysis and meta-regression of randomized controlled trials. *Critical Care.* 21 (1): 123.

Varon, J., Acosta, P. 2008. Therapeutic hypothermia. *Chest.* 133 (5): 1267–1274.

Vedio, A.B., Chinn, S., Warburton, F.G., *et al.* 2000. Assessment of survival and quality of life after discharge from a teaching hospital general intensive care unit. *Clinical Intensive Care.* 11 (1): 39–46.

Velissaris, D., Karamouzos, V., Ktenopoulos, N., *et al.* 2015. The use of sodium bicarbonate in the treatment of acidosis in sepsis: a literature update on a long term debate. *Critical Care Research and Practice.* Article ID 605830.

Venkatesh, B. 2014. Disorders of consciousness. *In* Bersten, A.D., Soni, N. (eds). *Intensive Care Manual.* 7th edition. Edinburgh. Butterworth-Heinemann Elsevier. 549–559.

Villata-Garcia, P., López-Herránz, M., Mazo-Pascual, S., *et al.* 2017. Reliability of blood test results in samples obtained using a 2-ml discard volume from the proximal lumen of a triple-lumen central venous catheter in the critically ill patient. *Nursing in Critical Care.* 22 (5): 298–304.

Vincent, J.-L., Rello, J., Marshall, J., *et al.*, EPIC II Group of Investigators. 2009. International study of the prevalence and outcomes of infection in intensive care units. *JAMA.* 203 (21): 2323–2329.

Vincent, J.L., Taccone, F.S., He, X. 2017. Harmful effects of hyperoxia in postcardiac arrest, sepsis, traumatic brain injury, or stroke: the importance of individualized oxygen therapy in critically ill patients. *Canadian Respiratory Journal.* 2017. Article ID 28349526.

Vogler, J., Breithardt, G, Eckardt, L. 2012. Bradyarrhythmias and conduction blocks. *Revista Española de Cardiología (English Edition).* 65 (7): 656–667.

Vyas, M.V., Garg, A.X., Iansavichus, A., *et al.* 2012. Shift work and vascular events: systematic review and meta-analysis. *BMJ.* 345 (3451): 15.

Wade, D., Hardy, R., Howell, D., Mythen, M. 2013. Identifying clinical and acute psychological risk factors for PTSD after Intensive Care: a systematic review. *Minerva Anesthesiolica.* 79 (8): 944–963.

Wagstaff, A.T.J. 2014. Oxygen therapy. *In* Bersten, A.D., Soni, N. (eds). *Intensive Care Manual.* 7th edition. Edinburgh. Butterworth-Heinemann Elsevier. 327–340.

Wainberg, M.A. 1999. HIV resistance to antagonists of viral reverse transcriptase. *In* Dalgleish, A.G., Weiss, R.A. (eds). 1999. *HIV and the New Viruses.* 2nd edition. San Diego. Academic Press. 223–250.

Wake, D. 1995. Ecstasy overdose: a case study. *Intensive and Critical Care Nursing.* 11 (1): 6–9.

Wallace, C.I., Dargan, P.I., Jones, A.L. 2003. Paracetamol overdose: an evidence based flowchart to guide management. *Emergency Medicine Journal.* 19 (3): 202–205.

Wallen, K., Chaboyer, W., Thalib, L., Creedy, D.K. 2008. Symptoms of acute posttraumatic stress disorder after intensive care. *American Journal of Critical Care.* 17 (5): 534–543.

Wallentin, L., Ärnström, E., Husted, S., *et al.*, for the FRISC-II study group. 2016. Early invasive versus non-invasive treatment in patients with non-ST-elevation acute coronary syndrome (FRISC-II): 15 year follow-up of a prospective, randomised, multicentre study. *Lancet.* 388 (10054): 1903–1911.

Walsh-Irvin, C. 2013. Cardiovascular alterations. *In* Sole, M.L., Klein, D.G., Moseley, M.J. (eds). *Introduction to Critical Care Nursing.* 6th edition. St Louis, MO. Elsevier Saunders. 289–344.

Walter, E.J, Carraretto M. 2016. The neurological and cognitive consequences of hyperthermia. *Critical Care.* 20: 199.

Walter, E.J., Hanna-Jumma, S., Carraretto, M., Forni, L. 2016. The pathophysiological basis and consequences of fever. *Critical Care.* 20: 200.

Walter, T. 1997. Secularization. *In* Parkes, C.M., Laungani, P., Young, B. (eds) *Death and Bereavement Across Cultures.* London. Routledge. 166–187.

Wang, F., Bo, L., Tang, L., *et al.* 2012. Subglottic secretion drainage for preventing ventilator-associated pneumonia: an updated meta-analysis of randomized controlled trials. *Journal of Trauma & Acute Care Surgery.* 72 (5): 1276–1285.

Wang, G., Wen, J., Xu, L., *et al.* 2013 Effect of enteral nutrition and ecoimmunonutrition on bacterial translocation and cytokine production in patients with severe acute pancreatitis. *Journal of Surgical Research.* 183 (2): 592–597.

Wang, J., Xu, E., Xiao, Y. 2014. Isotonic versus hypotonic maintenance IV fluids in hospitalized children: a meta-analysis. *Pediatrics.* 133 (1): 105–113.

Ward, D.S., Karan, S.B., Pandit, J.J. 2011. Hypoxia: developments in basic science, physiology and clinical studies. *Anaesthesia.* 66 (supplement 2): 19–26.

Waring, W.S. 2017. The acute management of poisoning. *Medicine.* 45 (2) 104–109.

Washington, G.T., Matney, J.L. 2008. Comparison of temperature measurement devices in post anesthesia patients. *Journal of PeriAnesthesia Nursing.* 23 (1): 36–48.

Waterhouse, C. 2005. The Glasgow Coma Scale and other neurological observations. *Nursing Standard.* 19 (33): 56–64.

Waterlow, J. 2005. *Pressure Sore Prevention Manual.* Taunton. Waterlow.

Waterlow, J.A. 1985. A risk assessment card. *Nursing Times.* 81 (48): 49–55.

Watkins, L.D. 2000. Head injuries: general principles and management. *Surgery.* 18 (9): 219–224.

Watson, J.B. 1924/1998. *Behaviourism.* New Brunswick, NJ. Transaction.

Watson, R. 2001. Assessing gastrointestinal (GI) tract functioning in older people. *Nursing Older People.* 12 (10): 27–28.

Webb, G., Phillips, N., Reddiford, S., Neuberger, J. 2015. Factors affecting the decision to grant consent for organ donation: a survey of adults in England. *Transplantation.* 99 (7): 1396–1402.

Weetman, C., Allison, W. 2006. Use of epidural analgesia in post-operative pain management. *Nursing Standard.* 20 (44): 54–64.

Weich, S., Pearce, H.L., Croft, P., *et al.* 2014. Effect of anxiolytic and hypnotic drug prescriptions on mortality hazards: retrospective cohort study. *BMJ.* 348: g1996. doi:10.1136/bmj. g1996.

Weil, D., Levesque, E., McPhail, M., *et al.* METAREACIR Group. 2017. Prognosis of cirrhotic patients admitted to intensive care unit: a meta-analysis. *Annals of Intensive Care.* 7: 33.

Weinberger, J., Cipolle, M. 2016. Mechanical prophylaxis for post-traumatic VTE: stockings and pumps. *Current Trauma Reports.* 2 (1): 35–41.

Weiss, M., Dullenkopf, A., Fischer, J.E., *et al.*, European paediatric endotracheal tubes in small children. 2009. Prospective randomised controlled multi-centre trial of cuffed or uncuffed endotracheal tubes in small children. *British Journal of Anaesthesia.* 103 (6): 867–873.

Wellnius, G.A., Mukamal, K.J., Kulshreshtha, A., *et al.* 2008. Depressive symptoms and the risk of atherosclerotic progression among patients with coronary artery bypass grafts. *Circulation.* 117 (18): 2312–2319.

Welsch, D., Tilley, R., Rhodes, A. 2001. Cardiovascular complications of cocaine. *Clinical Intensive Care.* 12 (5,6): 241–244.

Wen, Y.-M., Klen, H.-D. 2013. H7N9 avian influenza virus – search and re-search. *Emerging Microbes and Infections.* 2: e18. doi:10.1038/emi.

Wenger, N.K. 2012. What's new in antiplatelet and anticoagulant therapy recommendations for unstable angina/non–ST-elevation myocardial infarction. *Clinical Cardiology.* 35 (11): 669–672.

Wenham, T., Pittard, A. 2009. Intensive Care Unit environment. *Continuing Education in Anaesthesia, Critical Care & Pain.* 9 (6): 178–183.

West, E., Mays, N., Rafferty, A.M., *et al.* 2009. Nursing resources and patient outcomes in intensive care: a systematic review of the literature. *International Journal of Nursing Studies.* 46 (7): 993–1011.

Weston, D. 2013. *Fundamentals of Infection Prevention and Control: Theory and Practice.* 2nd edition. Chichester. John Wiley & Sons.

Whitehouse, T., Snelson, C., Ground, M. 2014. *Intensive Care Society Review of Best Practice for Analgesia and Sedation in the Critical Care.* London. Intensive Care Society.

W.H.O. 2005. *Clean Care is Safer Care.* Geneva. World Health Organization.

W.H.O. 2007. *Ethical Considerations in Developing a Public Health Response to Pandemic Influenza.* WHO/CDS/EPR/GIP/2007. 2. Geneva. World Health Organization.

W.H.O. 2009. *Nurses and Midwives: A Force for Health.* Copenhagen. World Health Organization.

W.H.O. 2014a. *Consolidated Guidelines on HIV Prevention, Diagnosis, Treatment and Care for Key Populations.* Geneva. World Health Organization.

W.H.O. 2014b. *Antimicrobial Resistance. Global Report on Surveillance.* Geneva. World Health Organization.

W.H.O. 2016a. *Global Report on Diabetes.* Geneva. World Health Organization.

W.H.O. 2016b. *Global Tuberculosis Report 2016.* Geneva. World Health Organization.

W.H.O. 2017. *Pandemic Influenza Risk Planning.* Geneva. World Health Organization.

Wiener, R.S., Wiener, D.C., Larson, R.J. 2008. Benefits and risks of tight glucose control in critically ill adults: a meta-analysis. *JAMA.* 300 (8): 933–944.

Wilcox, A. 2012. Meningococcal B disease: assessment and management. *Nursing Standard.* 26 (26): 50–55.

Wilkes, A.R. 2011. Heat and moisture exchangers and breathing system filters: their use in anaesthesia and intensive care. *Anaesthesia.* 66 (1): 31–39.

Williams, A.M., Irurita, V.F. 2004. Therapeutic and non-therapeutic interpersonal interactions: the patient's perspective. *Journal of Clinical Nursing.* 13 (7): 806–815.

Williams, J.M.L., Williamson, R.C.N. 2010. Alcohol and the pancreas. *British Journal of Hospital Medicine.* 71 (10): 556–561.

Williams, T.E., Baker, K., Evans, L., *et al.* 2016. Registered Nurses as professionals, advocates, innovators, and collaborative leaders. *The Online Journal of Issues in Nursing.* 21 (3).

Willison, H.J., Jacobs, B.C., van Doorn, P.A. 2016. Guillain-Barré syndrome. *Lancet.* 388 (10045): 717–727.

Wilson, L.A. 2005. Urinalysis. *Nursing Standard.* 19 (35): 51–54.

Wilson, S.R., Hirsch, N.P., Appleby, I. 2005. Management of subarachnoid haemorrhage in a non-neurosurgical centre. *Anaesthesia.* 60 (5): 470–485.

Winkeleman, A., Hilton, G. 2018. Patient management: nervous system. *In* Morton, P.G., Fontaine, D.K. (eds). *Critical Care Nursing: A Holistic Approach.* 11th edition. Philadelphia. Wolters Kluwer. 640–674.

Winslow, E.H., Jacobson, A.F. 1998. Dispelling the petroleum jelly myth. *American Journal of Nursing*. 98 (11): 16.

Winstock, A.R., Mitcheson, L. 2012. New recreational drugs and the primary care approach to patients who use them. *BMJ*. 344 (7844): 35–40.

Wittenberg, M.D., Kaur, N., Walker, D.A. 2010. The challenge of HIV disease in the intensive care unit. *Journal of the Intensive Care Society*. 11 (1): 26–30.

Wolberg, A.S., Aleman, M.M., Leiderman, K., Machlus, K.R. 2012. Procoagulant activity in hemostasis and thrombosis: Virchow's triad revisited. *Anesthesia and Analgesia*, 114 (2): 275–285.

Wolters, A.E., Slooter, A.J.C., van der Kooi, A.W., van Dijk, D. 2013. Cognitive impairment after intensive care unit admission: a systematic review. *Intensive Care Medicine*. 39 (3): 376–386.

WOMAN Trial Collaborators. 2017. Effect of early tranexamic acid administration on mortality, hysterectomy, and other morbidities in women with post-partum haemorrhage (WOMAN): an international, randomised, double-blind, placebo-controlled trial. *Lancet*. 389 (10084): 2105–2116.

Wong, L.Y., Bellomo, R., Robbins, *et al*. 2016. Long-term outcomes after severe drug overdose. *Critical Care and Resuscitation*. 18 (4): 247–254.

Wong, P., Liamputtong, P., Koch, S., Rawson, H. 2015. Families' experiences of their interactions with staff in an Australian Intensive Care Unit (ICU): a qualitative study. *Intensive and Critical Care Nursing*. 31 (1): 51–63.

Wong, T., Schlichting, A.B., Stoltze, A.J., *et al*. 2016. No decrease in early ventilator-associated pneumonia after early use of chlorhexidine. *American Journal of Critical Care*. 25 (2): 173–177.

Woodcock, T.E., Cook, T.M., Gupta, K.J., Hartle, A. 2014. Arterial line blood sampling: preventing hypoglycaemic brain injury. *Anaesthesia*. 69 (4): 380–385.

Woodcock, T.E., Woodcock, T.M. 2012. Revised Starling equation and the glycocalyx model of transvascular fluid exchange: an improved paradigm for prescribing intravenous fluid therapy. *British Journal of Anaesthesia*. 108 (3): 384–394.

Woodford, H. 2015. *Essential Geriatrics*. 3rd edition. Boca Raton, FL. CRC Press.

Woodrow, P. 2016. *Nursing Acutely Ill Patients*. London. Routledge.

Wren, M. 2009. *Clostridium difficile*: How big? How bad? *In* Ridley, S. (ed.). *Critical Care Focus 16: Infection*. London. Intensive Care Society. 46–55.

Wright, A.D., Flynn, M. 2011. Using the prone position for ventilated patients with respiratory failure: a review. *Nursing in Critical Care*. 16 (1): 19–27.

Wright, B. 2007 *Loss and Grief*. Keswick. M&K Update.

Wright, B.J. 2015. Inhaled pulmonary vasodilators in refractory hypoxemia. *Clinical and Experimental Emergency Medicine*. 2 (3): 184–187.

Wu, B.U., Hwang, J.Q., Gardner, T.H., *et al*. 2011. Lactated Ringer's solution reduces systemic inflammation compared with saline in patients with acute pancreatitis. *Clinical Gastroenterology & Hepatology*. 9 (8): 710–717.

Wu, C.L., Raja, S.N. 2011. Treatment of acute postoperative pain. *Lancet*. 377 (9784), 2215–2225.

Wu, Y.-K., Tsai, Y.-H., Lan, C.-C., *et al*. 2010. Prolonged mechanical ventilation in a respiratory-care setting: a comparison of outcome between tracheostomized and translaryngeal intubated patients. *Critical Care*. 14 (2): R26.

Wyffels, P.A.H., Sergeant, P., Wouters, P.F. 2010. The value of pulse pressure and stroke volume variation as predictors of fluid responsiveness during open chest surgery. *Anaesthesia*. 65 (7): 704–709.

Xavier, G. 2000. The importance of mouth care in preventing infection. *Nursing Standard*. 14 (18): 47–51.

Xie, Y., Bowe, B., Li, T., *et al*. 2017. Risk of death among users of proton pump inhibitors: a longitudinal observational cohort study of United States veterans. 7: e015735. doi:10.1136/bmjopen-2016-015735.

Yang, S., Wang, Z., Liu, Z., *et al*. 2016. Association between time of discharge from ICU and hospital mortality: a systematic review and meta-analysis. *Critical Care*. 20 (390).

Yaran, J. 2012. Trends in intensive care in patients over 90 years of age. *Clinical Interventions in Aging*. 7: 339–347.

Yassin, J., Wyncoll, D. 2005. Management of intractable diarrhoea in the critically ill. *Care of the Critically Ill*. 21 (1): 20–24.

Yealy, D.M., Kellum, J.A., Huang., D.T., the ProCESS Investigators. 2014. A randomized trial of protocol-based care for early septic shock. *New England Journal of Medicine*. 2014; 370 (18): 1683–1693.

Yıldırım, F., Kara, I., Demirel, C.B. 2016. Airway management of "at-risk extubation" in Intensive Care. *Eurasian Journal of Pulmonology*. doi:10.5152/ejp.2016.00922.

Yki-Järvinen, H. 2014. Non-alcoholic fatty liver disease as a cause and a consequence of metabolic syndrome. *Lancet Diabetes & Endocrinology*. 2 (11): 901–910.

Ympa, Y.P., Sakr, Y., Reinhart, K., Vincent, J.-L. 2005. Has mortality from acute renal failure decreased? A systematic review of the literature. *American Journal of Medicine*. 118 (8): 827–832.

Yoshida, T., Rinka, H., Kaji, A., *et al.* 2009. The impact of spontaneous ventilation on distribution of lung aeration in patients with acute respiratory distress syndrome: airway pressure release ventilation versus pressure support ventilation. *Anesthesia and Analgesia*. 106 (6): 892–900.

Young, D., Harrison, D.A., Cuthbertson, B.H., Rowan, K., TracMan Collaborators. 2013. Effect of early vs late tracheostomy placement on survival in patients receiving mechanical ventilation. *JAMA*. 309 (20): 2121–2129.

Young, J., Stiffleet, J., Nikoletti, S., Shaw, T. 2006. Use of a behavioural pain scale to assess pain in ventilated, unconscious and/or sedated patients. *Intensive & Critical Care Nursing*. 22 (1): 32–39.

Young, P., Bailey, M., Beasley, R., *et al.*, SPLIT Investigators and the ANZICSCTG. 2015. Effect of a buffered crystalloid solution vs saline on acute kidney injury among patients in the Intensive Care Unit. *JAMA*. 314 (16): 1701–1710.

Young, P.J., Saxena, M. 2014. Fever management in intensive care patients with infections. *Critical Care*. 18: 206.

Young, P.J., Saxena, M., Beasley, R., *et al.* 2012. Early peak temperature and mortality in critically ill patients with and without infection. *Intensive Care Medicine*. 38 (3): 437–444.

Yuki, N., Hartung, H.-P. 2012. Medical progress: Guillain-Barré Syndrome. *New England Journal of Medicine*. 366 (24): 2294–2304.

Zarbock, A., Kellum, J.A., Schmidt, C., *et al.* 2016. Effect of early vs delayed initiation of renal replacement therapy on mortality in critically ill patients with acute kidney injury. The ELAIN Randomized Clinical Trial. *JAMA*. 315 (20): 2190–2199.

Zhang, J., Ho, K.-Y., Wang, Y. 2011. Efficacy of pregablin in acute postoperative pain: a meta-analysis. *British Journal of Anaesthesia*. 106 (4): 454–462.

Zhang, X., Xuan, W., Yin, P., *et al.* 2015. Gastric tonometry guided therapy in critical care patients: a systematic review and meta-analysis. *Critical Care*. 19: 22.

Zhang, Z., Lu, B., Ni, H. 2012. Prognostic value of extravascular lung water index in critically ill patients: a review of the literature. *Journal of Critical Care*. 27: 420.e1–420.e8.

Zhou, F., Peng, Z.-Y., Bishop, J.V., *et al.* 2014. Effects of fluid resuscitation with 0.9% saline versus a balanced electrolyte solution on acute kidney injury in a rat model of sepsis. *Critical Care Medicine*. 42 (4): e270–e278.

Zhou, Y., Jin, X., Lv, Y., *et al.* 2017. Early application of airway pressure release ventilation may reduce the duration of mechanical ventilation in acute respiratory distress syndrome. *Intensive Care Medicine*. 43 (11): 1648–1659.

Zilberstein, J., McCurdy, M.T., Winters, M.E. 2014. Anaphylaxis. *The Journal of Emergency Medicine*. 47 (2): 182–187.

Zimmer, S.M., Burke, D.S. 2009. Historical perspective – emergence of *influenza A* (H1N1) viruses. *New England Journal of Medicine*. 361 (3): 279–285.

Zimmerman, J.E., Kramer, A.A., McNair, D.S., Malila, F.M. 2006. Acute Physiology and Chronic Health Evaluation (APACHE) IV: hospital mortality assessment for today's critically ill patients. *Critical Care Medicine*. 34 (5): 1297–1310.

Zimmerman, J.L., Shen, M.C. 2013. Rhabdomyolysis. *Chest*. 144 (3): 1058–1065.

Zirakzadeh, A., Patel, R. 2006. Vancomycin-Resistant *Enterococci*: colonization, infection, detection, and treatment. *Mayo Clinical Proceedings*. 81 (4): 529–536.

Index

Page numbers in *italic* type indicate relevant figures and tables.

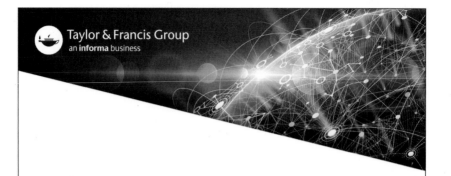